PRACTICAL PATHOLOGY

INCLUDING

Clinical Haematology, Microscopic Pathology, Pathological Specimens, Cytopathology, FNAC, Clinical Pathology, Applied Clinical Chemistry, Histopathological Techniques and Autopsy

THIRD EDITION

PRACTICAL PATHOLOGY

INCLUDING

Clinical Haematology, Microscopic Pathology, Pathological Specimens, Cytopathology, FNAC, Clinical Pathology, Applied Clinical Chemistry, Histopathological Techniques and Autopsy

THIRD EDITION

P Chakraborty
MBBS, MD (Path & Bact)
Formerly Associate Professor of Pathology, Govt Medical College Surat and North Bengal Medical College; Professor of Pathology and Microbiology, Medical College, Kolkata; Pathologist, Tata Hospital and DVC Central Hospital

New Central Book Agency (P) Ltd

Co-Published by

Bijay Publications

E-mail : bijaypublications@gmail.com

Exclusively Distributed by

Bijay Pustak Bhandar (P) Ltd

90/6A M. G. Road, Bhawani Dutta Lane, Kolkata-700007

✆ : (033) 4605-7856, 8777898576, 8274916104

E-mail : bijaypustakbhandar@gmail.com

NCBA

REGD OFFICE
8/1 Chintamoni Das Lane, Kolkata 700 009, India
email: ncbakolkata@gmail.com

OVERSEAS
NCBA (UK) Ltd, 149 Park Avenue North, Northampton, NN3 2HY, UK
email: ncbauk@yahoo.com

CORPORATE OFFICE
212 Shahpur Jat, New Delhi 110 049
email: delhincba@gmail.com

BIJAY PUBLICATIONS
90/6A M. G. Road, Bhawani Dutta Lane, Kolkata-7
E-mail : bijaypublications@gmail.com

BIJAY PUSTAK BHANDAR (P) LTD
90/6A M. G. Road, Bhawani Dutta Lane, Kolkata-7
E-mail : bijaypustakbhandar@gmail.com

PRACTICAL PATHOLOGY • P Chakraborty

First Published: 1998
Reprinted: 2000, 2002, 2005, 2008, 2009
Thoroughly revised, enlarged & updated Second Edition: 2010
Reprinted: 2011, 2012, 2013, 2015, 2016
Third Edition: 2017
Reprinted: 2018, 2019, 2020, 2022, 2024, **2025**

PUBLISHER • TYPESETTER • PRINTER
New Central Book Agency (P) Ltd
8/1 Chintamoni Das Lane, Kolkata 700 009

CO-PUBLISHED BY
Bijay Publications
90/6A M G Road, Bhawani Dutta Lane, Kolkata 700007

TECHNICAL EDITOR
Mita Sen, MBBS

PROJECT COORDINATORS
N Radhakrishnan, Prabhat Jas and Subir Pal

ISBN: 81 7381 332 9

Price ₹ 835.00

Dedicated

to the unforgettable and lingering blissful memories of

the author's daughter

Late Dr Maitrayee Chakraborty (Moulik), MBBS, DNB(I) (India), WBHS

(25-1-1967 — 20-12-1997)

and

the divine

Acharya Shrimat Swami Pranabanandaji Maharaj

of Bharat Sevashram Sangha

Foreword

I consider it to be a matter of unique pleasure and proud privilege to write a foreword of this useful and much sought-after handbook of *Practical Pathology* by Prof. P. Chakraborty and Dr Gargi Chakraborty.

It needs no mention that in the backdrop of explosive and phenomenal advances in the different fields of medicine including pathology in the current century, the challenge the students face to keep themselves updated is becoming increasingly difficult more than ever before.

To my mind, this handbook has come up to our expectations and has admirably summed up the different fundamental technique of Haematology, Clinical pathology, Morbid anatomy, Exfoliative cytology, Clinical biochemistry, Autopsy, Fine needle aspiration cytology, etc. in a concise and comprehensive manner. 200 attractive colour plates and the different illustrations have added a new feather to its colourful cap.

The users of this book would obviously be the best judges to assess to what extent the objectives of the book have been purposefully realised but shortfalls, if there be any, certainly do not stem from lack of sincere trying. Admittedly, the book will come up as a boon and blessing to all those it is intended for—the medical student in particular by providing him a ready version of the practical course of instructions which he receives only once during his student career. The book will be equally useful to the laboratory technologists and budding pathologists.

I can well imagine the untiring efforts and meticulous care the authors have put into in the preparation of the book. I wish it a successful voyage which it deserves on all accounts.

Prof. K K Bhattacharyya
MBBS, PhD (London), FRC (Path) (London), FSMF (WB)
Ex-Professor-Director of Pathology and Principal of Calcutta Medical College
Ex-Director of Medical Education and Ex-officio Secretary
Government of West Bengal

Calcutta
April 15, 1998

Preface to the Second Edition

I am delighted that this book has been widely received and there have been four reprints since the same was first published in 1998. Our primary goal has been to provide a comprehensive book on practical pathology for UG and PG medical students, teachers, pathologists, practising physicians, as also medical technologists. Medical college curricula are changing and often pathology is integrated with immunology, microbiology, and clinical subjects. Nowadays, stress is being given on topic- or problem-based curricula.

The current edition has been thoroughly revised and meticulously updated. These clearly reflect the remarkable advances made in the field of different branches of pathology. The general organisation of the book remains similar to that of the previous edition.

Some of the many more significant changes are :

- Chapters have been reorganised to be in tune with the practical demonstration classes.
- In addition to revision and reorganisation of the text, many valuable and significant changes in illustrations have been made.
- A new feature—highlighting important points in boxes—have been added.
- Histopathological descriptions of additional sections and gross appearance of additional specimens have been added along with necessary and clarifying photographs.
- In many cases of microscopic study, diagrammatic features along with microphotographs added, enrich the book.
- Majority of the chapters end with important questions—mostly case-based—which are useful in UG and PG medical examinations.
- Students are especially entreated to meticulously give their attention to the valuable appendices. They will be highly benefitted.

I am thankful to Prof. S. K. Sinha, Prof. and Head, Department of Pathology, Medical College, Kolkata, Prof. Pradip Mitra, Prof. of Pathology and Director of IPGMER, Kolkata, Prof. N. K. Pal of IPGMER, Kolkata, for revising the book. I am also indebted to Prof. Chandrasekhar Mukherjee, Head of the Department of Biochemistry, Medical College, Kolkata, for revising and editing the sections on Clinical Biochemistry. I am specially thankful to Dr Mita Sen for thoroughly editing the book. I am also thankful to Sri Nochiel Radhakrishnan, Sri Prasenjit Halder, and Sri Suman Dutta for their masterly design and pin-pointed computer-graphics. Once again I thank Sri Amitabha Sen, Director of New Central Book Agency, and other production staff members of NCBA for their constant cooperation.

EC 63, Salt Lake, Kolkata 64
February 3, 2010
Vyas Puja Tithi

P. CHAKRABORTY

Preface to the First Edition

This convenient handbook of practical manual containing various sections of practical pathology (Clinical pathology, Haematology, Macroscopic and Microscopic pathology, Cytopathology, FNAC) with more than 200 colour plates and 50 illustrations sets out the basic facts and principles clearly and briefly which is essentially visual in its impact.

The major portion of the book (Chapters 1-33 and 41) is intended for medical students studying for the professional examination in Pathology based on the course of Asian and African universities; Chapters 34-36 for postgraduate students and Chapters 37-40 (Applied Clinical Chemistry) for medical technologists.

We hope that the book will be useful for those who are beginning to specialise in pathology, to the technical staff working in the medical laboratories, as well as to the pathologists and clinicians.

We are deeply indebted to the authors of many text and reference books which we have frequently consulted —but their references have not been cited.

There is, no doubt, always room for improvement. We shall welcome suggestions and comments from all quarters.

Calcutta
April 15, 1998

P. Chakraborty
Gargi Chakraborty

Acknowledgements

We are grateful to Prof. (Mrs) S Sanyal for permission to take photographs of specimens and histopathological sections. We are again thankful to colleagues who have helped with discussions and advices. In Kolkata—Drs Sabitri Sanyal, Sulekha Das, Alpana Bose, S K Sinha, Rita Basu, Aparna Bhattacharya, Pranab Biswas, Madhumita Mukherjee, Sukanta Sinha, Krishna Basu, Manideepa Sengupta, Anup Roy, Keya Basu, Mrinal Choudhury, S Mandal, R N Ghosh, C C Paral, Asit Ghosh, Gayatri Gupta, Ashis Chakraborty, Pradip Mitra and S P Patra; in Burdwan—Drs Manimala Roy, Sreeparna Banerjee; in Bankura—Drs Monoj Choudhury, Ranjit Biswas and Bani Kumar Bhattacharya; in Imphal—Dr Y M Singh and Dr S N Singh; In Gauhati—Dr Panna Deka and Dr Rekha Sangma; in Patna—Dr R S Jha; and many others whose names could not be mentioned due to shortage of space.

Our special thanks to Dr (Mrs) Mita Sen, Dr Sujit K Chaudhuri (ex-Professor and Head of the Department of Physiology), Medical College, Kolkata; Dr P K Sikdar and Dr Monalisa Majumdar for revising the manuscript. For the photography, our thanks to Mr Sudarshan Chakraborty of Landsdown Studio and for the text diagrams to Mr Narayan Sur. The authors express their sincere gratitude to Mr Nochiel Radhakrishnan for computer graphics and supervising the process of this book. We are grateful to him for accommodating every whim of ours with a broad grin. We are also thankful to Mr Subir Pal for composing the text matters.

It was again a pleasing experience to work with Mr Amitabha Sen, BCom, MBA, LLB, of New Central Book Agency (P) Ltd, who was always ready to cooperate with his limitless energy and boundless enthusiasm. Indeed, we thank every member of the publishing house, not the least Mr J N Sen and Mr Arunabha Sen, for their sustained efforts in publishing the book.

We owe a particular debt to Prof. K K Bhattacharya — not only for writing the foreword to the book but also for his constant encouragement. We are specially indebted to Prof. Mukul Roy Choudhury, Professor of Pathology, University College of Medicine, Kolkata, for his suggestion and guidance. The authors are also indebted to Late Dr Maitrayee Chakraborty (Moulik), MBBS, DBB(I), WBHS, and Miss Atreyee Chakraborty, BE (E & C), ME (Biomedical) (Jadavpur University); for revising the manuscript and offering valuable suggestions.

Finally, we like to mention the sustained but silent inspiration provided by Smt Geeta Chakraborty (wife of the senior author and mother of the junior author).

P. Chakraborty
Gargi Chakraborty

Contents

Introduction

Although automated mechanisms are widely used in biochemistry, haematology and other related fields, the basic manual methods continue to be used in many laboratories. Hence, the laboratory personnel should be conversant with the following general principles.

PERSONAL CARE

Universal precautions

All health-care workers should routinely use appropriate barrier precautions to prevent skin, mucous membrane contact with blood or other body fluids of patients.

1. Use of gown or aprons.

2. Gloves should be worn for touching blood, body fluids, mucous membranes, non-intact skin of all patients, and for handling items or surfaces soiled with blood or body fluids. Gloves should be changed after contact with each patient.

3. Masks and protective eyewear or face-shields should be used during procedures that are likely to generate droplets of blood or body fluids to protect the mouth, nose and eyes.

4. Precautions should be taken to prevent injuries caused by needles, scalpels, etc.

5. Health-care workers with exudative lesions of skin should refrain from direct contact with patients.

6. Pregnant health-workers should take extra precaution to avoid perinatal infection (e.g., HIV) resulting from transmission.

7. Disposables, e.g., syringe, needles, are preferred.

8. Use of properly sterilised and disinfected equipments is mandatory.

Safe disposal of specimens

Decontamination of contaminated materials is most effectively done by autoclaving (sterilisation). In Table 3, a list of important disinfectants and the concentrations in which they are to be used in clean contaminated and grossly contaminated conditions are given.

UNITS OF WEIGHT AND MEASUREMENT

[Standard International (SI) Units]

Weight : [unit gram (gm/g)]

$\times 10^{3}$ kilogram (kg)

$\times 10^{-3}$ milligram (mg)

$\times 10^{-6}$ microgram (μg)

$\times 10^{-9}$ nanogram (ng)

$\times 10^{-12}$ picogram (pg)

contd. next page

Volume : [unit: litre (l) = dm^3]

× 10^{-1} decilitre (dl) (formerly 100 ml)

× 10^{-3} millilitre (ml) = cm^3 (formerly cc)

× 10^{-6} microlitre (μl) = mm^3

× 10^{-9} nanolitre (nl)

× 10^{-12} picolitre (pl) (formerly μμl)

× 10^{-15} femtolitre (fl) = $μm^3$

Length : [unit: metre (m)]

× 10^{-1} decimetre (dm)

× 10^{-2} centimetre (cm)

× 10^{-3} millimetre (mm)

× 10^{-6} micrometre (μm) (formerly μ)

× 10^{-9} nanometre (nm) (formerly mμ)

× 10^{-12} picometre (pm) (formerly μμm)

ATOMIC WEIGHTS AND MOLECULAR CONCENTRATIONS

The concentration of a substance in solution can be expressed either in g/l or in mol/l or N (normal). The practice of expressing in term of N solution is almost replaced by the use of two other terms.

Molar Solutions

A molar solution contains the molecular weight of the substance (including water of crystallisation if present in the chemical form) expressed as g/l which is equivalent to 1 mol (or 1,000 m mol/l).

Thus, e.g.,

Mol wt of NaCl = 58.5

∴ 1 mol/1 = 58.5 g/l

9 gm/l .... = 9/58.5 = 0.154 mol/l

= 154 m mol/l

The atomic weight and equivalent weight of some chemicals are given in Table 1.

Substance concentration [unit : moles/litre (mol/l) (formerly M)]

1 mol of NaCl = 58.5 g,

1 m mol of NaCl = 58.5 mg.

Thus

× 10^{-3} millimole per litre (m mol/1)

× 10^{-6} micromole per litre (μ mol/1)

Dalton

The dalton (Da) is a unit of mass equal to $\frac{1}{12}$ the

Table 1

SYMBOLS, ATOMIC WEIGHTS AND EQUIVALENT WEIGHTS OF SOME COMMONLY USED ELEMENTS

Element	Symbol	Atomic Weight	Valency	Equivalent Weight
Carbon	C	12.01	4	3.00
Chlorine	Cl	35.45	1	35.45
Hydrogen	H	1.00	1	1.00
Nitrogen	N	14.00	3	4.66
Oxygen	O	16.00	2	8.00
Phosphorus	P	30.97	3	10.32
Potassium	K	39.10	1	39.10
Silver	Ag	107.88	1	107.88
Sodium	Na	22.99	1	22.99
Sulphur	S	32.00	2	16.00

Table 2
SYMBOLS, MOLECULAR WEIGHTS, VALENCY AND EQUIVALENT WEIGHTS OF SOME COMPOUNDS

Name	Symbol	Molecular weight	Replaceable H atoms	Hydroxyl groups	No. of cation	Value of cation	Eq. wt.
Acid							
Acetic acid	CH_3COOH	60.08	1	–	–	–	60.08
Hydrochloric acid	HCl	36.468	1	–	–	–	36.468
Sulphuric acid	H_2SO_4	98.082	2	–	–	–	49.041
Alkali							
Ammonium hydroxide	NH_4OH	35.05	–	1	–	–	35.05
Calcium hydroxide	$Ca(OH)_2$	91.104	–	2	–	–	45.552
Sodium hydroxide	NaOH	40.005	–	1	–	–	40.005
Salt							
Sodium chloride	NaCl	58.454	–	–	1	1	58.454
Sodium sulphate	Na_2SO_4	142.060	–	–	2	1	71.030
Sodium carbonate	Na_2CO_3	106.004	–	–	2	1	53.002

mass of an atom of Carbon – 12, and 1,000Da = 1 kilodalton (kDa). The kilodalton, which is simply expressed as K, is a useful unit for the molecular mass of proteins. Thus, a 64K protein indicates the molecular mass of protein is 64,000 Da.

Solution

A normal solution is one which contains the gram equivalent weight (equivalent weight in grams) of a substance per litre of solution.

The *equivalent* weight is the number of units of the substance which will combine with or replace one unit of hydrogen, 35.5 units of chlorine, 8 units of oxygen etc. — or the number of units of that substance which will contain 1 unit of hydrogen, 35.5 units of chlorine, 8 units of oxygen, etc. (Table 2).

(i) *Equivalent weight of an element* is obtained by dividing the atomic weight by the valency. The *valency* is the number of atoms of hydrogen (or its equivalent) that one atom of a chemical element can hold in combination or displace in a reaction.

(ii) *Equivalent weight of an acid* is the weight of it in grams that contains one atomic weight (11.008 g) of replaceable hydrogen. It is found by dividing mol wt. by the number of replaceable hydrogen atoms in the molecule.

(iii) *Equivalent weight of an alkali* is that weight of it which will neutralise the equivalent weight of an acid. It is obtained by dividing the mol. weight by the number of hydroxyl (OH) groups in the molecule.

(iv) *Equivalent weight of a salt* is found by dividing its molecular weight by the number of metal ions, or radicals per molecule, multiplied by the valency of the ion or radical.

SPECIMENS OF BLOOD

Although capillary or venous blood is used in laboratory investigations, venous blood is most often collected for blood chemistry. Arterial blood is used for blood gas determination.

Most chemical determinations are performed on serum or plasma. For chemical analysis, serum is more widely used because of the potential interference of anticoagulants used while preparing plasma.

Haemolysis interferes with many investigations

and should be avoided by proper precautions. Serum should be separated and tests should be done as soon as possible after collection of blood since certain constituents of blood (e.g., glucose) are lost on storage.

Blood specimens for different analysis

1. ***Whole blood*** : For glucose, urea, NPN and pH estimation.

2. ***Serum*** : Total protein, albumin, globulin, bilirubin, cholesterol, creatinine, phosphates, PBI, uric acid, transaminase (SGOT, SGPT), etc.

3. ***Plasma*** : Chloride, fibrinogen, ascorbic acid and bicarbonate estimation.

Changes in the blood on keeping

1. *Loss of CO_2* : It diffuses from plasma to air.

2. *Conversion of glucose to lactic acid* by glycolysis.

3. *Increase in plasma inorganic phosphates* which form from ester phosphate present in cells.

4. *Formation of NH_3 from nitrogenous substances* like urea.

5. *Passage of substances through* red cell membrane, e.g., potassium passes from plasma to cell.

6. *Conversion of pyruvate* into *lactate*.

TIME OF COLLECTION OF BLOOD

1. Since most satisfactory specimen(s) are post-absorptive, it is preferable that blood for analysis be taken after a night's fast (without food for 12 hours). Post-prandial hyperlipidaemia interferes with some investigations due to turbidity.

2. When unexpected results are obtained during drug therapy, the test should be repeated at a suitable interval after withdrawal of drug.

DIAGNOSTIC REAGENT KITS

Diagnostic reagent kits are now commercially available from Ortho, Span, J. Mitra, Stangen and many other companies. These kits are now widely used. Only the principles of different biochemical tests will be discussed in the relevant section.

Table 3

DIFFERENT ANTISEPTICS AND THE CONCENTRATIONS IN WHICH THEY ARE USED

Disinfectants	Clean contaminated	Gross contaminated (dirty)
Chlorine		
1. Sod. hypochlorite	0.1%	1%
2. Liquid bleach (5% available chlorine)	2 m/dl	20 ml/dl
3. Chloramine (60% available chlorine)	2 g%	20 g%
Iodine		
1. Tincture of iodine (Iodine 0.5% + alcohol 70%)	2.5%	2.5%
2. Polyvidone iodine (PVI), Betadine (1% iodine)	2.5%	2.5%
3. Glutaraldehyde (*Cidex* : 2% glutaraldehyde)	2.5%	2.5%
4. Formalin (40% soln. formaldehyde)	5%	10%
Alcohol		
1. Ethyl (70%)	70%	70%
2. Isopropyl/methyl (70%)	70%	70%
Phenolic compounds		
1. Phenol (carbolic acid)	5%	10%
2. Cresol	2.5%	5%
3. Lysol (saponified cresol)	2.5%	2.5%
Chloroxytenols		
1. Dettol (4.8% v/v)	4%	6%
2. Dettol + 1% EDTA	3%	6%
Diguanide		
1. Chlorhexidine (1.5% v/v, e.g., Hibitane)	5%	10%
2. Chlorhexidine + cetrimide (savlon)	5%	10%

Chapter 1

Microscopy

Microscope is an instrument by which an object of minute size can be largely magnified.

Simple Microscope : It consists of a single biconvex hand lens that can magnify object about 200 times.

Compound Microscope : Compound Microscope utilises a battery of lenses, one type is placed near the object (objective lens) and the other type is fitted close to the eye of the observer known as eye piece lens. The objective and the eye piece lenses possess different magnification. There are mainly two types of compound microscope — monocular having single eye piece (Fig. 1.1) and binocular having two eye pieces (Fig. 1.2). These microscopes are called light microscopes and are used in most laboratories. The light microscope has a resolution power of approximately 2,000. There is, however, also electron microscope which has got a resolution power of approximate 100,000 (1 lakh). Electron Microscope is discussed at the end of the chapter.

LIGHT MICROSCOPE

A light microscope consisting of the following parts :

- Stand
- Body
- Optical system
- Light / illumination system

The stand gives stability to the microscope. The body consists of a limb that arises from the joint and by means of which the microscope can be moved in both upward and downward directions. The stand and the limb carry the body tubes, stage and knobs for coarse and fine adjustments.

Body has 2 tubes — one external tube carrying a revolving nose piece, fitted with objective lenses of different magnification and another internal tube known as draw tube that carries at its upper end one or two eye pieces depending upon whether it is a monocular or binocular.

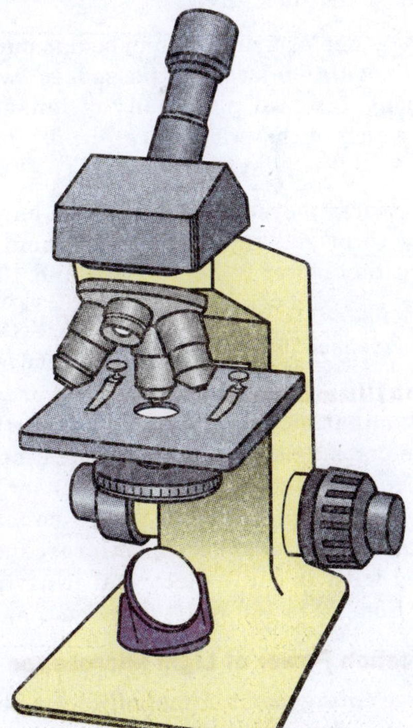

Fig. 1.1. Monocular light microscope (*mirror type*)

The stage consists of a metallic platform for accommodating glass slide having mounted object on it for examination. There is an aperture just below the level of the objectives in the centre of the stage that allow the light to reach the object. The slide on the stage can move horizontally or vertically by two knobs fitted to the slide holder just below the stage, a condenser is fitted through which light reaches the object. The substage fitted on the condenser can be moved up and down and contains an iris diaphragm, closing and opening of which controls the amount of light reaching the object.

Knobs for coarse and fine adjustment : Knobs are provided on either side of the body for coarse and fine adjustments. There are two bigger knobs for coarse adjustment and by movement of the same the body tubes can be moved with its lenses. For fine adjustment there are two smaller knobs on either side of the body. The fine focus is graduated and by each division objective moves by 0.002 mm.

Optical system : It contains eye piece, objectives and condensers.

There is one eye piece in monocular microcope while binocular microcope possesses two. Eye piece contains two planoconvex lenses. The magnification of those lenses can be 5×, 10×, 12× or 15×.

The objective system is made of a battery of lenses with prisms incorporated in them. Their magnification power is 4×, 10×, 40× and 100×.

Condenser is made up of two simple lenses which condenses light on to the object.

Light/Illumination system : For use of day light illumination, one mirror is fitted which is plane on one side and concave on the other side. The mirror is fitted under the condenser. Plane mirror is used in sunlight while concave in artificial light. Most of the microscopes are provided with in-built electrical illumination varying from 20 to 100 watts (Fig. 1.2).

Magnification Power of Light Microscope

The image enlargement or magnification power of a microscope depends on the length of the optical tube, magnifying power of objective, magnifying power of eye piece. Thus, the magnification power of a microscope = Magnifying power of objective × magnifying power of eye piece.

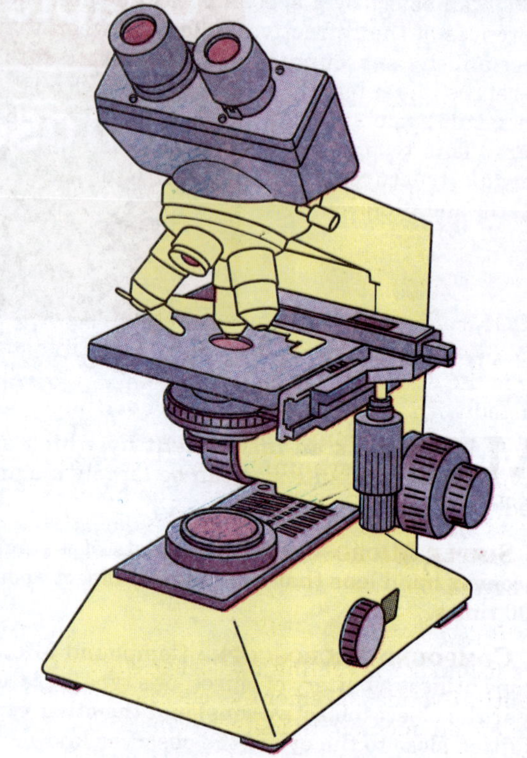

Fig. 1.2. Binocular light microscope *(base illumination type)*

Use of Light Microscope

- The microscope is to be kept in a comfortable position.
- Use appropriate illumination by adjusting the mirror or intensity of light.
- During examination of colourless objects, condenser should be at the lowest position and iris diaphragm is closed or partially closed.
- When using oil immersion, 100 × objective should dip in oil.
- Oil immersion lens of the objective should be cleaned with tissue paper or soft cloth after use.

OTHER TYPES OF MICROSCOPY

PHASE CONTRAST MICROSCOPE

A special condenser and objective are used in a light microscope. The different parts of a cell and its surrounding environment have got different refractive indices. When a beam of light is passed through an object by a special optical device, the differences of the refractive indices between the object and its surroundings are converted into differences into intensity of light (*phase contrast*). As a result some structures appear darker than others. This technique is applied in studies of internal structures of unstained living tissue, bacteria and protozoa.

Dark ground (dark field) illumination (DGI)

In DGI, *reflected light* is used instead of *transmitted light*. A dark field condenser with circular stop is the essential part of the microscope which is fitted with a light microscope. The condensor lens system is arranged in such a way that no light reaches the eye unless reflected from the object on the microscope stage. The bacteria or objects look luminous against a dark background. This method is employed to detect extremely slender organisms, such as, *Spirochaetes*.

Interference microscopy

It is useful for revealing cell organelles and for quantitative measurement of chemical constituents of cell such as, lipids, proteins and nucleic acids.

Fluorescence microscopy technique

In this, ultraviolet light is used. Bacteria stained with fluorescent dye (e.g., *auramine*) alter the wave length and become visible as bright objects against a dark background.

Immunofluorescne : Immunofluorescence combines serology with fluorescence microscopy by using immunoglobulin (antibody) labelled with fluorescent dyes for detection of specific antigens and bacteria. Fluorescent dyes commonly used are *fluorescein isothiocyanate, lissamine* and *rhodamine.*

Electron microscopy

In electron microscope, a beam of electrons is focused by a circular electromagnet (magnetic condenser) comparable to the lenses of light microscope. When an electron beam passes through an object, the electrons get scattered producing an image in the built-in fluorescent viewing screen. The wavelength of electrons employed is approximately 0.005 nm (cf. 500 nm with visible light). The resolving power is about 0.01–0.02 nm.

Shadow casting is an important technique in electron microscopy and that is achieved by depositing a thin layer of metal (e.g., platinum) on the object. Such metal-coated object is placed in the path of a beam of metal ions. The electron beam is directed on the object in such a way that a shadow is formed in the uncoated area on the other side and negative image is made. A positive image is made from negative image on a fluorescent viewing screen.

Negative staining with phosphotungstic acid is useful in studying the fine structure of object. **Scanning electron microscope** is a recent development and provides a three dimensioal image of the surface of the object.

Autoradiography

Cells are first treated with radioactive atoms and then covered with a photographic emulsion and stored in the dark for an optimal period of time. In the developed film, tracks appear from the sites of radioactive disintegration. This technique is employed to follow the DNA replication with the help of tritium-labelled thymidine as a specific tracer.

Chapter 2

Histopathology Techniques and Staining

Histopathology deals with microscopic diagnosis of various lesions of the organs. In a disease process, cellular elements exhibit considerable variation in structures and arrangements. Histopathological techniques deal with preparation of tissue either by biopsy or autopsy for microscopic viewing. This can be observed on suitably prepared material, cut into sections of single cell thickness and stained to differentiate the individual tissue elements. Tissue sent by surgeon should be kept in a preservative to prevent its decay and autolysis. The preservative is called fixative. The preparation of tissue for microscopy involves the following steps :

1. Fixation
2. Tissue processing
3. Blocking
4. Section cutting and fixing on slide
5. Staining with appropriate stain
6. Mounting.

FIXATION

A fixative is an agent that preserves the cells most closely to the original form present in the body. Most fixatives act by denaturation of proteins of tissues. The amount of fixative should be at least 10 times the volume of tissue. Tissue should be cut into small pieces (76 × 25 mm) for fixation. Several hours are needed for fixation.

Functions

1. Prevents autolysis of tissue.
2. Coagulates and renders insoluble various tissue elements.
3. Facilitates the staining reaction by acting as a mordant.

An ideal fixative should be effective, cheap, nontoxic and should facilitate all types of staining.

Types of fixatives

Fixatives may be primary and secondary. *Primary fixatives* include 10% formalin, Zenker's fluid, Helly's fluid and Bouin's fluid. *Secondary fixatives* are those which are used after the tissue has first been fixed for 3–4 hours in formalin. Formol sublimate and Helly's fluid can be used as secondary fixative.

Primary fixative

1. ***Formalin***

A 10% formol saline (formalin 10 ml + saline 90 ml) solution is the most commonly used fixative. Tissue is fixed in formalin usually in 12-24 hours. 10% neutral formalin (neutralized by calcium carbonate) in water is also used. Formalin is cheap, preserves most tissues well, and its only disadvantage that it is allergenic.

2. ***Zenker's fluid***

Preparation :

Mercuric chloride	...	5 g
Potassium dichromate	...	2.5 g
Water	...	100 ml

Add 5 ml glacial acetic acid immediately before use.

Advantage : It preserves nuclear and connective tissue very well. Fixation in Zenker's fluid facilitates metachromatic staining. Fixation time is 10–20 hours.

Disadvantage : Only thin pieces of tissue can be fixed (can penetrate up to 5 mm). It is expensive and has to be preserved only in special bottles made of nickel alloy. It deteriorates fast. If the tissue is left in the fluid for 3–4 days, it becomes hard and brittle.

Tissue requires to be washed for half an hour to one hour in running tap water after fixation in Zenker's fluid or several changes in 70% alcohol for same period of time.

3. ***Helly's fluid***

Composition : Stock solution is same as Zenker's fluid; add 5–10% of formalin immediately before use. It is similar in function as Zenker's fluid.

4. ***Bouin's fluid***

Picric acid saturated aqueous solution — 9 gm%)	....	75 ml
Formalin	....	25 ml
Glacial acetic acid	....	5 ml

Advantage : Rapid penetration, preserves glycogen, improves greatly staining of nuclei and connective tissue.

The tissue takes up yellow colour of picric acid, hence small piece of tissue can easily be spotted.

Disadvantage : It over-hardens the tissue if left in the fixative for more than 24 hours. It lyses red cells. Tissue fixed in Bouin's fluid should be directly transferred to 70% alcohol. It must not be washed in water because it forms water-soluble picrates.

Secondary fixative

The staining of tissue that has been fixed in formalin can be improved by placing in Helly's fluid or formol sublimate for 4-24 hours. The main advantage of secondary fixative is that, when further sections of tissue stored in formol saline for a long period be needed, the staining will show a marked improvement using secondary fixative.

Formol sublimate

Mercuric chloride (saturated aqueous solution — 8.3%)	....	90 ml
Formalin	....	10 ml

Staining is improved especially with acid dyes. Metachromatic staining is also brighter and good for secondary fixation.

Decalcification

The preparation of bone specimens presents special problems because of the necessity of decalcification of tissue before sections can be cut. Decalcification is the process by which bony tissue is softened and processed so that they can be cut.

1. ***Nitric acid method***

Nitric acid	....	5 ml
Distilled water	....	95 ml

Small pieces of bony tissues are left in aqueous nitric acid solution for 1–5 days. The solution is preferably changed every day and the tissue is to be tested to see if it has become soft enough to cut. This is done by bending the tissue or by piercing a knife or needle.

2. ***Formic acid method***

Formic acid (S.G. 1.2)	....	5-10 ml
Distilled water to	....	100 ml

It takes a longer time (5–14 days) for decalcification. The method is very satisfactory where speed is not essential.

The acid from the tissue must be removed with 70 per cent alcohol giving three changes during 24 hours.

3. ***Electrolyte method***

The method makes use of special electrolytic apparatus. The electrolyte used was equal parts of 8% HCl and 10% formic acid in distilled water and decalcification is completed in 1–4 hours. The method requires special supervision and cannot be recommended for routine laboratory work.

PROCESSING OF TISSUES

Thin sections of tissue have to be cut for microscopic examination for which the tissue should be embedded in medium that allows the section to be cut. Processing of tissue involves the following :

(a) Dehydration, (b) Clearing and
(c) Impregnation

Dehydration

Most of the tissue fixatives in use are aqueous solution. It becomes necessary to remove water from the tissue (*dehydration*) in order to embed the tissue in paraffin wax. This is achieved by immersing the fixed tissue in increasing strength of alcohol, 70%, 85% and 100%. The tissues are transferred from a solution of lower to higher concentration to prevent shrinkage of tissue which occurs by rapid dehydration. It takes 3–12 hours for dehydrating a tissue. The following dehydrating agents are in use :

1. *Ethyl alcohol* — most commonly used.
2. *Isopropyl alcohol.*
3. *Acetone* : It is sometimes used as dehydrating agent where speed is essential but it causes shrinkage and hardening of tissues.

Clearing

Since alcohol and wax are not miscible, the alcohol which occupies the tissue spaces is to be replaced with a solvent of the wax in which the tissue is to be later embedded before it can be cut. Majority of wax solvents make the tissue more or less transparent, and this effect has led to the use of the term *clearing.* The clearing agents are :

1. *Xylene,* most commonly used.
2. *Toluene,* next commonly used.
3. *Chloroform,* sometimes used.

Clearing in xylene and toluene takes 1–3 hours. On no account, should the tissue be allowed to remain in xylene longer than necessary as this produces brittleness of tissue with subsequent difficulty in section cutting.

Impregnation with wax

After clearing, the tissue is transferred to molten wax in a paraffin embedding oven (58-60 °C) to impregnate the tissue completely with molten paraffin. Tissue should be left in molten paraffin wax for 2–10 hours. Good quality paraffin wax (melting point 54–56 °C), free from dust and other foreign matter should be used. 10–20% bees wax is added to improve the texture of wax and harden it. Volume of wax should be 20–50 times the volume of the tissue. The paraffin wax should be replaced periodically as it becomes saturated with the clearing agent.

Routine manual processing schedule

1. Formalin (10%) — 12-24 hours
2. Alcohol (80%) — 1–4 hours
3. Alcohol (90%) — 2–4 hours
4. Absolute alcohol — 2–4 hours
5. Xylene (1) — 1–2 hours
6. Xylene (2) — 1–2 hours

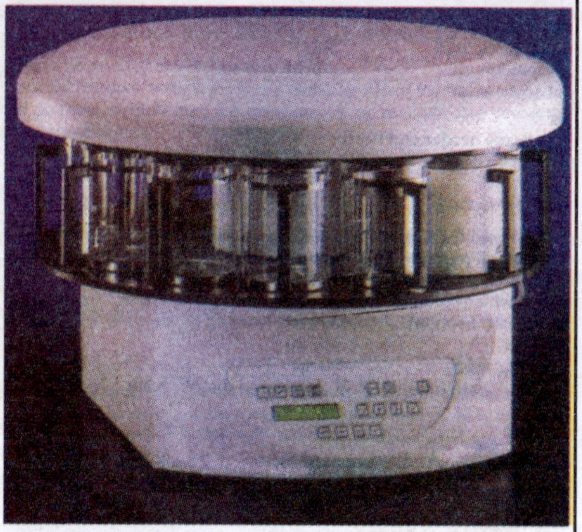

Fig. 2.1. Automatic tissue processor (*The model of that of Leica, Germany, Model No. TP 1020)*

7. Melted wax (1) — $1^1/_2$–2 hours
8. Melted wax (2) — $1^1/_2$–2 hours
9. Melted wax (3) — $1^1/_2$–2 hours.

Automatic tissue processor

The processing of tissue in the above mentioned manner can be done by automatic tissue processor (e.g., *autotechnicon*) (Fig. 2.1).

Advantage

1. Automatised, hence no supervision needed.
2. Large number of tissues can be processed with considerable ease.
3. Processing is uniform and reliable.
4. Rapid method : Processing begins after grossing of the day's specimens in afternoon and the processing is completed next morning after which the machine halts on its own.

Change of solution

After using the fluid for two days, the first jar containing the alcohol of lowest strength is discarded and the remaining jars are moved up, so that the jar which was at number two now becomes number one jar. A new jar filled with absolute alcohol now takes the position of previous last jar.

BLOCKING

Paraffin wax used for blocking is kept in a beaker in molten state in the wax oven.

1. The moulds are adjusted to suitable size and then filled with molten wax (Fig. 2.2).

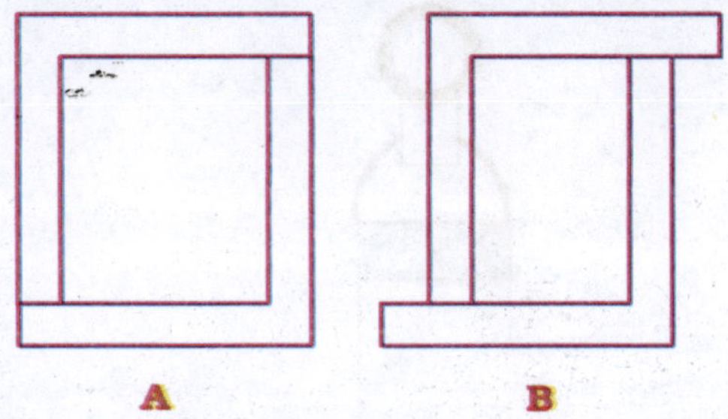

Fig. 2.2. Leukart's L blocks *(embedding moulds)*

2. Take the container with tissue out of the oven and place the tissue using forceps in this molten wax in such a manner that the surface to be cut faces downwards.

3. Press the tissue with tip of the forceps as far as it will go in the wax and allow to harden.

L–blocks or L–moulds are L–shaped pieces made of brass. By simple manipulation of two L-blocks, the size can be altered as per the need of the tissue. It is advisable to block out in a piece of plain glass. Besides the commonly used L-blocks, other types of mould include disposable polystyrene plastic trays (Fig. 2.3) with 8 or 10 moulds each.

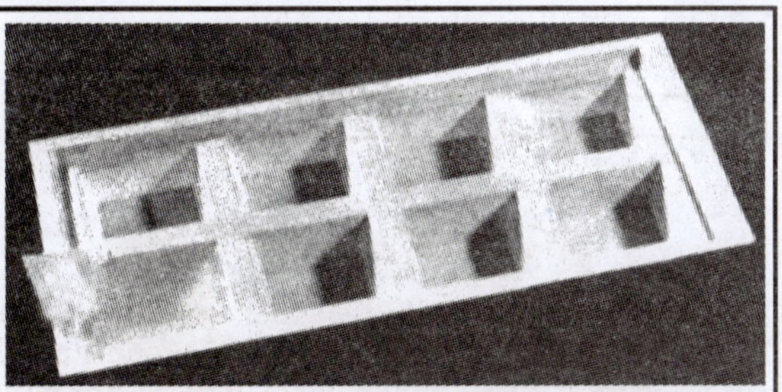

Fig. 2.3. Disposable polystyrene *(plastic)* moulds

Certain other substances can also be used for embedding, e.g., water soluble waxes, gelatin and celloidin.

SECTION CUTTING

The tissue block prepared in paraffin wax is cut into fine sections which involves the use of a precision instrument called *microtome.*

Microtome

There are five types of microtomes : *rotary, sliding, rocker, frozen section* and microtome for *ultra-thin sections.*

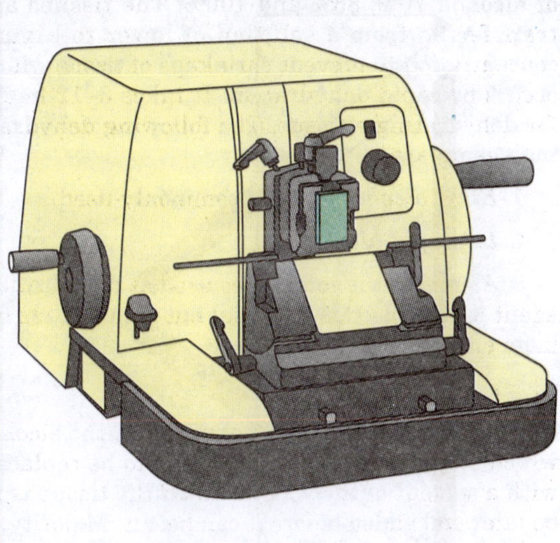

Fig. 2.4. Rotary microtome

1. ***Rotary microtome***

It is the most commonly used type and gives sections 3–4 µm thickness (Fig. 2.4). It has got a stationary knife holder and a moving ball joint block holder clamp. Knife is placed blade up. The length of the knife is small and can be used to cut small tissues and cutting serial sections. Large blocks cannot be cut out. Knife requires frequent sharpening. The machine has a relatively complex design.

2. ***Sliding microtome***

It has a simple design. The machine operates with a fixed object holder and a moving knife and with a vertical object fed to the cutting plane. Large sections like whole brain can be cut. Knife does not require sharpening regularly but because of its large size, sharpening becomes difficult.

Microtomes for cutting ulta-thin sections are available. Frozen section microtome is dealt in frozen section.

Microtome knife

The knife is perhaps the most important part of microtome. Standard knives are made of good grade steel with high carbon content and may be *biconcave, planoconcave* or *planowedge* (both surfaces are flat and tapered). Handles of knives are removable.

Sharpening

Handles are fitted and knives sharpened from

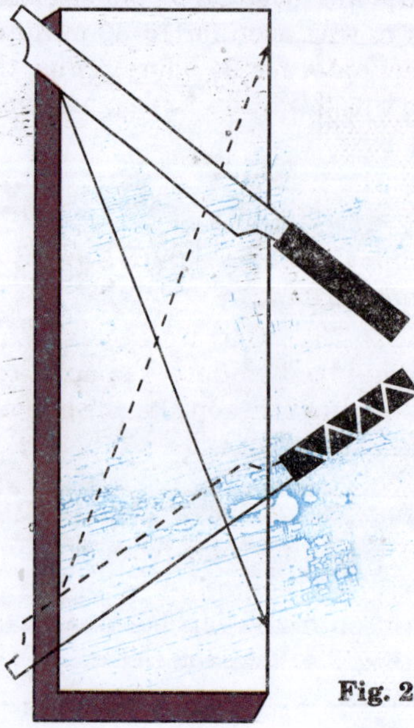

Fig. 2.5. Honing

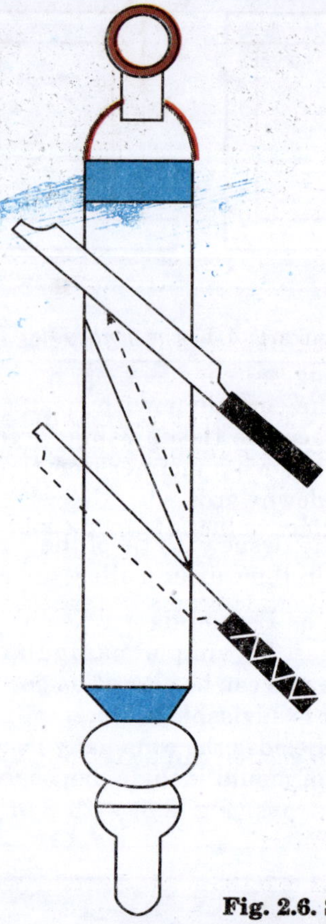

Fig. 2.6. Stropping

time to time by using *"hones"*. There are two types of hones : (i) *naturally occurring* ones called oil stones (e.g., Arkansas stone, yellow Belgian glass stone, green Belgian glass stone, Belgian black vein stone); (ii) *artificial stones* (e.g., plate glass carborundum).

Spread a little lubricant (e.g., olive oil, liquid paraffin) on the surface of hone. Knife is fitted with handle. Draw the knife edge first along the whole length of the hone, i.e., heel to toe (Fig. 2.5). Then the knife is turned on its thick edge and the movement on its other surface is repeated.

Automatic microtome knife sharpeners are also used for sharpening knife (Fig. 2.7).

Stropping

After honing, the knives are *stropped* on horse leather mounted on solid wooden block strops (measure 18" × 3-4") (Fig. 2.6). While stropping, the knife is moved from toe to heel, the *reverse of honing*. At the end of each stroke the knife is turned over on its back and the movement is repeated.

Block-holder

1. Excess paraffin on all sides of the block are removed by a scalpel keeping 3 mm paraffin around it (*trimming*).

2. The block is then fitted with a block-holder (Fig. 2.8) and kept in refrigerator for 5-10 minutes.

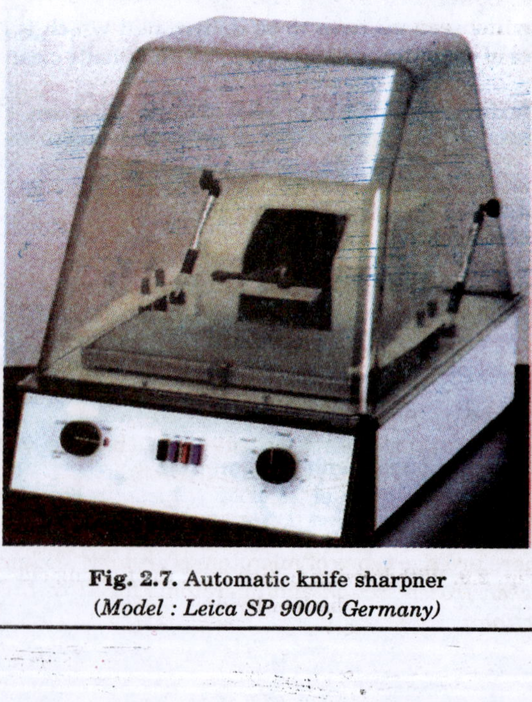

Fig. 2.7. Automatic knife sharpner
(Model : Leica SP 9000, Germany)

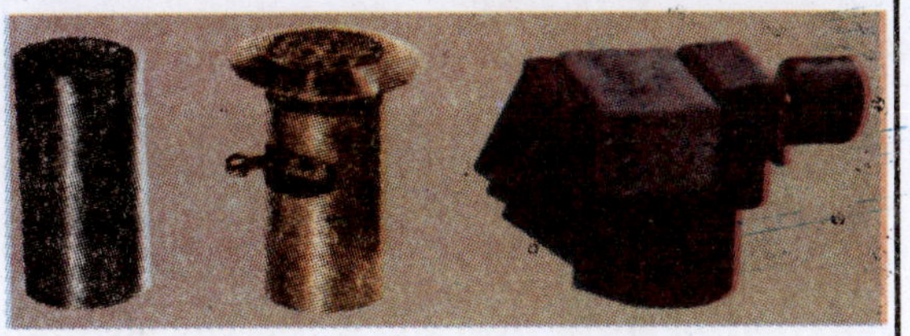

Fig. 2.8. Types of block holders

3. The block-holder is fixed to the microtome and the cutting knife is inserted.

4. The block is first trimmed setting the microtome to 20-25 μm until the actual tissue is exposed.

5. The surface of block is made cold on a piece of ice.

6. Adjust the microtome to required thickness of sections (3 5 μm).

7. Section is cut by applying regular and even forward strokes.

8. A ribbon section can be obtained with considerable practice.

Floating sections

1. Sections are then lifted gently using a fine brush in a hot water bath kept to temperature below the melting point of wax.

2. Lower a clean new slide gently into the water to which egg albumin has been applied and the section will glide off (Fig. 2.9).

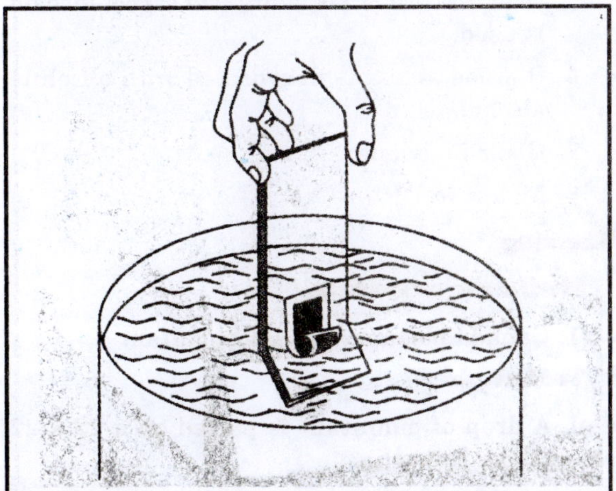

Fig. 2.9. Withdrawing section from the floating out bath or bowl

3. The slides are dried off by placing them on a tray in paraffin wax oven for 15-30 minutes or at 37°C in an incubator for 24 hours. Thus, the sections are fixed to the slide firmly and ready for staining.

STAINING OF SECTION

(a) *Haematoxylin* and *Eosin (HE)* : HE stain is most commonly used.

(b) *Special stains* : Certain special stains are sometimes employed to detect special features e.g., PAS, Reticulin, Masson's trichrome and Van Giesson's stains.

Haematoxylin and Eosin staining

Haematoxylin is obtained from a tree called *Haematoxylon campechianum* found in Mexico. Haematoxylin on oxidation becomes haematin which is the essential staining element. Cell nuclei take up haematin.

Preparation of stains

1. ***Harris's alum haematoxylin***

Haematoxylin	....	1 g
Absolute alcohol	....	10 ml
Aluminium potassium sulphate (Potash alum)	....	20 g
Distilled water	....	200 ml
Mercuric oxide	....	0.5 g

Dissolve the haematoxylin in the alcohol, the alum in water by the aid of heat, and the two solutions are then mixed. Bring rapidly to the boil. Remove from the heat and add the mercuric oxide. The solution is again reheated until it assumes a dark purple colour. As soon as the colour forms, the flame is removed and the container of stain is then plunged into bowl of water. It is now ready for use.

The staining of the nuclei improves if 4% glacial acetic acid is added to the stain.

2. ***Eosin aqueous***

Stock solution	5% in water, add a crystal of thymol or 1% formalin.
Working solution	Dilute to 1% with water.

Procedure of staining

1. Treat the section with xylene to deparaffinise it (two changes).

2. Wash off the xylene with graded alcohol (100%–90%–70% and water).

3. Wash in tap water and drain well.

4. Stain with Harris's haematoxylin for 10-20 minutes.

5. Tip off stain and wash thoroughly with tap water (15–30 seconds).

6. Differentiate in 1% acid alcohol (HCl 1 ml + 70% alcohol 99 ml) for 10-20 seconds.

7. Wash off the 1% acid alcohol with tap water.

8. *Blueing* : The term blueing is applied to a process when a section is transferred from an acid solution to an alkaline fluid. After step 7, the sections are placed in cold tap water (slightly alkaline) for 10-20 minutes. Alternatively, blueing can be done by placing the section in 2% ammonia water for 5-15 seconds.

9. Counterstain with 1% aqueous eosin (yellowish) for 1-5 minutes.

10. Wash in tap water, the length of time depends on the amount of eosin that is desired to be left in the section.

11. Wash with 95% alcohol for a few seconds.

12. Dehydrate with absolute alcohol for a few seconds.

13. Clear by washing with xylene (2 changes).

14. Mount in Canada balsam or DPX.

Result : Cell nuclei – blue
Muscle fibres – red
Collagen fibres – pink
RBCs – bright red

Special stains

Periodic and Schiff (PAS) stain

Use : Demonstration of glycogen, mucin, hyaluronic acid, colloid droplets, hyalin of arteriosclerosis.

Result : Nuclei – blue
Fungi – red
Glycogen – pink to red

Masson's trichome stain

Use : Demonstration of muscle, collagen, etc.

Result : Nuclei – black
Collagen, mucus – blue
Cytoplasm,
Keratin, muscle – red

Van Giesson's stain

Use : Demonstration of collagen fibres.

Result : Collagen – red
Muscle, cornified epithelium – yellow
Nuclei – blue to black

Reticulin stain (Gordon & Sweet's method)

Use : Demonstration of reticulin, elastic and nerve fibres.

Result : Reticulin fibres – black to brownish black
Nerve fibres – black
Elastic fibres – jet black
Nuclei – almost colourless
Collagen fibres – red (if stained with Van Geisson)

Other special stains

Congo red staining : Amyloid stains red, nuclei stain blue.

Sudan III or Sudan IV : Neutral fats stain orange, nuclei stain blue.

Staining bacteria in tissue

1. Treat paraffin section with xylene.
2. Wash off xylene with alcohol.
3. Wash in distilled water.
4. Blot with Whatman No. 1 filter paper until the section is dry.
5. Secton is now stained by appropriate method. In case of ZN stain, cold carbol fuchsin is used.
6. Stained smear is dehydrated with absolute alcohol.
7. Clear in xylene.
8. Mount in DPX.

Mounting

Media for mounting

1. Canada balsam 2. DPX mountant

Technique

1. A drop of mountant is placed on a 22 × 22 sq. m clean coverslip.

2. A slide with section is now placed on the coverslip in such a way that the section comes in contact with the mountant.

3. As soon as the mountant begins to spread, turn the slide over.

4. If the coverslip has not been quite square on the slide, gently adjust with a fine glass rod.

5. The mounted slide is kept in paraffin wax oven for 12-18 hours or in incubator at 37 °C for 24 hours.

FROZEN SECTION

Advantage

1. It becomes necessary at times to make frozen section of tissue when a quick diagnosis is needed so that the biopsy and surgery can be performed at the same sitting.

2. It is an essential technique in demonstration of lipids as the same is dissolved in routine processing.

3. Minimum amount of shrinkage occurs as compared to paraffin-wax technique.

4. Practically every method of staining can be performed on most frozen sections.

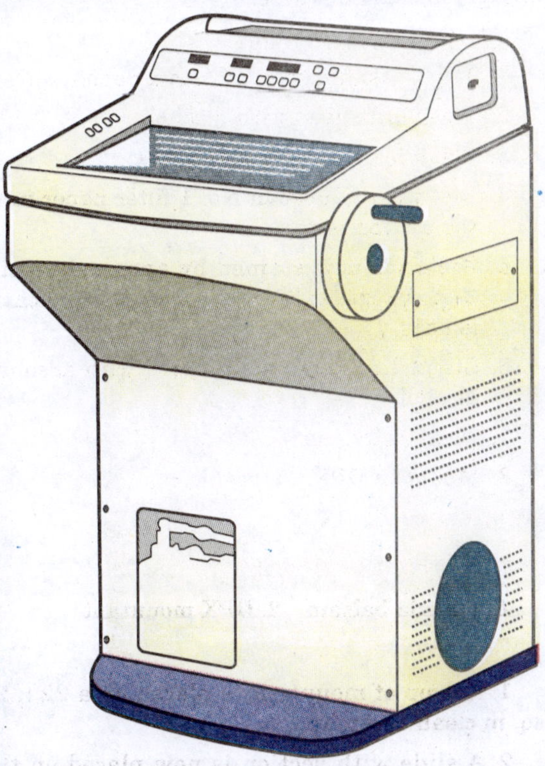

Fig. 2.10. Cryostat

Disadvantage

1. Thickness of sections obtained is 7–10 microns (μm) and thin sections are difficult.

2. Correlation of serial sections is practically not possible.

3. Moreover, interpretation of frozen biopsies needs especially trained pathologists.

Methods of preparing frozen sections

Two types of freezing microtomes are mainly used for taking frozen sections :

(a) *Freezing microtome* : A freezing microtome (Fig. 2.10) with carbon dioxide gas is in use for many years and is still a very popular technique.

(b) *Refrigerated microtome* (cryostat) : The microtomes that are in use with the cryostat are standard rotary microtomes or standard cambridge rotary rocker.

Processing

1. *Fixation* : Hot 10% formol saline is used as fixative. Tissues to be sectioned should not exceed 3 mm in thickness.

2. *Freezing* : Tissue is frozen with bursts of CO_2.

3. *Section cutting* : Sections are cut at 8-10 μm in thickness (6–8 sections are cut).

4. *Float* in distilled water and collect the section on a slide.

5. Cover the section with absolute alcohol.

6. *Rapidly transfer to a petridish* containing 0.5–1% celloidin, keep for 5–10 seconds.

7. *Drain excess celloidin* and allow the section to dry partially.

8. *Harden* the celloidin by 70% alcohol, 10-20 seconds.

9. *Staining* : By Coles haematoxylin for one minute.

10. *Wash* in tap water.

11. *Differentiate* with 1% acid alcohol.

12. *Rinse* in tap water.

13. *Counter-stain* with 0.3% aqueous eosin.

14. Wash eosin with tap water.

15. Rinse in 95% alcohol for 2 to 3 seconds.

16. Dehydrate with absolute alcohol.

17. Remove celloidin film by washing carefully with alcohol-ether mixture.

18. Rinse with absolute alcohol.

19. Clear with xylene.

20. Mount in DPX.

Cole's haematoxylin

Haematoxylin	...	1.5 g
Iodine (1% in 95% alcohol)	...	50 ml
Ammon. alum (saturated solution)	...	700 ml
Distilled water	...	250 ml

Dissolve the haematoxylin in warmed distilled water. Add the solution of iodine and mix well. Next add the alum solution and bring to the boil. Cool and filter.

Egg albumin mixture

Egg white	...	50 ml
Glycerine	...	50 ml
Sodium salicylate	...	50 ml

Mix thoroughly and filter through wet lint.

Section I

HAEMATOLOGY

Section I contains

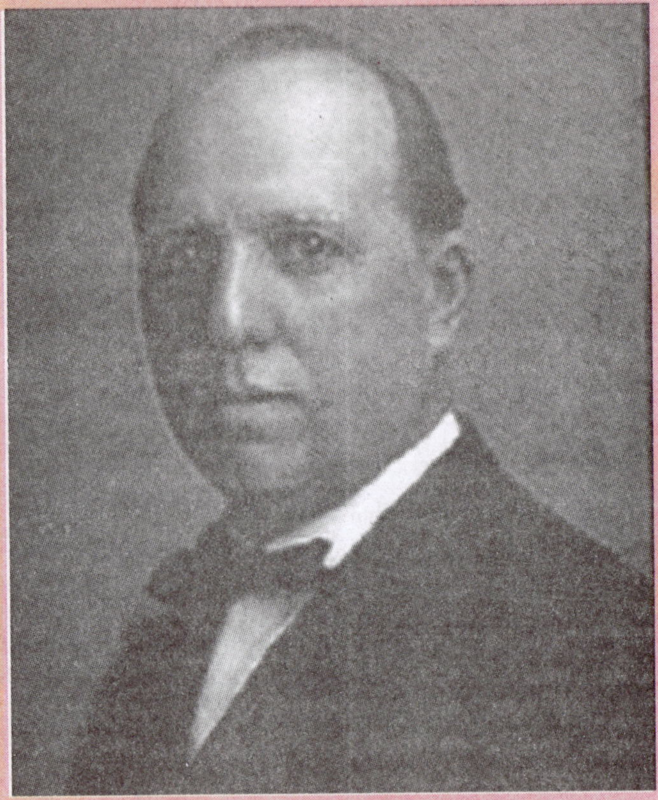

MM Wintrobe (1901–1986)

Wintrobe was an American Physician. *He devised Wintrobe haematocrit tube for estimation of PCV, ESR and that has enabled measuring red cell indices. He was a pupil of William Loyd, a pioneering teacher and eminent author of last century. William Loyd considered Wintrobe as a very stimulating teacher with keen interest in the development of museum.*

Chapter 3

Collection of Blood and Anticoagulants

BLOOD

Composition and function

Blood is a mesenchymal tissue consisting a liquid portion called plasma, in which there are formed elements such as Red Blood Corpuscles (RBCs), White Blood Corpuscles (WBCs) and platelets.

Plasma

Plasma contains all the clotting factors except calcium^{++} and is obtained by centrifugation of the anticoagulant added blood. *Serum* is obtained by allowing whole blood to stand at room temperature when it undergoes clotting. It lacks coagulation factors V, VII, VIII, IX, X, XI and that are used up in clotting.

The plasma proteins form an extraordinarily complex mixture, many of whch including albumin, fibrinogen and most globulins, are synthesised in liver; immunoglobulins are synthesised by reticuloendothelial system, the lymph nodules and plasma cells; the enzymes are released from various organs.

The three major types of plasma protein are as follows :

Albumin	....	4.5 gm%
Globulin	....	2.5 gm%
Fibrinogen	....	0.3 gm%

When blood is prevented from clotting in a penicillin vial or test tube by adding anticoagulant, the formed elements (cells) gradually sink to the bottom, leaving a clear yellow fluid above, which is called *plasma. Serum* is plasma minus some substances such as fibrinogen which have been used up for the formation of clot.

Functions of plasma

1. *Nutritive* : Carries food materials to tissues.

2. *Maintenance of correct body water distribution* : The colloid osmotic pressure of plasma proteins (primary function of albumin, to a lesser extent by other type of proteins) counteracts hydrostatic pressure and thus maintain the required circulatory volume.

3. *Buffers* : Proteins play a minor role in maintaining plasma pH by accepting hydrogen ions as they are negatively charged at body pH and so act as bases.

4. *Fluidity* : Keeps the blood fluid and carries formed elements.

5. *Transporting agents* : The albumin can transport a wide range of substances, while other proteins can carry only a particular one, e.g. transferrin for iron. The important substances thus transported include hormones (cortisol, thyroxine), lipids, fat-soluble vitamins and metals. Certain toxic substances are also rendered harmless by binding to protein.

6. *Blood coagulation* : Many of the coagulation factors are proteins.

7. *Protective* : Immunoglobulins are antibodies which give protection against infection.

8. *As enzymes* : The wide range of enzymes present in the plasma are proteins.

9. *Elimination* of waste materials from tissues is carried by protein to excretory organs.

Cellular elements

The RBCs, granulocytes (polymorphonuclear leucocytes), monocytes and platelets are derived from the bone marrow; white lymphocytes, though initially are derived from bone marrow, but are subsequenty derived from lymphoreticular system in adult life.

Functions

1. *Red blood cells* : (a) They carry oxygen from lungs to tissues and carbon dioxide from tissues to lung (for excretion). This is achieved by the haemoglobin in RBC which can loosely combine with oxygen and carbon dioxide. (b) They also help in maintaining acid base balance.

2. *White cells* : Their main function is to defend the body against infection.

Diseases produced

1. *Diseases involving red blood.*

Cells : (a) Deficiency of RBCs and haemoglobin — anaemia. (b Excess of red blood cells — polycythaemia.

2. *Diseases involving white blood cells.*

(a) Deficiency of WBCs— leucopenia and agranulocytosis. (b) Excess of WBCs—leucocytosis and leukaemia.

3. *Haemorrhagic diseases.*

COLLECTION OF BLOOD

Blood may be withdrawn by three methods :

(a) **Venous** blood from antecubital vein using a vacutainer/syringe.

(b) **Capillary** blood from a finger/heel.

(c) **Arterial** blood from an artery.

A. Method for Venous Blood

For haematological tests venous blood is preferred, usually from the ante-cubital fossa. A medium-sized needle of 19 or 20 gauge is preferable, with shaft about 15 mm long is particularly suitable for use in children. Use of thinner needle (23-24 gauge) may result haemolysis of blood. Congestion should be avoided during collection of blood as far as practicable, to prevent haemoconcentration. Use of tourniquet is a routine practice, but it should be loosened once the needle has been inserted into the vein. Instead of tourniquet, a sphygmomanometer cuff can be used, a pressure between systolic and diastolic is applied.

(a) Apply the tourniquet at the upper arm.

(b) Clean the skin over the antecubital area of the upper arm with 70% alcohol and allow it to dry. Patient closes the fist.

(c) Fix the vein in position by supporting patient's forearm with one hand.

(d) Holding the syringe with other hand, push the needle into the vein with a single direct puncture of skin and vein. Entrance of needle into vein is indicated by appearance of blood into the hub of the needle.

(e) Loosen the tourniquet if blood flows freely and the patient is asked to open the fist.

(f) When the desired amount of blood is obtained, release the tourniquet, withdraw the syringe and needle from the vein keeping a spirit swab at the skin puncture.

(g) Place one drop of blood each into three slides for preparing smears.

(h) Now pour the blood vial with anticoagulant (EDTA, citrate) as required.

B. Method for Capillary Blood

Finger Prick Method

(a) The site (e.g., tip of finger) is rubbed vigorously with a gauze or cotton pad moistened with 70% alcohol. Allow to dry.

(b) A rapid firm puncture is made with a sterile lancet or needle, 2-3 mm deep, on the lateral side of the tip of the finger. Above the puncture site gentle squeezing is allowable.

(c) The first two drops of blood containing tissue juices is to be discarded.

(d) Free flowing blood is collected in haemoglobinometer pipette, 0.02 ml each for Hb, TLC, platelet count, etc.

(e) Smears are made from the drops collected on the slides.

The finger prick method is generally less accurate because of dilution by tissue fluid, etc. However, in certain circumstances, for total and differential cell count and for haemoglobin estimation, blood can be collected by pricking from the following sites : palmar surface of tip of finger, ear lobe, and in infants, from plantar surface of hand or great toe. Ring finger is preferrable for collection of capillary blood. In case of finger prick should be adequately deep for free flow of blood or by applying gentle squeeze blood should flow. Tip of the finger should not be squeezed that dilutes blood with tissue fluid. Because the initial drops of prick become contaminated with the spirit, first few drops are to be thrown out. The ulnar side of the tip of finger is ideal for pricking since it is comparatively less innervated by nerve and hence less painful. Sometimes, blood may have to be obtained from femoral or jugular vein of infant.

After collection of blood, the syringe and needle is disposed of in antiseptic solution. *All samples of blood should be considered as potential sources of infection* and should not come in contact with the collector's body.

Containers for Venous blood

1. For *routine tests* of blood such as cell counts, estimation of haemoglobin, PCV, ESR, blood is collected in a penicillin vial or test tube containing suitable anticoagulant, e.g., EDTA.

2. *For tests using serum,* sample is collected in a clean dry sterile test tube or penicillin vial and allowed to clot.

3. *For bacteriological work,* sample is collected in sterile blood culture bottle containing glucose broth.

Heel Prick Method

Usually done in infants. In an infant, the heel is gently rubbed to warm it. Clean the lateral/ medial part of the heel (plantar surface) using alcohol. Give a prick on medial/lateral part of plantar surface. Blood is collected for Hb/TLC and make the peripheral smears.

C. Arterial Blood

It is usually collected from femoral artery for blood gas analysis. The pulsations of the femoral artery are felt below the inguinal ligament. Disposable needle and syringe are used for blood collection.

D. Vacutainer (Vacuum Tube) Method

- The first 2 steps of the method for venous blood is followed.
- An appropriate vacutainer tube is placed in a reusable plastic holder and thereafter a disposable needle is attached by screwing the threaded needle hub-top to the holder. Now insert the tube into the holder until the top of its stopper is levelled with the marked guideline which causes the tube to recede.
- Patient's arm is placed in slightly vertical position. When a vacutainer is to be used for venipuncture, one should be careful not to make a venipuncture in a horizontal plane which may cause black flow of blood.
- Needle is inserted into the vein just as a syringe is done and the base of the collection tube is pushed forward breaking the vacuum seal. Allow time for the vacuum tube to fill.
- Ask the patient to open the fist and remove the tourniquet and withdraw the needle with the syringe.
- When samples of blood are to be collected in multiple vials, the tourniquet is released before collection of each tube. The needle retained in the vein, the vial with blood is removed and the other vials/tubes are attached as needed.

ANTICOAGULANTS

A number of different anticoagulants are used for various purposes (Table 3.1).

1. ***EDTA*** : Sodium and potassium salts of ethylenediamine tetraacetic acid (EDTA) also called sequestrene, are specially suitable for routine haematological investigation.

Action : It is a powerful calcium chelating (binding) agent and acts by binding the calcium molecules in blood.

Concentration : Dipotassium salt of EDTA is routinely used in a concentration of 1.5 ± 0.25 mg/ ml blood. Usually a 10% solution is made and dried in incubator or oven. At this concentration of the salt, some shrinkage of RBCs occur which results in 2 to 3% decrease in PCV.

Disadvantage : Excess of EDTA (more than 2 mg/ml) causes shrinkage of both RBCs and WBCs and degenerative changes; decreased in PCV and increase in MCHC. EDTA is unsuitable for coagulation studies.

2. ***Trisodium citrate*** : A 3.8% aqueous solution of trisodium citrate ($Na_3C_6H_5O_7, 2H_2O$) is the anticoagulant of choice in studies of ESR and coagulation. It binds with calcium of blood.

Uses :

(a) ESR : 4 volumes of venous blood are diluted with 1 volume of 3.8% Sod. citrate solution (4 : 1).

Table 3.1 : Some anticoagulants and their use

Anticoagulants (per ml blood)	*Principle of action*	*Laboratory tests done*
NIL	—	Serum : Lipid profile (cholesterol, triglyceride, HDL, LDL), liver function tests (bilirubin, protein, SGOT, SGPT, alkaline phosphatase), creatinine, etc.
EDTA (1–1.5 mg/ml)	Binds Ca^{++}	TCDC, Hb, PCV, Platelet, Parasite (MP, microfilaria).
Heparin (0.1 to 0.2 mg/ml)	Inhibits thrombin action	Osmotic fragility of red cells, estimation of plasma iron.
Trisod citrate (3.8% aqueous solution)	Binds Ca^{++}	ESR, Prothrombin time.
Sod/Pot oxalate (2 mg/ml)	Binds Ca^{++}	Hb, Blood urea, Sp. gr. of blood.
Double oxalate (Ammon and Pot oxalate 2 mg/ml)	Binds Ca^{++}	TCDC, Hb, ESR, MCV.
Sod/Pot fluoride (6 mg/ml)	Glycolytic inhibition for glucose	Sugar (glucose).

(b) Prothrombin time : 9 volumes of blood are added to 1 volume of 3.8% Sodium citrate solution (9 : 1).

3. *Oxalates*

Potassium, sodium and ammonium oxalates act as chelating agents. They interact with blood calcium resulting in formation of calcium oxalate.

(a) *Potassium and Sodium oxalates* are used in a concentration of 2 mg per ml blood most often for chemical analysis.

(b) *Double oxalate* (Wintrobe's mixture) : The two oxalates are combined in a mixture with the ratio of 3 parts of NH_4 oxalate and 2 parts of K oxalate. It is used in a concentration of 2 mg. per ml blood and the vials are prepared as follows :

Ammonium oxalate	....	1.2 gm
Potassium oxalate	....	0.8 gm
Distilled water	....	100 ml

The solution contains 20 mg of oxalates per ml and 0.1 ml of this solution is pipetted into container and dried in an incubator or oven. The resultant powder is sufficient for 5 ml blood.

Uses : (i) Hb estimation and total cell count, (ii) Haematocrit value, (iii) Determination of sp. gr. of whole blood or plasma.

Double oxalate causes alteration of morphology of WBC and RBC. Smear made from anticoagulant added blood is unsuitable for morphological study. It is not much used nowadays.

4. *Sodium fluoride*

It forms calcium fluoride. It is used in a concentration of 30 mg powder per 5 ml blood. It is the anticoagulant of choice for blood sugar determination as it not only forms calcium fluoride but also prevents glycolysis by blocking phosphorylase enzymes in red cells. When estimation is likely to be delayed, thymol is added as a preservative along with sodium fluoride.

5. ***Heparin*** : Heparin powder or liquid acts by inhibiting thromboplastin formation and secondly as an antithrombin i.e. inhibiting the action of thrombin on fibrinogen. It is used in a concentration of 10-20 iu (0.1 to 0.2 mg) per ml blood.

Uses : Heparin is an effective anticoagulant and does not alter the size of RBCs and is specially useful in osmotic fragility tests, for studies of red cell enzyme (G–6–PD and PK deficiency) and for chemical estimations e.g. plasma iron.

Disadvantages : It is expensive. Heparinised blood is unsatisfactory for blood films and counts as it tends to cause leucocytes and platelets to clump. It is inferior to EDTA for general use.

QUESTIONS

1. *What is the composition of blood ?*
2. *How does plasma differ from serum ?*
3. *What is the composition of plasma ?*
4. *Which size of needle is used for collection of venous blood ?*
5. *Name the different containers for collection of blood.*
6. *Why initial 1–2 drops of blood are discarded after collecting blood by finger prick method ?*
7. *Name some anticoagulants and their use.*
8. *Why Wintrobe's mixture (double oxalates) are less frequently used ?*

Chapter 4

Estimation of Haemoglobin: Haemoglobinometer

HAEMOGLOBIN

Haemoglobin is the main component of red cells and is a conjugated protein in which four haem molecules are attached to one large molecule of globin (Fig. 4.1). The main function of haemoglobin is to transport oxygen from lungs to tissues. Four principal forms of Hb include :

(a) Oxyhaemoglobin (HbO_2)

(b) Carboxyhaemoglobin (HbCO)

(c) Sulphmethaemoglobin (SHb)

(d) Methaemoglobin (Hi)

ESTIMATION OF HAEMOGLOBIN

Most of the techniques described are colour or light intensity matching techniques. The iron content or oxygen combining capacity of blood (1.34 ml O_2 per gram Hb) is hardly practicable to estimate in clinical work.

Methods

1. Colorimetric or spectrophotometric method
   (a) Cyanmethaemoglobin method
   (b) Oxyhaemoglobin method
2. Acid–haematin (Sahli) method
3. Alkaline—haematin method
4. Tallqvist method
5. Haematology analysers

Of the different procedures, cyanmethaemoglobin (HiCN) method is most widely used because of the availability of a stable and reliable reference preparation. Sahli's acid – haematin method is less accurate as the colour which develops is unstable and begins to fade almost immediately after it has reached its peak.

Reading of result

Haemoglobin content is expressed in terms of grams per 100 ml of blood or grams per cent. Since different methods of estimation use different levels of Hb as equivalent to 100%, expression by percentage is not advisable. However, 14.5 gm per cent (Hellige) is widely accepted as normal level of Hb in an adult as equivalent to 100%.

Findings

1. *Normal level*

   In male : 14–16 gm %.

   In female : 13–15 gm %.

   In newborn baby : 16–18 gm %.

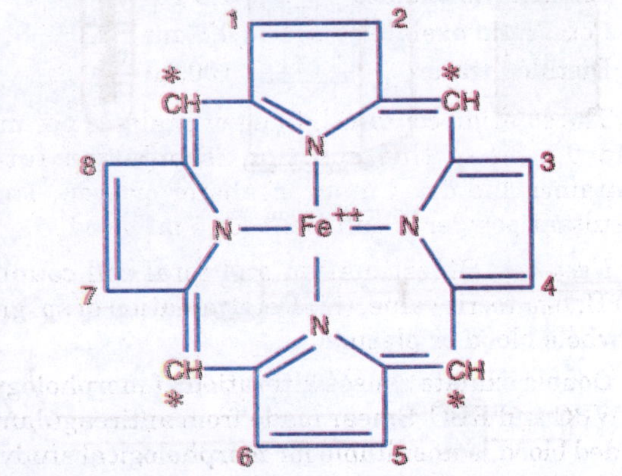

Fig. 4.1. Basic structure of the haemoglobin molecule, showing one of the four haeme complexes bound with the central globin core of the haemoglobin molecule

2. *Abnormal level*

(a) *Diminished level* : In anaemia (usually less than 10 gm %).

(b) *Increased level* : In polycythaemia and haemoconcentration due to dehydration.

I. Acid-haematin Method (Sahli method)

Although Acid-haematin method of estimation of haemoglobin is not very accurate, yet it is practised by some rural laboratories.

Principle : Haemoglobin is converted into acid haematin by adding N/10 hydrochloric acid (0.1 N) and the resulting brown colour is compared with standard brown glass reference blocks. Acid haematin, being a colloidal suspension, cannot be read in colorimeter which requires optically clear solution.

Instruments required

The Sahli haemoglobinometer consists of a standard brown glass mounted on a comparator and a graduated tube. A special pipette with a single mark 20 cu.mm is supplied with the instrument.

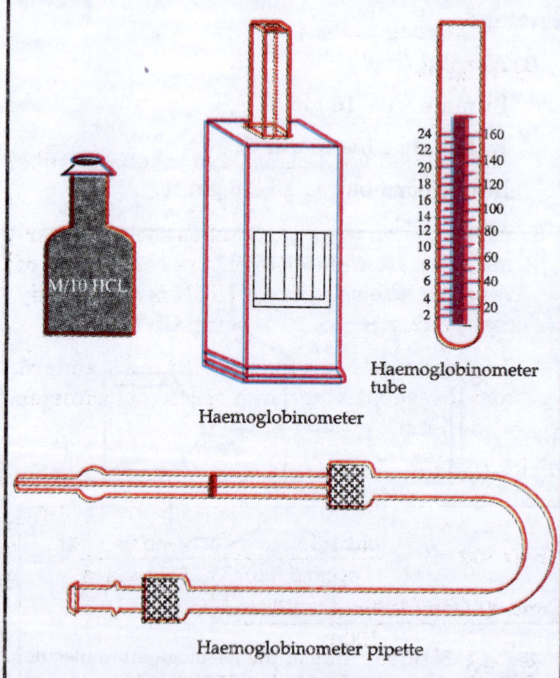

Fig. 4.2. Sahli haemoglobinometer : comparator, haemoglobinometer tube and haemoglobinometer pipette

1. ***Haemoglobinometer tube***

Identification : It is a graduated tube marked on ascending order on both sides — on one side (left side Fig. 4.2) shows grams per 100 ml and the opposite side indicates percentage. Graduation on tubes varies with different modifications. The recent Hellige's tubes are square and give 14.5 gm as 100 per cent when compared with the brown colour of the comparator glass. When the colour of the solution of acid haematin in square Hb tube is compared with flat brown surface of the comparator, the reading is taken easily eliminating error resulting from curvature of round tube.

Use : It is used for quantitative estimation of Hb by acid-haematin method.

2. ***Haemoglobinometer pipette***

Identification : It is a slender special pipette with a single mark of 20 cu.mm.

Use : (i) The pipette is used for quantitative estimation of haemoglobin in blood. (ii) *Other uses* : WBC count (0.4 ml fluid +0.02 ml blood, 1 : 20), RBC count, platelet count, cell count of other fluids and sperm count.

3. ***Haemoglobin comparator***

It is used for matching the colour of acid haematin formed in haemoglobinometer tube.

Procedure

The graduated haemoglobinometer tube is filled to the lowest mark (20) with N/10 HCl. Draw blood up to 20 cu.mm in the pipette after finger prick or from EDTA or double oxalate mixed blood and transfer it to acid in the tube. The pipette is rinsed well by drawing up some of the acid and re-expressing it. The acid and blood are mixed by shaking the tube well. The tube is then allowed to stand in the comparator on the table for at least 10 minutes for full conversion of haemoglobin to acid haematin (development of brown colour). About 95% of the total colour develops at the end of 10 minutes, 98% at the end of 20 minutes.

The brown solution is then diluted drop by drop with distilled water and stirred with a stirrer until the colour matches with the glass plates in the comparator. The matching should be done only against natural light.

Reading : The level of the fluid at its upper meniscus and the reading corresponding to this level on the label of scale of comparator is read in grams per cent.

Note : Reading is taken from upper meniscus of the coloured test solution (c.f. in colourless solution like water, the reading is made from the lower meniscus of the solution). The stirrer is not withdrawn from the Hb meter tube because small quantity of acid haematin sticking to the glass rod may be lost giving a lower haemoglobin value. During reading, the stirrer is to be lifted in the upper part of the tube.

Limitations : Acid-haematin technique is not a very accurate method of determination and the error is 5-20 per cent.

The carboxy Hb, carbamino Hb and sulphaemoglobin are not converted into acid haematin.

N/10 HCl : It is prepared by mixing 3.6 gm or 3 ml concentrated HCl and 996.4 gm or 997 ml of distilled water.

II. Cyanmethaemoglobin Method

This is the most accurate and most widely used method of estimation of haemoglobin in most parts of the world. It is the internationally recommended method for best quality control.

Principle :

When blood is mixed with a solution containing potassium cyanide and potassium ferricyanide, haemoglobin (Hb), methaemoglobin (Hi) and carboxyhaemoglobin (HbCo) (but not sulphmethaemoglobin, SHb) are converted into cyanmethaemoglobin (HiCN). Cyanide (CN) ions provided to the solution by pot. cyanide combines with haemoglobin forming cyanmethaemoglobin. The absorbance of the solution is measured in a photoelectric colorimeter/spectrocolorimeter at a wave length of 540 nm or using a yellow-green filter (Ilford 625) (Fig. 4.3).

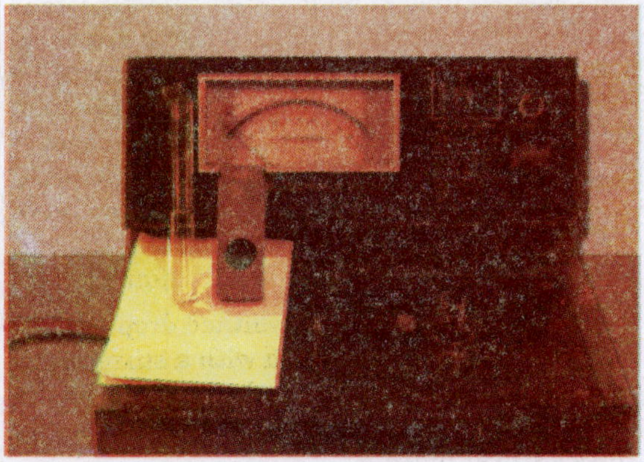

Fig. 4.3. Photoelectric colorimeter. In cyanomethaemoglobin method of Hb estimation green filter or at wavelength 540 is used.

Reagents

1. ***Drabkin's cyanide-ferricyanide solution***

The original Drabkin's solution had a pH of 8.6 but that of modified solution is 9.6, which is less likely to cause turbidity of solution by precipitated plasma proteins.

Composition :

Pot. ferricyanide	....	200 mg
Pot. cyanide	....	50 mg
Sod. bicarbonate	....	1 gm
Distilled/deionised water to	....	1000 ml

The solution is clear, pale yellow and keeps for months when stored in a brown bottle at room temperature. The solution should be discarded if it turns turbid.

2. ***Reference solution***

The standard reference solution conforming to the international specification of 550 to 850 mg Hb per litre, dispensed in 10 ml sealed vial/ampoule is commercially available.

Techniques

1. Pipette 4 ml of diluent into a test tube.
2. Add 0.02 ml whole blood and invert the tube several times.
3. Allow the mixture to stand at room temperature for 10 minutes to ensure completion of reaction, the solution of HiCN is then ready for reading.
4. Test solution is compared with the standard and a reagent blank in a spectrocolorimeter at 540 nm.

Calculation :

$$\text{Hb g / 100 ml} = \frac{\text{optical density of blood sample}}{\text{optical density of standard}} \times \frac{\text{Conc.std(mg / 100ml)} \times \text{dilution factor}}{1000}$$

$$= \frac{75 \times 200}{1000}, \text{when conc. of std is 750 mg / L}$$

$$= 15.$$

Table 4.1
OD–Hb table on Cyanmethemoglobin method

OD	Hb	OD	Hb	OD	Hb	OD	Hb
		0.221	7.0	0.395	12.6	0.572	18.2
		0.227	7.2	0.402	12.8	0.579	18.4
		0.233	7.4	0.409	13.0	0.586	18.6
0.063	2.0	0.239	7.6	0.415	13.2	0.593	18.8
0.069	2.2	0.246	7.8	0.421	13.4	0.599	19.0
0.075	2.4	0.253	8.0	0.427	13.6	0.606	19.2
0.081	2.6	0.259	8.2	0.434	13.8	0.613	10.4
0.088	2.8	0.265	8.4	0.441	14.0	0.619	19.6
0.095	3.0	0.271	8.6	0.447	14.2	0.625	19.8
0.101	3.2	0.278	8.8	0.453	14.4	0.632	20.0
0.107	3.4	0.285	9.0	0.459	14.6		
0.113	3.6	0.291	9.2	0.465	14.8		
0.120	3.8	0.297	9.4	0.471	15.0		
0.127	4.0	0.303	9.6	0.477	15.2		
0.133	4.2	0.310	9.8	0.483	15.4		
0.139	4.4	0.317	10.0	0.489	15.6		
0.145	4.6	0.323	10.2	0.496	15.8		
0.151	4.8	0.329	10.4	0.503	16.0		
0.157	5.0	0.335	10.6	0.509	16.2		
0.163	5.2	0.341	10.8	0.515	16.4		
0.169	5.4	0.347	11.0	0.521	16.6		
0.175	5.6	0.353	11.2	0.527	16.8		
0.182	5.8	0.359	11.4	0.534	17.0		
0.189	6.0	0.365	11.6	0.540	17.2		
0.195	6.2	0.371	11.8	0.546	17.4		
0.201	6.4	0.377	12.0	0.552	17.6		
0.207	6.6	0.383	12.2	0.558	17.8		
0.214	6.8	0.389	12.4	0.565	18.0		

OD-Hb Table (Table 4.1)

For preparation of OD-Hb table the standard haemoglobin solution is diluted with distilled water in 1 in 2, 1 in 4, 1 in 8 taking the OD against blank–Drabkin solution. A graph is plotted between OD and the corresponding Hb value that gives rise to a straight line. From the standard curve thus obtained, a table of OD with corresponding Hb value is prepared. After recording OD of the test samples in a colorimeter/spectrometer the corresponding Hb value is recorded from the table. The readings of the table should be checked with a new standard every week preparing a new table.

Advantages :

(i) It is being a colorimetric procedure, chances of personal error of matching colour (as in acid haematin technique) is not there.

(ii) All forms of Hb except sulphaemoglobin can be estimated.

(iii) Standard of cyanomethaemoglobibn is very stable, commercially available and does not undergo alteration with time.

Disadvantages :

(i) Pot. cyanide is a very potent toxin and requires careful handling. Reagent bottle should be labelled as POISON.

(ii) Drabkin solution should be fresh and clean because any turbidity in the Drabkin solution gives high OD value giving inaccurate results.

(iii) Results of Hb value are affected due to hyperbilirubinemia.

Precautions :

(i) Use of suction bulb or auto disper in pipetting Drabkin solution is a MUST.

(ii) Hb standard should be of international quality.

III. Tallqvist Method

A drop of blood collected from finger is absorbed on a piece of blotting paper and dried for a few seconds and then compared with reference standards of coloured paper made by the manufacturer. It is an easy, quick and very inaccurate method, and of some use to remote villages without any medical facility.

IV. Electronic Counter Method

It is a multi-parameter determining electronic equipment.

Principle : The method is based on electrical impedance principle. An accurately diluted suspension of blood is made in an isotonic conductive solution (e.g., Isoton). A non-ionic detergent is included to ensure rapid lysis of red cells and to reduce turbidity developing from cell membranes and plasma lipids. Now measurement of absorbance is made by the inbuilt colorimeter at 540 nm at a set time interval after mixing the active reagents and blood but before the reaction is completed. Now, H_1 CN (cyanmet haemoglobin) has been replaced with a nontoxic chemical, sodium lauryl sulphate to reduce possible environmental hazards.

Disadvantage : High leucocyte count (> 30,000/µl) causes false elevation of Hb.

V. Direct Reading Electronic Haemoglobinometers

There are inbuilt filters in these instruments. An accurately diluted suspension of blood. The result of haemoglobin per cent is displayed on the screen by the light-emitting diode of the instrument. Procedure of test is on the principle of cyanmet Hb or oxy-Hb method.

Disadvantage : The calibration of the instrument should be checked as it can be faulty.

VI. Other Methods of Estimation of Hb

1. ***Oxyhaemoglobin method***

Take 0.02 ml of blood and mix with 4.0 ml (accurately 3.98 ml) of 0.04% liquor ammonia (ammonium hydroxide). It is mixed by inverting the tube several times. Ammonium hydroxide is used to lyse the red cells and release the haemoglobin. The solution of oxyhaemoglobin (HbO_2) is now matched in a colorimeter at 540 nm or with yellow-green filter. The result is calculated comparing with the reading of known standard.

HbO_2 method is more accurate than acid-haematin method and is used in many laboratories now. The range of error is 2 to 3 per cent.

2. ***Alkaline-haematin method***

Strong alkali (N/10 NaOH) when added to blood, haemoglobin is converted to alkaline haematin. Although carboxy-haemoglobin, meth-aemoglobin and sulf-haemoglobin are converted to alkaline-haematin, certain forms of haemoglobin, such as foetal (HbF) and Barts, are resistant to alkali denaturation.

This ancillary method is less accurate than HiCN or HbO_2 methods, but it is useful to detect the foetal haemoglobin.

Technique : Add 0.05 ml blood into a tube containing 4.95 ml of 0.1 mol/7N NaOH and heat in a boiling water-bath for exactly 4 minutes. By heating solution, HbF and Hb Barts are converted to acid haematin. The brown solution is then read against comparator standards or in a colorimeter by using a suitable standard.

3. ***Chemical method (Iron content)***

Iron content of Hb is 0.347%. Total iron content of blood is estimated chemically and Hb content is found out by dividing the result by 3.47. This is an elaborate method.

QUESTIONS

1. *Define haemoglobin.*
2. *Name the methods of estimation of Hb.*
3. *Name the different uses of Hb pipette.*
4. *Which method of Hb estimation is still practised in village level laboratories?*
5. *Which is the most accurate method of Hb determination and why?*
6. *What is the principle of cyanomethaemoglobin method?*
7. *All haemoglobins except one are converted to cyanmet Hb in cyanomethaemoglobin method. Name the haemoglobin.*
8. *What are the limitations of acid haematin method?*
9. *Why Hb tube is allowed to stand in comparator (in Sahli's method) after mixing blood with acid?*
10. *Why the Hb tube is square?*
11. *Why N/10 HCl is used?*

Chapter 5

Haemocytometer: Cell count

Cellular elements consisting of red cells, white cells and platelets constitute 45% of blood volume. These cells get altered in various diseases.

The Haemocytometer

It is an instrument used for counting the blood cells and consists of two pipettes (one for WBC, other for RBC) and a counting chamber (Fig. 5.1). The smaller pipette with a smaller white bulb is the WBC pipette, whereas larger one with the larger red bulb is the RBC pipette (Fig. 5.4).

Counting chamber

I. Improved Neubauer Chamber

The *Neubauer* and *improved Neubauer* chambers are in general use. The most commonly used counting chamber is the Levy chamber with **Improved Neubauer** ruling (Fig. 5.1). A thick coverslip is provided with the chamber.

Identification

The chamber has usually two ruled stages separated by a small gutter. The two stages in turn are separated from two ridges by gutters, one on each side. The surface of the two ridges is $^1/_{10}$ mm above the surface of the stage, so that when the cover glass is placed on the platform of the counting chamber, the space between the bottom of the coverslip and the base of the grooved area measures $^1/_{10}$ mm in depth.

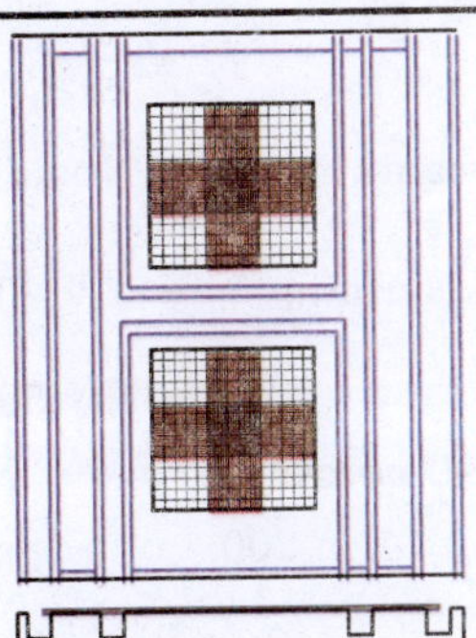

Fig. 5.1. Open counting chamber. The lower figure shows the chamber in cross section with coverglass in place

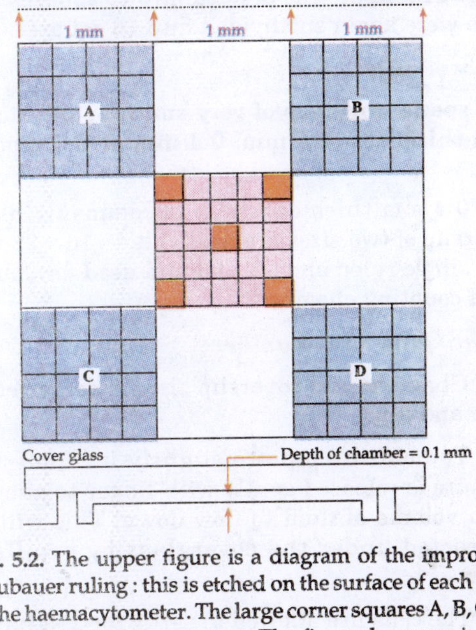

Fig. 5.2. The upper figure is a diagram of the improved Neubauer ruling : this is etched on the surface of each side of the haemacytometer. The large corner squares A, B, C, D are used for leukocyte count. The five red squares in the centre are used for red cell counts or for platelet counts. Actually, each of the 25 squares within the central sq. mm has within it 16 smaller squares for convenience in counting (Fig. 5.3).

The lower figure is a side view of the chamber with the coverglass in place.

Ruled area (Fig. 5.2)

There is a large ruled area of 3 mm × 3 mm on each chamber stage which is divided into 9 squares (Figs. 5.1 and 5.2). The big squares at four corners measures 1 mm × 1 mm each. Each of the four corner squares are divided into 16 smaller squares ($^1/_4$ mm × $^1/_4$ mm each) and are used for counting white cells.

The central 1 mm × 1 mm square in the **Improved Neubauer** chamber is divided into 25 squares (Fig. 5.2), each of which in turn is divided into 16 small squares (Fig. 5.3). The area of each 25 small squares measures $^1/_{25}$ sq. mm ($^1/_5$ mm × $^1/_5$ mm) and five of these medium squares (or a total of 80 small squares) are used for total red cell count.

Since the depth of the grooved area is $^1/_{10}$ mm, the total volume of each big square of the corner measures 1 mm × 1 mm × $^1/_{10}$ mm = $^1/_{10}$ cu. mm and that of medium square in the central area is $^1/_5$ mm × $^1/_5$ mm × $^1/_{10}$ mm = $^1/_{250}$ cu. mm.

The central ruled area in the original **Neubauer chamber** was divided into 16 squares and these were again subdivided into 16 squares.

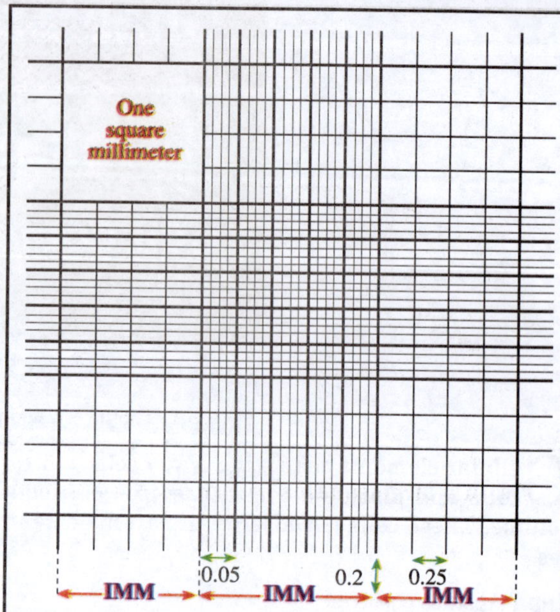

Fig. 5.3. Improved Neubauer ruling on a haemocytometer

Cover slip

A special coverslip of very smooth surface and even thickness (0.3 mm, 0.4 mm or 0.5 mm) is used.

A 0.4 mm thick coverslip is commonly used. Coverslip of two sizes are available — 16 × 22 mm for a single ruled and 22 × 23 mm used for double ruled counting chamber.

Charging the chamber

1. Chamber and coverslip should be perfectly clean and dry.

2. To hold the pipette slightly inclined and pressure is released gently with finger to allow a small volume of fluid to flow down. This will be contracted under the coverglass by capillary action.

3. The cells are allowed to settle for 2–3 minutes so that they all may be seen in the same plane of focus.

Counting

Cell count is made under **high power** (40 ×) objective; **low power** (10 ×) is used first to focus the ruling. Only cells within the square are counted and cells lying on the lines of any two adjacent sides (top and right, or bottom and left) are included in the total count :

Calculation

(using Improved Neubauer ruling)

1. *Total WBC count*

Dilution .... 1 in 20

Depth .... $\frac{1}{10}$ mm

No. of WBCs in 4 large corner square : N

Vol. of 4 large squares $= 1 \times 1 \times \frac{4}{10}$ cu. mm

$= \frac{2}{5}$ cu. mm

2/5 cu. mm contains = N × dilution

∴ 1 cu. mm contains $= N \times 20 \times \frac{5}{2}$ RBCs

= N × 50.

2. *Total RBC count*

Dilution .... 1 in 200

Depth .... $\frac{1}{10}$ mm

No. of RBCs in 5 medium squares in central large square : N

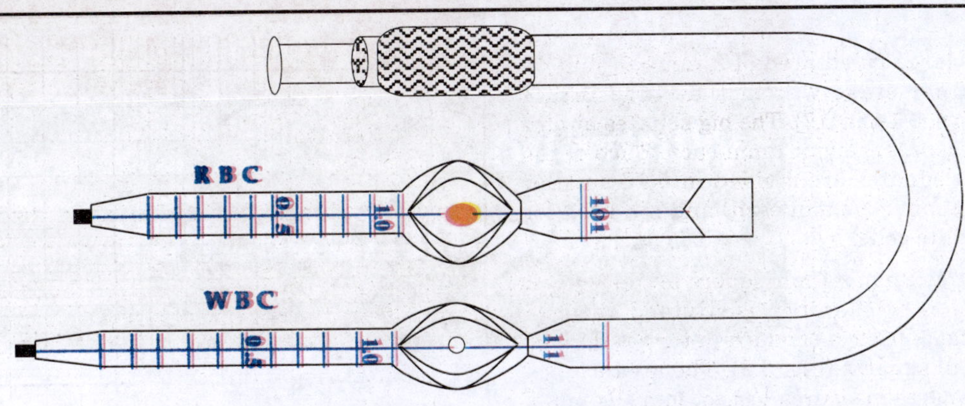

Fig. 5.4. Thoma red and white cell diluting pipettes

Vol. of 5 large squares $= \frac{1}{5} \times \frac{1}{5} \times \frac{1}{10} \times 5$ cu.mm

$= \frac{1}{50}$ cu.mm

$\frac{1}{50}$ cu. mm contains $= N \times$ dilution

$= N \times 200.$

$\therefore$ 1 cu. mm contains $= N \times 200 \times \frac{50}{1}$

$= N \times 10000$

3. Total platelet count

Dilution ..... 1 in 20

Depth ..... $\frac{1}{10}$ mm

No. of platelets in 5 medium sq. in central large square : N

Vol. of 5 medium sq. $= \frac{1}{5} \times \frac{1}{5} \times \frac{1}{10} \times 5$ cu. mm

$= \frac{1}{50}$ cu. mm

$\frac{1}{50}$ cu. mm contains $= N \times$ dilution

$\therefore$ 1 cu. mm contains $= N \times 20 \times 50$
$= N \times 1000.$

Uses of improved Neubauer's Chamber

1. Blood cell count : RBC, WBC, Platelet.
2. Cell count of different body fluids such as CSF, pleural, peritoneal, pericardial and synovial fluid.
3. Sperm count of semen.

II. Fuch's Rosenthal chamber

The ruled area of the chamber is 16 sq. mm and depth is 0.2 mm (Neubauer chamber depth is 0.1 mm) and hence more amount of mixture of blood/ CSF and diluting fluid can be examined, giving an accurate result. The chamber is often used in absolute eosinophil count (AEC) and in cell count of CSF in nonpyogenic meningitis.

Cleaning pipettes

At first the pipettes are cleaned by filling them with water and blowing out. Next, acetone is sucked inside the pipette and blown it out. Water is removed by acetone. Acetone dries the pipette in which the bead rolls freely.

Cleaning Neubauer chamber

The chamber is rinsed in water after use. Then it is wiped clean with lint free cloth and dried. Chamber should not be cleaned by lint or gauze which may cause scratch on the chamber. Chamber should be held from sides and ruled area is not to be touched.

QUESTIONS

1. *What is a haemocytometer?*
2. *Give the measurement of ruled area in modified as well as in the original Neubauer chambers.*
3. *Name the different squares in which cells are to be counted in WBC, RBC and platelet count.*
4. *How do you clean the pipettes?*
5. *How do you charge the chamber?*
6. *What is the advantage of Fuch's Rosenthal chamber?*

Chapter 6

Wintrobe Haematocrit Tube: PCV

ESTIMATION OF PCV

The term 'haematocrit' literally means blood separation. Wintrobe haematocrit tube is used for measurement of packed cell volume (PCV) as a screening test for anaemia. It is also useful for evaluating absolute values (MCV, MCHC) and determination of ESR.

Haematocrit or PCV may be defined as the volume of packed Red Blood Cells in a given sample of blood, which is expressed as a percentage of the total volume of the blood sample. The methods of measurement of PCV include :

(a) **Direct method**

1. A *macro-method* using Wintrobe tube.
2. A *micro-method* using Capillary tube.

(b) **Electronic method**

1. Wintrobe's Method (see Figs 6.1, 6.2 and 6.4)

Wintrobe haematocrit tube

Identification :

1. It is a special, thick-walled glass tube 11 cm long, with an internal diameter of 2.5 mm and a flat inner base.

2. It is calibrated at 1 mm intervals to 100 mm and holds about 1 ml of blood.

3. The tube is marked in reversed directions, ascending marking for determination of PCV and descending marking for estimation of ESR.

Uses :

1. Primarily for PCV of blood.

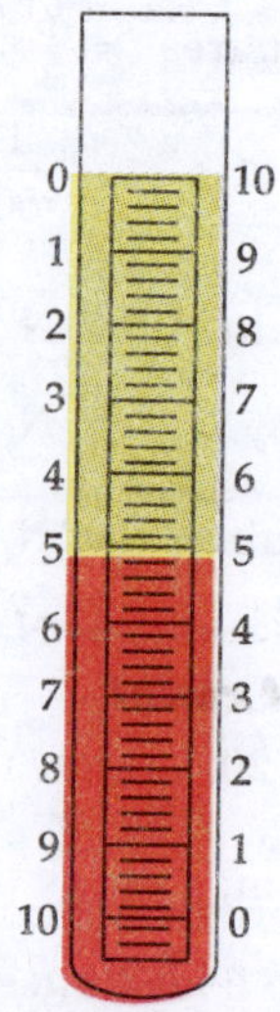

Fig. 6.1. Wintrobe haematocrit tube

2. Determination of ESR.

3. Buffy coat smear preparation for LE cell phenomenon and studies of abnormal cells in aleukaemic leukaemia.

Anticoagulant :

Venous blood, anticoagulated with EDTA, double oxalate or heparin.

Method :

1. Two ml venous blood is collected and mixed immediately with anticoagulant in the vial. The Wintrobe tube is filled with the thoroughly mixed blood with the help of a long Pasteur pipette (Fig. 6.4) from the bottom up to the mark '0' or '10' above.

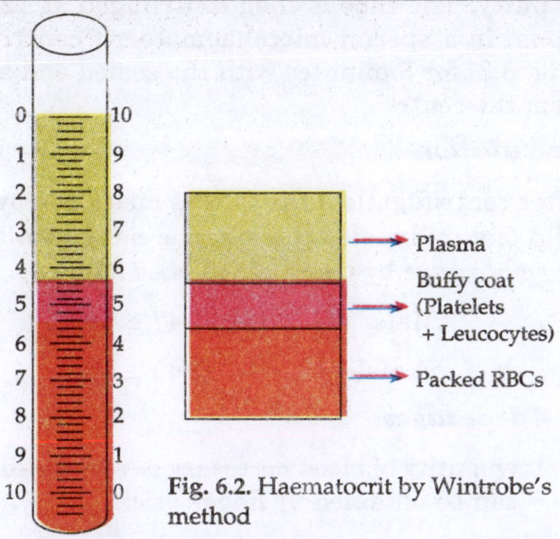

Fig. 6.2. Haematocrit by Wintrobe's method

2. Centrifuge the tube in a centrifuge machine of 15 cm radius at 3000 r.p.m. for 30 minutes.

PCV : Then read the upper level of the column of packed red cells by the markings in ascending order which is expressed as percentage of the total volume of blood.

ESR : For simultaneous determination of ESR and PCV, the haematocrit tube after filling with blood is kept vertically over the stand (Fig. 6.4) for one hour and ESR is noted by measuring the free plasmatic zone above — by noting the marking on tube in descending order. After an hour, the tube is centrifuged for half an hour at 3000 r.p.m. for 30 minutes for determining PCV.

Zones separated after centrifugation (Fig. 6.2)

1. The layer of *packed red cells* (PCV) is lowermost — normally, 45 to 50%.

2. A thin intermediate layer of WBC and platelets which is just above the red cells. This greyish layer is called *buffy coat* — normally varies between 2 to 3%.

Uses of buffy coat smear :

(i) LE cell preparation.

(ii) Subleukaemic leukaemia : Morphology and cytochemisty of abnormal blast cells can be studied.

3. Uppermost layer of plasma is 48 to 52%. When colour of plasma is orange, green or yellow, it indicates jaundice. Increase in buffy coat layer is indicative of severe degree of leucocytosis or leukaemia.

Advantages :

Only a small volume of blood is necessary that can be collected from finger prick/heel prick in infants.

Precautions :

1. Reading should be taken quickly as slanting of red cell column occurs if tube is kept horizontally for more than 5 minutes.

2. Do not include buffy coat while recording PCV.

3. While filling the capillary tube from a finger prick, squeezing the finger to be avoided.

Sources of error

1. Prolonged stasis of blood occurs due to use of tourniquet which leads to haemoconcentration and false high results may be obtained.

2. Muscular activity may cause increase in number of red and white cells and platelets leading to higher haematocrit reading than the actual.

3. Excess EDTA concentration.

Normal range of PCV

Men	—	40 to 54 per cent
Women	—	36 to 47 per cent
At birth	—	44 to 62 per cent
1 year	—	35 per cent (approx)
10 years	—	37.5 per cent (approx)

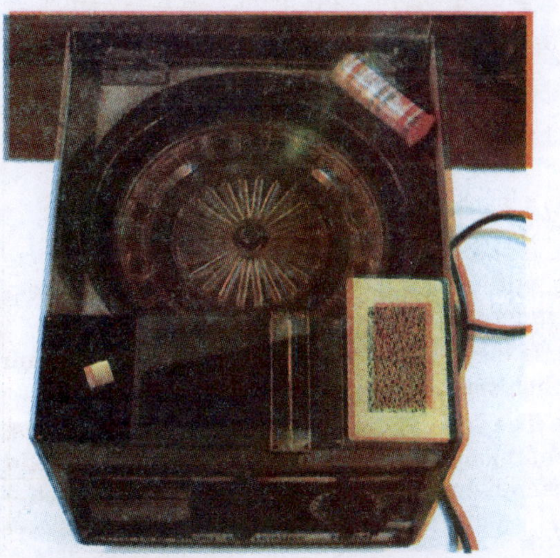

Fig. 6.3. Microhaematocrit centrifuge machine. The capillary tubes are placed in the machine after filling with blood.

Abnormal PCV

1. *Diminished* : Anaemia (usually less than 30%).
2. *Increased* : Polycythaemia, severe degree of dehydration, cholera, acute gastroenteritis.

Sources of error

1. Inadequate mixing of blood.
2. Inadequate duration and speed of centrifugation.
3. Irregularity of the bore of Wintrobe tube.
4. Trapping of leucocyte-platelet clumps.
5. Excess anticoagulant.

2. PCV by Microhaematocrit method (Fig. 6.3)

The use of capillary tube of 75 mm in length and about 1 mm internal diameter is very convenient for estimation of PCV as routine procedure in laboratory work. It is advantageous to use heparinised capillary tubes (rinsed in 1:1000 heparin, dried at 56°C and stored) since blood from finger prick is then adequate. For EDTA mixed venous blood, plain capillary tube is used.

About $^3/_4$ th of the tube is filled with blood and the empty end is sealed with a microburner, wax or putty. The tube is then centrifuged at 12,000 r.p.m. in a special microhaematocrit centrifuge (Fig. 6.3) for 5 minutes with the sealed end away from the centre.

Calculation

After centrifugation, the PCV is measured by the help of a millimeter rule commercially available. *Normal range* by this method is as follows :

Male	—	47 ± 7%
Female	—	43 ± 5%

Advantages

1. Quantity of blood necessary is very small and can be obtained by finger prick.
2. Time required for centrifugation is short.
3. Convenient as a routine work.

3. Automatic electronic analyser

In multi-channel Coulter counter, PCV can be estimated with other haematologic indices in 40-50 seconds.

LE CELL TEST

Antibodies of various types are demonstrable in auto-immune diseases, such as SLE, Rheumatoid

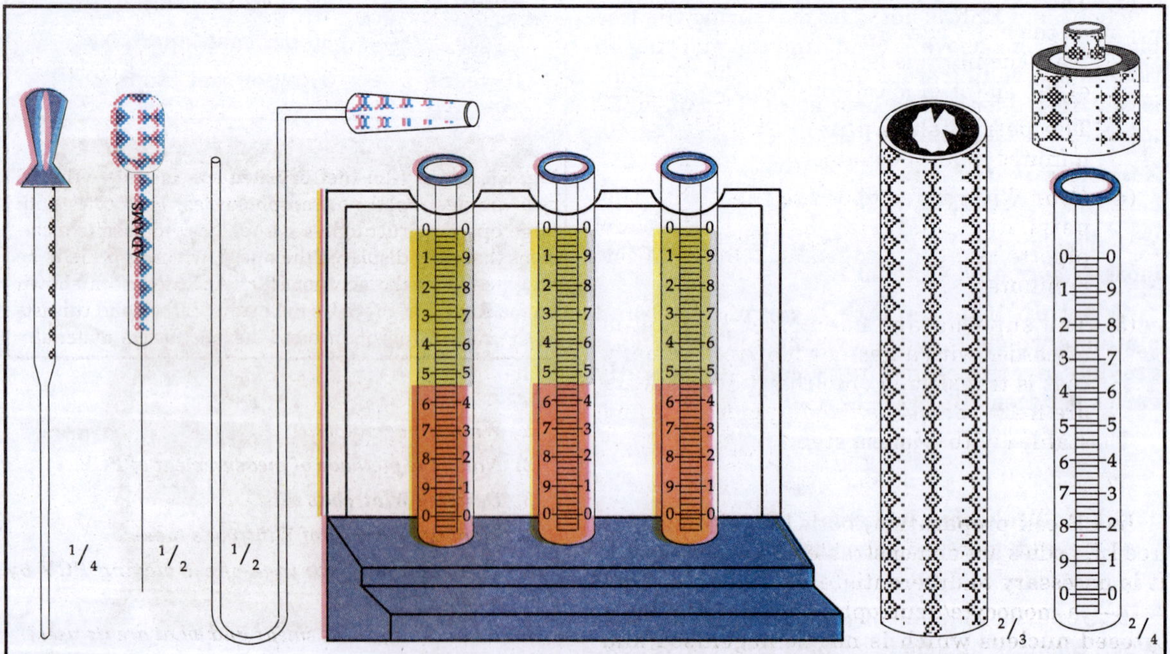

Fig. 6.4. Wintrobe haematocrit tube and accessories : left to right — pipette, all glass; pipette with stainless steel capillary; tube cleaner; Wintrobe rack with charged haematocrit tubes; adaptor for centrifuge shield to hold Wintrobe tube; Wintrobe haematocrit and sedimentation tube with rubber cap

arthritis and other diseases. Of these — LE factor is an IgG antibody directed against deoxyribonucleoprotein. This antinuclear antibody reacts with the damaged nucleus causing swelling and homogenisation of nuclear material which are called **LE bodies**. These LE bodies are recognised by neutrophils. Neutrophils phagocytose LE bodies in the presence of complement and this is known as **LE cell.** In LE cell preparations, LE bodies are surrounded by neutrophils. The **LE rosettes** are also demonstrated in figure 6.5.

Principle

In making LE cell preparation, the nuclear membrane of neutrophils is damaged by glass beads/passing through sieve. Thus nucleoproteins of neutrophilis are exposed and then interact with LE factor (antinuclear antibody) in patient's serum. This results in its homogenisation forming a LE body which is phagocytosed by neutrophil — LE cell (Fig. 6.5).

Method

(1) A volume of 6 ml blood is taken in a plain test tube and kept it at 37°C for 1 hour for clot to retract. The serum is separated from clot. Serum can be utilised for other serological tests.

(2) The clot is grinded with a penicillin bottle on the mesh of the sieve (used for preparing tea). The fibrin is left on the mesh and rest of the material is collected in a petri dish.

(3) The petri dish is placed at 37°C for 30 minutes in an incubator.

(4) Four Wintrobe's tubes are filled with the petri dish material using a Pasteur pipette and centrifuged at 1000 RPM for 5 minutes.

(5) The supernatant haemolysed serum is discarded with a Pasteur pipette. The buffy coat is transferred onto the slides. Smears are made. Smear is fixed in methanol and stained with Giemsa stain.

Result

In LE cell preparation, both LE cell and also free LE bodies are demonstrable in a positive case. It is necessary to differentiate LE cell from **Tart cell** — a monocyte/neutrophil containing phagocytosed nucleus which is not homogenised and retains its chromatin pattern. Significance of tart cell is not known and it may be observed in healthy individuals.

Significance

LE cells are detectable in SLE, lupoid hepatitis, rheumatoid arthritis, penicillin sensitivity and other collagen diseases.

Glass bead method

This is a better technique for defibrination of blood and causing damage to neutrophils. Take 2 ml heparinised blood in a test tube and place 5-6 glass beads inside it. The blood in the tube is shaken vigorously for 10 minutes closing the tubes with a tightly fitting rubber cork. Then place the tube in a water bath at 37°C and keep for 10 minutes. The contents are transferred to a Wintrobe tube and centrifuged at 1000 RPM for 5 minutes. Smears are prepared from the buffy coat, fixed in methanol and stained by Giemsa stain. The air-dried smear is examined for LE cell phenomenon.

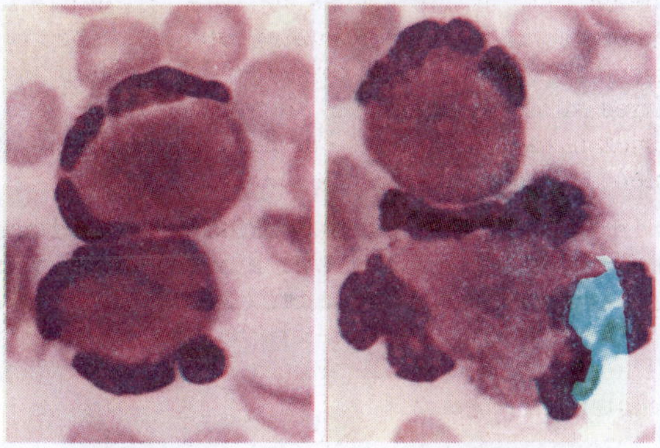

A (Lt) B (Rt)

Fig. 6.5. Blood film (defibrinated specimen) — The LE cells are neutrophil polymorphonuclear leucocytes with large opaque structureless basophilic cytoplasmic inclusions that have displaced the nuclei, which appears to be wrapped round the inclusions **(Left A)**. Rosette form shown on the **Right (B)**, precedes the mature LE cell and consists of several polymorphs around the free nuclear material.

QUESTIONS

1. *What is haematocrit?*
2. *Name the methods of measurement of PCV.*
3. *Describe Wintrobe's tube.*
4. *What are the uses of Wintrobe's tube?*
5. *What is the advantage of estimating PCV by micromethod?*
6. *What is buffy coat smear and what are its uses?*
7. *What is LE cell and what does it indicate?*
8. *Name diseases in which LE cell phenomenon are seen.*

Chapter 7

Westergren Tube: ESR

TEST FOR ACUTE PHASE RESPONSE

Inflammatory response to tissue injury (acute phase response) includes alteration in the concentration of serum protein, especially with a rise in fibrinogen and C-reactive protein (CRP); and a fall in albumin. Such a change occurs in acute inflammation as well as during active phases of chronic inflammation. Some useful tests to measure the extent of inflammation include estimation of fibrinogen, CRP and measurement of the erythrocyte sedimentation rate (ESR). In acute phase response, all three are increased in blood. The rise in ESR results from increased fibrinogen content in blood.

Erythrocyte Sedimentation Rate (ESR)

There are two commonly used methods for measuring ESR :

1. *Westergren method.* 2. *Wintrobe method.*

Westergren Method

This is a more sensitive and accurate method as compared to Wintrobe's method and most widely used. In this technique a 200 mm long column of blood is studied instead of a short column of blood 100 mm long blood as in Wintrobe method. This is the cause of sensitiveness.

Westergren tube

Westergren tube is actually a thick-walled pipette (open at both ends), 300 mm long, of which 200 mm is graduated and upper 100 mm portion is ungraduated. The tube has an inner diameter of 2.5 mm and resembles a 1 ml pipette (Fig. 7.1A) Hence it is also known as *Westergren's pipette.*

Anticoagulant

A solution of 3.8% trisodium citrate is used in the proportion of blood : anticoagulant = 4 : 1. The citrate solution is filtered after preparation and stored in a sterile container. The solution can be stored for several months at 4°C but it should be discarded when it becomes turbid due to growth of moulds. However, it is preferable to prepare the solution every week. To eliminate some work, 1.9 g reagent powder can be weighed into each of a large number of plastic vials at one sitting. On the day of use, the powder is added to 50 ml distilled water and dissolved, which is discarded after a week's use. Thus, 1.6 ml venous blood is mixed with 0.4 ml of 3.8% sod. citrate solution.

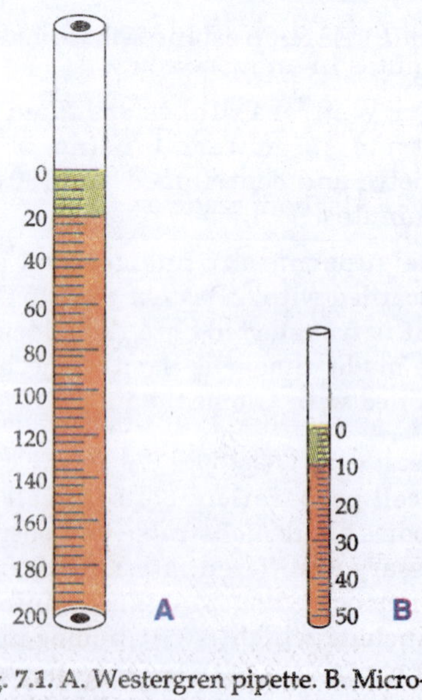

Fig. 7.1. A. Westergren pipette. B. Micro-ESR

Method

The usual practice is to collect the blood (2 ml) directly into the citrate solution (0.5 ml). However, it can also be carried out with blood anticoagulated with EDTA, provided that 4 volumes of blood is mixed with 1 volume of sod. citrate solution before the test is performed.

The test should be performed within 2 hours after collection, although a delay up to 6 hours is permissible provided the sample is preserved at 4°C. ESR is reduced in stored blood.

To a 0.4 ml of 3.8% sod. citrate in a test tube, 1.6 ml blood is added and immediately mixed. The blood sample is thoroughly mixed and is drawn up into Westergren tube up to the 200 mm mark with the help of a teat or mechanical device; mouth suction should be avoided. The tube is now set exactly vertical in a Westergren stand in which a spring clip, pressing on the top, holds the point firmly against a piece of rubber at the lowest end. The tube is now left to stand (Fig. 7.2) free from vibrations for 60 minutes to 120 minutes and not exposed to sunlight.

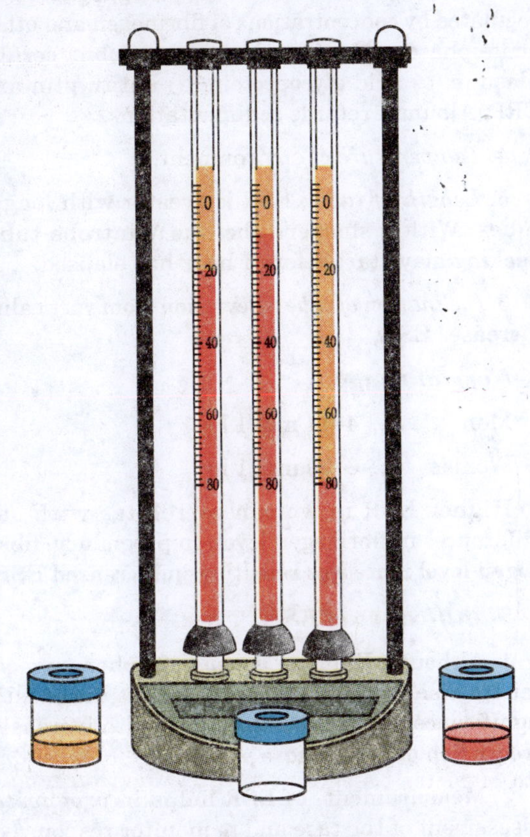

Fig. 7.2. Westergren blood sedimentation apparatus

Recording result

The red corpuscles begin to settle down leaving a clear plasma above. The upper level of the red cell column is read at the end of one hour. This measurement in mm is ESR (Westergren, 1 hour).

ESR result after one hour gives more accurate result. The earlier tendency of finding out mean ESR is now discouraged.

Example : ESR (Westergren method),
at the end of one hour 40 mm
at the end of two hour 72 mm

$$\text{Mean ESR} = \frac{\text{1st hour reading} + \frac{\text{2nd hour reading}}{2}}{2}$$

$$= \frac{40 + \frac{72}{2}}{2} \text{ mm} = 38 \text{ mm},$$

when 1st hour reading is 40 and 2nd hour reading is 72. Mean ESR does not give accurate result.

Stages of sedimentation

Sedimentation is observed to take place in four stages :

1. *Rouleaux formation* : Red cells form rouleaux in first fifteen minutes phase during when minimum sedimentation occurs.

2. *Formation of fine threads* by fibrinogen and globulin resulting in network formation occurs during 2nd 15 minutes. The rouleaux of red cells get trapped in the mesh of fibrin and globulin network and becomes heavier which starts settling rapidly.

3. *Rapid fall of protein network* : The protein network along with red cell mass is maximum during the third 15 minute phase.

4. *Phase of packing of red cells* : The sedimented protein-red cell mass undergoes rapid packing during fourth 15 minute phase.

Factors influencing sedimentation

The rate of fall of erythrocytes is influenced by a multitude of inter-reacting factors :

1. *Difference in specific gravity* between red cells and plasma.

2. *Ratio of red cells to plasma,* i.e., the PCV, plasma viscosity.

3. *Rouleaux fromation* and aggregation is regulated by concentrations of fibrinogen and other acute phase proteins such as haptoglobin, ceruloplasmin, α_1 acid glycoprotein, α_1 antitryptin and CRP. Albumin retards sedimentation.

4. *Temperature* of environment.

5. *Length of tube* : ESR is greater with longer tubes. With a shorter tube like Wintrobe tube, packing may start before 1 hour has elapsed.

6. *Inclination of tube* : Deviation from verticality increases ESR.

Normal range

Men .... 4–14 mm/1 hr

Women .... 6–20 mm/1 hr

Higher ESR in women correlates with sex differences in fibrinogen level. In pregnancy, fibrinogen level increases resulting in increased ESR.

Significance of ESR

1. Although ESR is a *nonspecific* phenomenon, yet its rise is suggestive of indirect diagnostic significance in diseases associated with increased production of *acute phase proteins.*

2. Measurement of ESR helps in *prognostic* assessment of the case and to monitor response of the disease to treatment. For this purpose, measurement of ESR is repeated at intervals of a fortnight/month.

Abnormal levels of ESR

(a) *Rapid ESR found in* :

1. *Chronic infection* : Tuberculosis, chronic osteomyelitis, chronic bronchiectasis, chronic lung abscess.

2. *Auto immune diseases* : SLE, rheumatoid arthritis, acute rheumatic fever.

3. *Acute inflammation* : Acute myocardial infarction, any extensive inflammation.

4. *Neoplasm* : Hodgkin's disease, leukaemia, carcinomatosis, multiple myeloma.

(b) *Slow ESR* is usually seen in : Polycythaemia, congestive cardiac failure, hypofibrinogenaemia and abnormal red cell disorders such as poikilocytosis, spherocytosis or sickle cell anaemia. These abnormalities of red cells prevent rouleaux formation.

Other method of ESR determination

1. ***Wintrobe method*** : The blood (anticoagulated with EDTA) after thoroughly mixing is transferred by a Pasteur pipette into Wintrobe's tube so as to fill up to the '0' mark. The pipette is then vertically placed in its stand. After one hour, reading at the top of the red cell layer is noted and that reading in mm corresponds to ESR.

In anaemic patients correction of the reading was previously recommended by the help of a special chart printed in most standard text books. Nowadays, actual values are preferred.

Normal range

Men .... 0–9 mm/1 hr

Women .... 2–20 mm/2 hrs

2. ***Zeta sedimentation rate (ESR)*** : EDTA blood filled in a special capillary tube is centrifuged in a zetafuge (Coulter Electronics) for four times each for 45 seconds. It requires only 0.2 cc blood and does not need dilution. The capillary tube is mechanically rotated at 180 degrees and centrifuging is done in reverse direction at every 45 seconds for 4 times. Formation of red cell rouleaux occurs which travel down the tube by alternate compaction and dispersion.

Recording of result :

ZSR is expressed in terms of percentage. Normal range in adult male and female varies between 40-54%.

Zetacrit is the rise of the height of red cells to the total height of blood column.

Advantages :

(a) Requires small amount of blood (0.2 ml) and obviates dilution.

(b) Requires minimum time.

(c) Eliminates effects of anaemia.

(d) Believed to be more sensitive than Westergren ESR.

Limitations : (a) Requires special and relatively expensive apparatus. (b) ZSR has not yet been fully standardized. It has not replaced the universally used routine practice used in ESR.

3. ***Micro ESR method (Barret 1980)*** : A capillary tube of 230 mm long with 1 mm inner diameter is filled with 0.2 ml EDTA mixed blood

and kept vertically on a stand and the result is read after one hour.

The method can be used wth both venous and capillary blood and is of great advantage, specially in paediatric cases.

QUESTIONS

1. *What are acute phase proteins?*
2. *Describe Westergren tube.*
3. *Why Westergren tube is also called Westergren's pipette?*
4. *Name the stages of sedimentation of blood.*
5. *Which are the factors that influence sedimentation of blood?*
6. *How do you record ESR?*
7. *Where ESR rapidly rises?*
8. *When do you find slow ESR?*
9. *What is zeta sedimentation?*
10. *What is micro ESR method?*
11. *Why ESR estimation by Westergren method is preferable?*
12. *What is normal range and significance of ESR?*

Chapter 8

RBC Pipette: Total RBC count, Red cell absolute values (MCV, MCH, MCHC)

RED CELL COUNT

The red cell count is defined as determination of the number of RBCs per µl of blood.

Methods

Total red cell count is done by 2 methods :

1. **Electronic cell counter** : Electronic cell counter for cell count (RBCs, WBCs, Platelets) is now widely used. It has greatly improved speed and counting precision. Some counters are limited to particle counting, while others use inter-related systems by which size of the red cells can be measured, so as to provide values for PCV and MCV; estimation of haemoglobin can also be done on the same samples, which provide results for MCH and MCHC.

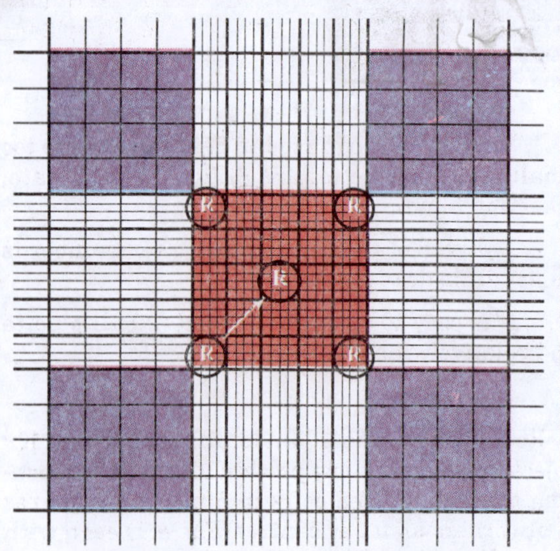

Fig. 8.1. Areas used for red cell count

2. **Counting RBCs by visual haemocytometer method** : A visual direct method, however, is adopted in laboratories which do not have electronic cell counters and, also, in many laboratories for leucocyte and platelet counts.

Materials required :

(i) RBC pipette,

(ii) RBC diluting fluid,

(iii) Improved Neubauer's chamber.

RBC pipette

Identification :

It is a small pipette with a bulb with marking 0.5, and 1 on the stem and 101 on the top above the bulb (Figs. 5.1, 5.2). It often contains a red glass bead inside.

Use s :

(1) For total RBC count.

(2) For total platelet count.

(3) For total leucocyte count in cases of leukaemia with a very high count.

(4) For total count of sperm in seminal fluid.

Red cell diluting fluid

Two types of RBC diluting are there :

(a) *Hayem's fluid* :

Mercuric chloride	0.25 g
Sodium chloride	0.5 g
Sodium sulphate	2.5 g
Distilled water	100 ml

After filtering the solution, it is kept at room temperature. Addition of mercuric chloride prevents bacterial growth, while sodium chloride and sodium sulfate provide iso-osmolality. However, red cells tend to agglutinate in this fluid especially in cases of dysproteinaemia. Hence, Dacie's fluid is preferred.

(b) *Dacie's fluid*

Trisodium citrate	—	5 g	Stock solution
Formalin	—	1.0 ml	
Distilled water to	—	100 ml	

Stock solution is diluted 1 in 10 before use. The formalin acts as preservative by fixing the red cells and prevents bacterial or fungal growth in the fluid.

Method for total red cell count

Blood from finger prick or EDTA/double oxalate mixed blood is drawn up to the mark 0.5 (to the mark 1, if the patient is very anaemic) into RBC pipette (Fig. 5.1). The side of the pipette is wiped clean by wet cotton and then diluting fluid is sucked up to the mark 101. The pipette is rotated rapidly between the fingers for allowing the fluid to mix well. The presence of glass bead inside the pipette helps better mixing.

Then, thorough mixing of blood and fluid is accomplished either by closing the end of the pipette with a finger while rotating or by keeping the pipette perfectly horizontal during mixing.

Charging chamber : Since the capillary end of the pipette is entirely occupied by the diluent, first few drops are discarded by flow. Take a clean dry counting chamber with its cover-glass in position. One end of the pipette is sealed with index finger and the tip is placed on the platform adjacent to the edge of the coverslip. The pipette is held slightly inclined and pressure of the finger is gently released allowing a small volume of fluid to flow in. The fluid moves under the cover-glass by capillary action. The chamber is left undisturbed on a bench for 2-3 minutes for allowing the cells to settle so that they all may be seen in the same plane of focus. If it is left for longer, drying at the edges initiates currents that cause movement of cells after they have settled.

Bulk dilution method

1. A volume of 3.98 ml of diluting fluid is placed in an ordinary 75 × 12 mm clean dry tube.

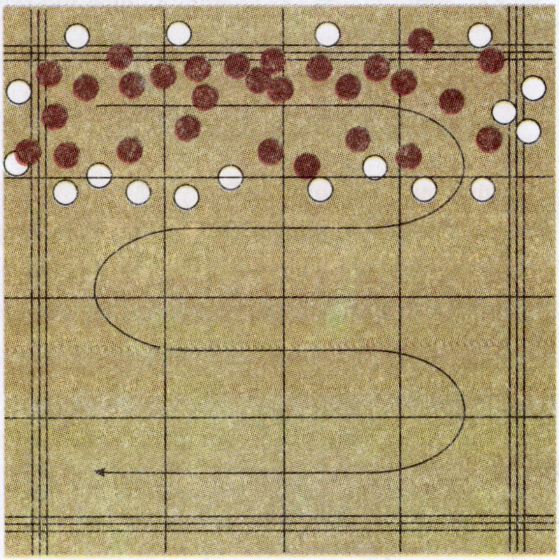

Fig. 8.2. Cells touching top and left centre boundary lines are counted. Cells touching bottom and right centre boundary are not counted

2. Add 0.02 ml blood by a haemoglobinometer pipette washing into the diluent.

3. Mixing is done either by a mechanical mixture after sealing the tube with a rubber bung, or alternatively by hand rotating for at least 2 minutes. In the tube method, blood is diluted 1 in 200 as in the bulb diluting pipettes. The fluid is delivered to the chamber without delay by means of a Pasteur pipette.

Advantage of bulk dilution

1. Volumes of blood used in RBC pipette are too small and the pipettes are difficult to calibrate, label and handle.

2. Delivery of fluid from pipette to chamber is an art difficult to master.

3. It is easy to calibrate 0.02 ml (20 μl) pipette and relatively inexpensive.

Counting

Red cells are counted under the high dry or 40× objective using the low power (10×) first for focusing the ruling. Red cells in 5 medium squares (4 at corners and 1 at centre) (Fig. 8.1) each with 16 small squares (Fig. 8.2), in the central 1 mm^2 area of improved Neubauer chamber are counted.

Let N number of red cells are counted in 80 small squares (total volume = $^1/_{25} \times 5 \times 0.1$ cu. mm

= 0.02 μl) and the blood is diluted 1 : 200, the red cell count comes to :

$$\frac{N}{0.02} \times 200 \text{ per cu. mm}$$

$$\text{or, } N \times 10{,}000 \text{ per cu. mm.}$$

Normal range of total RBC

Adult : 4.5 to 5.5 millions per cu. mm of blood ($4.5 - 5.5 \times 10^{12}$/L).

New born baby : 6 to 8 million per cu. mm blood (6 to 8×10^{12}/L).

Variation of RBC level in blood

(a) *Increase* : Polycythaemia, central cyanotic disease, haemoconcentration (e.g., cholera), congestive cardiac failure and in infants.

(b) *Decrease* : Anaemia.

Errors of RBC count

The errors are of two main kinds :

1. *Technical errors* : This includes defective apparatus and /or technique. Technical errors can be minimised by the use of accurately calibrated apparatus and by a careful technique.

2. *Inherent error* : The distribution of the red cells is of an irregular (random) pattern in the counting chamber. This affects the accuracy of visual count and the error is in the tune of ± 20%, which can be minimised by counting a large number of RBCs.

ERYTHROCYTE INDICES
(Red cell absolute values)

Based on the results of *Haemoglobin, Packed Cell Volume* and *Total Red Cell* count, Wintrobe introduced the calculations which give quantitative information about the red blood cell in respect of its size, content and haemoglobin concentration. These are called *RBC Indices,* which are also known as *absolute values.* Since the tests, on the basis of which these calculations are made, are not absolute but have some error, the term *Indices* is preferred. Utmost care should be taken to get accurate results on these three basic tests to make the calculations of *Indices* meaningful.

1. MCV (Mean Corpuscular Volume)

The MCV is the average volume of the individual red cells.

Calculation :

$$\text{MCV} = \frac{\text{PCV (per cent)} \times 10}{\text{Red cell count (millions per cu. mm)}} \text{ cu. micron (cu. } \mu)$$

Examples :

1. PCV = 20%, Red cell count = 1,500,000/cu.mm

$$\text{MCV} = \frac{20 \times 10}{1.5} = 133 \text{ cu. micron (cu. } \mu)$$

(*Macrocytic anaemia*)

2. PCV = 20%, Red cell count = 3,000,000/cu. mm

$$\text{MCV} = \frac{20 \times 10}{3} = 67 \text{ cu. } \mu$$

(*Microcytic hypochromic anaemia*)

Normal range : 87 ± 5 cu. μ per cell

Result is also expressed in femto-litres (fl).

Abnormal level

(a) *Decrease* : Microcytic anaemia, sometimes as low as 50 cu. μ.

(b) *Increase* : Macrocytic anaemia, sometimes as high as 150 cu. μ.

2. MCH (Mean Corpuscular Haemoglobin)

It is the amount (weight) of haemoglobin in average red cell or the average content of haemoglobin per cell in all the red cells.

Calculation :

$$\text{MCH} = \frac{\text{Hb gm per cent} \times 10}{\text{RBC count (in millions per cu. mm)}} \text{ picogram (pg)}$$

Examples :

1. Haemoglobin = 7 gm%; red cell count = 1,400,000/cu. mm

$$\text{MCH} = \frac{7 \times 10}{1.4} = 50 \ \mu\mu\text{g (pg)}$$

(*Macrocytic anaemia*)

2. Haemoglobin = 5 gm%; red cell count = 2,400,000/cu. mm

$$\text{MCH} = \frac{5 \times 10}{2.4} = 21 \ \mu\mu\text{g (pg)}$$

(*Microcytic hypochronic anaemia*)

In most anaemias, changes in the average size of red cells (MCV) parallel similar alterations in the weight of haemoglobin in red cells MCH. Hence variations in MCV and MCH are similar.

Normal range

27–32 (29.5 ± 2.5) pico-g (micro micro-g)

Abnormal level

(a) *Decrease* : Hypochromia due to decrease in cell haemoglobin.

(b) *Increase* : MCH may be somewhat increased in macrocytic anaemia.

3. MCHC (Mean Corpuscular Haemoglobin Concentration)

The MCHC is the average haemoglobin concentration per 100 ml of packed red cells in per cent.

Calculation :

$$\text{MCHC} = \frac{\text{Hb gm \%} \times 100}{\text{PCV (per cent)}} \%$$

Examples :

1. Haemoglobin = 7.2 g%;
   PCV (haematocrit) = 20%.

$$\text{MCHC} = \frac{7.2 \times 100}{20} \% = 36 \text{ gm per cent}$$

(Macrocytic anaemia)

2. Haemoglobin = 5.0 g%; PCV = 20%.

$$\text{MCHC} = \frac{5 \times 100}{20} \% = 25 \text{ gm per cent}$$

(Hypochromic anaemia)

Normal range : 32–36% (34 ± 2)

Abnormal level

(a) *Decrease* : Hypochromic anaemia (may be as low as 20%).

(b) *Increase* : In macrocytic states, although MCH may be increased, but MCHC usually remains normal or slightly decreased. However, MCHC may be elevated in spherocytosis.

Other red cell values (see also Table 8.1)

(1) *Colour index* : It is the average amount of haemoglobin in each red cell in comparison to normal amount.

$$\text{Colour index} = \frac{\text{Hb\% (of normal)}}{\text{RBC\% (of normal)}}$$

Norrmal red cell count and normal haemoglobin are assumed as follows :

Hb 14.5 g as 100%

RBC 5 million/cu. mm as 100%

Example :

When a patient has haemoglobin of 12.0 g% and RBC count of 4.3 million, his

$$\text{Hb\% of normal} = \frac{100 \times 12}{14.5} = 83\%$$

$$\text{RBC \% of normal} = \frac{100 \times 4.3}{5.0} = 86\%$$

$$\text{Colour index} = \frac{83\%}{86\%} = 0.97$$

Table 8.1 : Haematological values in health

	Different age groups				
	Men	*Women*	*Children (10–12 years)*	*Children (1 year)*	*Infant*
Red cells (millions/cumm)	4.5–6.5	3.9–5.6	5–7	5–7	6–8
Haemoglobin (g %)	13.5–18	11.5–16.5	11.5–14.5	11–13	12.5–19.5
PCV (%)	47 ± 7	42 ± 5	41 ± 4	38 ± 6	54 ± 10
MCV (cμ)	85 ± 8	85 ± 8	84 ± 7	78 ± 8	106
MCH (pico-g)	29.5 ± 2.5	29.5 ± 2.5	—	—	—
MCHC (%)	33 ± 2	33 ± 2	—	—	—
MCD (μm)	6.7–7.7	6.7–7.7	—	—	—
Reticulocytes (%)	0.2–2.0	0.2–2.0	—	—	2–6

Normal range :

0.85 – 1.15

< hypochromic anaemia

> megaloblastic anaemia

(2) *MCD (Mean Corpuscular Diameter)*

MCD of red cells are measured by :

Calibrated eyepiece micrometer : It is done by the help of a slide placed on the eyepiece of microscope, on which a scale, usually 1 mm in 0.01 mm (10 μm) intervals, has been engraved.

About 200-500 cells are studied and the individual diameter of all cells are added, and the total divided by the number of cells measured on a blood film gives the mean diameter of a red cell. This is known as Price-Jones curve.

Normal range :

7.4 ± 0.2 μm (micrometre).

QUESTIONS

1. *Describe RBC pipette and mention its uses.*
2. *How does red cell diluting fluid act?*
3. *What is bulk dilution method of RBC counting?*
4. *Name the causes of increase as well as decrease of RBC count.*
5. *How do you clean the sides of pipette after drawing blood?*
6. *Why first few drops from counting pipette are discarded?*
7. *Define PCV, MCV, MCH and MCHC.*
8. *Name the conditions with abnormal MCV, MCH and MCHC.*
9. *Define colour index and MCD. How do you determine them?*

Chapter 9

WBC Pipette: Leucocyte counts

LEUCOCYTE COUNT

White blood corpuscles are present in much smaller number than red cells and hence the dilution required is much less. The total leucocyte count by visual method is achieved by the help of special bulb dilution (WBC pipette) (Fig. 5.1) or by bulk dilution. Electronic counters are used in many laboratories.

TOTAL COUNT

A. Manual Method

1. *WBC pipette*

Identification

The WBC pipette is smaller than RBC pipette and is marked 0.5, 1 below and 11 above the bulb (Figs. 5.1 & 5.2). There is a white bead in the bulb.

Uses :

1. Total WBC count of blood.
2. Total cell count of body fluids such as CSF, peritoneal, pleural, pericardial and other aspirated fluids.
3. Total sperm count of semen (when count is low).
4. Total platelet count specially when the count is low.

Technique

Blood is drawn up to 0.5 mark and diluting fluid up to 11 mark and the same procedure is adopted as in the case of RBC. The presence of glass bead in the bulb helps in better mixing of blood and diluent. This results in a dilution of blood to 1 : 20.

2. *Bulk dilution method*

The WBC pipette for total WBC count is nowadays less commonly used and Dacie & Lewiss do not recommend its use. Bulk dilution is better than the use of WBC pipette and is also reliable.

Technique

1. Place 0.38 ml of diluting fluid into a small test tube.
2. Measure 0.02 ml (20 µl) blood with a haemoglobinometer (Sahli) pipette and transfer to the diluting fluid. This makes a dilution of 1 in 20.
3. The tube is sealed with a clean rubber stopper and the content is mixed well by rotating the hand for two minutes.

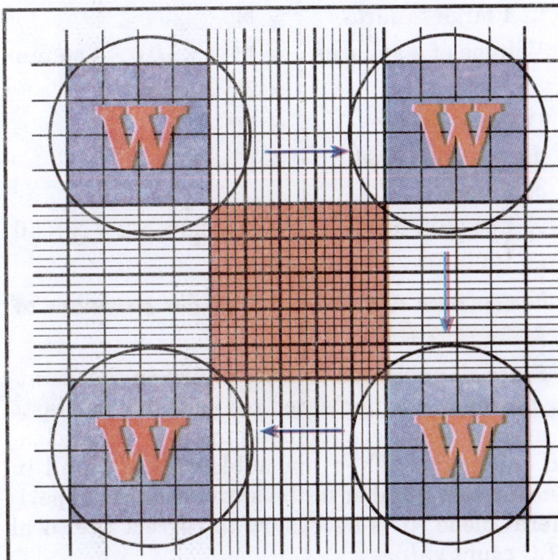

Fig. 9.1. Improved Neubauer ruling : areas for white cell count

4. Counting chamber is charged with a capillary pipette.

WBC diluting fluid

Turk's fluid :

Glacial acetic acid	1.5 ml
Sodium chloride	0.9 gm
1% aqueous solution of gentian violet (or methyl violet)	0.5 ml
Distilled water to	100 ml

Glacial acetic acid causes lysis of red cells. Gentian violet or methyl violet slightly stains the nuclei of leucocytes. The fluid should be filtered frequently to remove yeasts or moulds. A pinch of thymol may be added to prevent the growth of moulds.

Sources of error

The possible sources of error in WBC counting is the same as for the RBC count.

Counting of leucocytes

Cells in large 4 corner squares (1 × 1 mm each) of the Improved Neubauer chamber are counted using either the *Low power* (10 × objective) lens and a 10 × eyepiece or high power (40 × objective) lens and a 5 × eyepiece.

Calculation

Number of leucocytes in 4 large squares	= N
Volume of 4 squares	= 1 × 1 × 1/10 × 4 cu.mm
	= 2/5 cu. mm
Dilution factor	= 20
2/5 cu. mm blood contains	= N × 20
∴ 1 cu. mm blood contains	= N × 20 × 5/2 = N × 50

Correction of WBC count in the presence of nucleated RBC

Since all nucleated cells look alike on the counting chamber, the nucleated red cells (normoblasts or megaloblasts) are included in the total nucleated cell count. When normoblasts are found in considerable number in the stained smear of peripheral blood, it is necessary to correct the total WBC count values.

When nucleated red cells are present in peripheral blood smear, number of such cells seen per 100 WBC are counted.

Reporting on nucleated cells

(1) When 1 or 2 present in whole slide.	— *Rare*
(2) When 1 or 2 present but less than 1 per 100 WBC	— *Occasional*
(3) When more than 2 per 100 WBC	— *To correct the total WBC.*

Correction

$$\text{Total WBC} = \frac{100 \times \text{Total cells}}{100 + \text{Normoblasts per 100 WBC}}$$

Example :

Stained blood smear shows 10 normoblasts per 100 leucocytes.

Total cell including nucleated cell count = 11000/cu. mm.

$$\text{Total WBC} = \frac{100 \times 11000}{100 + 10} = \frac{100 \times 11000}{110}$$
$$= 10000 / \text{cu. mm.}$$

Normal range :

4,000 to 6,000/cu. mm (4 – $10^{9/L}$)

Note : (i) In cases where the total leucocyte count is very high (e.g., leukaemia), TLC is made by RBC pipette. (ii) When TLC is low, blood is drawn up to the mark 1 of WBC pipette and diluting fluid up to the mark (dilution 1:10) and accordingly calculation is made (dilution factor 100).

B. Electronic method

Several manufacturers have manufactured automated blood counter and instruction manuals are provided by them.

Haematology autoanalyser (cell counter— Fig. 9.2) is capable of providing rapid and precise report on various parameters such as Hb, PCV, TLC, platelet, DLC, MCV, MCH, MCHC, red cell diameter and platelet diameter. Most of the cell counters utilize a cyanide-free biodegradable reagent :

(i) RBCs and platelets are counted using the DC–detection method. (ii) WBCs are estimated by flow cytometry using a semiconductor laser. (iii) Haematocrit is determined by cumulative pulse height detection method.

ABNORMAL LEUCOCYTE COUNT

Leucocytosis

When increase in total WBC count to more than

Table 9.1
Causes of leucocytosis

Sub types		Diseases
A. Physiological		
1. *Age* — at birth – total WBC – 18000/cu. mm (approx), drops gradually to adult level.		
2. *Pregnancy* — WBC 12000–15000/cu. mm, count rises immediately after delivery and then gradually drops to normal.		
3. *Muscular exercise, high temperature, severe pain, great emotion.*		
B. Pathological		
1. *Neutrophilic leucocytosis*	:	Lobar pneumonia, bronchopneumonia, lung abscess, myocardial infarction, acute pyogenic meningitis, acute appendicitis, acute peritonitis, myeloid leukaemia.
2. *Lymphocytosis*	:	Whooping cough, infectious mononucleosis, chronic lymphocytic leukaemia, lymphocytic choriomeningitis, tuberculosis, syphilis, influenza, measles.
3. *Eosinophilia* (when total eosinophil count > 500 per cu. mm blood)	:	Tropical eosinophilia, parasites (filaria, hookworm), bronchial asthma, hay fever, Hodgkin's disease, eosinophilic leukaemia.
4. *Monocytosis*	:	Tuberculosis, syphilis, malaria, kala-azar, monocytic leukaemia, infectious mononucleosis.
5. *Basophils*	:	Measles, basophilic leukaemia.

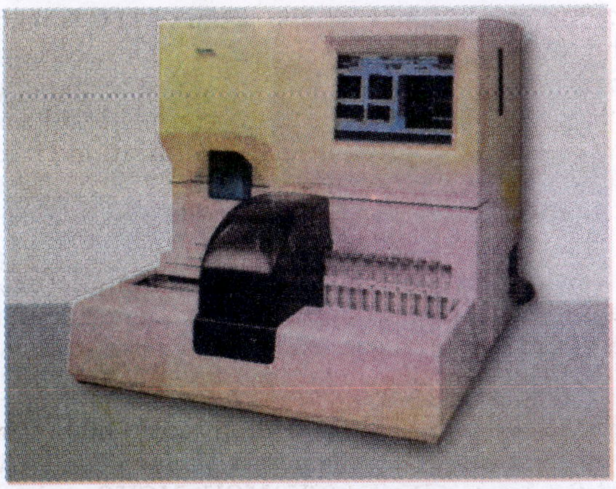
Fig. 9.2. Haematology autoanalyser employed for estimation of Hb, counting total leucocytes and platelets, and determining MCV, MCH, MCHC and DLC

10,000/cu. mm ($10 \times 10^{9/L}$) of blood, it is known absolute leucocytosis.

Causes of leucocytosis

The causes may be physiological or pathological (Table 9.1). Of the pathological causes infections and leukaemia are more important.

Relative leucocytosis

The condition where total WBC count is either normal or decreased, due to decrease in most instances of the polymorphs, the differential count shows as increase of a particular type of leucocyte (lymphocyte or monocyte).

(1) *Leucopenia with relative lymphocytosis,* e.g., enteric fever, malaria.

(2) *Leucopenia with relative monocytosis,* e.g., Kala-azar.

Table 9.2 : Causes of Leucopenia

Group	Diseases
A. Infection	(i) *Bacterial* : Enteric fever, tuberculosis. (ii) *Viral* : Influenzae, dengue, measles. (iii) *Protozoal* : Malaria, chronic Kala-azar.
B. Anaemia	Megaloblastic, iron deficiency.
C. Bone marrow depression	(i) *Primary* : Aplastic anaemia. (ii) *Secondary* : Drugs (chloramphenicol, anticancer drug, heavy metal); radiation effect.
D. Miscellaneous	Aleukaemic leukaemia, myelofibrosis, hypersplenism.

Leukopenia

Decrease in the total WBC count usually to less than 4000/cu. mm blood is called leucopenia (Table 9.2).

ABSOLUTE EOSINOPHIL COUNT (AEC)

Sometimes it is necessary to do a direct total or absolute eosinophil count to get an accurate count even though it can be done by calculating the number of eosinophils from total and differential white cell counts.

Diluting fluid

Eosin (2% aqueous soln.)	10 ml
Acetone (Graded reagent)	10 ml
Distilled water	80 ml

The solution after filtration is kept in a refrigerator at 4 °C. The fluid keeps well for about a month.

The fluid stains the eosinophils distinctly and lyses red cells and leucocytes other than eosinophils. Water serves as lytic agent and acetone as preservative of configuration of eosinophils.

Method

The blood is diluted either in WBC pipette as described before or in a test tube. The tube method is preferable.

Take 0.38 ml of diluting fluid in a small test tube and 0.02 ml of EDTA mixed blood is added. Mix well and leave for 10–15 minutes before charging the counting chamber.

The eosinophils are counted as per technique of counting total WBC, i.e., when cells in 4 large corner squares of an Improved Neubauer chamber are counted, the formula is N × 50/cu. mm blood as in WBC.

AEC using Fuch's Rosenthal chamber

Since the ruled area in Fuch's Rosenthal chamber is larger (16 sq. mm) and depth is also larger (0.2 mm) than the Neubauer chamber, greater number of cells can be found in this chamber (vide ch. 42).

Normal count

50-450 Eosinophils/cu. mm of blood.

Eosinophilia

When the absolute eosinophil count is more than 500 per cu. mm. of blood, the condition is called eosinophilia. See Table 9.1 for causes of eosinophilia.

Eosinopenia

When the total eosinophil count is less than 50 per cu. mm of blood, the condition is called eosinopenia.

Causes

Cushing syndrome, corticosteroid therapy, ACTH therapy.

QUESTIONS

1. *How do you identify WBC pipette? What are its uses?*
2. *How do you correct WBC count in presence of nucleated RBC?*
3. *How do you make total WBC count when count is very high?*
4. *Name the causes of Leucocytosis and leucopenia.*
5. *How do you make an absolute eosinophil count?*

Chapter 10

Platelet Count

PLATELET COUNT

The principal function of thrombocytes or platelets is to stop bleeding when a blood vessel is cut. The counting of platelet is an important component of blood cell count.

Platelet count using electronic *Coulter counter* has greatly improved counting precision, but visual methods are still widely used.

Greater care necessary in platelet count

1. Platelets are very small in size (diameter, 2–4 μm).
2. They agglutinate and break up easily.
3. They adhere to glasswares and particles in the diluting fluid.
4. False high count may be obtained if dust and bacteria and fragments of RBC are present in the diluting fluid, which may be mistaken for platelets. Platelets exhibit brownian movement and stain light blue by vital stain (e.g., brilliant cresyl blue) while the dust particles are not.
5. Syringes and containers of blood should be perfectly clean.
6. Diluting fluid should be freshly prepared each week, kept in refrigerator at 2-4 °C and filtered daily before use.

Diluting fluid

The RBCs are haemolysed in diluting fluid leaving platelets.

1. *Brecher-Cronkite fluid*

Ammonium oxalate	— 1 g
Fresh glass-distillled or deionized water	— 100 ml

To be prepared in small amout of 100 ml each week (preferably everyday) and filtered, preferably, through a micropore (0.22 μm) and kept at 2–4°C. Before use, the fluid is to be refiltered.

2. *Rees-Ecker fluid*

Sodium citrate	3.8 g
Brilliant cresyl blue	50 mg
Formalin	0.2 ml

Distilled water to make 100 ml.

Brilliant cresyl blue stains platelet pale blue.

3. *Dacie's fluid*

Sodium citrate dihydrate	5 g
Formalin	1 ml
0.2% brilliant cresyl blue	0.1 ml
Distilled water to	100 ml

Stock solution is diluted 1 in 10 before use.

Methods

A. Visual method

(1) ***Direct method*** : Blood is withdrawn with a clean venepuncture and it should flow into the syringe with minimum suction. After detaching the needle, requisite amount of blood is delivered without frothing into a vessel containing EDTA. Blood is mixed gently. The dilution of blood may be postponed for up to 3-4 hours if the collection has been satisfactory.

The direct method is preferred for total count of

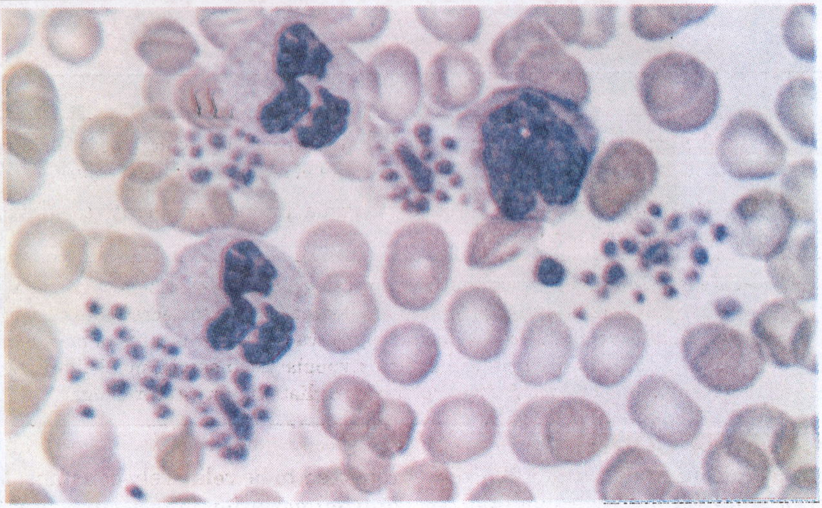

Fig. 10.1. Blood film : Platelet aggregates— Two areas of platelet aggregates are evident. Note the variation in size of the platelets. Platelets clump readily and may be seen in blood films as aggregates. *May–Grunwald-Giemsa stain* × 1200

platelets. The diluent ammonium oxalate, causes lysis of RBCs and WBCs leaving platelets.The blood is diluted 1 in 20 in the diluent by adding 0.1 ml blood to 1.9 ml diluent in a test tube. Blood may also be diluted in WBC pipette. The suspension is mixed well for 2 minutes before charging the improved Neubauer counting chamber.

The chamber is charged with the suspension using a Pasteur pipette or by a WBC pipette as the case may be, and it is left for 10 minutes in a Petridish containing moist filter paper. The moist filter paper keeps the air inside the Petridish moist and prevents drying during this time. Ten minutes standing allows the platelets to settle on the surface of counting chamber.

Using high power objective (40 ×) lens and 10 × eyepiece with condensor racked down, the platelets appear as highly refractile paticles.

The number of platelets in one or more areas of 1 mm^2 are counted. For greater accuracy, at lest 200 platelets to be counted. When the number of platelets is less than 200 in one or two large squares, then platelets in all the four squares are to be counted.

Calculation

If N is the number of platelets counted in an area of 1 mm^2 (0.1 cu. cm/µl in volume), the number of platelets :

$$\text{Per cu. mm } (\mu l) \text{ blood} = N \times 10 \times 20 \text{ (dilution)}$$
$$= N \times 200.$$

If N number of platelets in 2 squares are counted, then count/cu. mm = N × 200/2 = N × 100.

(2) ***Indirect method*** : This is an inaccurate method and only approximate count is possible as platelets are probably always lost by clumping and adhesion at the site of puncture.

After cleaning the finger tip with ether, place a drop of 2% sodium citrate in normal saline on dry surface of the finger. The finger tip is then pricked through the drop to dilute the blood at once in order to prevent breaking and clumping platelets. A thin smear is prepared by using a drop. The smear after drying in air is stained by Leishman's stain. At the same time, total RBC count is performed using another drop of blood after wiping the finger dry.

One thousand RBCs on the stained smear are counted while noting down the number of platelets (Fig. 10.1) seen during red cell counting.

Calculation

Thus, if RBC count is 5 million/cu. mm and N be

Table 10.1
Conditions with abnormal platelet count

Type	Disease
Thrombocytosis	(a) *Benign* : Immediately after severe haemorrhage (bleeding), post-operative phase, pregnancy, post-partum phase, in stage of shock, after burn injury. (b) *Malignant* : Essential thrombocythaemia, primary proliferative polycythaemia, chronic myeloid leukaemia.
Thrombocytopenia	Acute leukaemia (both lymphatic and myelogenous) — commonest cause, aplastic anaemia — where all three cellular elements are decreased due to decreased production by the bone marrow, idiopathic thrombocytopenic purpura (ITP), some cases of megaloblastic anaemia, thrombotic thrombocytopenic purpura, hypoplastic anaemia, myelofibrosis, chloramphenicol toxicity, hypersplenism, radiation, anticancer drugs.

the number of platelets counted around 1000 red cells, the number of platelets per cu. mm of blood,

$$= \frac{N}{1000} \times 5 \text{ million platelets / cu. mm.}$$

B. Electronic method

Platelet counting by electronic counter requires degree of resolution which is available with recently developed counters. Count is made either directly from the blood or platelet rich plasma that provides more reliable result. The platelet containing plasma is obtained by gravitational sedimentation of blood.

Normal range of platelet count

1. 150,000–400,000/cu. mm of blood.

2. Platelet counts in individual subjects are reported to be relatively constant, although slight diurnal variation may occur.

3. Women during menstruation may show slighly lower count.

Abnormal platelet count

A decrease in the number of platelets in blood is called thrombocytopenia and an increase, thrombocytosis (Table 10.1).

QUESTIONS

1. *Name the method of platelet count.*
2. *Which is the preferred method for platelet count and why?*
3. *Name the conditions with abnormal platelet count.*

Chapter 11

Blood Film: Preparation and Staining method, Examination of Stained film

A suitably prepared peripheral smear (peripheral blood film, PBF) is an essential part of haematological investigation, hence the film must be well spread, well stained and examined with care. PBF provides the following informations :

1. *Information on red cells* : Their number, shape, size and variations in morphology for diagnosing different types of anaemia and other haematologic disorders.

2. *Differential leucocyte count* (DLC) : DLC is useful in diagnosis of many diseases.

3. *Assessment of platelet* : The approximate number of platelets, their aggregates and morphological appearances are very useful in diagnosis of various bleeding disorders. Abnormal cells are also detected.

4. *Blood parasites* : Malarial parasites and sometime trypanosomes are detected in PBF.

Collection of blood

1. Syringe should be sterile. Slides should be clean and should not be greasy. Smear made on greasy slide has blank oval areas.

2. Sample of blood may be collected from the antecubital vein for haematological and biochemical studies at a time.

PREPARATION OF BLOOD FILMS

A drop of blood is placed in the centre line of a slide about 1-2 cm from one end. Almost immediately place a glass slide (spreader) with a smooth edge at an angle of about 45° to the slide and move it back to make contact with the drop of

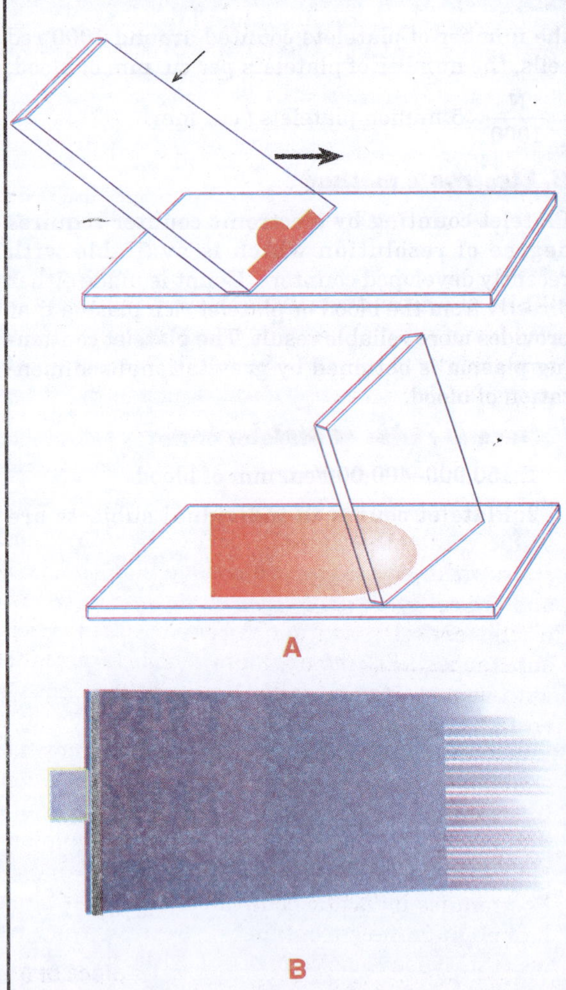

Fig. 11.1. Method of making peripheral blood smear : (A) good film, (B) bad film.

blood. The drop is to be spread out quickly along the line of contact of the spreader with the slide. Ensure that the "drop of blood is pulled by the spreader but it is not pushed ahead of the spreader". The amount of blood in the drop should be just adequate for a film of 3 or 4 cm length (Fig. 11.1). Ideally, the thickness of the film should be such that there is some overlap of red cells throughout much of the film's length with separation and lack of distortion towards the tail of the film. Recognition of the white cells should be possible throughout the length of film, although they can be recognised at the head of the film (thicker part) with some difficulty (Fig.11.1A & B).

Labelling : Patient's name and date is to be written by pencil on the head or thick end of the smear.

Sources of error : When the edge of spreader is not smooth, ragged tail of smear is produced which is known *tailing* of the smear. Most of the neutrophils and platelets are found in that area.

Thick smear preparation

While the film described above is suitable for studies of cellular morphology, sometimes thick smears are prepared for detection of malarial parasites and microfilaria which is shown in Fig. 12.2.

Staining of blood films

Some structural components of blood cells are acidic while others are basic. Acidic substances stain with basic stain (methylene blue, Azure B) and are callled *basophilic,* e.g., nucleic acids. The nuclei are also stained by basic stain. Basic substances like haemoglobin which are stained with acid stains are called *acidophilic*. Most use eosin as acid stain. Stains which are made up of combinations of acid and basic dyes are known as *"Romanowsky" stain* that make subtle distinctions in staining of cell, and of staining the granules differentially. Neutrophilic granules in cytoplasm get weakly stained by azure complexes, eosinophilic granules by acidic component of dye, whereas basophilic granules contain acid heparin which has an affinity for basic component of the dye.

Various modifications of the original Romanowsky combination of methylene blue and eosin now in use include *Wright's, Leishman's, Giemsa's* and *Jenner's stains*. Leishman's stain is mostly used in the routine staining of blood film.

Leishman's Stain

Leishman powder
(eosin-methylene blue powder) — 0.5 g
Methyl alcohol (acetone free) — 100 ml

The powder is transferred to a conical flask to which methyl alcohol is added. The mixture is warmed to 50 °C for 10–15 minutes. It is then filtered. The dye is ripened by keeping the filtrate in sunlight for 3–4 days or in an incubator at 37 °C for 7 days.

Buffer water (Sorensen's phosphate buffer)

Solution A :
Pot. dihydrogen phosphate — 9.08 g/litre
Solution B :
Dibasic Sod. phosphate — 9.47 g/litre

Mix solutions A and B in the following proportion to make 100 ml buffer water for pH 6.8 :

Solution A — 50.8 ml
Solution B — 49.2 ml

Method

The smear gets fixed by methyl alcohol present in stain. The air dried smear is covered with the stain for 1–2 minutes. Then buffered water (alternatively, distilled water) about double the volume of stain is added drop by drop over the smear and left for 10 minutes and then washed with tap water and dried in air.

Other Stains

(1) ***Wright's Stain***

Wright's stain powder — 0.2 g.
Methyl alcohol (acetone free) — 100 ml

The solution is kept at 37°C for a few days before use.

Method

The same as in Leishman's staining. When the stain is ripe, a scum of film is formed over the surface of the stain.

(2) ***Giemsa's Stain***

Giemsa powder — 0.6 g
Glycerol — 50.0 ml
Acetone-free methyl alcohol — 50.0 ml

0.6 g of powdered dye is transferred to a conical flask of 250 ml capacity to which 50 ml glycerol is added. The mixture is warmed at 50°C for 15 minutes with occasional shaking and then 50 ml methanol is added to the mixture. It is then filtered and made ready for use. The stain is to be diluted 1 : 10 before use.

Method

Blood film is first dried in air and then fixed with methyl alcohol for 8 to 10 dips in a Coplin jar and dried. Diluted stain (1:10) is poured on the fixed smear and kept for 20–25 minutes. Wash the smear with neutral water and dry.

(3) *Field's Stain*

It is sometimes used for staining thick film for malarial parasites and offers rapid staining.

Stain A (polychrome methylene blue) :

Methylene blue	0.26 g
Azure B	0.1 g
Disodium hydrogen phosphate	2.5 g
Potassium dihydrogen phosphate	1.25 g
Water	100 ml

Stain B (eosin) :

Eosin	
(Yellow eosin, water soluble)	0.26 g
Disodium hydrogen phosphate	2.5 g
Potassium dihydrogen phosphate	1.25 g
Water	100 ml

Table 11.1

Peripheral blood smear study on morphology of red cell

Condition	Cause
Red cell morphology	
Size	
Normocyte	Normal red cell (7–7.5 μm) diameter.
Macrocytosis	Increase in size of RBC, e.g., megaloblastic anaemia.Macrocytes are generally oval in appearance vit B_{12} and folic acid deficiency (Fig. 16.4).
Microcytosis	Decrease, in size of RBC, results from fragmentation of normocytes or macrocytes, e.g., iron deficiency anaemia and thalassaemia major, and hereditary spherocytosis.
Anisocytosis	Irregular in size (both macro and microcytes).
Biconcave	Shape of normal red cell.
Spherocytosis	Both sides are bulged out giving a spherical shape to RBC.
Elliptocytosis	Red cells are elliptical, e.g., hereditary elliptocytosis.
Ovalocytosis	Oval red cells.
Poikilocytosis	Irregular in shape of red cells.
Target cell	Red cells with centrally placed haemoglobin and a thin rim of haemoglobin along the cell wall and a clear space in between. They are mainly found in sickle cell anaemia, thalassaemia major; and variable numbers in haemolytic anaemias, in iron deficiency anaemia, post-splenectomy and hepatic disease.
Burr cells	Periphery of red cells is provided with cytoplasmic prolongation like beak of a bird.
Appearance and colour reaction	
Normochromia	Normal red cells look pinkish brown due to haemoglobin. Peripheral part appears deep brown while the central part is faint because of biconcave shape of RBC.
Hypochromia	When red cells contain less haemoglobin, they appear faintly brown; indicates anaemia.
Polychromasia	Literally means many colour, but in practice red cells appear bluish grey — these are the reticulocytes.
Anisochromasia	Some but not all of the red cells stain palely after haematinics.

Table 11.1 contd. from previous page

Condition	Cause
Immature red cells	Their presence indicate highly active marrow.
Early and intermediate normoblasts	Excessively active marrow, regenerating blood in a normal manner.
Early normoblast	Severe anaemia, polycythaemia.
Late normoblast	Moderate anaemia, thalassaemia.
Megaloblasts	Pernicious anaemia, tropical malnutrition, liver damage.
Erythroblasts	Erythroblastosis foetalis.
Intracorpuscular structures	
Cabot ring	Stains reddish purple, appears as either round or figure of eight (8), found in pernicious anaemia, lead poisoning and leukaemia.
Howell-Jolly bodies	These are true nuclear fragments, stain reddish blue. Found in secondary anaemia, pernicious anaemia, leukaemia, after splenectomy, splenic atrophy.
Rouleaux formation	
Rouleaux	Multiple myelomatosis, macroglobulinaemia.

Table 11.2

Peripheral blood smear study on leucocytes, platelets and parasites

Condition	Cause
Differential leucocyte count	
Differential leucocyte count	Incidence of neutrophils, eosinophils, basophils, lymphocytes and monocytes in different conditions.
Leucocytosis or leucopenia	Indirect evidence can be obtained from peripheral smear.
Immature cells	Presence of primitive blast cells or partly mature myelocytes and promyelocytes indicate leukaemic blood picture.
Study on platelets	
Thrombocytopenia *Thrombocytosis*	Peripheral smear gives an approximate idea on the number of platelets present.
Morphology	Can be identified.
Thrombasthenia	Big sized giant platelets are indicative of diminished functional activity of platelets.
Parasites	
Extracellular	Microfilaria, Trypanosomes.
Intracellular	Malaria parasites within RBC and occasionally LD bodies in monocytes.

Preparation of solution :

The phosphates are disssolved in warm freshly boiled water. Azure B is ground in a mortar with phosphate solution to dissolve it well. The dyes are added in phosphates solution and mixed well and filtered.

Method

(i) Dip the blood film in Stain A for one second.

(ii) Remove the film from Stain A and rinse immediately waving very gently in clean

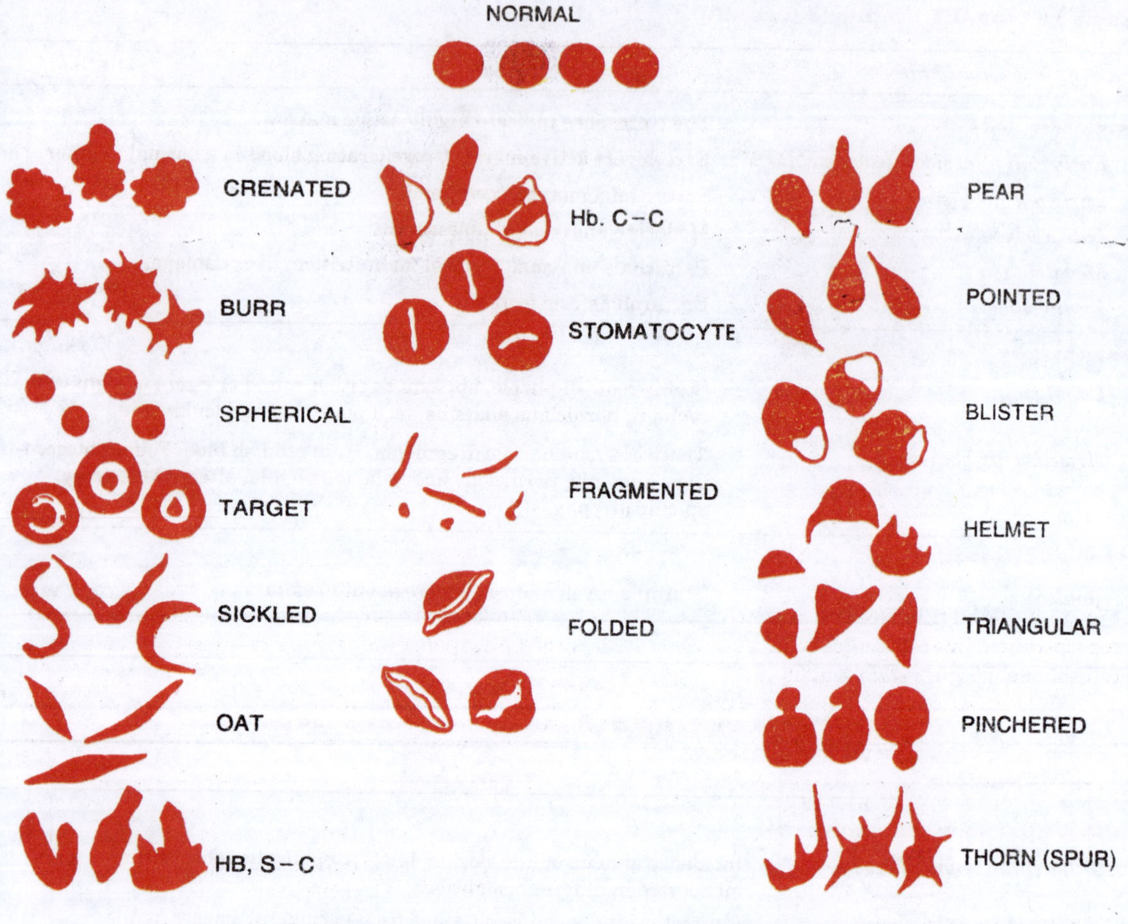

Fig. 11.2. Shapes of erythrocytes in dried blood smear

water for 5-10 seconds until the stain ceases to flow from the film and the slide becomes free from the stain.

(iii) Dip for 1 second in solution B.

(iv) Rinse in clean water for 2-3 seconds.

(v) Place vertically against a rack, drain and dry.

(4) *May-Grunwald-Giemsa's Stain*

It stains well films of blood, bone marrow and aspirated material.

May-Grunwald's Stain :

May-Grunwald powder	0.3 g
Acetone-free methyl alcohol	100 ml

Dissolve the dye in 100 ml methanol warming at 50°C for 10 minutes, shaking time to time. Filter after 24 hours.

Method

(i) Smear fixed in methanol as in Giemsa.

(ii) Stain the film with dilute dye solution (1:10) for 5 minutes.

(iii) Then stain the film with dilute (1:10) Giemsa's stain for 10-15 minutes.

(iv) Wash with buffered water and dry in the air.

EXAMINATION OF STAINED FILM

Examination of peripheral blood smear provides valuable information on morphology of RBCs

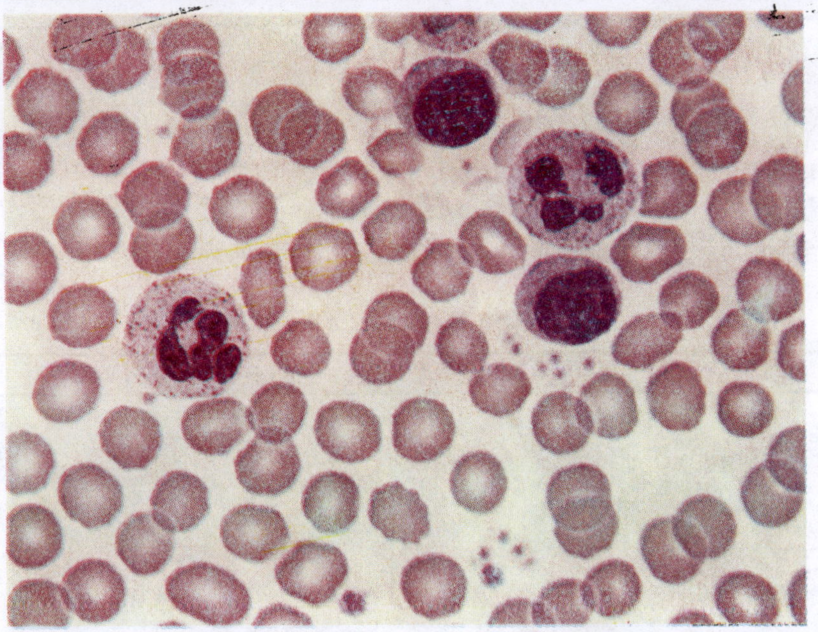

Fig. 11.3. Blood film Normal erythrocytes— Cells are of uniform size and shape with a normal haemoglobin concentration. One cell, centre of field, reveals a small are of central pallor which is less than one-third of the total cell volume. *Wright's stain* X 1200

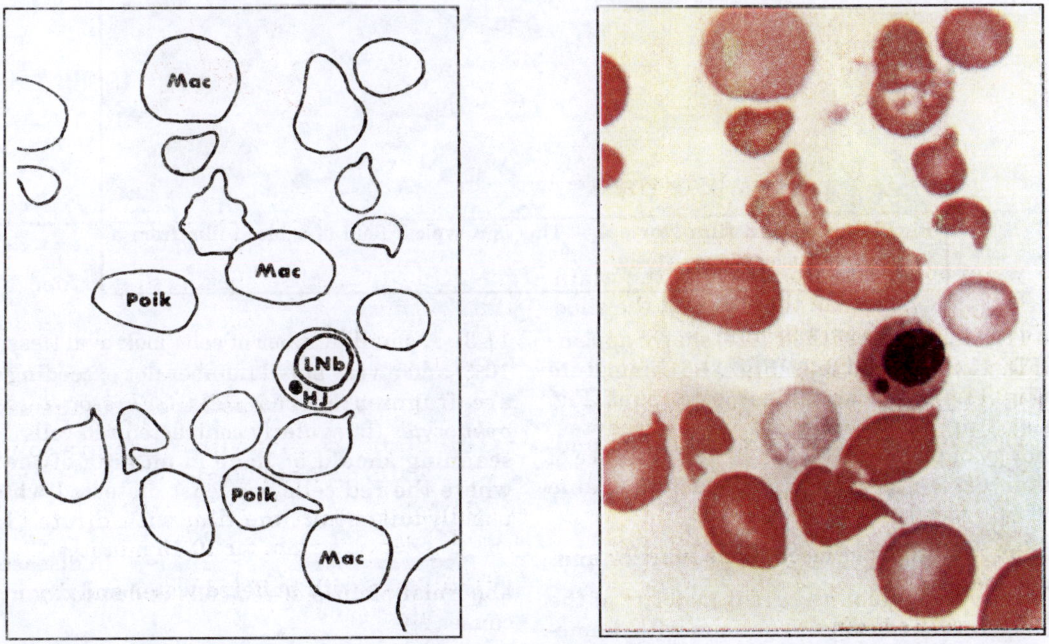

Fig. 11.4. Abnormal erythrocytes (in pernicious anaemia) : Anisocytosis +, poikilocytosis +, macrocytosis +; and a late normoblast containing a Howell-Jolly body.

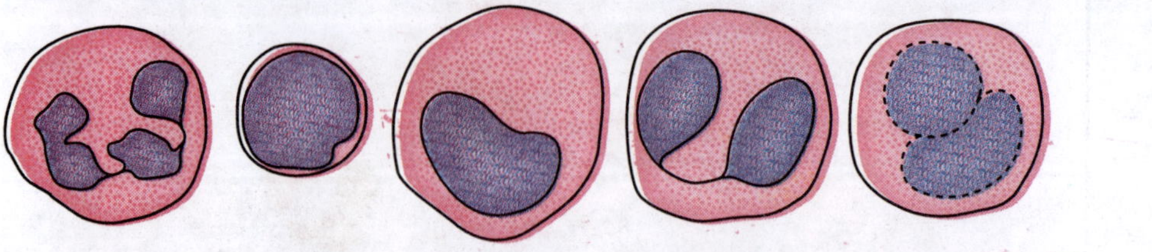

Fig. 11.5A. Morphology of leucocytes

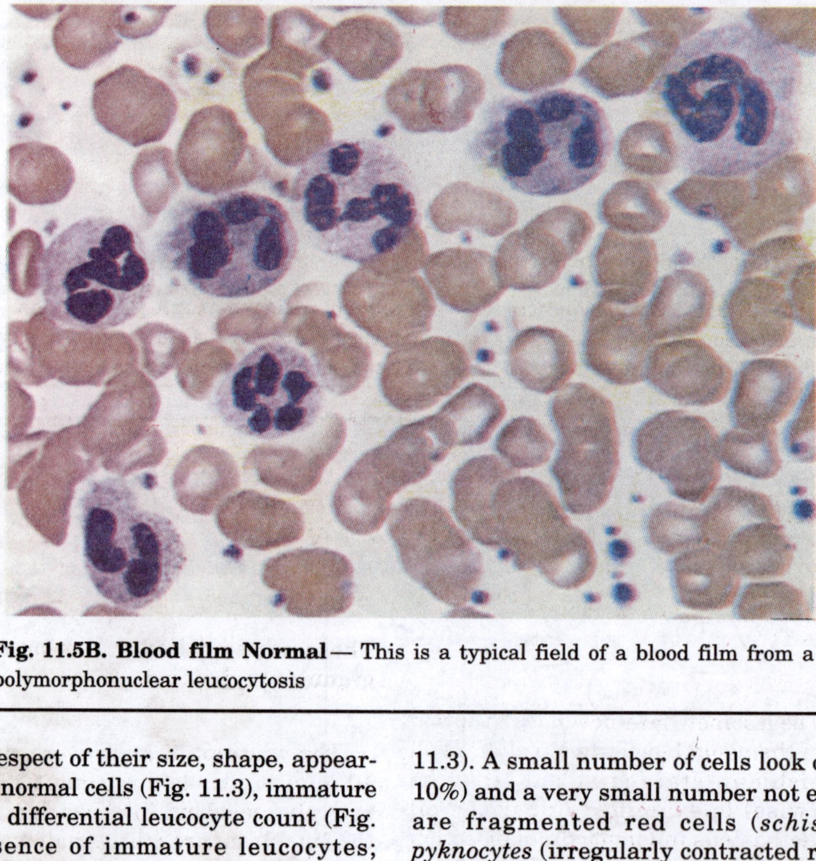

Fig. 11.5B. Blood film Normal— This is a typical field of a blood film from a polymorphonuclear leucocytosis

(Table 11.1) in respect of their size, shape, appearance (Fig. 11.2), normal cells (Fig. 11.3), immature cells (Fig. 11.4); differential leucocyte count (Fig. 11.5) and presence of immature leucocytes; morphology of platelets (Fig. 11.3) and presence of megakaryocytes; presence of parasites (Table 11.2).

Red cell morphology

In a healthy individual, the great majority of the red cells have round smooth contours with diameters of 6–8.5 µm. They deeply stain at the periphery with the eosin component of Romanowsky dyes due to normal biconcavity of the cell (Fig. 11.3). A small number of cells look oval (less than 10%) and a very small number not exceeding 0.1% are fragmented red cells (*schistocytes*) and *pyknocytes* (irregularly contracted red cells). RBC scanning should be done in an area of the film where the red cells are least distorted which is usually tail end of film.

Abnormal RBC morphology: In disease, the abnormal picture of red cells is due to four main causes :

1. *Abnormal erythropoiesis* which may be effective or ineffective.
2. *Inadequate haemoglobin synthesis.*

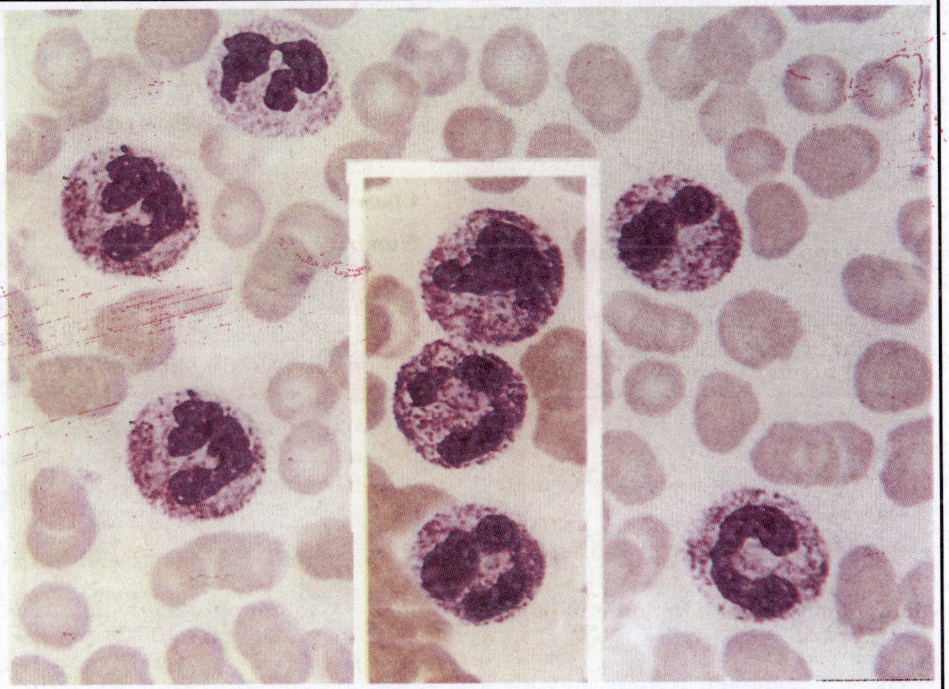

Fig. 11.6. Blood film Polymorphonuclear leucocytosis with toxic granulation— There is an increase in the number of polymorphonuclear leucocytes, some of which are not fully developed. Note also that the granules are much coarser and that their staining reaction is more acidophilic than in normal neutrophil leucocytes

3. *Changes affecting, or damage, to erythrocytes* after leaving the bone marrow.

4. *Increased erythropoiesis*—attempts made by bone marrow to compensate for anaemia.

The various changes of morphology of red cell is shown in Table 11.1.

White cell morphology

There tends to be a somewhat uneven distribution of leucocytes in the usual blood film on slide. Well dried and Leishman stained smear (may be stained otherwise) is examined under the oil immersion objective lens in longitudinal direction from head to tail of the film avoiding the margins of the smear. Counting of different types of leucocytes is done at 2–3 lengthwise strips till at least 200 cells are counted, although counting of 500 cells at different strips are preferable. The error is of the order of ± 7% when 200 cells are counted.

Differential count : The differential leucocyte count on the basis of size, cytoplasm with or without granules, and type of nucleus of WBCs include (Table 11.2) :

Granulocytes : Neutrophils, eosinophils, basophils.

Agranulocytes : Lymphocytes, monocytes.

A. Granulocytes

These are so called due to presence of specific granules in their cytoplasm.

I. Neutrophil polymorphonuclears

The neutrophils have average diameters of 10-12 mm, multilobed nucleus (1-4 lobes) and are actively amoeboid in character. The granules in the cytoplasm are quite small and stain pale pink or faintly violet (neutral stain). Number of nuclear lobes increases with age of cell (Figs.11.5A&B). Neutrophils constitute 40–70 per cent of WBCs of all leucocytes in adult.

Certain other informations can be obtained from morphologic features of neutrophils, eg., (i) in megaloblastic anaemia, hypersegmentation of nucleus (5 or more lobes) occurs, (ii) second X chromosome (corresponding to Barr body) : presence of drum stick on the nucleus is seen.

Following abnormalities may be observed in neutrophils :

1. *Toxic granules* : These are large deeply staining blue to purple basophilic granules. (Fig. 11.6) found in cytoplasm of neutrophils in severe bacterial infections or toxaemias. These granules may be small and scattered in between the neutrophil granules or may be large and coarse that have completely replaced the normal pinkish granules.

Large reddish staining granules are often found in aplastic anaemia and sometimes in myelosclerosis.

Large, dark staining granules are a characteristic feature of the genetic disorder, *"Alder abnormality"* in which coarse granules may also be found in lymphocytes and monocytes.

2. *Vacuoles* : Along with toxic granules some neutrophils contain phagocytic vacuoles known as *Toxic vacuoles* in severe bacterial infections and toxaemia.

3. *Dohle bodies* : Some neutrophils may also contain bluish staining round or oval 2–3 μm diameter patches, usually in the periphery of the cytoplasm, called *"Dohle bodies"*. They are mostly found in bacterial infections.

Measurement of body's response to infection

Immature neutrophils have fewer nuclear lobes or divisions or some with nuclei that have not yet divided. Because in an infection there is leucocytosis with an increase in the number of less mature cells in the blood, two techniques were developed to try to measure quantitatively the body's response to infection, which include *Arneth count* and the *Schilling count.*

(a) ***Arneth count*** : Neutrophils are graded from 1 to 5 according to the number of lobes in their nuclei.

Group I	Unilobed (one lobe) but deeply indented nucleus.
Group II	Two lobes connected by one thin segment.
Group III	Three lobes connected by two thin filaments.
Group IV	Four lobes connected by four thin filaments.
Group V	Five or more lobes connected by 5 or more thin filaments.

One hundred neutrophils are counted and the number in each is expressed as a percentage (Table 11.3) :

Table 11.3
Arneth count

Class	I	II	III	IV	V
Number	6	35	40	17	2

Since there appears an increasing number of younger cells (Group I and II) in blood in acute infection, thre is a *"shift to the left"*. In megaloblastic anaemia and other clinical conditions where bone marrow is less active, the production of neutrophils is low, circulating leucocytes are older with hypersegmented nuclei. There is a *"shift to the right"*.

Arneth index : Percentage of cells in Group I, II and 1/2 of III is about 60 (normal range 51–65). Only about 2–5% fall in Group I.

(b) *Schilling count* : Here all the granular leucocytes are divided into four groups and the number of each of these group of cells are expressed as a percentage of the WBCs and merely of the granulocytes.

The four groups are :

1. Myelocytes
2. Juveniles or metamyelocytes
3. Stab cells or band forms
4. Segmented cells.

Differential count as seen normally is given below (Table 11.4).

A *shift to left* occurs when the number in per cent increases to the left of the dividing line.

The *Arneth* and *Schilling counts* are not followed now as they are too complicated for ordinary use. However, a *"shift to the left"* with band and stab forms and perhaps with a few myelocytes are found in severe bacterial infections and septicaemia accompanied by toxic granulation. On the other hand, a *"right shift"* can help in the diagnosis of megaloblastic anaemia and uraemia.

II. Eosinophil

They are 14-16 μm in diameter and constitute 2–4% of all leucocytes. As the name indicates, their cytoplasm contains large, oval or round, orange-

Table 11.4
Schilling Count

Total	Percentage							
	Basophil	Eosino	Myelo	Juve	Stab	Seg	Lymph	Mono
5,000–8,000	0–1	2–4	0	0–1	3–5	51–67	21–35	4–8

red (eosinophilic) granules. The granules fill the cytoplasm usually completely and sometimes are found over the nucleus. The nucleus has got fewer lobes, on an average only two, so called "spectacle arrangement".

III. Basophil (or Mast cell)

Count of basophils vary from 0.5–1% of all leucocytes and the diameter is 8-10 µm. They contain large, round coarse, deep purple to bluish black (basophilic) granules and most often are found overlying the nucleus. The nucleus is, therefore, not very clearly seen. The nucleus is kidney-shaped or slightly lobulated.

B. Agranulocytes

Although lymphocytes and monocytes do not show granules by ordinary stain, granulation may be demonstrated with azure blue. Lymphocytes contain a few azurophilic granules and monocytes show numerous, fine azurophilic granules.

1. Lymphocytes

Lymphocytes constitute 25-35% of total leucocytes in adults and 40-60% in infants. Normally, majority of circulating lymphocytes are small cells and only 10% are large cells.

(a) **Small lymphocyte** : They are small round cells, about the size of red cells, with only a scant rim of cytoplasm in which there are a few scattered azurophil granules. The nucleus stains dark with condensed chromatin (smudgy or pyknotic), sometimes slightly indented (Fig. 11.5A).

(b) **Large lymphocyte** : They are 12-15 mm in diameter with abundant cytoplasm and a large round or slightly indented nucleus. Their cytoplasm frequently contain azurophil granules.

2. Monocytes

They form 2–7% of total leucocytes. Monocyte is a large cell with 16–22 µm diameter, although smaller forms may occur. The cytoplasm is plentiful, staining sky-blue and contains a few very fine azurophil granules. The nucleus is situated at one side, lobulated, kidney-shaped or horse-shoe shaped with loosely arranged chromatin. Rarely, monocytes of very large size with abundant, flowing, vacuolated cytoplasm, which have acted as macrophages are seen in peripheral blood films, e.g., bacterial endocarditis.

Agranulocytosis : In this condition, there is severe neutropenia. As a result the patient is susceptible to bacterial infections.

Virocytes

In certain infectious states like infectious mononucleosis, influenza and measles, transformed mononuclear cells (lymphocytes) having an appearance of blastoid/monocytoid/plasmacytoid cells appear in peripheral blood. These are called virocytes. In infectious mononucleosis, white cell count may reach one lakh per cu. mm with 90-95% virocytes. There is thus leukaemoid reaction produced in infectious mononucleosis.

QUESTIONS

1. *How do you prepare a peripheral blood smear?*
2. *What is tailing of smear?*
3. *What do you look for in peripheral blood smear in respect of erythrocytes, leucocytes, platelets and parasites?*
4. *Name the various shapes of erythrocytes.*
5. *What are toxic granules and Dohle bodies?*
6. *What observation on platelets can be made from peripheral smear?*
7. *How do you make a measurement of body's response to infection?*
8. *What is agranulocytosis?*
9. *What are abnormal mononuclear cells (virocytes)?*

Chapter 12

Examination for Haemoparasites

Indian subcontinent is endemic for parasitic diseases, particularly malaria and filaria, and these parasites are frequently encountered in peripheral blood smear.

MALARIA

Clinically the patient suffers from high fever with chill and rigor. These paroxysms of fever lasts for 4-16 hours followed by afebrile period with either a 48-hour (tertian : days 1 and 3) or 72-hour (quartan : days 1 and 4) periodicity.

Stages of parasite seen: All stages of *P. vivax* trophozoites, schizonts and gametocytes are present in peripheral blood. In case of *P. falciparum* only ring stage (trophozoite) and gametocytes are present in peripheral blood and schizonts are not found since schizogony occurs in tissues.

Plasmodium vivax (Fig. 12.1)

(a) *Trophozoite* (Fig. 12.1) : The early trophozoite looks like a ring and also known as ring form. The diameter of the ring is 2.5 to 3 µm, about a third of the size of erythrocyte. Nucleus is usually seen as a single red chromatin dot. Cytoplasm is blue and nucleus is red. In a growing trophozoite, the ring becomes irregular in a large red cell with development of Schuffner's dots.

(b) *Late trophozoite* (Fig. 12.1) : It is an amoeboid form and almost fills an enlarged RBC. It contains malarial pigment. *Mature erythrocytic Schizont contains 12-24 (average 16) merozoites.*

(c) *Gametocyte* : Both male and female gametocytes are large (9-12 mm) nearly filling the enlarged red cell (Fig. 12.1). The cytoplasm is pale blue and contains pinkish Schuffner's dots. The nucleus is pale red and diffuse and accentric.

Plasmodium falciparum (Fig. 12.3)

(a) *Early trophozoite or ring form* (Fig. 12.3) : It is very delicate inside RBC and tiny, measures 1.25 to 1.5 µm in diameter, about a sixth of red cell diameter. There are usually two nuclear chromatin.

(b) *Gametocyte* : Gametocytes are crescentric within RBC and only a thin red cell border can be made out. Male gametocyte is paler in colour,

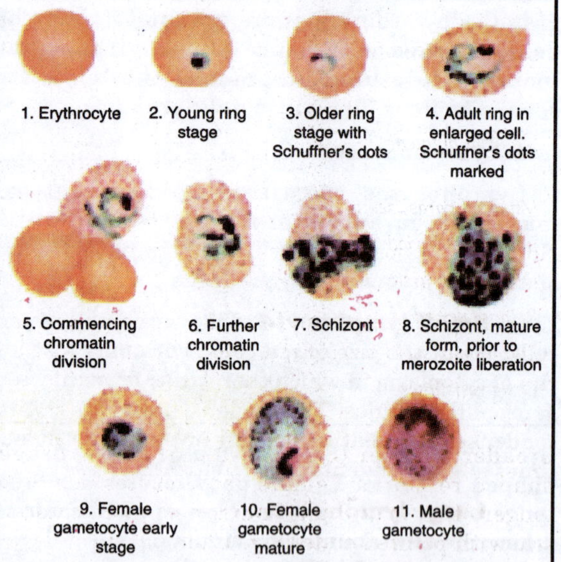

Fig. 12.1. *Plasmodium vivax* : Erythrocytes stages. 1. Normal red cell; 2. Ring form (early trophozoite); 3. Older ring form, red cell contains Schuffner's dots; 4. Amoeboid trophozoite; 5, 6, 7. Early schizont; 8. Mature schizont; 9. Female gametocyte (early); 10. Female gametocyte (mature); 11. Male gametocyte.

Table 12.1 : Differential characters of the two parasites

Collection of blood	*P. vivax*	*P. falciparum*
Erythrocytic schizogony (duration)	48 hours	48 hours
Forms of parasite in peripheral blood	Trophozoites, schizonts, Gametocytes.	Only ring and crescents (gametocytes).
Ring form in a RBC	Large 2.5 µm, single, prominent chromatin.	Delicate, small, 1.5 µm, Double chromatin and multiple rings common. Accole forms found.
Late trophozoite	Large, irregular with a prominent vacuole. Actively amoeboid.	Compact, seldom seen in blood smear.
Schizont	9-10 µm, large, fills an enlarged red cell.	4-5 µm, fills two-thirds of a red cell which is not enlarged. Usually not seen in blood smear.
Number of merozoites	12-24, arranged in irregular grape-like cluster.	18-24, arranged in grape-like cluster.
Gametocytes	Spherical or globular. Size – much larger than a red cell, male 9 µm, female 10-11 µm. Host cell enlarged with Schuffner's dots.	Crescentic. Larger than a red cell, male 9-11 µm, female 12-14 µm. Host cell hardly recognizable.
Infected erythrocyte	Enlarged, pale, Schuffner's dots present.	Normal size, Maurer's dots (large red spots) sometimes basophilic stippling.
Malarial pigment	Yellowish brown, fine granules.	Dark brown or blackish, one or two solid blocks.
Maximal parasitaemia	25,000/µl	100,000/µl
Incubation period	14 days	12 days
Duration of first attack (untreated)	18-20 years	10-20 days
Relapse period	2–5 years	Recrudescence
Duration of sporogony in mosquito at 25 °C	9-10 days	10-12 days
Drug resistance	No	Yes

broader, shorter (8-10 × 2-3 µm) and sausage-shaped reniform. Female gametocytes are blue, longer (10-12 × 2-3 µm), narrower, more crescentric with pointed ends (Fig. 12.3).

Table 12.1 shows differential characters of the two parasites.

Laboratory diagnosis

Peripheral blood smear

Blood is collected at or just after the height of febrile paroxysm. Since erythrocytic schizogony occurs in peripheral blood, all stages of *P. vivax*, *P. ovale* and *P. malariae* are found in peripheral blood. In case of *P. falciparum* infection, early trophozoites (ring form) and gametes are only found in peripheral blood since the growing trophozoites and schizonts remain in capillaries of internal organs.

Method : Examination of blood film is the most important method of diagnosis. It is a good practice to prepare one thin and other thick smear at a time. Smears must be collected before administration of antimalarial drugs.

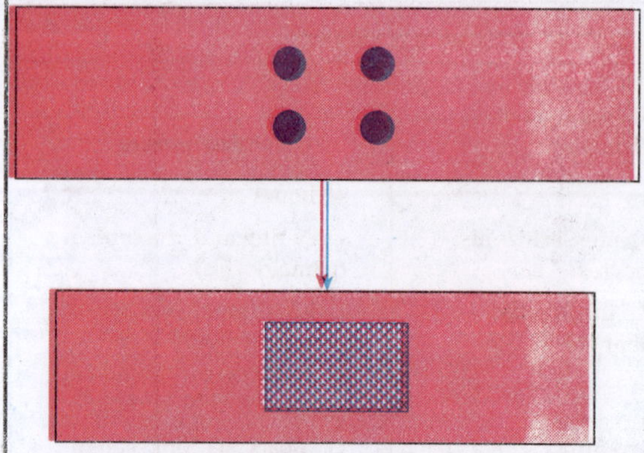

Fig. 12.2. Preparation of thick smear for MP

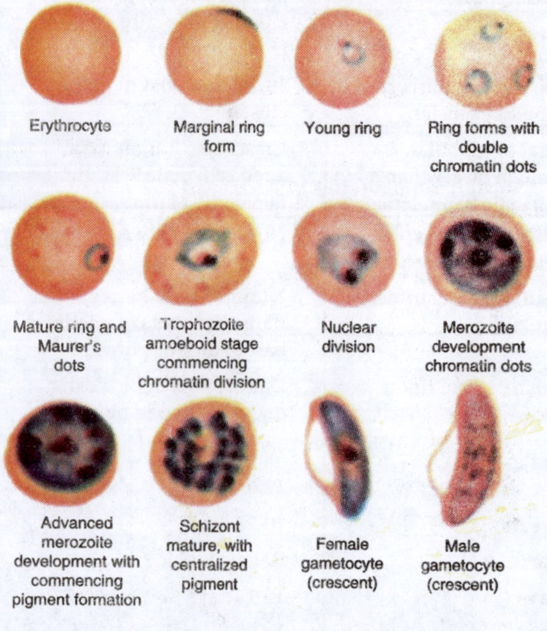

Fig. 12.3. *Plasmodium falciparum* : Erythrocyte stage

(i) *Thin smear* prepared as usual is stained by Leishman stain.

(ii) For *thick smear*, 4 drops of blood are placed at 4 corners of a 2.5 cm × 1.25 cm = 3.2 sq cm (half sq in) area at the middle of the glass slide and are joined by a needle (Fig. 12.2). Thick smear is dried in air and dehaemoglobinised by placing the film in vertical position in distilled water for 5-10 minutes. The film is dried in air and stained by Leishman stain and examined under oil immersion objective.

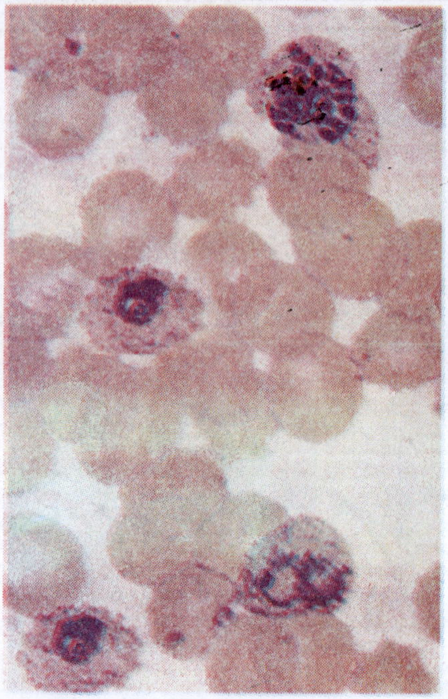

Fig. 12.4. Blood film of *P. vivax* infection (BT malaria): Merozoites (top left), trophozoites (bottom); Schuffner's dots are present in infected red cells

Thick smear preparation helps quick detection of M.P. and thin smear helps to study the morphology. In Romanowsky (Leishman) stained smear trophozoite of plasmodia appear to consist of a blue cytoplasmic ring within RBC and a red nucleus (chromatin dot). *P. vivax* primarily infects young erythrocytes and reticulocytes which are larger mature red cells, so red cell is longer in *P. vivax* infection. *P. falciparum* infects red cells of all ages. Gametocytes of *P. vivax* are globular and much larger than a red cell and host cell contains Schuffner's dots.

FILARIASIS

Most important species of filarial nematodes — *Wucheria bancrofti* and *Brugia malayi* parasitise the lymphatics. *W. bancrofti* is largely confined to tropical and subtropical countries. Mosquitoes (*Culex, Aedes* and *Anopheles*) introduce infective larvae into the skin that slowly develops long thin adult worm found in the lymph node and lymphatics of limbs (usually lower) and groin. In chronic infection, repeated episodes of lymphangitis cause obstruction to lymph flow resulting in lymphoedema and elephantiasis. Embryos (microfilaria) of *W. bancrofti* pass through lymph nodes,

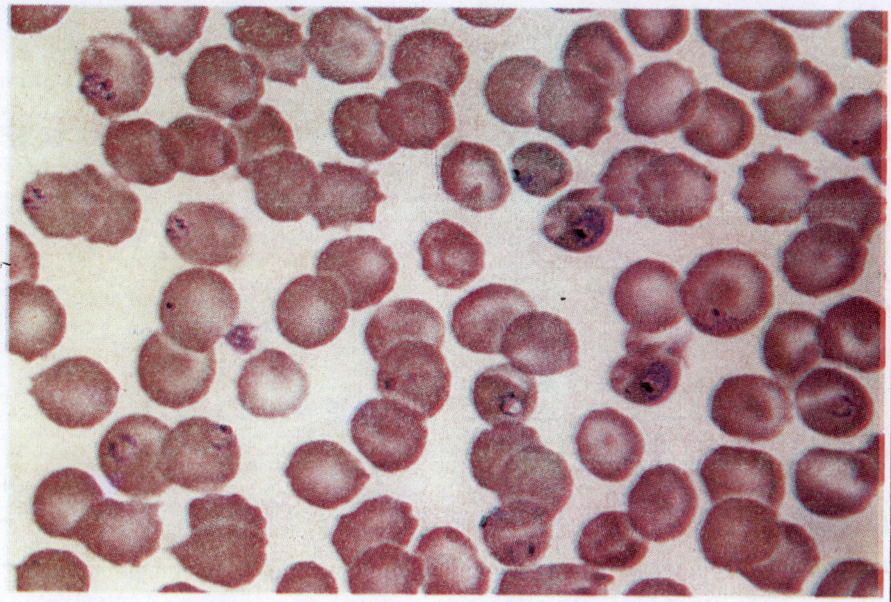

Fig. 12.5. Blood film of *P. falciparum* (MT malaria) : Trophozoites in ring form

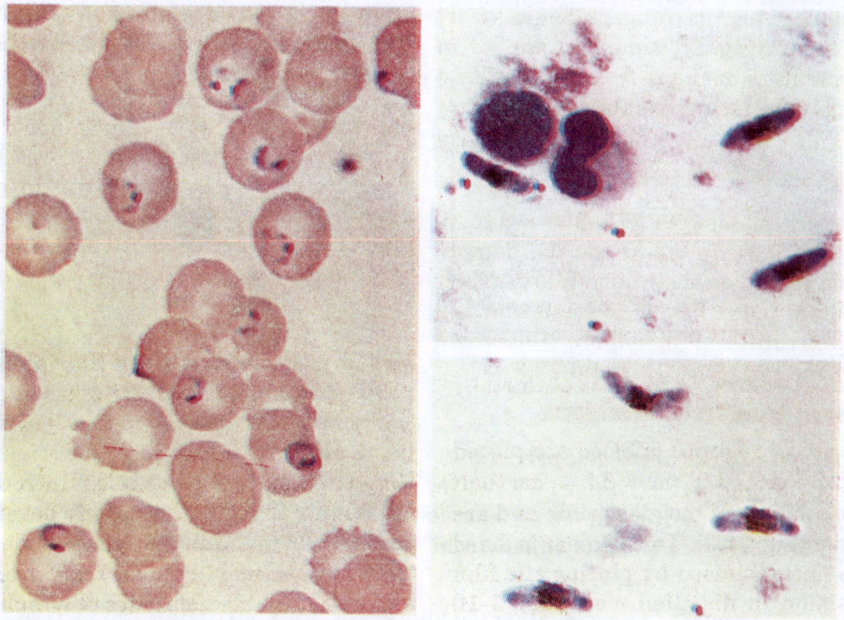

Fig. 12.6. Blood film of *P. falciparum malaria* : Thick film (dehaemoglobinised) with ring form of Trophozoite and macrogametocytes (*May-Grunwald-Giemsa stain*)

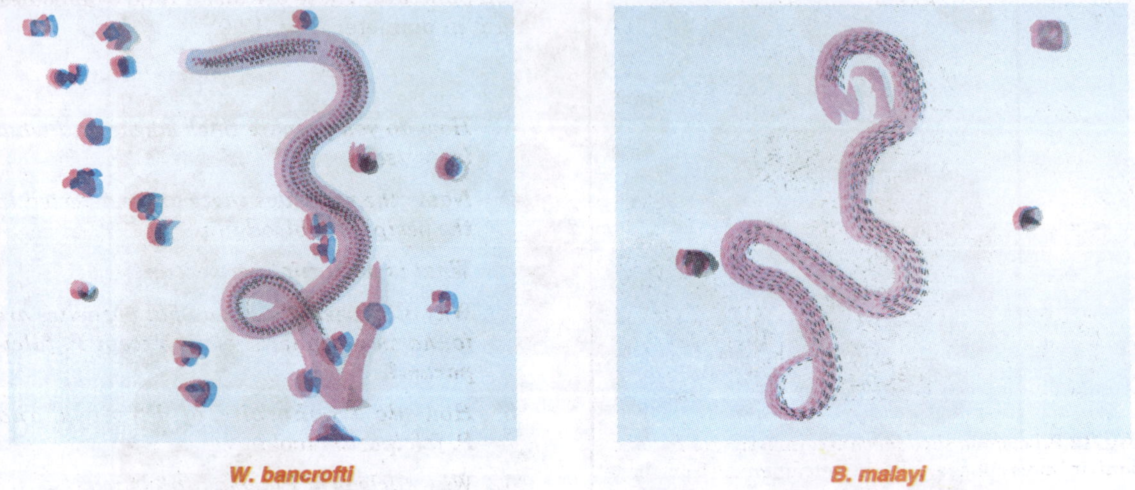

Fig. 12.7. Microfilariae of *W. bancrofti* and *B. malayi* seen in human blood smear

lymphatics and reach circulating blood. Demonstration of microfilaria in peripheral blood is diagnostic of filariasis (Fig. 12.7).

Nocturnal periodicity

Microfilariae typically exhibit *nocturnal periodicity,* i.e., they remain confined in the capillary bed of deep organs (lungs, kidneys, heart and big arteries) during day time and appear in peripheral circulation at night from 10 p.m. to 4 a.m., coinciding with the biting habits of the vector mosquito.

Morphology of microfilaria

The larval body measures 275–300 × 8 to 10 μm. *W. bancrofti, B. malayi* and *Loa loa* demonstrate a hyaline sheath on their microfilaria. Their diffe rentiation is made based on head and tail structures of microfilariae.*W. bancrofti* does not have nuclei in the tail (Figs. 12.7 and 12.8).

Examination of blood for microfilaria

Since the parasite shows *nocturnal periodicity,* blood is collected at midnight (10 p.m.-4 a.m.) or keeping the patient in a dark room for at least 2 hours. About 5-6 ml venous blood is collected in anticoagulant (pot. oxalate or EDTA).

1. **Stained blood smears** : Occasionally microfilaria can be demonstrated in peripheral blood smear. Thin and thick smears prepared as for malarial parasite may sometimes show the microfilaria.

2. **Concentration method** : 5-6 ml of oxalated blood is mixed with 2% formalin and centrifuged at 2000 r.p.m. for 5 minutes.

(a) *Staining* : Smear prepared from the sediment is air-dried and stained by Leishman stain.

(b) *Unstained wet preparation* : Two drops of deposit is mixed with equal volume of water to lyse the red cells on a slide. Place a coverslip and examine microscopically.

Alternatively use 2% acetic acid solution in place of formalin, keep the blood overnight, and

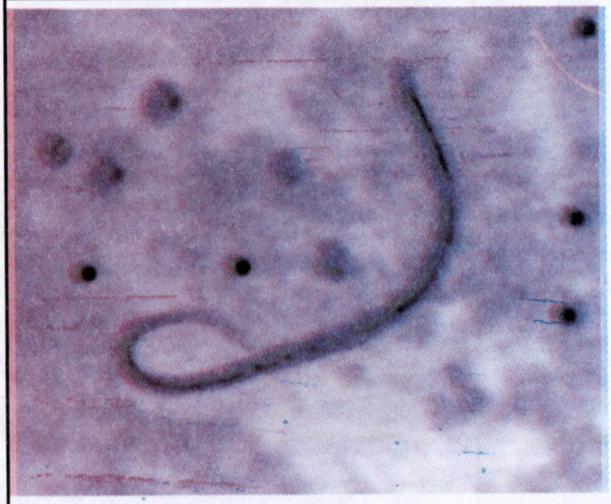

Fig. 12.8. Microfilaria *(W. bancrofti)* in peripheral blood

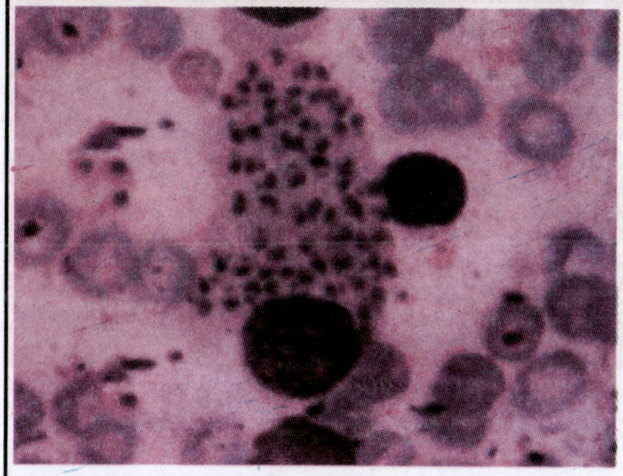

Fig. 12.9. *Leishmania donovani* : Amastigotes *L. donovani* in macrophage cells in smear made from bone marrow aspirate (Giemsa skin)

then centrifuge. Smear made from the deposit is stained as usual. Unstained coverslip preparation of centrifuged deposit of blood when examined under low power objective of microscope, also reveals microfilaria.

LEISHMANIA DONOVANI

Kala-azar is endemic in Northern Bihar. *Amastigotes* of *L. donovani* are found in groups of the reticuloendothelial cells of bone marrow and spleen puncture. These are small roud oval bodies, 2-4 μm in diameter (Fig. 12.9).

QUESTIONS

1. *How do you prepare thick smear and what is its use?*
2. *Name the parasites that can be detected in the peripheral blood film.*
3. *What is nocturnal periodicity?*
4. *Why all stages of all malarial parasites are found in peripheral blood except P. falciparum?*
5. *How do trophozoite of P. vivax and P. falciparum look?*
6. *Why nucleus of Plasmodium is red?*
7. *How do you differentiate P. vivax from P. malaria?*
8. *Why red cell is longer in P. vivax infection?*
9. *How do gametocytes of P. vivax and P. falciparum differ?*
10. *Name the complication of P. falciparum infection.*
11. *Name the vector of microfilaria.*
12. *How to differentiate microfilaria of W. bancrofti and B. malayi?*

Chapter 13

Blood Formation:

Cellular Haematopoiesis

SITES OF HAEMATOPOIESIS

Haematopoiesis is the process of production of blood cells. Blood cells are formed both in foetal liver and spleen up to 5th month of intra-uterine life and thereafter in the bone marrow and from birth onwards is restricted to these sites.

The whole of the marrow cavity is utilised for haemopoiesis at birth. There is a progressive diminution in the amount of red marrow during childhood, so that in the young adult it is confined to the head of the femur and humerus, to flat bones (sternum, ribs, iliac crest and vertebrae). Fat occupies rest of the marrow cavity. However, during increased demand for blood formation, the red marrow reappears in the shafts of the long bones replacing the fat.

CELL HIERARCHY

Cell hierarchy consists of three levels of cells :

1. Haemopoietic stem cells (precursor cells)
2. Progenitor cells
3. Maturing cells

Stem cells : The bone marrow contains *pluripotential stem cells.* All the circulating cells of blood are descendants of these **pluripotential stem cells**. These cells comprise one in every thousand bone marrow cells, which reside among the small and intermediate sized lymphoblasts. They are capable of completely replacing bone marrow when injected into a host whose own bone marrow has been completely destroyed.

Progenitor cells : At the initial stages of development, the uncommitted *pluripotential stem cells* differentiate into committed stem cells (progenitors) of the lymphoid and myeloid system termed *lymphoid stem cell* and *myeloid stem cell* respectively (Fig. 13.1). These committed progenitors are destined to produce the differentiated, recognisable precursors of different cell lineages.

The pluripotent uncommitted stem cells can reproduce themselves slowly for indefinite self-renewal, whereas the committed progenitor cells are not capable of indefinite self renewal. They "die by differentiation" and their numbers depend on the influx from the pluripotential stem cell pool.

Maturing cells : The pluripotential stem cells have the ability to differentiate to produce more mature cells like neutrophils, monocytes, lymphocytes, platelets and erythrocytes (Fig. 13.1). Stem cell is not morphologically identifiable but can be identified by the specialised tissue culture technique for their capacity to produce clones of cells belonging to one or more blood cell series. These haematological units are called colony forming units (CFU) or burst forming units (BFU). The CFU which generate only neutrophil granulocyte series (CFU-G), granulocyte-monocyte series (CFU-GM), monocyte series (CFU-M) exist in the bone marrow and blood.

Regulation of haematopoiesis

Colonies of pluripotential stem cells do not occur unless their formation is stimulated by materials known as *stem cell stimulating factor* (SCF); myeloid colony stimulating factor (M-CSF), granulocyte-macrophage colony stimulating factor (GM-CSF), eosinophil colony stimulating factor (Eo-CSF), and erythrocyte colony stimulating factor (E-CSF). These factors are derived from various tissues, monocytes and macrophages.

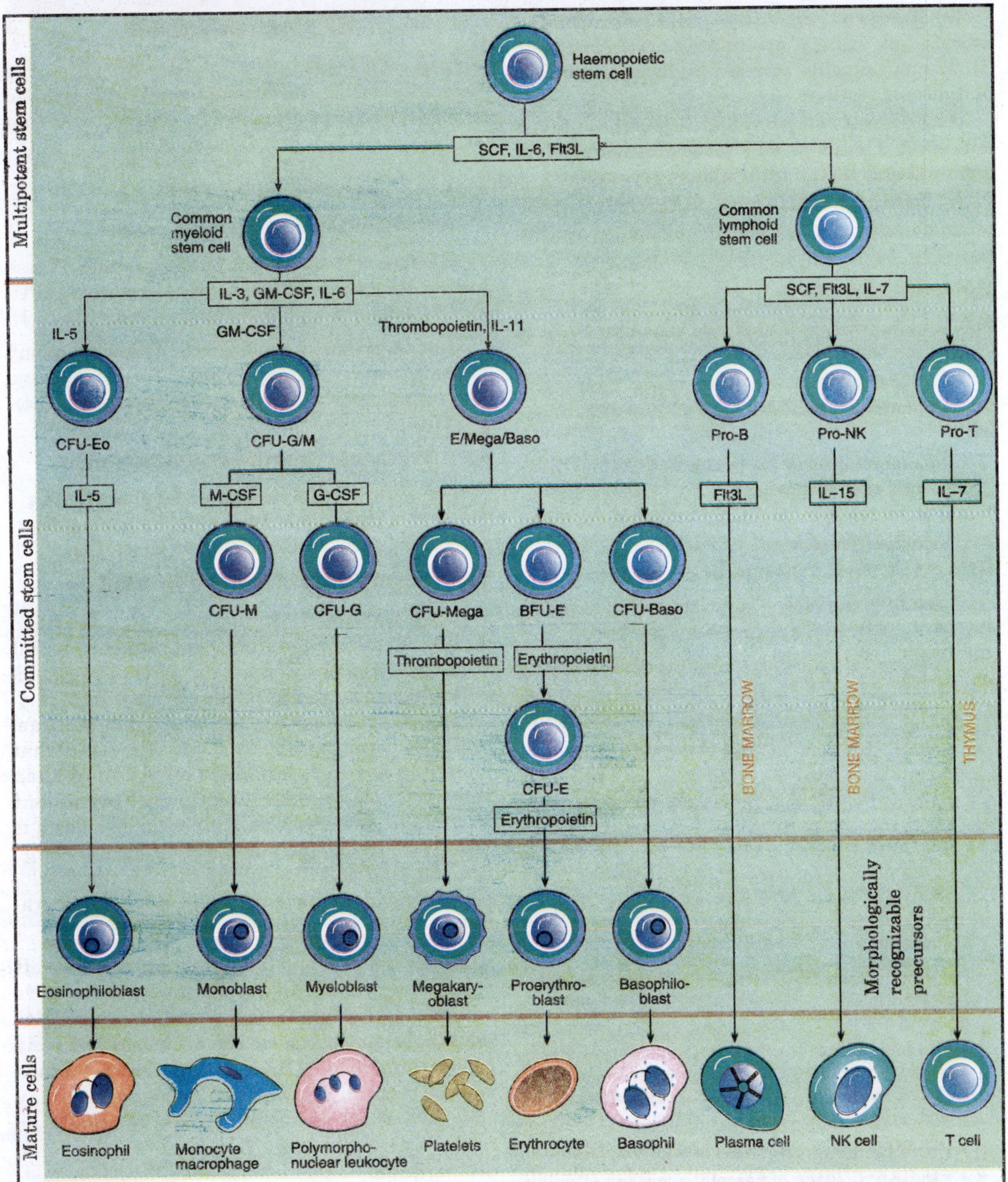

Fig. 13.1. Differentiation of haematopoietic cells. SCF, stem cell factor; Flt3L ligand; GM-CSF, granulocyte-macrophage colony-stimulating factor; M-CSF, macrophage colony-stimulating factor; G-CSF, granulocyte colony-stimulating factor.

(a) *Humoral regulation* : (i) Erythropoietin, secreted by kidney, stimulates erythropoiesis. (ii) Thrombopoietin, secreted by liver, stimulates platelet production.

(b) *Stromal cell products* : Cytokines : Interleukins 1, 3, 6 act as CSF for trilineage myeloid stem cell and IL-1, 6 for lymphoid stem cell.

(c) *Role of inhibitory mechanisms* : (i) They control over production of cells. (ii) Role of apoptosis.

Bone marrow pools

The bone marrow contains two separate pools of progenitor stem cells :

1. **Trilineage myeloid stem cells**: These cells form committed precursor cells of four cells lineages :

   (i) *Proerythroblast* — precursors of erythrocytes and platelets.

   (ii) *Myeloblast* — precursors of polymorphonuclear leucocytes.

   (iii) *Monoblast* — precursors of monocytes.

   (iv) *Megakaryoblast* — precursors of platelets.

2. **Lymphoid stem cells**: The lymphoid stem cells develop into pre-B cell and pre-T cell, which mature in primary lymphoid organs, i.e. bone marrow and thymus, respectively. Pre-NK cells also originate from lymphoid stem cell.

KEY OF SOME TERMS

- **Colony**: A colony consists of 40 to a few hundred cells.
- **Cluster**: Contains 3-40 cells.
- **CFU**: Colony forming units are the colonies of these cells.
- **CFU-GEMM or CFU-MIX**: Earliest units giving rise granulocyte, erythroid, monocytic and megakaryocytic cells.
- **CFU-GM**: A unit of progenitor cells of granulocytic-monocytic series. The biologic activity of GM-CSF is measured by its ability to stimulate haemopoietic progenitor cells.
- **CFU-EO**: Colonies of eosinophilic myeloid cells.
- **CFU-BAS**: Colonies of basophilic myeloid cells.
- **CFU-MG**: Colonies of megakaryocytic cell series.
- **BFU-E**: These are the earliest erythroid progenitor cells (BFU–E, Burst forming units).
- **CFU-E**: These are more differentiated cells of erythroid progenitors.

ERYTHROPOIESIS

Erythropoiesis is the process by which the progenitor cell in the bone marrow proliferate and differentiate into normoblast, reticulocytes that are released into circulation. About 1% of the erythrocytes are replenished daily. There are two major compartments in erythropoiesis.

1. **Progenitor cell compartment**

(a) *More primitive erythroid progenitors* : These are burst-forming units termed as erythroid (BFU-E). They exhibit high proliferative rate (Fig.13.1).

(b) *Late primitive progenitors* : These are colony forming units called erythroid (CFU-E) and have lower proliferative activity and synthesize erythropoietin.

2. **Erythroid-precursor compartment**

The cells can be recognised by morphologic features in this compartment and include : proerythroblasts, early normoblasts and so on (Fig. 13.2).

Normoblastic maturation (Fig. 13.2)

Proerythroblast (pronormoblast) : It is the earliest identifiable erythrocyte precursor present in the bone marrow. It has a diameter of 14-20 μm, and a basically round outline with minor peripheral protruberances. The nucleus has a fine, uniform, chromatin pattern which is somewhat more distinct and more intensely staining than that of myeloblast, one or several prominent nucleoli are present. The peripheral cytoplasm is usually only a narrow rim around relatively large nucleus and more basophilic than in the myeloblast. It divides rapidly and does not contain granule.

Early normoblast (basophilic normoblast) : It is a round cell, 12–16 μm diameter, has a more basophilic cytoplasm (owing to abundance of RNA) than the proerythroblast. The nucleus is relatively large, stains deeply and the chromatin strands may be partially clumped and the pattern may suggest a wheel with broad spokes. Generally, no nucleoli are to be seen. It also undergoes rapid proliferation.

Intermediate normoblast (polychromatic normoblast) : It is a round cell between 10 and 14 μm in diameter. The characteristic polychromatic appearance of the cytoplasm is derived from the mixture of the basophilic RNA and acidophilic haemoglobin thus giving a purple tint which

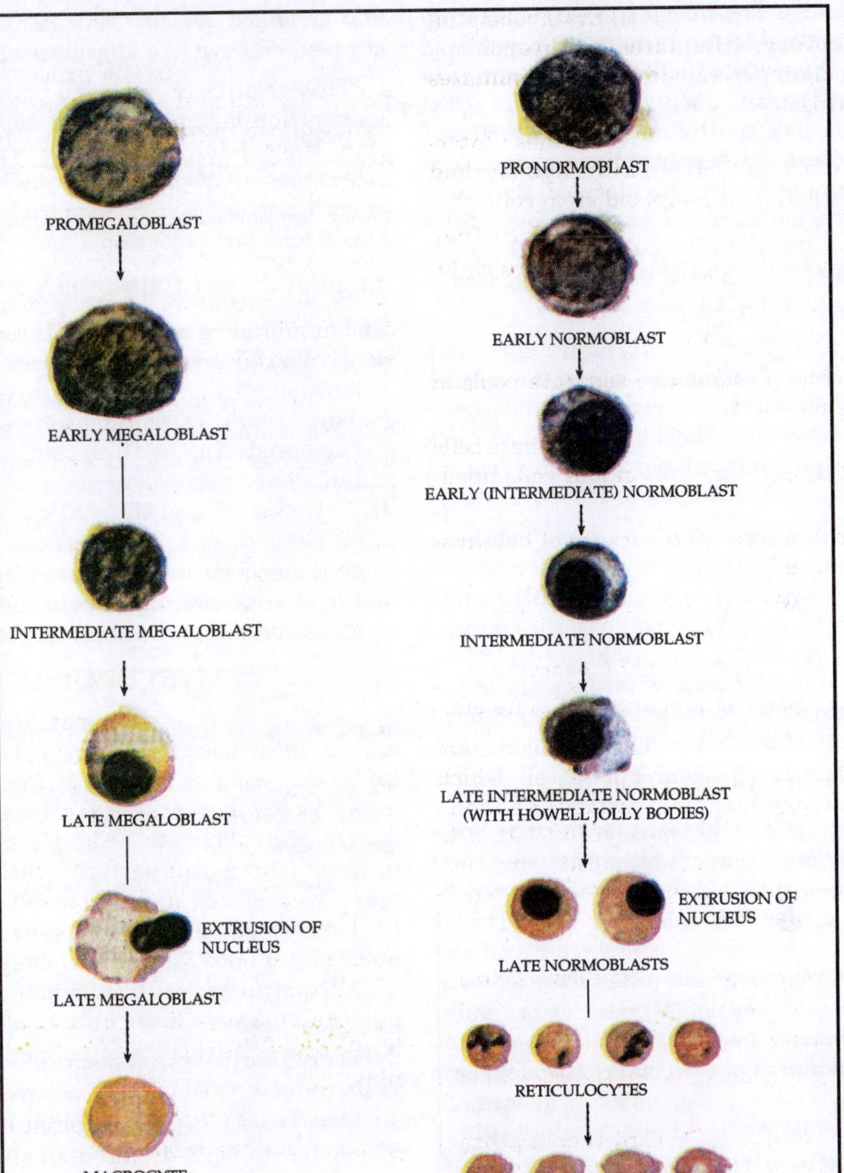

Fig. 13.2. Maturation sequence of normoblast and megaloblast

becomes more acidophilic as the cell matures, due to haemoglobinisation. The nucleus occupies about half the area of the cell, stains intensely, and has moderately condensed chromatin which is sharply distinct from the deep parachromatin. The nucleus decreases in size as the cell ages. It undergoes one or two mitotic divisions.

Late normoblast (orthochromic normoblast) : It constitutes the next and final stage of maturation of the nucleated red cell series. It is 8–12 µm in diameter; cytoplasm may show a faint polychromatic tint. Nucleus is small and dense (pyknotic). As the cell matures, nucleus becomes eccentric, occasionally lobulated.

Reticulocyte : The nucleus is extruded from the late normoblast to form the reticulocyte. It is a young erythrocyte which still contains fine basophilic reticulum. When stained by vital staining with new methylene blue or brilliant cresyl blue, there are deeply stained granules or chains of granules in the reticulocytes. By Leishman stain reticulocytes exhibit a pale blue basophilia. Reticulocyte count is 0.2% to 2% normally. Reticulocytes have the same biconcaved discoid shape like the RBCs.

Erythrocyte : Red cells normally enter the blood at the stage of reticulocytes or of the mature red cell. Reticulocytes slowly synthesize haemoglobin within marrow for a day followed by one more day in the peripheral blood and thereafter mature into erythrocytes. Its life span is 120 days.

Erythrocyte is a circular biconcave cell, size varies between 6.7–7.7 μm in diameter with a mean of 7.2 μm. It appears eosinophilic when stained by the Romanowsky methods, the staining is deep at the periphery but gradually lessening towards the centre because of biconcavity of the cell. Central pale area occupies less than one-third of the diameter of the cell.

Megaloblastic maturation (Fig. 13.2)

Megaloblasts are not present in normal bone marrow. Their occurrence results from abnormal maturation of erythroid precursors that occurs in vitamin B_{12}, and/or folic acid deficiency. This is known as *megaloblastic maturation* and the abnormal erythroid cells are called *megaloblasts.* The maturation of megaloblastic series is similar to that of normoblastic series but there are morphological differences at each stage. Megaloblastic erythropoiesis is often accompanied by abnormalities in the development of the myeloid (giant metamyelocyte and large atypical granulocytes) and megakaryocytic (decreased/atypical) series. A moderate increase in the number of progenitor stem cells also occurs.

Cells in the megaloblast series are named as their normoblastic counterparts, the primitive cell is *promegaloblast,* from which a series of maturing cells develop through *early, intermediate and late megaloblast* to the macrocytes. Megaloblasts differ from normoblasts in the following respects :

(i) *Cell size* — Large with increase in cytoplasm and nucleus at every stage of development.

(ii) *Nucleus*—Chromatin network is more open and arranged in a fine reticular fashion to give a stippled or seive like appearance.

This results in enlarged cells, with nuclear maturation lagging behind cytoplasmic maturation. Howell-Jolly bodies may be present in the late stages. In megaloblastic anaemia, almost 50% of erythroid series in bone marrow are promegaloblasts and early megaloblasts.

Regulation of Erythropoiesis

The formation of red blood cells (erythropoiesis) is controlled by circulating glycoprotein hormone erythropoietin, produced mainly in the kidneys (tubular cells). These cells respond to hypoxia in tissues producing erythropoietin. Erythropoietin stimulates erythropoietic stem cells to proliferate. IL-1, IL-3, IL-6 and GM-CSF also stimulate erythropoietic stem cells. Moreover, red cell production is subject to a feed-back control — i.e., inhibited by a supernormal circulating red cell count and is stimulated by anaemia.

MYELOPOIESIS

Myelopoiesis leads to the production of mature neutrophils, eosinophils, basophils, monocytes, macrophages and dendritic cells (Figs.13.1 and 13.3). The various stages of development in myelopoiesis are :

1. **Haemopoietic stem cells**

These haemopoietic stem cells proliferate and differentiate into multipotent stem cells.

2. **Pluripotential (multipotential) stem cells (Progenitor cells)**

These pluripotential stem cells are committed cells to form various cells of myeloid/monocytic linages. These stem cells differentiate into various colony forming units.

3. **Colony forming units (CFUs)**

The following CFUs are the precursors of granulocyte/monocyte pathway :

(a) CFUS — granulocytic, monocytic (CFU-GM)
(b) CFU — granulocyte (CFU-G)
(c) CFU — monocyte (CFU-M)
(d) CFU — eosinophil, basophil (CFU-EB)

Regulation of Myelopoiesis

Myelopoiesis is regulated by : (1) ***GM-CSF*** : It activates functions of neutrophils and monocytes/macrophages. (2) ***G-CSF*** : It stimulates granulocyte production.

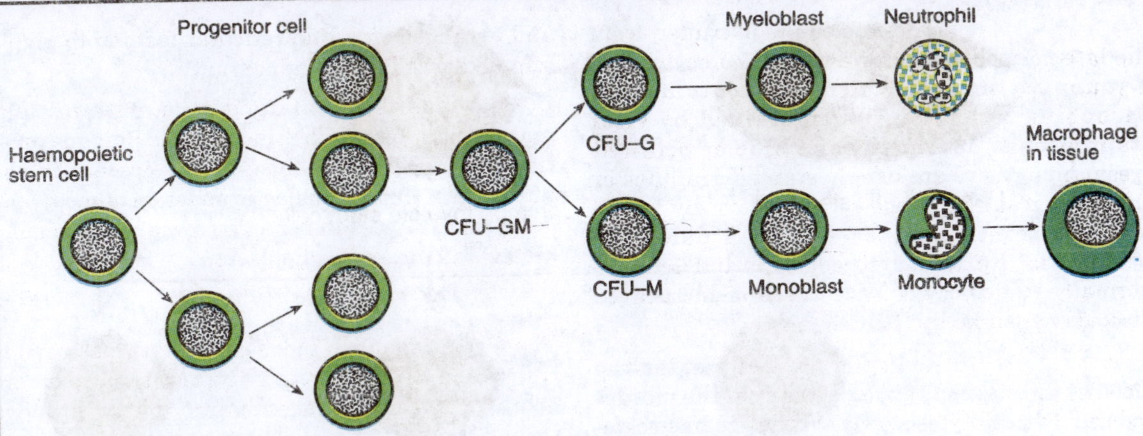

Fig. 13.3. Maturation of granulocyte and monocyte

Cells of myeloid (granulocytic) series (Fig. 13.4)

The first recognisable cell of granulocyte series is *myeloblast,* from which the *promyelocyte,* and then by progression the *myelocyte, metamyelocyte,* the *nonsegmented* (stab) forms, and finally the *mature segmented* to polymorphonuclear granulocytes develop (Figs.13.1,13.4). Specific azurophil granules that determine the nature of mature cell, i.e., neutrophil, eosinophil or basophil begin to appear at the promyelocyte stage and become fully differentiated in the myelocyte. Mitotic division takes place up to the myelocyte stage and the normal metamyelocyte is incapable of mitosis.

Myeloblast (Fig. 13.4)

Myeloblast is a large cell, 15-20 μm in diameter, with a round to oval nucleus which occupies about four-fifths of the total cell area. Cytoplasm is moderately deep blue in staining reaction, nongranular or may contain a fine azurophil granule in the late stage. Nuclear chromatin is arranged in fine strands which stain reddish purple with occasional aggregates. Nucleoli are typically prominent, while two to four are usual, there may be up to six nucleoli. Histochemically they are peroxidase, PAS and Sudan Black reactions positive.

Promyelocyte (Fig. 13.4)

Promyelocyte is slightly larger (20–25 μm) than myeloblast and the features of the cell are similar to those of myeloblast, except that the cytoplasm contains blue to reddish purple azurophil granules and a slightly more coarse appearance of the chromatin. Nucleoli are still present but less well-defined.

Myelocyte : The differences between this cell and promyelocyte include :

(a) cytoplasmic granules have now assumed their specific neutrophilic character,

(b) no nucleoli are visiblle,

(c) cell size — 18 to 20 μm in diameter,

(d) cytoplasm stains light blue and the cytoplasmic nuclear ratio is increased and

(e) cytoplasm progressively acquires a pinkish blue and in the mature form is predominantly or completely pink.

(f) Nucleus is round or oval. The nuclear chromatin is fine and dispersed in the early stage but in the late stage, neutrophil myelocyte has a somewhat more condensed chromatin pattern.

Metamyelocyte : This cell is distinguished from myelocyte by an indented, kidney-shaped smaller nucleus with more condensed chromatin. The cytoplasm is pink and contains fine neutrophilic granules resembling the myelocyte. The size of cell varies from 14-20 μm.

Juvenile (non-segmented) neutrophil leucocyte

The cell is usually smaller than metamyelocyte and the degree of indentation of the nucleus is greater than 50 per cent of the nuclear diameter. Nuclear chromatin is coarse and clumped. Cytoplasmic granules are identical to those in the mature segmented form.

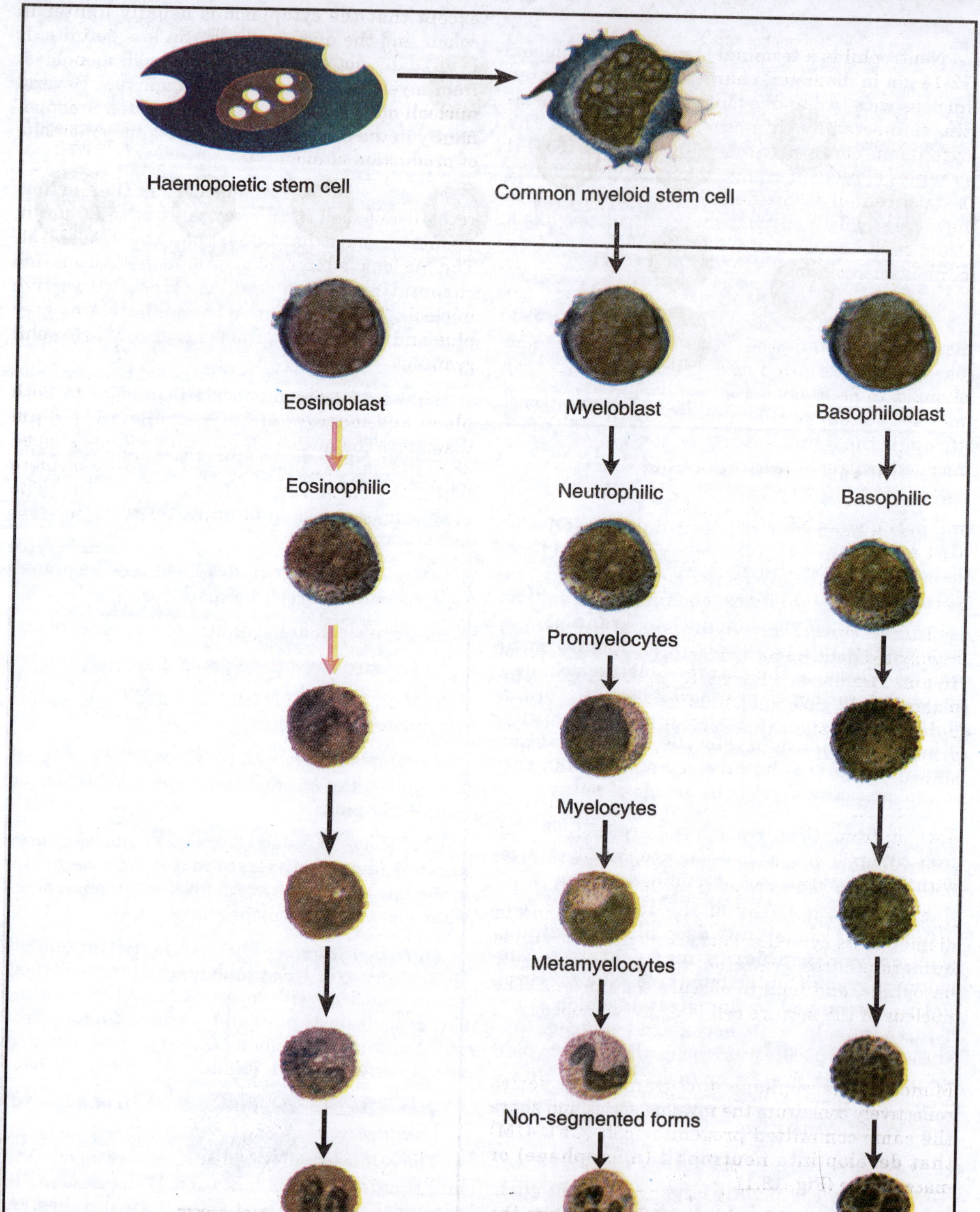

Fig. 13.4. Maturation of granulocyte cell

Mature (segmented) neutrophil

Neutrophil is a terminal stage of development, 12-14 μm in diameter, characterised by lobulated nucleus with two to five lobes of clumped chromatin, connected by thin chromatin strands. The cytoplasm contains numerous fine neutrophil granules of reddish orange colour. Approximately 1–3 per cent of segmented neutrophils in females have clearly defined bead-shaped structure like a drum-stick attached to one nuclear lobe by a thin chromatin strand.

Eosinophil-Basophil series Figs. 13.1, 13.4

Knowledge on the production of eosinophils and basophils are limited and still developing. It is thought to be produced in the bone marrow in a manner similar to the production of neutrophils through the same stages as the polymorphonuclear neutrophil series.

Eosinophil series : The eosinophilic cytoplasmic granules are usually reddish orange in colour that are apparent at the myelocyte stage, the cells have the same morphological characteristics as their neutrophil counterparts.

Mature eosinophil : It is slightly larger than segmented neutrophil with an average diameter of 16 μm. The nucleus is usually bilobed. The cytoplasm stains pink and contains many large granules (larger than those of neutrophils). These granules stain bright orange with Romanosky stains.

Basophil series : Basophils are thought to develop from a cell resembling myeloblast. The first recognisable stage is a basophil myelocyte, with the appearance of basophilic granules.

Mature basophil : It varies from 14-16 mm in diameter, its cytoplasm stains pink and contains numerous large granules, which are intensely basophilic, and tend to obscure the nucleus. The nucleus of the mature cell is usually bilobed.

Monocyte-Macrophage series (Fig. 13.4, 13.5)

Monocyte macrophage and granulocyte series collectively constitute the myeloid series and share the same committed progenitor cell (CFU-GM) that develop into neutrophil (microphage) or macrophage (Fig. 13.1).

Monoblasts : Monoblasts (18-22 μm) are the least mature of morphologically recognisable members of the monocyte macrophage series and are very similar in appearance to myeloblasts except that the cytoplasm is usually lighter in colour and the nuclear chromatin less definite. It is virtually not possible to distinguish monoblast from myeloblast in normal bone marrow. Several nucleoli may be visible. They are located predominantly in the bone marrow, which is the major site of production of monocyte.

Promonocyte : Promonocyte is the earliest recognisable cell in this series. It is 15-20 μm in diameter, somewhat larger than the myeloblast. The nucleus is large, oval or indented with a fine chromatin pattern and contains two to five nucleoli. The cytoplasm is basophilic, stains grey blue and contains a variable number of azurophil granules.

Monocyte : The monocyte is present in both blood and marrow, slightly smaller, 15-18 μm diameter. The nucleus is generally kidney-shaped or round, but may be lobulated with two or more lobes, the chromatin being relatively fine. The cytoplasm stains grey-blue colour as ground glass

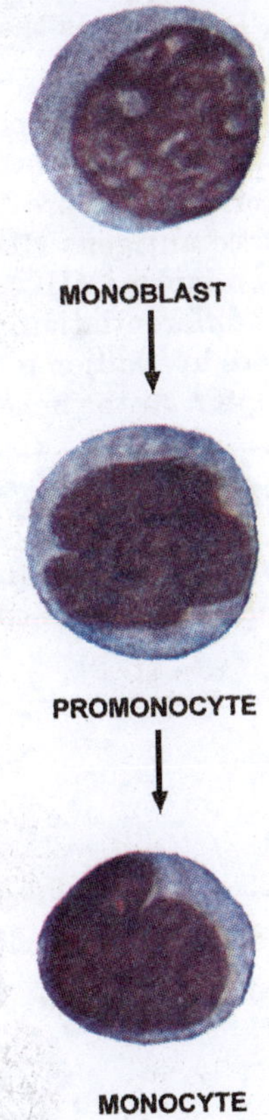

Fig. 13.5. Maturation of monocytes

appearance and contains some fine azurophilic granules.

LYMPHOPOIESIS

Originating from pluripotent *stem cells* in the bone marrow, the uncommitted *lymphoid stem cells* develop into two types of committed stem cells, *B stem cell* and *T stem cell* in the primary lymphoid organs, bone marrow and thymus, respectively (Figs. 13.1,13.6,13.7,13.8). Recent evidences suggest that committed stem cell of NK cell also originates from the uncommitted lymphoid stem cell (Fig. 13.1).

1. Development of B lymphocytes

Maturation of B cell : B stem cells remain within the bone marrow and divide into functional stages, pre-B cell (lymphoblast) and mature (resting) B cell. In chickens and birds, B lymphocytes mature in the cloacal bursa (lymphoepithelial organ). It is now established that bursal equivalent in man is bone marrow, which is the site for both B stem cell proliferation and development of pre-B cell, as well as the maturation of B lymphocytes.

Pre-B cells lack surface immunoglobin but display intracytoplasmic mu (μ) chains but no light chains. Majority of the pre-B cell, however, contain cell surface antigens CD 19 and major histocompatibility complex (MHC) class II (Ia). In the early stage of differentiation, B cells express IgM on their surface in addition to C3 (for complement) and Fc receptor. At the next stage of differentiation, B cells bear IgM alone or in combination with IgA or IgG and IgD, which marks the entrance of B cells into mature phase. These mature B lymphocytes are called *virgin cells* as they have not yet been exposed to antigen. These cells express CD 19 and CD 20 surface antigens.

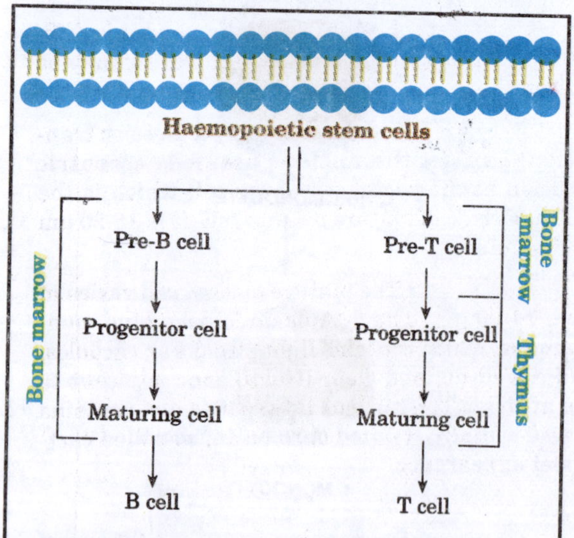

Fig. 13.6. Development of lymphocyte (schematic)

The mature *virgin* B lymphocytes circulate around the body and are exported into peripheral (secondary) lymphoid organs, such as spleen, lymph nodes and mucosal associated lymphoid tissues.

Activation of B lymphocytes : The virgin B cells reside in the secondary lymphoid organs and are now ready to respond to antigenic stimulus. Following triggering with antigen, the resting B cells are activated and subsequently proliferate. The activated proliferating B cell divide into functional stages, *differentiating B cell,* secretory B cell (plasma cell) and memory cell (Fig. 13.7).

The activation of resting B cell is accompanied by sequential changes of surface antigen. They loose IgD and CD 21 but acquire new antigens and play important roles in localisation and binding of activated B cells in the microenvironment. B cells are responsible for synthesis of antibody.

2. Development of T lymphocytes (Figs. 13.6 and 13.7)

Maturation of T cell : The committed T stem cells migrate from the bone marrow to thymus during early embryonic and early postnatal development. The thymic microenvironment provides a setting and eventual development and functionally competent T cells in stages, pre T cell (lymphoblast) and mature (resting) T cell. The mature virgin T cells are exported into peripheral lymphoid organs and circulate in blood. During intrathymic differentation, a sequence of changes in the cell surface antigens of these cells occur and they acquire new antigens. When these T cells leave the thymus, they are segregated into cells expressing either CD 4 (helper T cell), CD 8 (cytotoxic/suppressor T cell), constituting about 65 and 35% of peripheral T cells, respectively.

Activation of T cell : T cell has got an antigen receptor consisting of a heterodimer composed of α and β chain in association with CD 3 complex. The virgin T cells are activated on exposure to antigen and differentiate into functional stages, *differentiating T cell,* effector and memory T cells. T cells are responsible for cell-mediated immunity.

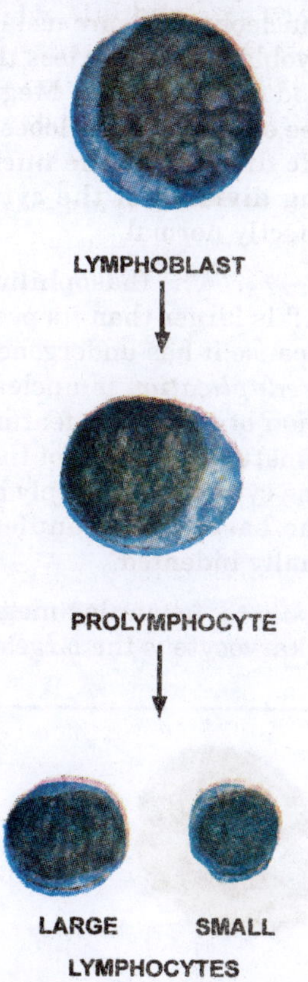

Fig. 13.7. Maturation of lymphocytes

Memory B and T lymphocytes are cells that have been exposed to an antigen and becomes readily converted to effector cells by a subsequent encounter with the same antigen. Unlike other lymphocytes, memory cells persist in the body for months or years.

Cells of lymphoid series (Fig. 13.7)

Lymphoblast : A lymphoid stem cell gives rise to first recognisable pre-B and pre-T cells which are the committed lymphoblasts. The pre-B and pre-T cells are morphologically similar in appearance.

Lymphoblasts are slightly smaller than myeloblast, about 15-20 μm in diameter. It resembles myeloblast in general structure, except that the ratio of the diameter of the nucleus to that of the cytoplasm tends to be greater, and the number of nucleoli tends to be fewer than in myeloblast.

The nucleus of lymphoblast is large, usually occupying four-fifths of the cell area with stippled and reticular chromatin. The cytoplasm is non-granular, stains deep blue at the periphery and a lighter colour centrally and contains generally one or two nucleoli.

Large lymphocyte : It is 12-16 μm in diameter, and is round in outline. The nucleus is dense staining, round or slightly indented, and the chromatin is more clumped than in the lymphoblast. The cytoplasm is fairly abundant than in lymphoblast, and is usually sky-blue and may contain a few sharply defined azurophil cytoplasmic granules.

Small lymphocytes : It varies from 9-12 μm in diameter, and are thus smaller than segmented granulocytes. The cytoplasm is scanty, a thin narrow rim, medium to deeply basophilic, around the round or marginally indented nucleus. The nucleus contains deeply staining, heavily clumped chromatin.

Plasma cells

Plasma cells represent the most well-differentiated progeny in the B cell series of activated lymphocytes. When triggered by antigen, B cell undergoes blastoid transformation which divides rapidly becoming successively *plasmablasts* (clone formation), intermediate transitional cells and plasma cells (Fig. 13.8).

Plasmablast : It is the most immature stage of development of plasma cell, closely resembling the lymphoblast in size, shape and staining reaction except for possessing more basophilic cytoplasm. It has an average size of 18 μm. There is no visible cytoplasmic granulation and it is difficult to identify nucleoli although up to six may be present.

Proplasma cell : In the intermediate or transitional stage, the nucleus assumes eccentric location at the periphery of the cell which is the characteristic of mature plasma cell. It is 15-20 μm in diameter.

Plasma cell : The mature plasma cell varies in size, 14-20 μm. The cytoplasm is deep blue, non-granular, which contains light streaks or vacuoles, and a well-defined clear (Golgi) zone adjacent to the nucleus. The nucleus is eccentric and contains coarse radially striated chromatin, so-called cart-wheel appearance.

MEGAKARYOCYTE SERIES (Fig. 13.9)

Megakaryoblast : The earliest recognisable megakaryoblast is 25-30 μm in diameter. The cytoplasm stains intensely blue, it is generally just an irregular rim to the large nucleus which is usually oval or kidney-shaped. The nuclear chromatin is ill-defined and contains several deep blue stained nucleoli which are usually indefinite. The megakaryoblasts number less than 1% of the total nucleated marrow cells. Megakaryoblasts with two, three or four nuclear lobes may be seen, due to mitotic division of the nucleus without corresponding division of the cytoplasm; this finding is perfectly normal.

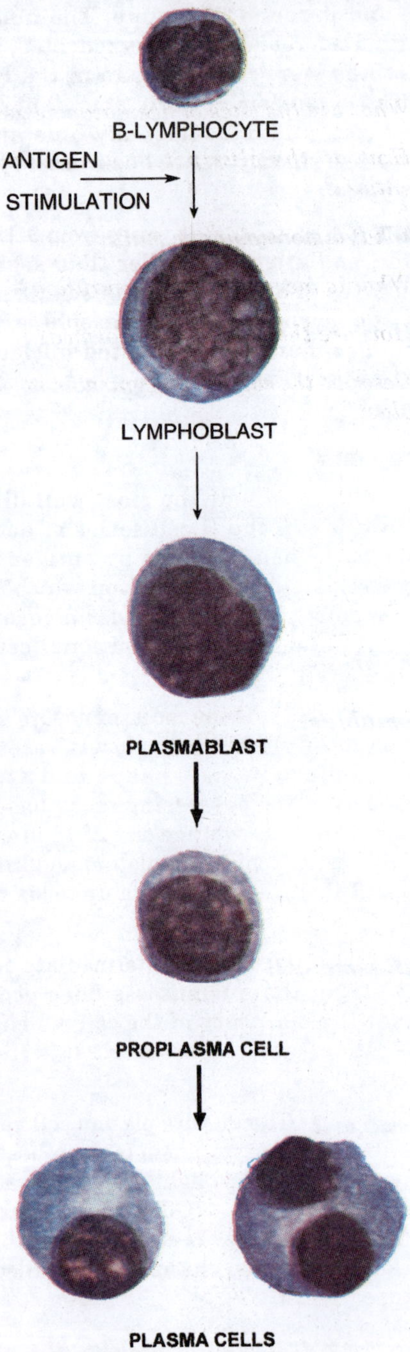

Fig. 13.8. Antigenic stimulation of B cell, development of plasma cell and effector cell

Promegakaryocyte (basophilic megakaryocyte) : This cell is larger than its precursor megakaryoblast because it has undergone endoreduplication. *Endoreduplication* is nuclear replication without division of the cell, a feature characteristics of more mature members of the megakaryocyte series. The cytoplasm is deeply basophilic and contains some basophilic granules. Nucleus is large and usually indented.

Megakaryocyte (granular megakaryocyte) : Mature megakaryocyte is the largest cell found in

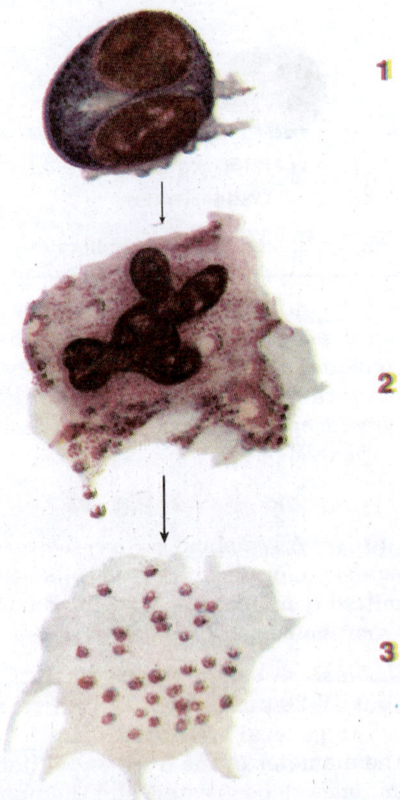

Fig. 13.9. Development of platelets : (1) Megakaryoblast. (2) Megakaryocyte. (3) Platelets

marrow and can be up to 100 μm in diameter (range 30-90 μm), contains 4-16 nuclear lobes with coarsely clumped chromatin. The cytoplasm is bulky in comparison with the volume of nucleus and contains many small red-purple azurophil granules. The cell margin is irregular and the late stages of maturation (budding megakaryocytes) shows differentiation of granular platelets in pseudopodia-like structures (Fig. 13.9).

Platelets appear to be formed by protrusion sinusoids of pseudopods of megakaryocyte cytoplasm, which detach into the blood stream and fragment to yield platelets.

Platelets : Platelets are small, anucleate, fragments of cytoplasm which have become detached from periphery of the megakaryocyte. They are discoid and have a diameter of 1-4 μm. The cytoplasm stains blue and contains small red purple granules which are located in the central area of platelet.

QUESTIONS

1. *What are the sites of haematopoiesis?*
2. *How do the pluripotent stem cells differentiate?*
3. *What is normoblastic maturation?*
4. *What is megaloblastic maturation?*
5. *How are the plasma cells formed?*
6. *Describe the earliest recognisable megakaryoblast.*

Chapter 14

Reticulocyte Count

Reticulocytes are juvenile or immature non-nucleated red cells. These cells take 2 days to mature in bone marrow and are in circulation for one day, during which they can be detected in blood. The number of reticulocytes present in the peripheral blood is a fairly accurate reflection of erythropoietic activity of bone marrow (formation of red cell).

Reticulocyte count

Principle : Reticulocytes contain remnants of ribosomes and RNA which were present in larger amounts in the cytoplasm of their precursors, i.e., normoblasts. This ribonucleoproteins have the property of reacting with certain basic dyes such as brilliant cresyl blue, new methylene blue or azure blue to form a blue precipitate of granules or filaments. This reaction takes place only when the reticulocytes are still alive (without fixing the cells), i.e., in vitally stained unfixed preparations. These stains are called supravital stains. They stain RNA of red cells. Largest amount of dark blue network or reticulin is found in the most immature reticulocytes, whereas only a few dots or short strands are seen in the least immature reticulocyte (Fig. 14.1).

Staining solution :

Brilliant cresyl blue or new methylene blue	....	1.0 g
Sodium citrate	....	2.0 g
0.85% saline (NaCl)	....	100 ml

At first sodium citrate is dissolved in saline and then the dye is added and dissolved. Sodium citrate is an anticoagulant. Sodium chloride provides iso-osmolarity as that of blood. When EDTA mixed blood is to be examined, there is no need of adding sodium citrate to the solution.

Method :

1. Deliver 2 or 3 drops of dye solution into a small glass test tube (75 × 10 mm) by means of a Pasteur pipette.

2. Add 2-3 drops of EDTA blood to the dye solution and mix well and keep at 37°C for 15-20 minutes. In severe anaemia with very low haemoglobin it is best to use a little more extra blood in the mixture. On the other hand, a little extra fluid may be required in blood from polycythaemia. Mix and make one of the following preparations :

(a) *Smear preparation* : Films are made on glass slides in the usual way using a well mixed drop of the mixture. The smear is dried in air and exa-

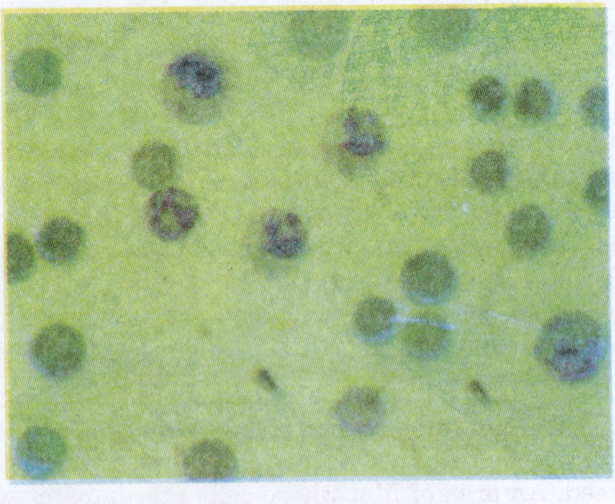

Fig. 14.1. Reticulocyte with fine reticular fibrils : Stained by *Brilliant Cresyl Blue*

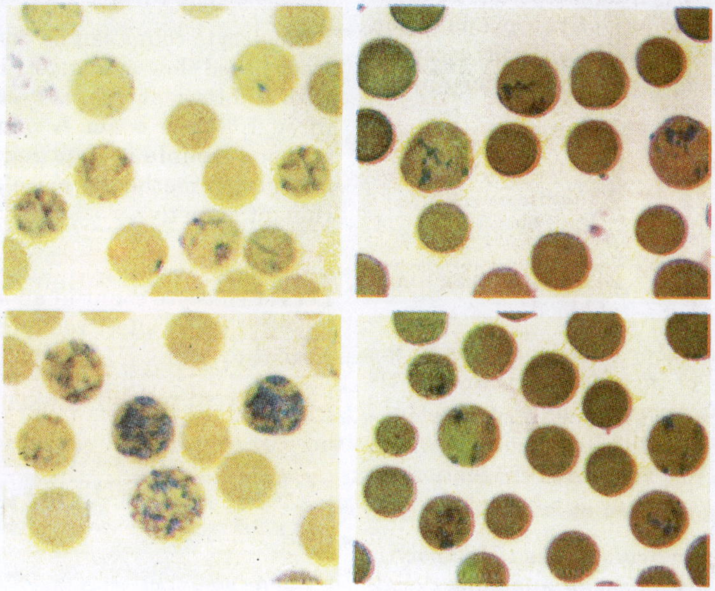

Fig. 14.2. Reticulocyte : Brilliant cresyl blue preparation of peripheral blood : Blood film stained with Brilliant Cresyl Blue and counterstained with Leishman

mined under the oil immersion objective without fixing or counter-staining. This technique is most widely practised.

(b) *Coverslip preparation* : Take a drop of the mixture on a slide and place a coverslip over it. The coverslip is pressed gently to make a thin film. The excess of fluid from the slide is wiped off with a blotting paper. This gives a cover-slip wet preparation.

Identification : Reticulocytes contain basophilic multiple granules or reticulation (Fig. 14.2) which have to be distinguished from red cells containing *Pappenheimer* bodies (iron containing after splenectomy) and *Heinz* bodies (due to denaturation of haemoglobin in primaquine and phenylhydrazine sensitivity). In the latter two cases, inclusion bodies also stain by vital stains and appear as a single blue dot (Fig. 16.12).

Counting : The reticulocytes are counted with an oil immersion objective and if possible, eyepiece provided with adjustable diaphragm to be used. An area of film where cells are undistorted with good staining is chosen.

Calculation : Reticulocyte count is expressed in percentage in terms of red blood cells. Thus, if the number of reticulocytes in 150 fields is 50 and number of red cells in 150 fields is 3000, then

Reticulocyte percentage = $\frac{50}{300} \times 100 = 1.6\%$. The standard error is about 10% by this technique.

For *absolute reticulocyte count,* total RBC count is done by usual method and expressed as (% Reticulocyte × RBC per cu. mm)/100.

When reticulocyte percentage = 0.5% and total RBC = 4.0 million/cu.mm, absolute reticulocyte count = (0.5 × 4.0 million)/100 = (0.5 × 40,00000)/100 = 20,000/cu. mm of blood.

Reticulocyte count by fluorescent microscope

Reticulocyte count by fluorescent microscopy gives a more precise value.

Preparation :

Acridine orange solution
(50 mg/100 ml of 9 g/L NaCl) .... 1 volume
Blood .... 1 volume

Mix gently for 2 minutes. Films are made on glass slides, dried rapidly and examined in a fluorescent microscope.

Counting

RNA shows orange-red fluorescence while

nuclear material (DNA) fluoresces yellow. Since the brightness and colour of the preparation quickly fades, a special fluorescent microscope is necessary. The method is not suitable for routine use.

Normal value :

Adults	...	0.2–2%
Infants	...	2–6%
Absolute count	...	24,000–48,000/cu. mm of blood.

Increase in the number of reticulocytes in the blood is indicative of increased erythropoietic activity of bone marrow leading to premature release in circulation, while their absence or low count denotes bone marrow suppression.

Abnormal reticulocyte count

(a) *Conditions for reticulocytosis* : Haemolytic anaemia, regenerative phase of anaemia, pernicious anaemia.

(b) *Conditions for reticulocytopenia* : Hypoplastic anaemia, myelofibrosis, cytotoxic drug therapy and radiation sickness.

Indications for reticulocyte count

1. *Assessment of erythroid activity of bone marrow.*
2. *Checking therapeutic response in anaemia.*

(a) Rise in reticulocyte consent occurs in iron deficiency anaemia following iron therapy.

(b) To check potency of drug : Reticulocyte response starts 2-10 days after initiation of therapy and attains its peak 3-10 days after the initial response. Thereafter, reticulocyte count gradually declines while RBC count rises steadily.

Automated method

Reticulocyte count can be done by using an argon laser based flow cytometer. Reticulocytes stained with fluorescent dye auramine – O are passed through a laser beam. A volume of 100 microlitre of blood sample is required. Although count by automated method is more precise but the instrument is costly.

Reticulocyte correction for anaemia

Let reticulocyte count in an adult having 6.5 g Hb is 2%, it does reflect real picture of bone marrow response.

Corrected reticulocyte count :

$$= \frac{\text{Patient's Hb} \times \text{Estimated Reticulocyte count}}{\text{Normal Hb value for that age}}$$

$$= \frac{6.5 \times 2}{15}$$

$$= 0.86\%$$

QUESTIONS

1. *What are the sites of haematopoiesis?*
2. *What is supravital stain?*
3. *During identification of reticulocytes, What precautions are to be taken?*
4. *Name the methods of reticulocyte count.*
5. *Where do you get abnormal reticulocyte count?*
6. *What are the indications of reticulocyte count?*

Chapter 15

Marrow Puncture Needle and Trephine Needle: Examination of bone marrow

The examination of bone marrow is indicated in any disease characterised by abnormalities of the blood when the usual clinical examination and laboratory tests fail to diagnose the condition. There are two methods of obtaining the marrow :

1. *Aspiration (Needle) biopsy* : It is a simple, safe and relatively painless procedure in which bone marrow is aspirated through a wide bore needle (marrow puncture needle) e.g., Salah's or Klima's needle (Fig. 15.1).

2. *Trephine biopsy* : It is a little less simple procedure in which specially made trephine (microtrephine) needle (Fig. 15.2) is used. Trephination of bone consists of removal of blocks or bits of tissue from the marrow cavity from which histological sections and smears are made. It can be performed on outpatients. Where aspiration is not possible, surgical biopsy may be necessary.

In most cases needle aspiration is the method of choice and only trephine biopsy is done in patients where repeated aspiration has failed to provide diagnostic information.

BONE MARROW ASPIRATION

Marrow puncture needle (*Sternal puncture needle*)

Types : Several types of needles are available for aspiration of bone marrow of which two types are commonly used (Fig. 15.1) :

1. Salah's needle
2. Klima's needle

Identification : Salah's needle is most frequently used. It is a stout wide-bore needle with a close-fitting stilette and a guard. The stilette prevents blockage of the mouth of the needle by skin or soft tissue tag during introduction. The guard is adjustable for the desired distance and prevents penetration of the needle further than is desired. Klima's needle is almost similar to Salah's needle except that the former is slightly shorter and stouter than the latter (Fig. 15.1).

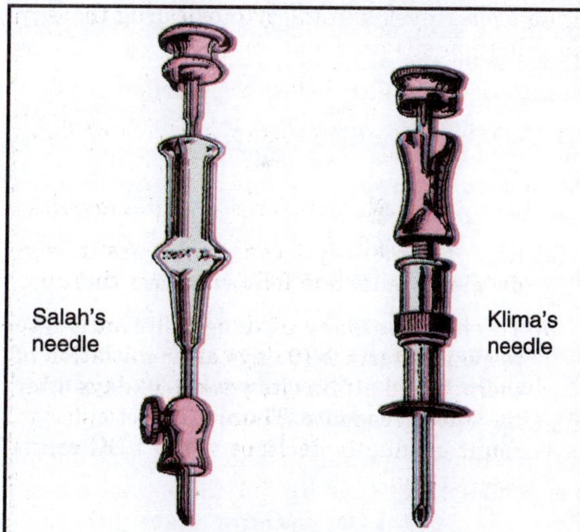

Fig. 15.1. Bone marrow aspiration needles — Salah and Klima

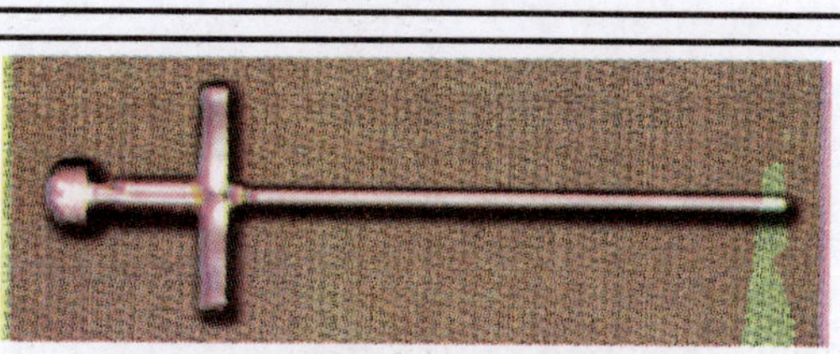

Fig. 15.2. Trephine biopsy needle

Sites for puncture

(a) *Adult* :

1. Sternum 2. Posterior iliac crest
3. Spinous processes of lumbar vertebra.

Sternum is preferred by most haematologists. It is ideal because the bone is near the surface, the cortical bone is thin and the marrow cavity contains numerous cells and relatively little fat and trabecular bone. Other sites are selected when sternum cannot be used or sternal puncture results a dry tap.

(b) *Infants* : The upper end of tibia is the site of puncture of choice for newborn, infants and children less than 1 year of age.

Method of sternal puncture

The usual site is the manubrium or the first or second piece of the sternum. Width of marrow cavity in adult is usually 1 cm and thickness of cortical bone is 1-2 mm. Patient lies on back on firm bed. After taking usual aseptic precautions such as cleaning with spirit, iodine and spirit again, the skin, subcutaneous tissues and periosteum over the sternum, opposite the second interspace, are infiltrated with a small quantity of 1% xylocaine. Then, the needle is inserted in the midline of the body of the sternum at the level of the second interspace. When the needle point reaches the periosteum, the guard is adjusted so as to allow the needle for about 5 mm further, and then the guard is fixed tightly in position.

Then the needle is pushed with a boring motion into the cavity of the bone. The resistance offered by the outer table of bone is released when the cavity of bone has been entered.

Then remove the stilette and with a well-fitting 2 or 5 ml syringe suck up (0.2 ml to 0.25 ml) not more than 0.3 ml of marrow material (bone marrow diluted with a variable amout of blood). Generally, material is sucked into the syringe without difficulty, but occasionally, it may be required to reinsert the stilette and push the needle a little further and to suck again.

Preparation of smear : Withdraw the needle and syringe together. Transfer the material without delay on slides as it tends to clot rapidly. Irregularly shaped marrow fragment adhere to the slide.

(a) Single drops of aspirated material is delivered onto slides 1 cm from one end and then most of the blood is quickly sucked off with a fine Pasteur pipette and placed to the edge of each drop. Films are prepared by pushing a spreader (glass slide). The marrow fragments are dragged behind the spreader and leaves a trail behind them. The differential count is made in these cellular trails.

(b) Remaining portion of material *(clot sections of the marrow)* is transferred in 10% formol saline for histopathological examination.

Marrow staining : After drying in air the films are immediately fixed in acetone-free methyl alcohol for 20 minutes and stained by Leishman, May-Grunwald or Giemsa stains.

(i) Smears are stained by *Leishman stain* routinely.

(ii) Few smears may be stained by *PAS* or *May-Grunwald stain.*

(iii) Prussian blue staining may be done to demonstrate iron in haemosiderin deposit (*Prussian blue reaction*).

Indications for marrow aspiration

(i) *Disorders of red cell* — Megaloblastic anaemia, pure red cell aplasia, pancytopenia.

(ii) *Disorders of white cell* — Subleukemic/ aleukemic leukemia, all acute blastic leukemias for FAB typing.

(iii) *Disorders of megakaryocytes* — ITP and other thrombocytopenias.

(iv) *Myeloproliferative disorders* — Polycythemia vera, chronic myeloid leukemia, idiopathic thrombocythemia.

(v) *Myelodysplastic syndromes*

(vi) *Storage disorders* — Gaucher's and Niemann-Pick's disease.

(vii) *Plasma cell disorders* —Multiple myeloma.

(viii) *For iron stores.*

(ix) *For metastatic deposits* — Ca breast, prostate, lung, kidney, etc.

(x) *Parasitic disorders* — Kala-azar.

Dry Tap : In certain states like aplastic anaemia and myelofibrosis, marrow is not obtained and the needle and syringe remain dry — called dry tap. Marrow has been replaced by fat in aplastic anaemia while in myelofibrosis, marrow is replaced by fibrous tissue.

Clot sections of the marrow

The clotted marrow material is to be placed in a vial containing adequate quantity of 10% formalin and processed like tissue biopsy. Sections made from paraffin block are stained with hematoxylin and eosin. These HE stained sections of marrow give additional information regarding the cellularity of marrow and topography of the cells similar to those of a trephine biopsy of the marrow.

Examination of aspirated bone marrow

Normal finding : At first, the bone marrow smears are screened with the help of a *scanner objective* to see the presence of *marrow particles.* In the tail of the smear, most of the bone marrow particles are present and trails made by the marrow particles provide adequate cells. Morphology of these bone marrow cells are studied for making a differential count on the smears. The yellow marrow contains mainly fat cells with a few strands of connective tissue. Red bone marrow is extremely cellular and contains islands of leucoblastic and erythroblastic elements in various stages of maturation. The immature white cells outnumber the immature red cells. The myeloid-erythroid ratio varies from 8:1 to 2:1 (A and B, Table 15.1) and the lymphoid erythroid ratio is similarly 0.2-4.0 : 1. A total of 300-500 nucleated cells are to be counted.

Reporting on bone marrow

A detailed myelogram report includes :

1. *General cellularity of the marrow,* e.g., differential count.
2. *Type of erythropoiesis,* e.g., normoblastic, megaloblastic or dyserythropoietic.
3. *Type of leucopoiesis.*
4. *Estimate of myeloid-erythroid ratio.*

Cellularity

An assessment of cellularity of the marrow is made by visual evaluation of the marrow particles. In children the bone marrow is highly cellular and with advancing age there is progressive increase in the content of fat with concomitant reduction in cells. There are about 75% marrow and 25% fat in children, while in adult there are about 40% fat and 60% marrow cells in a *normocellular* fragment of bone marrow.Marrow is reported as *hypercellular, normocellular (Table 15.1),* or hypocellular as assessed by the use of scanner and low power objectives of microscope. In a *hypercellular* fragment, amount of fat is either reduced or absent. The amount of fat is increased in *hypocellular* fragments. The *aplastic* fragments of bone marrow have hardly any cells.

Table 15.1
Normal range for differential count of bone marrow smears

	Percentage		
	Neutrophil	*Eosinophil*	*Basophil*
Polymorphonuclears	7–25	0.2–3	0–0.5
Metamyelocytes	10–25	0–2.5	–
Myelocytes	5–20	0.1–3	0–0.5 A
Promyelocytes		0.5–5	
Myeloblasts		0.3–3.5	
Lymphocytes		5–20	
Monocytes		0–5	
Plasma cells		0.1–3.5	
Megakaryocytes		0.1–0.5	
Late normoblasts		4–15	
Early and intermediate normoblasts		4–20	B
Proerythroblast		0.5–5	

Erythropoiesis

Type of erythropoiesis : In simple hyperplasia of *normoblastic* type which occur in simple anaemias (e.g., haemorrhage), differential cell count shows a good proportion of early normoblasts and larger number of intermediate and late normoblasts with "shift to the left", whereas in *megaloblastic* erythropoiesis, the proerythroblasts give rise to large number early, intermediate and late megaloblasts along with megalocytes (Fig. 13.2).

Activity and maturity : The activity of erythroid cells is measured by the number of erythroid cells present and by noting down myeloid erythroid ratio.

Bone marrow findings in iron deficiency and B-12/folate deficiency anaemia are shown in Table 15.2.

Table 15.2 : Bone marrow findings in iron deficiency anaemia and B-12/folate deficiency anaemia

	Iron deficiency anaemia	B-12/folate deficiency anaemia
Hyperplasia	Erythroid hyperplasia	Erythroid hyperplasia Hypercellular BM
Reaction	Micronormoblastic	Megaloblastic
Giant meta myelocyte	Nil	++
Iron store	Nil	Increased

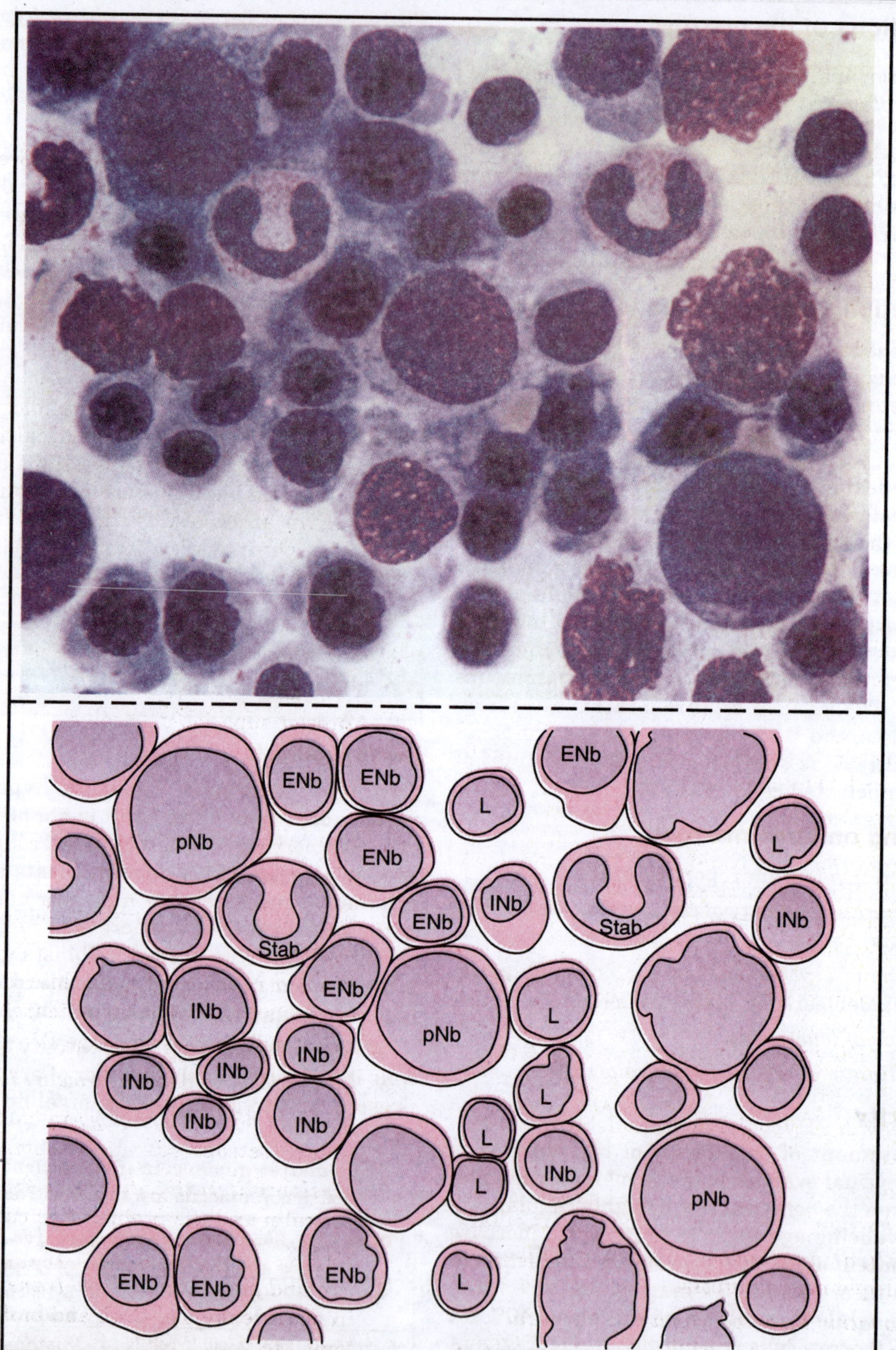

Fig. 15.3. Normoblastic hyperplasia (Marrow film). pNb—pronormoblasts; INb—intermediate normoblast; ENb—early normoblast; L—lymphocyte; Stab—non-segmented polymorphonuclar leucocyte. Majority of the cells are normoblasts in varying stages of development. Lymphocytes are useful for comparison of nuclear structure and intensity of staining. In this condition the myeloid-erythroid ratio is markedly decreased *(May-Grunwald-Giemsa stain)*

Leucopoiesis

1.Number and maturity of *granulocytes, lymphocytes, plasma cells* and *megakaryocytes* are noted.

2. *Myeloid* : *Erythroid* ratio is determined by counting 300–500 cells. In *simple hyperplasia,* which proceeds along physiological expansion, there is marked increase in the polymorphonuclear precursor cells (Fig. 15.2).

3. If the marrow is practically replaced by one cell type *leukaemia,* e.g., marrow is largely composed of young myelocytes and others in myelogenous leukaemia and by lymphocytes and their precursors in lymphatic leukaemia.

Megakaryopoiesis

In the cell trails of the marrow particles of the smear, megakaryocytes are looked for. In a normal marrow smear, there are a number of megakaryocytes. It is important to specially look for the budding of platelets from megakaryocytes in addition to noting down the relative number of promegakayocytes to megakaryocytes.

Foreign cells

Metastatic tumour cells, Gaucher's and Niemann-Pick cells may be present.

Parasites and bacteria

Leishman Donovan bodies in RE cell, malarial parasites in RBC, microfilaria, tubercle bacilli and lepra bacilli may be present.

Iron Stores

Iron stores in marrow material or in other organs are assessed by Perl's stain (vide Ch. 16 Laboratory Diagnosis of Anaemia).

Other indications of marrow aspiration

1. *Anaemia* : Hypoplastic, megaloblastic anaemia.
2. *Kala-azar.*
3. *Leukaemia* : Aleukaemic type in particular.
4. *Infiltrating disease* : Hodgkin's disease, multiple myelomatosis.
5. *Idiopathic thrombocytopaenic* purpura.
6. *Aplastic anaemia* : There is replacement of bone marrow by fat with marked reduction of all three haemopoietic elements, hence bone marrow aspiration often results in dry tap. In such cases trephine biopsy with Jamshide needle is done.

Contraindications of marrow aspiration

Haemophilia A and haemophilia B.

BONE MARROW TREPHINE BIOPSY

In bone marrow trephine biopsy, a core of bone with marrow spaces is obtained. Several types of needles are employed for obtaining bone marrow biopsy which include : Jamshidi needle, Westerman-Jensen needle and Islam needle. The core of the bone marrow obtained in this technique, is rolled between two glass slides to obtain marrow *imprint* smears. The imprint smears are representative of the marrow. These are very useful and excellent material for study of morphology and for special stains. Biopsy material is decalcified first and then processed. Multiple sections are made from the paraffin block. Sections are stained with Hematoxylin and eosin stain, reticulin stain, Masson's trichrome stain for fibrous tissue and immunocytochemical stains in acute leukemias.

Sites of trephining

1. Posterior superior iliac spine is the preferable site.
2. Anterior superior iliac spine.
3. Spinous process of vertebra.

Indications

1. *Red cell disorders* : Aplastic anemia
2. *Myelofibrosis* (Fig. 19.23).
3. *White cell disorders* : Hypoplastic acute leukemia.
4. *Metastasis in cancer cases* : Marrow positive for metastatic deposit indicates disseminated malignancy i.e. stage IV.
5. *Involvement of bone marrow by lymphoma.*
6. *Study of bone morphology* in chronic renal failure, osteoporosis and osteomalacia.
7. *Myeloproliferative disorders* for studying reticulin and the proliferative cell lines for typing.
8. *Pre and post bone marrow transplantation* in acute leukemia, CML and multiple myeloma etc.
9. *PUO* —for studying tuberculous granuloma.
10. Myelodysplastic syndrome (vide chapter 19).

QUESTIONS

1. *What are the types marrow puncture needle?*
2. *How does aspiration biopsy differ from trephine biopsy?*
3. *Name the usual sites for bone marrow aspiration.*
4. *What is dry tap?*
5. *How do you know that bone marrow aspiration is successful?*
6. *What are the normal BM findings?*
7. *What are marrow findings in iron deficiency anaemia and B12/folate deficiency anaemia? For answer, also refer to chapter 16 (Anaemia).*
8. *Describe BM picture in aplastic anaemia. For answer, also refer to chapter 16 (Anaemia).*
9. *Name the indications of marrow aspiration.*
10. *What are contraindication of marrow aspiration?*

Chapter 16

Anaemia

Definition

Anaemia is a pathological condition characterised by a decrease in oxygen carrying capacity of the blood. Anaemia is defined as reduction in the concentration of haemoglobin in the peripheral blood below normal for the age and sex of the patient. An adult man is said to be anaemic when the haemoglobin level falls below 12 g per cent and an adult female when her haemoglobin level falls below 10.5 g per cent (WHO).

Anaemia must, therefore, occur :

1. When the production of haemoglobin is poor in quantity or quality.

2. When the blood loss or blood destruction outstrips the available supply of the new cells.

Clinical features

Although certain pathological changes are more or less characteristic of anaemia as of particular types, but there are certain common features to all severe anaemias (Table 16.1).

Table 16.1 : Symptoms and signs of anaemia

Symptoms	*Signs*
Lassitude, Fatigue, palpitation, Breathlessness, on exertions, Dimness of vision, Insomnia, Angina, Paresthesia in finger and toes.	Pallor of skin, mucous membranes, palms of hand, conjunctiva, Tachycardia, cardiac dilatation, systolic flow murmur. Oedema

Classification

Anaemia may be classified on the basis of morphology of red cell (and the cell indices) or from the aspect of cause.

I. Morphologic classification

It is based on red cell indices, MCV, MCH and MCHC and morphology of red cell on a peripheral blood smear.

1. **Normocytic normochromic anaemia (Fig. 16.1)**

(a) RBC count : decreased

(b) Hb% : reduced

(c) PCV% : lowered

(d) Individual cell size (MCV) : normal

(e) Individual cell Hb (MCH, MCHC) : normal

(f) Smear : red cells more spread apart but individual RBC is relatively normal in appearance.

This type of blood picture is associated with *haemolytic anaemia, hypoplastic anaemia,* acute blood loss *(haemorrhage)* and anaemias associated with *leukaemia.*

2. **Microcytic hypochromic anaemia (Fig. 16.2)**

(a) RBC count : reduced

(b) PCV, MCV, MCH, MCHC : reduced below normal value.

(c) Smear : red cells appear pale with a larger area of central pallor (hypochromic) and many appear to be smaller than normal.

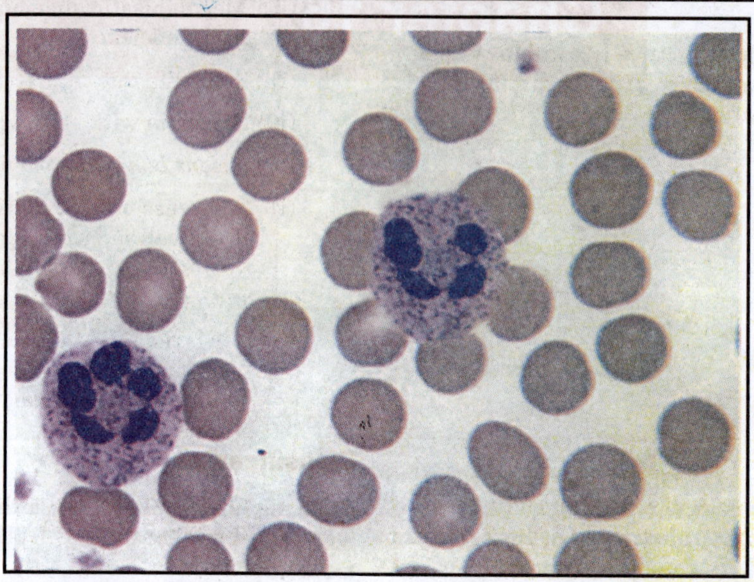

Fig. 16.1. Blood film Normal erythrocytes — Cells are of uniform size and shape with a normal haemoglobin concentration. One cell, centre of field, reveals a small area of central pallor which is less than one-third of the total cell volume *(Wright's stain)*

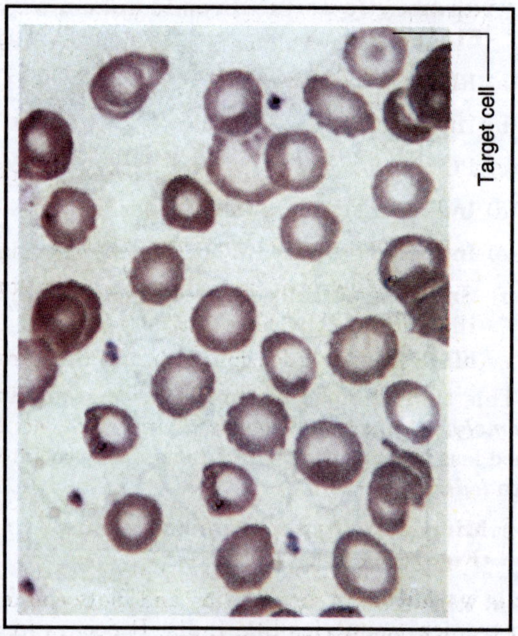

Fig. 16.2. Microcytic hypochromic red cells : Marked decrease in intensity of staining of red cells; central pallor with darker at the periphery of many erythrocytes. One target cell is seen at upper right of the field *(Leishman)*

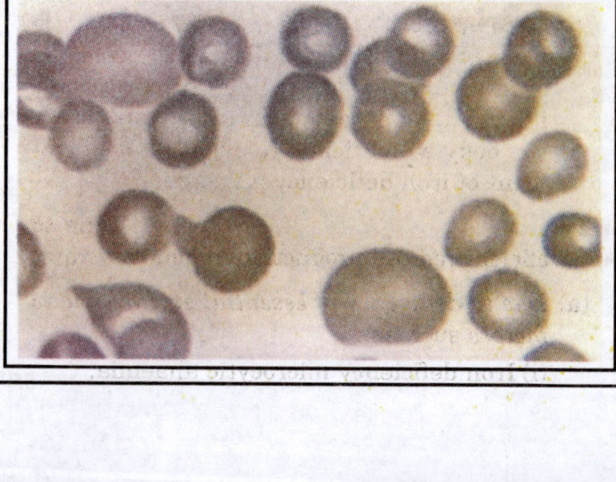

Fig. 16.3. Macrocytic anaemia of pregnancy : Marked oval macrocytosis, aniso and poikilocytosis marked. Similar picture is seen in pernicious anaemia *(May-Grunwald-Gienisa)*

Causes :

This type of blood picture is especially seen in *iron deficiency* anaemia. Hypochromic cells are also seen in *thalassaemia* but MCV is not so low and many of the red cells appear definitely macrocytic.

3. **Macrocytic normochromic anaemia (Fig. 16.3)**

(a) RBC count : greater decrease than Hb content.

(b) MCV, MCH : elevated.

(c) MCHC : normal.

(d) Smear : many macrocytes with normal staining and even an apparent hypochromia with loss of the usual pallor area.

This picture is largely associated with deficiency of vitamin B_{12} and/or folic acid (megaloblastic anaemia).

Dimorphic anaemia : When there is combined deficiency of iron, vitamin B_{12} and folic acid at a time, there may be found both macrocytes and microcytes (Fig. 16.5).

4. **Macrocytic normochromic anaemia (simple microcytic) (Fig. 16.4)**

This is mild degree (usually not marked) of reduction in MCV and MCH but the MCHC is within normal range and the blood picture does not show much hypochromia. This type of anaemia is found in some of the anaemias of *chronic infection* and some other chronic diseases.

II. Aetiological classification

1. **Haemorrhagic anaemia** : due to extracorpuscular blood loss.

(a) *Acute blood loss* : It results from accidental injury, surgery, gastrointestinal bleeding.

(b) *Chronic blood loss* : It is found in bleeding ulcer or gastrointestinal cancer, prolonged excessive vaginal bleeding and hookworm infection. This results in iron depletion in the body which leads to eventual development of iron deficiency anaemia.

2. **Dyshaemopoietic anaemia** : It is due to deficient red cell production in bone marrow :

(a) *Due to deficiency of essential erythropoietic factors* such as :

(i) Iron deficiency microcytic anaemia.

(ii) Megaloblastic anaemia due to B_{12} or folic acid deficiency.

(iii) Anaemia due to protein malnutrition.

(iv) Anaemia with scurvy.

(b) *Deficient bone marrow function* such as :

(i) In disease of bone marrow, the production of red cell is either diminished (*hypoplasia*) or nearly abolished *(aplastic anaemia)*, or

(ii) When red cell precusor are crowded out of the marrow by other cells or tissues, e.g., leukaemia, malignant lymphoma, myelosclerosis, myeloma.

3. **Haemolytic anaemias (Fig. 16.4)** : There is an increased cell destruction with shortening of life span of red cell due to :

(a) ***Intrinsic red cell abnormality***

(i) *Morphologic defects* : Ovalocytosis, elliptocytosis, hereditary spherocytosis.

(ii) *Haemoglobin defects* : (a) Thalassaemia, (b) haemoglobinopathies.

(iii) *Enzymatic defects* : Spherocytosis (G6PD deficiency), aldolase deficiency, pyruvate kinase deficiency, hereditary haemolytic anaemia, paroxysmal nocturnal haemoglobinuria.

(b) ***Extrinsic causes*** : extracorpuscular or environmental defects.

(i) *Autoimmune haemolytic anaemia.*

(ii) *Haemolytic disease of newborn* (erythroblastosis).

(iii) Parasitic infection with malarial organism.

(iv) Hypersplenism.

DYSHAEMOPOIETIC ANAEMIAS

Iron Deficiency Anaemia

It is worldwide in distribution and more common in tropical countries like India. It occurs in all ages. Iron deficient anaemia is asymptomatic in most instances. Nonspecific indications like weakness, listlessness and pallor may be present in severe cases. The red cells are microcytic hypochromic (Fig. 16.2). Although bone marrow shows normoblastic hyperplasia, it is limited by the availability of iron, consequently the volume of active marrow is usually only slightly increased.

Iron metabolism

Iron is an essential element for all higher organisms and also for many lower forms of life. It is present in several haem-protein complexes (haemoglobin, myoglobin) that transports oxygen or enzymes active in electron transport (cytochromes, cytochrome oxidase).

There is about 4 g of iron in the body of an adult male, 70% of which is incorporated into haemoglobin and myoglobin and 25% is stored in liver, spleen and bone marrow in combination with non-haem-proteins as ferritin or haemosiderin. Only a small amount, 0.2% of total body iron bound to β-globulin and transferrin circulates in plasma.

About 20-25 mg of iron is contained in aged red cells that are daily degraded in reticuloendothelial system, the same amount is required daily for the synthesis of new red cells which is accomplished by the re-utilisation of the released iron.

Sufficient iron is ordinarily derived from everyday food stuffs (5–10% of the 10–15 mg daily requirement of body) to balance the small daily excretion in faeces (mainly unabsorbed iron), urine, and perspiration in men, but the women

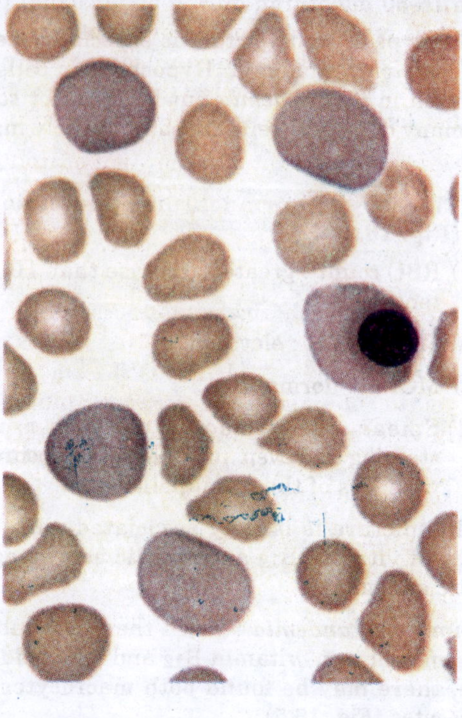

Fig. 16.4. Blood film Haemolytic anaemia : Polychromatic cells and microcytes are prominent. One late normoblast is present. *(May-Grunwald-Giemsa)*

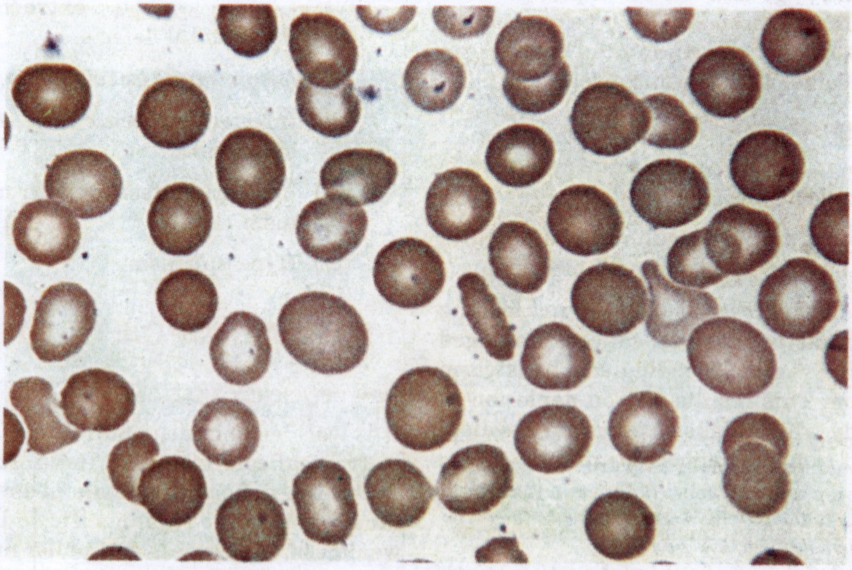

Fig. 16.5. Blood film : Dimorphic anaemia showing both macro and microcytes *(May-Grunwald-Giemsa Stain)*

lose 15-50 mg of iron during a menstrual period. The loss is about 400 mg in pregnancy due to the need of growing foetus and bleeding during delivery. Therefore, the requirement of more iron in diet for women is necessary than that in men.

Maximum amount of absorption of iron occurs in stomach and upper intestine as Fe^{++} (ferrous iron) and traverses the intestinal mucosa, where it is oxidised to Fe^{+++} (ferric form) and stored temporarily as ferritin. Iron balance is maintained by a regulation of absorption according to body needs rather than excretion of unwanted excess. The ferric iron (Fe^{+++}) is released from the mucosal cell to enter the blood stream bound to transferrin and then carried to bone marrow, liver and other tissue through plasma for storage (as ferritin) or utilisation.

The iron transport protein of plasma, transferrin, normally binds only about one-third of iron which is capable of combining. Normal serum iron averages 100 μg and the *total saturation capacity* (TSC) is 300 μg for 100 ml of serum. The *total iron binding capacity* (TIBC) is estimated after saturating the *transferrin* with iron and then removing the excess unbound iron with magnesium carbonate. The additional iron in excess of normal TIBC which is bound is called the *latent or unsaturated iron-binding capacity* (UIBC).

TIBC = UIBC + serum Fe. The concentration of iron in plasma in different states is shown in Table 16.2.

Plasma iron clearance

The rate of clearance of iron from plasma is influenced by the intensity of erythropoietic activity and also by the activity of the macrophages of the reticuloendothelial system, especially in spleen, liver and bone marrow where iron is stored. The rate is *increased* in hyperactive state of one or more of these mechanisms as found in iron-deficiency anaemias, haemorrhagic anaemias, haemolytic anaemias and polycythaemias; whereas the rate is decreased in aplastic anaemia.

Causes of iron-deficiency anaemia

Iron-deficiency anaemia is not a disease by itself but a symptom of some other clinical conditions which are enumerated below.

Table 16.2 : Serum concentration of iron in normal and pathological states

Pathological state	*Serum iron (μg%)*	*TIBC (μg%)*	*Per cent saturation*
Normal			
Neonate (steadily falls for 1st 4-6 months; reaches adult level by 3rd year)	190	—	—
Adult male	60 – 150	250–400	—
Adult female	50 – 130	—	—
Old age (above 70)	50 – 80	—	—
Increased			
(1) Bone marrow block *(refractory anaemias)*, (2) Iron excess *(haemochromatosis)*, (3) accelerated red cell destruction *(haemolytic anaemias)*, (4) decreased red cell formation *(aplastic anaemia)*	Increased	—	Increased
[**TIBC** : An increase in amount of transferrin raises TIBC : *Iron deficiency anaemias, haemolytic anaemias, refractory anaemias.*]	—	Increased	—
Decreased			
(1) Insufficient dietary intake of iron *(iron deficiency anaemia, malabsorption.* (2) Impairment in the release of iron from RE cells *(infection, neoplasia, rheumatoid arthritis).* (3) Accelerated loss *(acute or chronic haemorrhage, late pregnancy).*	Decreased	—	Decreased
[**TIBC** : TIBC is decreased when there is decreased synthesis of transferrin : *infection, neoplasia, uraemia.*]	—	Decreased	—

1. *Chronic blood loss* : Hookworm infection, gastrointestinal bleeding (peptic ulcer, gastric cancer, ulcerative colitis, oesophageal varices, anorectal piles), haematuria, vaginal bleeding (menorrhagia, cancer).

2. *Excessive body need* : Increased demands not met by normal dietary source occurs during growth, pregnancy or lactation.

3. *Inadequate absorption of iron* : This occurs in diarrhoea, vomiting, achlorhydria and resection of intestine, malabsorption with sprue and coeliac disease following gastrectomy.

4. *Inadequate intake of iron,* particularly in developing countries may occur.

5. *Defective utilisation of iron,* e.g., vitamin C deficiency and in toxic process such as nephritis, lead poisoning.

MEGALOBLASTIC ANAEMIA

The term megaloblastic anaemia is applied to those anaemias in which enlargement of proliferating erythroid precursor cells create megaloblasts and corresponding abnormally large red cells (macrocytes, megalocytes). Vitamin B_{12} and folic acid are the essential elements for proper synthesis of DNA. Both cause proliferations of cells having relatively rapid turnover, especially haematopoietic precursors and gastrointestinal epithelial cells. Lack of these two substances results in impairment of DNA synthesis, so that the proliferating cells laboriously synthesise DNA and enlarge their nuclei but the ultimate mitotic division is delayed, although the cytoplasmic development progresses normally. Thus the megaloblastic cells tend to be large, with an increased ratio of RNA to DNA, which is referred to as "nuclear-cytoplasmic asynchrony". Proliferation of erythroid precursor cells are particularly affected. Other proliferating cells include giant metamyelocytes, yielding hypersegmented neutrophils.

An accumulation of megaloblasts occur in bone marrow due to maturational derangements, yielding too few erythrocytes, hence the anaemia. Moreover, the situation is aggravated by two other concommitant processes :

1. *Ineffective erythropoiesis* : Megaloblastic erythroid cells are predisposed to undergo autohaemolysis in the marrow in excessive manner.

2. *Increased haemolytic destruction* of the abnormally large red cells.

Types :

There are two principal types of megaloblastic anaemia, one due to a deficiency of cobalamin (Vitamin B_{12}) and other by a lack of folic acid. In some other cases, there may be lack of both cobalamin and folic acid (Table 16.3).

Table 16.3 : Classificatin of megaloblastic anaemia

Deficiency	*Clinical states*
I. B_{12} *deficiency*	**A. Malabsorption :**
	(1) *Inadequate production of intrinsic factor (IF)*: Pernicious anaemia, gastrectomy, congenital absence or functional abnormality of IF (rare).
	(2) *Disorders of terminal ileum* : Tropical sprue, nontropical sprue, regional enteritis, intestinal resection.
	(3) *Competition for cobalamin* : Fish tapeworms, bacterial blind loop syndrome.
	B. Inadequate dietary intake : Virtually limited to strict vegetarians (rare).
II. *Folate deficiency*	**A. Inadequate intake** : Persons with marginal diets, alcoholics and drug addicts.
	B. Increased metabolic requirements : Pregnancy, during rapid growth (malignancy, infancy), chronic disease.
	C. Malabsorption : Tropical sprue, nontropical sprue, drugs (phenytoin, barbiturates).
	D. Impaired metabolism :
	(1) Inhibitors of dihydrofolate reductase, methotrexate; pyrimethamine, triamterene pentamidine etc.
	(2) Alcohol.

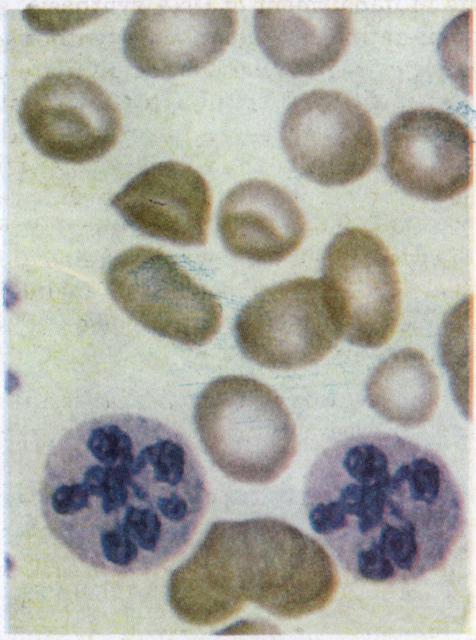

Fig. 16.6. Blood film Hypersegmented neutrophil leucocytes : Megaloblastic anaemia. *(May-Grunwald-Giemsa Stain)*

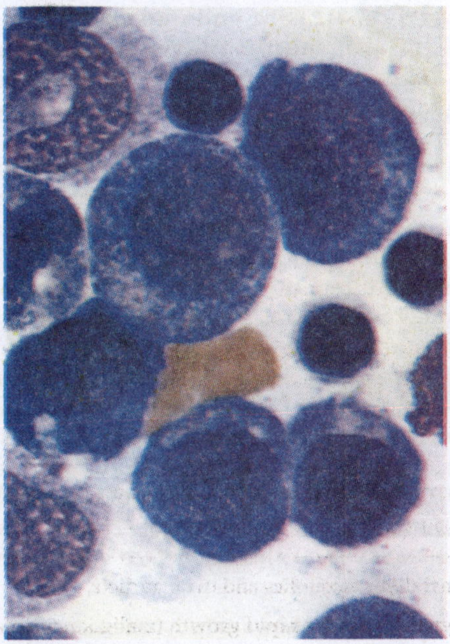

Fig. 16.7. Marrow film : Megaloblastic anaemia, early megaloblasts (several) and one promyelocyte, three late megaloblast *(May-Grunwald-Giemsa stain)*

Blood finding

Megaloblastic anaemia can be suspected when *peripheral blood film* (Fig. 16.6) shows macrocytic normochromic oval red cells, pear-shaped poikilocytes and polymorphonuclear leucocytes with hypersegmented nuclei (increased to five or six). An elevated MCV, often without anaemia, is the first indication in many cases. Confirmation may be made by examining bone marrow which contains megaloblasts (Fig. 16.7) and giant metamyelocytes.

The folate deficiency anaemia is distinguished from B_{12} deficiency anaemia by assays of serum folate and vitamin B_{12}, and red cell folate levels, which also confirm the diagnosis.

Pathogenesis

The various clinical conditions associated with megaloblastic anaemia are shown in Table 16.3.

Folate (Folic acid) deficiency anaemia

Folic acid is the common name of pteroylmonoglutamic acid and is found in fresh green vegetables and fruits, as well as liver, milk and yeast. The minimum daily requirement is normally 50 µg, which is increased to several fold during enhanced metabolic demand, e.g., pregnancy. Most dietary folates are heat-labile and destroyed by 10–15 minutes cooking. Hence, green vegetables should be eaten either uncooked or lightly cooked. Normal adults have 5–20 µg folic acid in various body stores, half in the liver.

Absorption : Food folates are predominantly in the polyglutamate form, and must be split into monoglutamate form for absorption. This conversion into monoglutamate form is done in the lumen of gut by *conjugates* (γ-glutamyl carboxy peptidases). The monoglutamates are then readily absorbed in the proximal jejunum (upper third of small intestine). Acidic foods and conjugate inhibitors present in beans and other legumes hamper absorption by inhibiting intestinal conjugates. Malabsorptive disorders (e.g., coeliac disease, tropical sprue) affect the upper third of small intestine and impair absorption of folates.

Metabolism : After absorption the monoglutamate is transported by blood to cell in which it undergoes conversion to several derivatives, but of principal importance is that it must be reduced to tetrahydrofolate (THF) by a reductase. (This reductase is inhibited by folate analogue, e.g., methotrexate, which deprives cells of folate and the capacity to divide rapidly. This principle is applied by using folic acid antagonists as antineoplastic agents). The primary function of THF is an acceptor and donor of one carbon unit to appropriate acceptor compound to form metabolic intermediates which are ultimately converted to building blocks such as purines, thymidylate, and, therefore, thymine. Thus, folate deficiency leads to slow DNA synthesis which accounts for megaloblastic anaemia.

Vitamin B_{12} (cobalamin) deficiency anaemia

Vitamin B_{12} is a large complex organometallic compound containing one molecule of cobalt per molecule. All vitamin B_{12} in nature is originally derived from bacteria. Animals including man cannot synthesise cobalamin (B_{12}) but can store it. It must be supplied in the diet. The only dietary source of B_{12} is animal products : meat and dairy foods and the minimum daily requirement is about 2.5 µg. Unlike folic acid, B_{12} is not destroyed by boiling. Normally, about 2 mg vitamin B_{12} is stored in the liver and another 2 mg elsewhere in the body. Since the daily requirement is minimum, it takes 3-6 years for a normal individual to become deficient in B_{12} if absorption ceases abruptly.

Since vegetables do not contain vitamin B_{12}, strict vegetarians are more apt to become B_{12} deficient than meat eaters.

Absorption

1. Peptic digestion releases dietary vitamin B_{12}, which then forms a stable complex with salivary and gastric B_{12} binding proteins called *R binders*.

2. On entering the duodenum, R–B_{12} complex are digested and split by pancreatic proteases, releasing B_{12}. The released B_{12} attaches to *intrinsic factor (IF)* secreted by the parietal cells of the gastric fundic mucosa.

3. The IF–B_{12} complex travels to the distal ileum, where it attaches to the specific epithelial IF receptors, followed by absorption within the mucosal cell. Within the epithelial cell, the IF is destroyed over the course of several hours and the cobalamin is transferred to another transport protein, *transcobalamin* II (TC II).

4. The cobalamin–TC II is then secreted into the circulation, from which it is delivered into the liver and other cells of the body.

Although TC II is the initial acceptor of absorbed cobalamin from epithelial cells, but most circulating cobalamin is bound to transcobalamin I (TC I), a glycoprotein (appears to be derived in part from leucocytes) closely related to gastric R binder. TC II bound to cobalamin is rapidly eliminated from blood (about 1 hour), while clearance of cobalamin bound to TC I requires many days. Function of TC I is not clear.

Mechanism

There are two metabolically active cobalamins in man, methyl cobalamin and adenosylcobalamin. Cyanocobalamin (also called vitamin B_{12}), administered therapeutically, must be converted to a biologically active form before it can be used by tissues.

Methyl cobalamin is an essential co-factor in the conversion of homocysteine to methionine. When this reaction is disturbed due to B_{12} deficiency, folate metabolism is deranged leading to an internal folate deficiency by affecting some critical step in folate metabolism. Although folates are abundant, they are not available in a metabolically useful form, so DNA synthesis is impaired.

Pernicious anaemia

There are many potential causes of a B_{12} deficiency anaemia, including inadequate diet, increased repairment and impaired absorption (Table 16.3) but only the vitamin B_{12} deficiency, in which **intrinsic factor** (IF) secretion ceases owing to idiopathic atrophy of much of the gastric mucosa which constitutes pernicious anaemia. IF is a glycoprotein (MW 45000). It is evident that IF plays a critical role in the absorption of vitamin B_{12}. It is a disease of the elderly. The derangement in synthesis of IF appears to be caused by an autoimmune reaction. Patients with pernicious anaemia have autoantibodies in serum and gastric juice against parietal cell and intrinsic factor. The acid and pepsin secreting portion of stomach is affected, antrum is spared. Megaloblastic changes of gastric and intestinal epithelium occur. Neurological changes of a demyelinating disorder involving the peripheral nerves and ultimately the spinal cord occur *(subacute degeneration* of spinal cord). *Atrophy* of epithelial surface is also common in the tongue and vagina.

Blood picture shows pancytopenia. Since this severe type of anaemia was first described by Addison, it is also called *Addisonian pernicious anaemia*. Patients with long-standing pernicious anaemia have 3–5 times greater risk of gastric carcinoma.

Clinical aspect

The megaloblastic anaemia is almost always

due to malabsorption of cobalamin and folic acid in most parts of the world. In India, nutritional deficiencies of cobalamin and folic acid and deficiencies due to problems of malabsorption in the intestine in sprue are the principal causes of megloblastic anaemia. The incidence of pernicious anaemia is very low.

Combined deficiencies of B_{12} and folic acid are not uncommon. Pernicious anaemia is not common in India. Nutritional deficiences of B_{12} and folic acid due to malabsorption in the intestine are the principal causes of megaloblastic anaemia in India.

APLASTIC AND HYPOPLASTIC ANAEMIAS

Anaemia is termed aplastic when little or no cellular marrow exists and hypoplastic when marrow is merely of reduced cellularity. Anaemia may result from suppression of the bone marrow which impairs the formation red cells. Most often there is a failure or suppression of stem cells associated with a hypocellular marrow, anaemia, thrombocytopenia and leucopenia *(pancytopenia).* The term *aplastic anaemia* should be restricted to conditions in which pancytopenia occurs due to a cellular or markedly hypocellular bone marrow.

Aetiopathogenesis

1. **Primary idiopathic aplastic anaemia** : In about half the cases, aplastic anaemia appears without any apparent cause. An autoimmune mechanism may be responsible for majority of these cases of *primary idiopathic acquired* aplastic anaemia. Fanconi's aplastic anaemia is an autosomal recessively inherited disease usually appearing in childhood.

2. **Secondary aplasia or hypoplasia** : Secondary pancytopenia may occur as a result of reaction to certain *drugs* (chloramphenicol, antithyroid drugs, indomethacin, sulpha-methoxypyridazine and tolbutamides, sulphonamides, anticonvulsants, antimalarials); certain *industrial chemicals* and *insecticides* chiefly benzene and

Table 16.4 : Classification of the causes of haemolytic anaemia

I. Congenital haemolytic disorders (Intracorpuscular defects)	
A. *Cell membrane defects* :	(1) Hereditary spherocytosis (2) Hereditary elliptocytosis (3) Hereditary xerocytosis (4) Hereditary stomatocytosis
B. *Enzyme defects* :	(1) Glucose–6–phosphate dehydrogenase deficiency (2) Pyruvate kinase deficiency (3) Pyrimidine–5–nucleotidase deficiency
C. *Haemoglobin defects* (haemoglobinopathies) :	(1) Structural haemoglobinopathies : Sickle cell disease (HbS), HbS C, D and E. (2) Synthetic failure e.g. thalassaemia
II. Acquired haemolytic disorders (Extracorpuscular defects)	
A. *Sequestrational haemolysis* :	Hypersplenism
B. *Immune-haemolytic disorders* :	(1) Alloimmune (2) Autoimmune (3) Drug-induced
C. *Paroxysmal nocturnal haemoglobinuria*	
D. *Toxins* :	Arsenic, copper, clostridial toxins, snake poison
E. *Metabolic abnormalities* :	Spur cell haemolytic anaemia
F. *Due to red cell parasites* :	Malaria, babesiosis, bartonellosis
G. *Due to red cell trauma* :	March haemoglobinuria, fragmentational haemolysis due to cardiac, large vessel of micro-circulation abnormalities.

its derivatives (trinitrophenol, trinitrotoluene, gamma-benzene hexachloride); majority of drugs used in the chemotherapy of malignant tumours; exposure to radiation; replacement of bone marrow by tumour cells or fibrous tissue and deficiency states, e.g., severe lack of vitamin B12 and folate. Certain viral infections (viral hepatitis, Epstein-Barr, cytomegalo and parvoviruses) are sometimes associated with aplastic anaemia.

In some instances, the cytopenia is more selective and involves only one cell line, most frequently the neutrophils; such finding is often incidental unassociated with ill health. The disease may have an immunological basis.

Diagnosis : Clinically, the patient presents with symptoms related to anaemia with a bleeding tendency or minor persistent infections.

1. **Peripheral blood** shows pancytopenia with reduction in reticulocyte count. Red cells are usually normocytic and normochronic. Lymphocyte count may be normal.

2. **Bone marrow** is hypocellular and fatty though islands of haemopoietic tissue persist.

HAEMOLYTIC ANAEMIA

The basic pathological change in all haemolytic anaemias is a reduction in the normal life span of 120 days of the red cells to 10–20 days. If the shortening of life span is minimal (20 days), the bone marrow production increases to 6–8 times and compensates the loss by producing enough additional red cells to keep up the haemoglobin and cell count. When the marrow output can no longer compensate the loss, anaemia develops.

Classification : Haemolytic anaemias may occur either due to production of inherently defective red cells or due to noxious factors present in the intravascular environment. Intrinsic abnormalities, mostly genetically determined, may occur in the red cell membrane or in its contained haemoglobin or enzymes whereas environmental abnormalities that prejudice red cell survival are almost always acquired. A classification of haemolytic anaemia is given in Table 16.4.

HEREDITARY DEFECTS IN THE MEMBRANE OF RED CELL

Hereditary spherocytosis (HS)

It is an inherited haemolytic anaemia characterised by osmotically fragile, partially spherical, spectrin deficient red cells in the peripheral blood which are slectively trapped by the spleen. Although it occurs in all races, particularly common amongst northern Europeans where the prevalence is 1 in 5000. The disease is autosomal dominant (familial) in 75% cases and the rest are nondominant (probably autosomal recessive).

Pathogenesis

The principal defect appears to be a deficiency of spectrin from all HS red cells, a red cell membrane protein. This allows excessive permeability by red cell membrane to glycolysis, red cells lose biconcave shape, become spherical, which are more susceptible to osmotic lysis. Since premature destruction of these erythrocytes occur almost exclusively in the spleen, splenomegaly is a constant association.

Clinical features

The disease may present at any age. Symptoms vary from none to those of severe anaemia with jaundice and splenomegaly. Complications of haemolytic crises are more frequent, aplastic crises are less prevalent. Megaloblastic crisis may occur when dietary consumption of folic acid is inadequate.

Cytoskeleton of red cell membrane is composed of a number of proteins, spectrin, ankyrin, actin, anion exchange protein and various glycophorins. These proteins form an interlocking underlying and attached to the red cell membrane. There is a qualitative or quantitative defect in the spectrin molecule in hereditary spherocytosis, which results in membrane defect. As a result, the red cell attain spheroidal shape with reduced plasticity and become trapped in the red pulp of spleen. Transfused cells survive normally in patients with hereditary spherocytosis following splenectomy.

Investigations

The diagnosis is suggested when haemolysis is associated with microspherocytes in the peripheral blood (Fig. 16.9) and is confirmed by an increased osmotic fragility of the red cells.

(1) Blood film : Spherocytosis; requires to be distinguished from other causes (Table 16.5).

(2) Reticulocyte count : Increased.

(3) MCHC : Increased.

(4) Osmotic fragility of red cell : Increased.

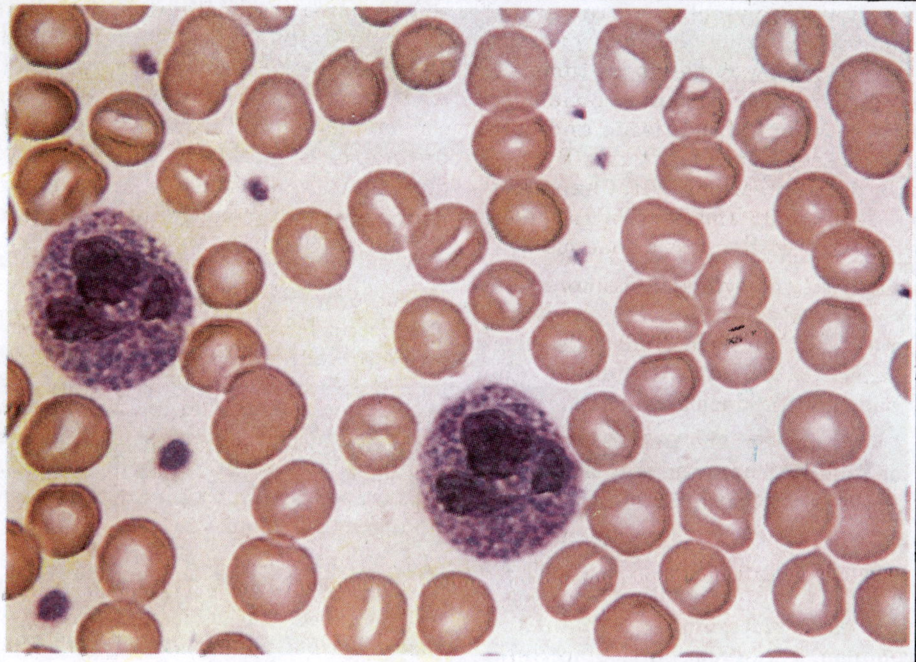

Fig. 16.8. Peripheral blood film : Hereditary stomatocytosis

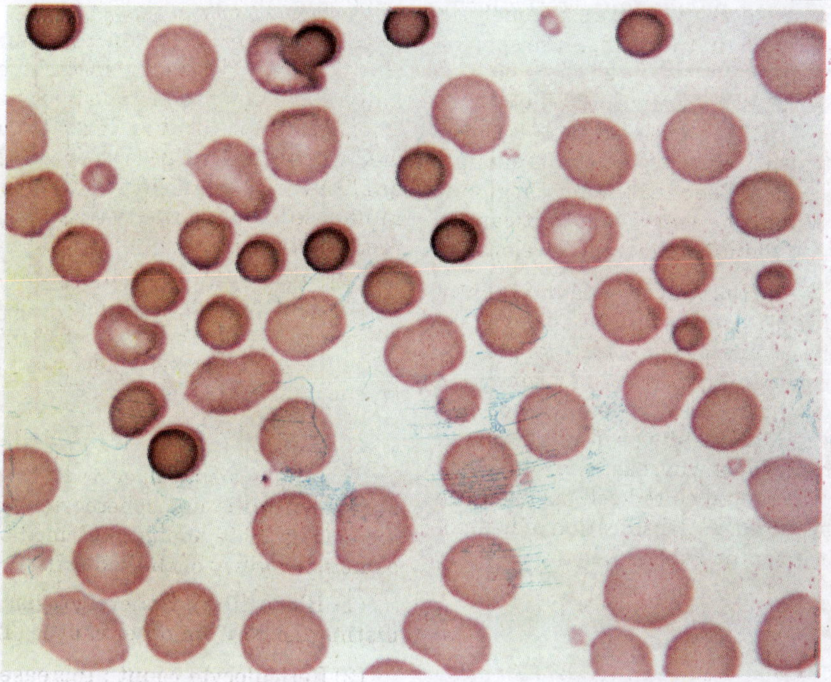

Fig. 16.9. Blood film : Hereditary spherocytosis showing spherocytosis and anisocytosis. Spherocytes have round contours

Table 16.5 Diseases associated with spherocytosis	
Type	*Diseases*
I. Common	(1) Hereditary spherocytosis (2) Immunohaemolytic anaemia (3) ABO incompatibility in neonates
II. Uncommon	(1) Haemolytic transfusion reaction (2) Severe burns and other red cell thermal injuries (3) Clostridial sepsis (4) Severe hypophosphataemia (5) Spider, bee and snake venoms

Hereditary elliptocytosis

It is inherited as an autosomal dominant trait relatively common, 1 in 4000, particularly in its non-haemolytic form. The defects lie either in the head end of spectrin that interfere with spectrin self association or by partial absence of membrane protein. Great majority of the patients have mild haemolysis and have no anaemia (reticulocyte count 1–3%). Blood film (Fig. 16.10) shows prominent elliptocytosis (usually > 40%, normal < 15%), osmotic fragility is normal. In a minority (10-15%) of cases, moderate haemolysis occurs with reticulocyte count of about 15–20%. The red cells are normocytic normochromic in both anaemic and nonanaemic individuals.

Hereditary stomatocytosis

Stomatocytes (Fig. 16.8) are red cells in which the central biconcave area appears as a slit rather than circular pallor in air dried films. Small numbers of stomatocytes may be found in many films, but large numbers of this type of red cell have been noted in an uncommon type of hereditary haemolytic anaemia. Their presence in large number is frequently seen in films of Australians of Mediterranean origin and has been attributed to a genetic factor.

HEREDITARY RED CELL ENZYME DEFECTS

The survival of normal red cells is dependent on the integrity of two enzyme-systems concerned in metabolism of glucose, (a) the hexose monophosphate shunt and (b) the Embden-Meyerhoff pathway (Fig. 16.13).

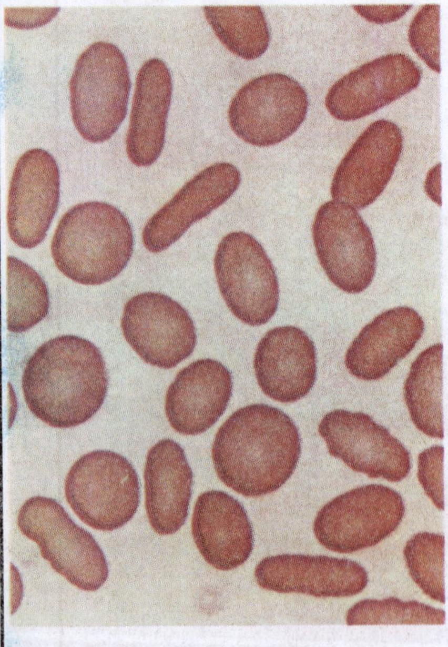

Fig. 16.10. Blood film : Hereditary elliptocytosis. Virtually all the red cells are elliptocytes

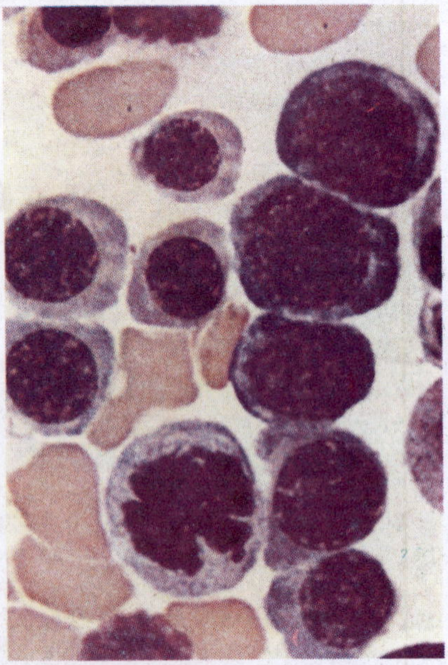

Fig. 16.11. Marrow film : Erythroblastic reaction following haemorrhage

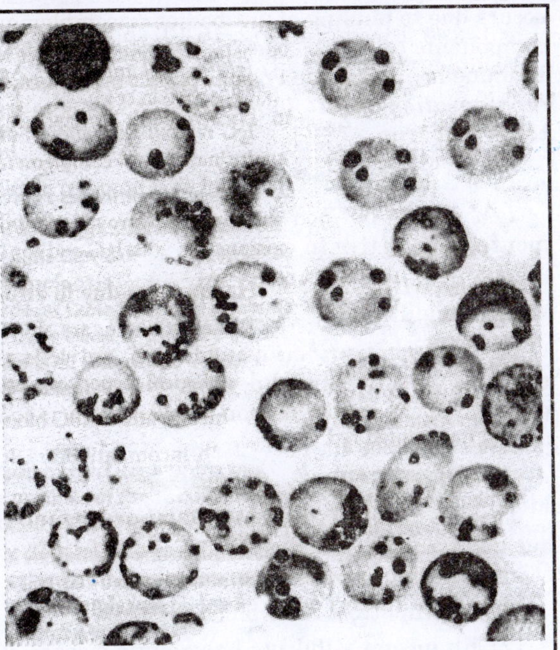

Fig. 16.12. G6PD deficiency. Blood exposed to acetyl phenylhydrazine. The majority of the cells contain several Heinz bodies. Stained supravitally by methyl violet

Glucose–6–phosphate dehydrogenase

Glucose–6–phosphate dehydrogenase (G6PD) is the first enzyme in the hexose monophosphate shunt EM glycolytic pathway from which erythrocytes derive most of their metabolic energy. Through this shunt, G6PD is to give service to the enzyme glutathione reductase and glutathione peroxidase which protect the erythrocytes aginst damage due to oxidation. NADH produced through the shunt contributes additional reducing power and mediates the production of reduced glutathione. Reduced glutathione is an important intracellular buffer that gives protection to red cell against exogenous and endogenous oxidants which would threaten to oxidise haemoglobin to methaemoglobin *(Heinz bodies)* (Fig. 16.12).

Glucose–6–phosphate dehydrogenase (G–6–PD) deficiency

Deficiency of G–6–PD is inherited as a X-linked disorder with a high frequency (up to 40%) among persons of Mediterranean, South East Asian and Negro ancestry. Since the deficiency is determined by a gene on the X-chromosome, full expression of deficiency is observed in male hemizygote. Partial expression may be found in heterogygote female who has two population of red cells, one normal and one deficient. The principal effect is a reduction of NADPH production resulting in decreased amount of reduced glutathione. As a result haemoglobin is readily oxidised to methaemoglobin which precipitates as a *Heinz bodies*.

Types : More than 150 isoenzymes of G–6–PD are identified which show variation in geographical distribution. There is a wide clinical spectrum of disease depending on the type of isoenzyme involved. The main variants : (1) type A (G–6–PD A^-) affects Negros, in which the enzyme is produced in normal amount, but being unstable, decreasing amounts are found in ageing red cells; and (2) type B (G–6–PD B^-) affects persons of Mediterranean and South East Asian countries. The B type deficiency is much more severe and destruction of red cells tends to be greater with higher incidence of haemolysis. G–6–PD deficiency is most common in areas where malaria occurs endemically, reflecting the protection which deficient cells afford against falciparum infection.

Clinical features and offending agents

Persons with G–6–PD deficiency normally enjoy good health, but are liable to haemolysis in response to oxidant stress, e.g.,

(1) Acute infections.

(2) Drugs — Primaquine, pamaquine and other antimalarials, nalidixic acid, nitrofurantoin, sulphonamides, tri-nitrotoluene, aspirin and vitamin K.

(3) Diet — Ingestion of fava bean (favism).

Spontaneous haemolysis occurs in about 5% individuals in Mediterranean countries. The

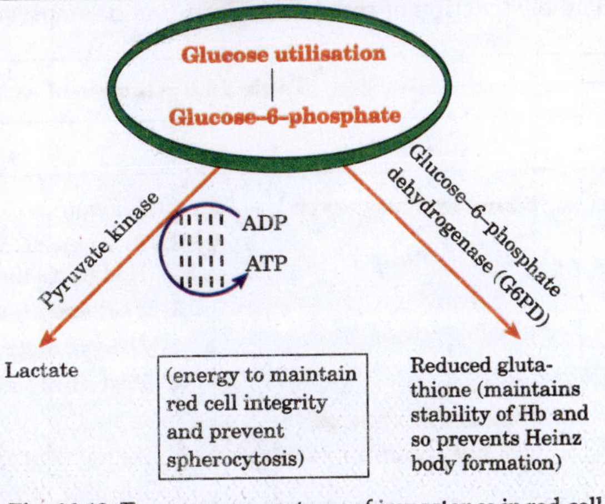

Fig. 16.13. Two enzyme systems of importance in red cell survival

haemolytic episode is self-limiting in milder cases since young red cells contain higher amounts of G-6-PD.

Diagnosis

(1) *Estimation of G-6-PD activity* gives confirmative diagnosis, but this is not absolutely diagnostic, if there is a considerable reticulocytosis (reticulocytes contain higher levels of G-6-PD than matured cells).

There is relatively severe G-6-PD deficiency in older red cells that are haemolysed on exposure to oxidant drugs, infections or chemicals. On the other hand, younger red cells with some amount of G-6-PD remain intact that limits the haemolysis of these cells.

(2) Blood film shows contracted and fragmented red cells along with *Heinz bodies.*

(3) A number of screening test (dye reduction test, ascorbate cyanide test, fluorescent spot test) are available.

Pyruvate kinase (PK) deficiency

PK deficiency is much less common than G-6-PD deficiency. Inheritance is autosomal recessive. It is a mild to moderately severe haemolytic anaemia that occurs in homozygous state. Patient tolerates the anaemia rather well because of rise in intracellular 2, 3-diphosphoglycerate, which occurs as a result of the block in glycosis. Reticulocyte counts may be very high. The diagnosis is made by measuring erythrocyte PK activity.

ACQUIRED HAEMOLYTIC ANAEMIA

Immune haemolytic anaemias

The destruction of red cells in immune haemolysis occurs due to binding of antibodies or complement components or both to the erythrocyte membrane. Immune haemolysis may occur as a result of *autoimmunisation,* or *alloimmunisation,* or exposure to certain drug.

Types of antibodies

IgM red cell antibodies : Agglutinating, complement-fixing, active in cold.

IgG red cell antibodies : Fully active at 37°C, weakly agglutinating and complement fixing.

IgA red cell antibodies : Have little complement fixing activity and destroy red cells poorly; usually appear in conjunction with IgG and/or IgM red cell antibodies.

Haemolysis due to alloantibodies

These antibodies are able to destroy transfused, but not autologous, red cells and are the products of immunological responses, such as :

(1) Incompatible ABO blood transfusion.

(2) Rh incompatibility : haemolytic disease of the newborn.

Autoimmune haemolytic anaemias

Autoimmune haemolytic anaemias are characterised by formation of anti-red cell antibodies with specificity for autologous red cell antigens. Mechanism of production of auto-antibody is not fully understood. There are two main types characterised on the basis of thermal characteristics of the antibody, *warm antibody type* and *cold antibody type* (Table 16.6).

Warm antibodies

Antibodies that react with protein antigens of red cells are usually IgG and react at body temper-

Table 16.6 : Causes of autoimmune haemolytic anaemia

Types	*Diseases*
A. Warm antibody type :	1. *Idiopathic* 2. *Lymphomas* : Chronic lymphocytic leukemia, non-Hodgkin's lymphomas, Hodgkin's disease (infrequent) 3. *SLE* and other collagen diseases 4. *Drugs* : Methyldopa, penicillin, quinidine 5. Post-viral infections
B. Cold antibody type :	
(i) *Cold agglutinin diseases*	1. Acute : Mycoplasmal infection, infectious mononucleosis 2. Chronic : Lymphomas
(ii) *Miscellaneous*	Paroxysmal cold haemoglobinuria

ature (37°C), occasionally, they are IgA. This type of autoimmune haemolytic anaemia occurs secondary to an underlying disease, usually neoplastic or collagen vascular disease (Table 16.6).

Cold antibodies

Most of these cold-reacting antibodies are usually IgM and react better at lower temperatures (4°C), hence the name cold-reacting antibodies. Naturally occurring antibodies tend to be IgM type and bind complement strongly. Cold agglutinins arise in two clinical settings :

(i) monoclonal antibodies as the product of lymphocytic neoplasia and

(ii) polyclonal antibodies in response to an infection.

Synthesis of polyclonal cold agglutinins may increase in response to certain infections especially in mycoplasma and infectious mononucleosis and in some lymphoproliferative disorders (Table 16.6). The antibody titre is usually too low in these cases to produce clinical symptoms but its presence is of diagnostic value; only occasionally is haemolysis present.

Mechanism

High thermal amplitude of cold agglutinins bind to the red cells in the cooler portions of the circulation (e.g., extremities, ears, nose) and initiate agglutination and complement activation by classical pathway. C_1 initiates the reaction and progresses up to binding of nascent C3b to the red cell membrane but the plasma C_3 inactivator (factor 1) cleaves EC3b so rapidly that the latter is unable to effectively support activation of the membrane attack components (C5-9). Other defence mechanism (factor H) also come into play in the mechanism of inactivation of C3b. Thus, significant intravascular haemolysis is prevented.

Clinical manifestations

Patients of all ages are affected. Symptoms differ from patient to patient with the severity of the disease and its underlying cause and are mainly those of anaemias. Splenomegaly and sometimes hepatomegaly may be found.

Laboratory findings

(a) ***Warm antibody type***

1. *Blood count* : RBC count variable; WBC, platelet normal.

2. *MCV, MCHC* : MCV—increased, MCHC—elevated when spherocytosis is prominent.

3. *Peripheral blood smear* : Rouleaux formation (+), moderate degree aniso and poikilocytosis with numerous microspherocytes, fair number of reticulocytes. Nucleated red cells may be present, particularly when haemolysis is rapid.

4. *Indirect antiglobulin test* : Result (±), positivity indicates excess production of red cell autoantibody.

(b) ***Cold antibody type***

1. *Spontaneous agglutination* : As the patient's blood is drawn, RBCs may clump so rapidly that the sample appears to clot even when mixed with anticoagulant. When the anticoagulated blood is warmed to 37°C, it rapidly restores the normal appearance.

2. *Reticulocyte count* : Slightly increased, suggestive of sub-optimal bone marrow compensation.

3. *Cold agglutinin titre* : Elevated, antiglobulin (Coombs') test positive.

Note : Electronically measured blood counts are frequently inaccurate due to autocoagulation of blood at room temperature.

Paroxysmal cold haemoglobinuria (PCH)

PCH is now an exceedingly rare autoimmune haemolytic disorder, more frequent at a time when tertiary syphilis was prevalent. It is caused by IgG cold-reacting antibodies (Donath-Landsteiner antibody) directed against the P blood group antigen which can induce complement-mediated lysis of red cells. Nowadays PCH is sometimes seen as a complication of some viral infections. Attacks are precipitated by exposure to cold and are associated with paroxysms of chills, fever, headache, backache and abdominal pain accompanied by haemoglobinuria.

Pathogenesis : Patients' serum contain cold haemolysin, nonagglutinating antibody which activates complement so efficiently that intravascular haemolysis occurs. The disease extends over many years.

Investigation : Diagnosis is made by demonstration of cold-reacting IgG antibodies by haemolysis test (when the titre is high) or by special antiglobulin test.

(1) *Haemolysis test* : Normal red cells are mixed with patient's serum and guinea-pig serum (source of complement) and chilled (0–4°C). The cell suspension is then incubated at 37°C. Positive result shows haemolysis.

(2) *Direct Combs' test* : Usually weakly positive.

(3) *Haemoglobinuria* : Intermittent.

Paroxysmal nocturnal haemoglobinuria (PNH)

PNH is an acquired intracorpuscular defect resulting from the proliferation of an abnormal clone of stem cells of erythrocytes whose progeny are uniquely sensitive to lysis by complement in the blood causing intermittent haemolytic anaemia, haemoglobinuria and thrombotic episodes.

Pathogenesis : PNH is an acquired clonal disease, probably arising from a single abnormal clone. It may occur in association with other stem cell disorders including aplastic anaemia (frequently), myelofibrosis and rarely with other disorders of myeloid series.

Normal red cell membranes contain a glycoprotein, called delay-accelerating factor (DAF), that inhibits assembly of C3 convertase. PNH red cells are deficient in DAF which is the principal cause of complement-mediated haemolysis. Similarly, platelets and granulocytes of PNH patients also lack DAF and show abnormal sensitivity to complement activation leading to aggregation of platelets (thrombosis) and thrombocytopenia. Most PNH patients show relative marrow hypoplasia.

Investigations :

(1) *Hb* : Anaemia variable.

(2) *Blood count* : Mild granulopenia and thrombocytopenia.

(3) *Red cell morphology* : Normocytic normochromic unless gross haemoglobinuria.

(4) *Urine* : Intermittent haemoglobinuria.

(5) *Acid haemolysis test* : Positive sensitivity of PNH red cells to complement.

LABORATORY INVESTIGATION OF ANAEMIA

In addition to history and detailed clinical examination of patient, some screening tests are necessary for diagnosis :

(i) Examination of peripheral blood film, haemoglobin estimation and quantitative cell count provides screening tests for accurate diagnosis.

(ii) Sometimes diagnosis cannot be made without bone marrow examination.

(iii) Special investigations are also sometimes necessary.

Table 16.7 : Bone marrow changes in anaemias

Condition	*Cellularity*	*Nature of cell reaction*	*Haemosiderin storage*
1. *Iron deficiency anaemia*	Hypercellular, erythroid hyperplasia	Normoblastic, erythroid cell increased over usual 20% of nucleated cells.	Nil
2. *B_{12}, folic acid deficiency anaemia*	Hypercellular with erythroid hyperplasia, ME ratio is reversed to 1 : 1, 1 : 2 or 1 : 3. Giant metamyelocytes and dysplastic megakaryocytes — present. Megakaryocytes are reduced in number.	Megaloblastic with predominance of early and intermediate megaloblasts.	Normal
3. *Pernicious anaemia*	Hypoplastic, often difficult to obtain bone marrow (paucity of all the three haemopoietic cell lines)	Megaloblastic with reduction of erythroid, myeloid and megakaryocytic cells.	Slightly increased
4. *Haemolytic anaemia*	Hypercellular	Normoblastic	Increased
5. *Hypoplastic anaemia*	Hypocellular	Scanty cells with adipose tissue replacement. Bone marrow aspirate is often dry.	Normal

Table 16.8
Laboratory findings in anaemia

	Iron deficiency anaemia	*Megaloblastic anaemia (B_{12}/Folate deficiency)*	*Pernicious anaemia/ aplastic anaemia*
Haemoglobin	Variably reduced	Often reduced	Reduced
MCV	Reduced (microcytosis)	Usually raised, commonly > 120 (macrocytic)	Raised (macrocytic)
RBC count	Normal or reduced, less than Hb level	Low for degree of anaemia	Low
WBC count	Normal	Low, normal/reduced	Low
Blood film	Hypochromia, microcytosis, oval and elliptical cells, poikilocytes in more severe cases	Oval macrocytosis, poikilocytosis, red cell fragmentation, neutrophil hypersegmentation	Similar to megaloblastic anaemia
Differential WBC count	Normal	Neutropenia	Neutropenia
Platelet count	Normal or raised	Low, normalor reduced	Reduced
Reticulocyte count	Normal or reduced, rises in response to therapy	Low for degree of anaemia	Low for degree of anaemia
ESR	Less elevated for degree of anaemia	Moderately raised	Moderately raised
Bone marrow	Micro/normoblastic with erythroid hyperplasia, iron store-empty	(i) Hypercelluarity of marrow along with erythroid hyperplasia with reversal of ME ratio to 1 : 1, 1 : 2 or 1 : 3. (ii) Marrow shows megaloblastic reaction with plenty of megaloblasts predominated by early and intermediate forms with irregular and or budding nuclei. (iii) Megakaryocytes — reduced in number. (iv) Giant metamyelocytes present. (v) Iron store — increased in pure B_{12}/folate deficiency.	(i) Bone marrow is replacedby fat in aplastic anaemia, hence BM shows marked paucity of all three haemopoietic cell lines (pancytopenia) and bone marrow aspirante is dry tap. (ii) Bone marrow shows megaloblastic reaction. (iii) Here bone marrow trephine biopsy with Jamshide needle is necessary for studying BM.
Plasma iron	Reduced	Elevated	Elevated
Serum iron-binding capacity (250–400 µg% with about 30% saturation)	Raised, saturation may be as low as 5%	Increased saturation	Increased saturation
Serum ferritin	Reduced	Elevated	Elevated
Red cell folate (16–64 µg%)	Normal	Reduced < 1–14 µg%	Reduced < 3-40 µg%

Table 16.8 : Laboratory findings in anaemia contd. from previous page

	Iron deficiency anaemia	*Megaloblastic anaemia (B_{12}/Folate deficiency)*	*Pernicious anaemia/ aplastic anaemia*
Serum vitamin B_{12} (16–76 μg%)	Normal	Very low	Very low
Serum folate (0.3–2 μg%)	Normal	Very low	Normal
Anti-intrinsic factor antibodies	—	—	+

I. Peripheral blood examination

1. **Blood smear examination** : It indicates :
   (i) *Nature of RBCs* : Morphological defects, size (macro or microcytosis), shape (spherical, oval, etc.), colour reaction (hypochromic or normochromic).
   (ii) *Abnormal cell* : Premature red cell (normoblasts, megaloblasts, polychromasia).
   (iii) *White cells* : Hypersegmented neutrophils (as seen in megaloblastic anaemia), leucopenia (aplasia, hypoplasia of bone marrow).
   (iv) *Thrombocytes* : Thrombocytopenia and pancytopenia in aplastic/megaloblastic anaemia.
   (v) *Parasites* : Malarial parasite.
2. **Quantitative measurement**
   (i) ***Haemoglobin, PCV, RBC.***
   (ii) Determination of ***red cell indices*** — MCV, MCH, MCHC.
   (iii) ***Micrometry*** for MCD.
   (iv) *Total leucocyte count* : Leucopenia (bone marrow hypoplasia), high leucocyte count (fulminant infections, leukaemia).
   (v) *Reticulocyte count* : Reticulocytes are increased (5–20%) as response to haemolysis, haemorrhage and regenerative phase of anaemia after proper therapy.
   (vi) *ESR* : Mild rise is often seen in anaemia and in old age but a significant rise is observed in chronic infection, malignancy, autoimmune diseases.

II. Bone marrow smear examination

Bone marrow smear is examined for cellularity, nature of cell reaction and haemosiderin deposits (Table 16.7).

III. Special tests

Following special tests are sometimes necessary for accurate diagnosis of the case (Table 16.8) but which can be done only in specialised laboratories :

1. *Plasma iron*
2. *Serum ferritin*
3. *Serum* and *red cell folate* level
4. *Serum vitamin B_{12}* level
5. *Urinary forminoglutamic acid* (FIGLU)
6. *Schilling test*
7. *Osmotic fragility test of RBC*
8. *Coombs' test*
9. *Perl's staining for siderocytes* and *sideroblasts*

The diagnostic features of different types of anaemia are shown in Table 16.8.

Osmotic fragility test for RBC

Principle

When red cells become thinner than normal (their volume to surface area is increased) as in iron deficiency anaemia and thalassaemia major, osmotic fragility of red cells is decreased, i.e., osmotic curve shifts to the right.

A 0.85% sodium chloride solution is isotonic with plasma. The test measures the ability of red cells to swell in a graded series of hypotonic solution. Spherocytes are osmotically fragile and haemolyse more readily than normal cells in hypotonic solution. However, target cells are osmotically resistant.

Heparinised or defibrinated blood (preferable than EDTA or oxalated blood) is added to buffered saline (pH 7.4) in each tube in a proportion of 1 to 100. The test is performed in room temperature and lysis of red cells is noted.

Reagents

Stock solution (10% NaCl) : A buffered stock solution of buffered sodium chloride (AR) osmotically equivalent to 10 per cent NaCl, is prepared as follows :

NaCl	....	90.00 g
Na_2HPO_4	....	13.65 g
$NaH_2PO_4, 2H_2O$	....	2.43 g
Distilled water to	....	1 litre

Working solution (1% NaCl) : 10 ml of 10% stock solution is diluted to 100 ml with distilled water. Dilutions equivalent to 1.0, 0.9, 0.8, 0.7, 0.6, 0.5, 0.4, 0.2 and 0.1 per cent NaCl solution are convenient test concentrations made for use.

Method

Take 10 small test tubes in a row in a rack. Distilled water and 1% buffered saline solution, are mixed in order to have the solution of graded dilution as follows (Table 16.9) :

Table 16.9

DW in ml	1% saline in ml	NaCl %
9	1	0.1
8	2	0.2
7	3	0.3
6	4	0.4
5	5	0.5
4	6	0.6
3	7	0.7
2	8	0.8
1	9	0.9
0	10	1.0

To each tube 0.1 ml blood is then added and mixed well. The tubes are allowed to stand at room temperature for 30 minutes. Remix and centrifuge for 5 minutes at 2000 r.p.m. The amount of lysis of red cells in each tube is measured with that in 0.1% saline tube (100% lysis) with the help of a colorimeter using a green (Ilford 625) fiter.

Factors influencing osmotic fragility

1. *Relative volume of blood and saline* : Optimum result is obtained with 1 volume blood to 100–200 volumes of saline.

2. *Final* pH *of blood-saline suspension* : A shift of 0.1 of a pH unit is equivalent to altering the saline concentration by 0.1%. Hence a fall in pH increases osmotic fragility.

3. *Temperature at which test done* : Haemolysis is usually complete within 30 minutes at 0.1% hypotonic saline at 20°C.

Interpretation of results

Since the spherocytes are already round with increased volume to surface area ratio, they are unable to swell much. They rupture even when a small amount of water enters the cell.

Note the *three* tubes, *first* showing a trace of haemolysis (starting point), *second* with 5% haemolysis (median corpuscular fragility, MCF) and the *third* with 100% haemolysis. Their concentration is noted. When osmotic fragility is normal, red cells begin to haemolyse at 0.5% saline, reaches MCF at 0.4–0.42% saline and 100% lysis occurs in 0.30% saline. The results of haemolysis are plotted on a probability scale against concentration of saline and the fragility curve is obtained (Fig. 16.14).

Significance

1. *Increased osmotic fragility* : It is highly increased in hereditary spherocytosis. Lysis of red cells begins at 0.75% saline and complete lysis occurs at 0.45% saline. After splenectomy, red cells become more homogenous and fragility curve returns to normal.

Osmotic fragility is also increased in acquired spherocytosis (Table 16.5). If the acquired spherocytosis is of autoimmune origin, then direct Coombs' test is positive.

2. *Decreased osmotic fragility* : It is seen when volume to surface area ratio is decreased with low MCV and MCH, e.g., iron-deficiency anaemia, leptocytosis and thalassaemia.

Coombs' test

In immune haemolytic anaemias, the destruction of red cells results from the binding of auto-antibodies or complement components or both to the red cell membrane. IgM antibodies cause prompt red cell agglutination at room temperature, e.g., warm autohaemolytic anaemia. IgG antibodies are non-agglutinating.

The *direct antiglobulin (Coombs')* test is done to demonstrate antibodies (immunoproteins) present on the red cell membrane, e.g., examination of cord blood in erythroblastosis foetalis. The *indirect*

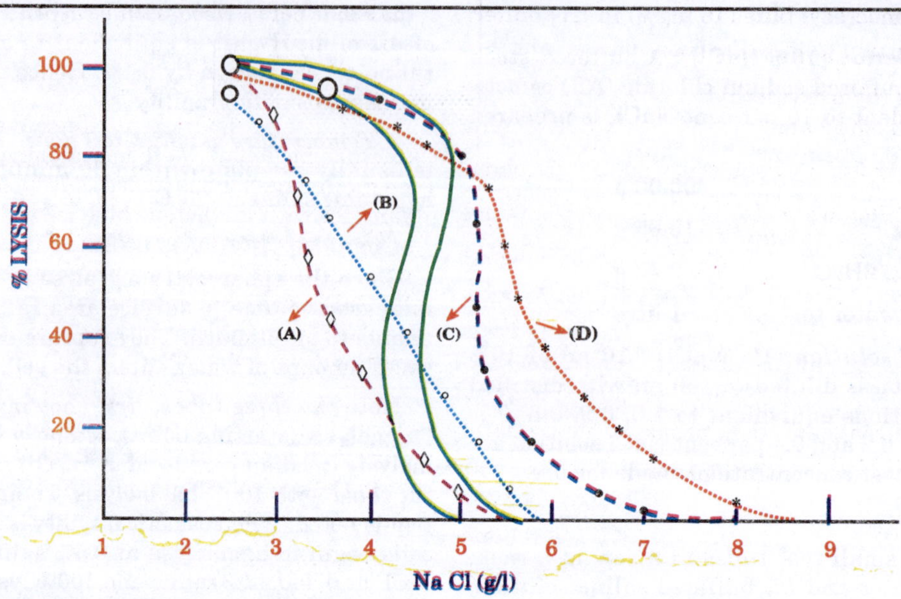

Fig. 16.14. Osmotic-fragility curves. Osmotic fragility curves of patients suffering from : (A) sickle cell anaemia ◊......◊. (B) β–thalassaemia major °........°. (C) hereditary spherocytosis •........•. (D) 'idiopathic' warm autoimmune haemolytic anaemia *........*. The normal range is indicated by the unbroken lines.

antiglobulin test is used to detect serum antibodies capable of attaching to normal red cells, e.g., autoimmune haemolytic anaemia.

Glucose–6–phosphate dehydrogenase (G6PD) deficiency assay

(Screening test)

The *Mediterranean type* (type A) G6PD deficiency found in black population of West Africa and USA show primaquine sensitivity. Both group A and group B types of G6PD deficiency are susceptible to haemolysis produced by oxidant drugs and infections. G6PD deficiency may be detected by one of the screening tests : *fluorescent spot test* or *a dye reduction test*. Confirmation is made with a quantitative assay.

1. Fluorescent spot test

Principle : Normally NADPH is an important reducing compound that converts oxidised glutathione (GSSG) to glutathione (GSH). GSH in red cell detoxifies low level of H_2O_2 and also maintains integrity of the red cell.

Whole blood (haemolysate) is added to a mixture of glucose–6–phosphate (G6P), NADP, saponin and buffer, and a spot of the mixture is placed on filter paper and examined under long wave (UV) light. G6PD present in the haemolysate converts NADP to NADPH which fluoresces under UV light. In G6PD deficiency there is an inability to produce sufficient NADPH which results in a lack of fluorescence.

2. Dye reduction test

(A) ***Bromocresyl blue test***

Principle : A mixture of glucose–6–phosphate, NADP and bromocresyl blue dye (in buffer) is incubated with haemolysate. NADP will be reduced to NADPH when G6PD is present in the haemolysate, which, in turn, will reduce the blue dye to its colourless form. The time required for this reduction to take place is inversely proportional to the amount of enzyme (G6PD) activity and is prolonged in individuals with G6PD deficiency. The reaction can be represented as :

(i) $\text{G–6–phosphate} + \text{NADP} \xrightleftharpoons{\text{G 6PD}} \text{6–phosphogluconolactone} + \text{NADPH}$

(ii) $\text{NADPH} + \dfrac{\text{Bromocresyl blue}}{\text{(Blue colour)}} \rightarrow \text{NADPH} + \dfrac{\text{Reduced dye}}{\text{(Colourless)}}$

Reagents

Commercial test kits are now available.

*1. Bromocresyl blue (16 mg%) in tris buffer.

Tris-HCl buffer (pH 8.5) :

Tris (hydroxymethyl aminomethane	....	2.42 gms
100 mol/L hydrochloric acid	....	54.00 ml
Distilled water to	....	100.00 ml

*2. $NADP^+$ .... 1.67 mg/ml

*3. G6P .... 152 mg anhydrous disodium salt, (mol. wt. 304.1) in 10 ml.

4. Dye reagent—It is prepared immediately before use by mixing :

Dye	....	8 volumes
$NADP^+$	....	1 volume
G6P	....	1 volume

Procedure

Step 1 : Preparation of red cell haemolysate :

Distilled water	....	2.50 ml
Fresh blood	....	0.05 ml

Mix well and allow to stand for 5 minutes at R.T.

Note : Use of fresh blood is preferable. However, anticoagulated blood (EDTA or heparin) may be used. If patient is anaemic, 0.1 ml blood is to be added in 2.5 ml distilled water.

Step 2 : Qualitative assay of enzyme :

(a) Add 1 ml of haemolysate to 0.5 ml of dye reagent and mix gently.

(b) Cover with 2 ml liquid paraffin or mineral oil immediately.

(c) Close the vial/tube, and incubate in water bath at 37°C.

Observe : The time required for the colour change from initial deep blue to reddish purple colour of reduced haemoglobin. Follow up to a maximum of 6 hours with 30 minutes intervals.

Results (Decolourisation time) :

(a) Normal subjects : 30–60 minutes.

(b) G6PD deficient subjects : 140 min–24 hours (heterozygous males, homozygous females).

(c) G6PD carriers (heterozygous females) : Some give results which overlap with normal males; others decolourise between 90 minutes to several hours.

(B) *Methaemoglobin reduction test*

Principle : Sodium nitrite converts Hb to Hi (methaemoglobin). Methaemoglobin persists when no methylene blue is added, but incubation of the samples with methylene blue leads to stimulation of pentose phosphate pathway in subjects with normal G6PD levels resulting in reduction of Hi. In G6PD deficient individuals, the block in the pentose phosphate pathway prevents the Hi reduction.

Reagents

1. *Sodium nitrite* — 180 m mol/l

2. *Dextrose*—280 m mol/l. Dissolve 5 g dextrose and 1.25g $NaNO_2$ in 100 ml water.

3. *Methylene blue* — 0.4 m mol/l. Dissolve 150 mg methylene blue chloride (methylthionine chloride) in 1 litre of distilled water.

Preparation of reagent : Mix equal volumes of sodium nitrate-dextrose with methylene blue, and 0.2 ml of the combined reagent is pipetted into each of several glass tubes. The tubes with the reagent are allowed to evaporate to dryness either at room temperature or at 37°C in an incubator. The reagents keep well at room temperature for six months.

Method

Test is done with anticoagulated blood (EDTA, heparin or ACD) within one hour of collection. Sample collected in ACD can be stored in refrigerator up to 1 week. In severely anaemic patient, adjust the PCV to 0.40 ± 0.05.

1. Add 2 ml blood to the tube containing 0.2 ml combined reagent (freshly prepared or dried).

2. The tube is closed by a stopper and gently inverted 15 times for mixing the contents.

3. Control tubes are prepared by adding 2 ml blood to a similar tube without reagents (normal reference tube) and to a tube containing 0.1 ml nitrite-dextrose mixture without methylene blue (deficient reference tube).

4. Samples are incubated at 37°C for 3 hours.

5. After incubation, 0.1 ml amounts from test sample, normal reference tube and deficient reference tube, are transferred into 10 ml amount of water in separate clear glass tubes of identical

diameter. The contents are mixed gently and colour in the different tubes are compared.

Interpretation

1. *Normal* : Colour similar to that in normal reference tube (clear red).

2. *Deficient subject* : Colour similar to that in the deficient reference tube (brown).

Prussian blue reaction for iron *(Pearl's stain)*

Principle **:** The dietary iron is absorbed in blood from stomach, duodenum and small intestine and then carried to its storage sites-bone marrow, liver and other tissues in the ferric form as haemosiderin (*vide Iron metabolism,* p.88) present in the reticuloendothelial cells as well as free in the marrow. Iron is demonstrated by prussian blue reaction.

Test procedure

(i) Bone marrow smear should be freshly collected and should contain marrow fragments because iron is demonstrable only in marrow particles.

(ii) The smear is fixed in methanol for 15 minutes and dried.

(iii) Equal volumes of 2% potassium ferrocyanide and N/5 HCl are mixed in a Coplin jar. The stain is warmed to 55°C just before use.

(iv) The fixed marrow smear is placed in the Coplin jar containing staining solution and kept for 30 minutes.

(v) The slide is then washed in running tap water for 15 minutes which is followed by washing in distilled water.

(vi) The smear in the slide is counterstained with 1% nuclear fast red or 0.1% neutral red that stain the nuclei red.

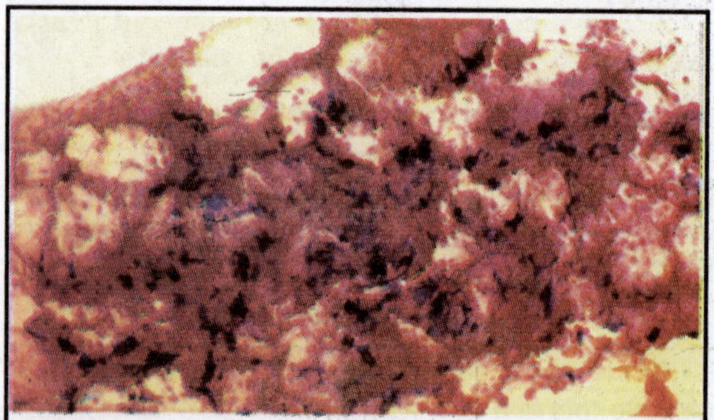

Fig. 16.15A. Pearl's stain (*Prussian blue reaction*) : Bone marrow fragment showing increased iron stores

Findings

(i) The smear on the slide is examined and looked for marrow particles with the help of a scanner objective.

(ii) The marrow particles are at first examined in low power objective and then using high power objective for presence of iron granules in reticuloendothelial cells and also for free iron.

Gradation of iron stores

The grading of iron stores is done in the following method :

(a) *Nil* — There is no iron containing macrophage/no free iron. This is indicative of iron deficiency anaemias.

(b) *Decreased* — Occasional macrophage containing granules are found on high power objective which is the main feature in *iron deficiency anaemias.*

(c) *Normal*—There are hemosiderin granules present in reticulum cells in marrow fragments/ free iron amongst marrow cells. It is detected under low power.

(d) *Increased* — When there is increased stored iron, hemosiderin granules are abundant inside the reticular cells and extracellularly (Fig. 16.15A), as found in *hemolytic anaemia*, in *anaemia of chronic renal failure, multitransfused patients* e.g., in thalassemia, aplastic anaemia (hemosiderosis), *megaloblastic anaemia* and *sideroblastic anaemia.*

The normoblasts are examined for iron granules. These are called *sideroblasts* and can be seen by oil immersion lens.

(a) *Normal sideroblasts* — There are 1-3 haemosiderin granules of pinpoint size in cytoplasm of late normoblasts.

(b) *Abnormal sideroblasts* — 1-10 pinhead size in late and intermediate normoblasts *e.g., megaloblastic anaemia.*

(c) *Ring sideroblasts* — These are coarse granules, 2-5 in number, arranged in a perinuclear ring pattern *e.g., sideroblastic anaemia.*

In all cases of deficiency anaemia bone marrow should be examined because it is a rapid and simple (Table 16.10) method of assessing iron stores. It is a very useful guide for chelation therapy in thalassemics and for differentiating thalassemia from iron deficiency anaemia.

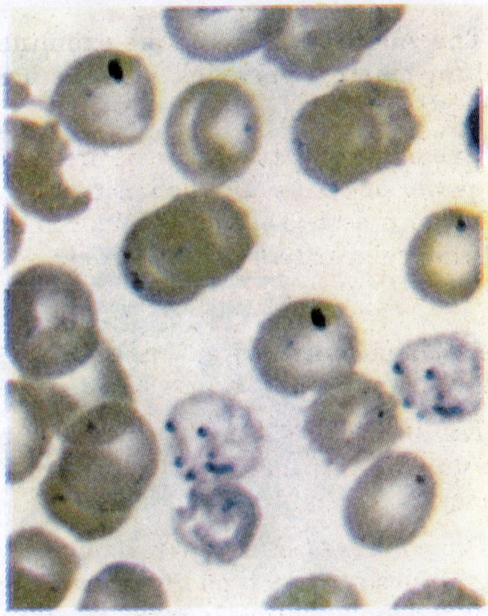

Fig. 16.15B. Siderocytes (Pappenheimer bodies) in blood film : Many erythrocytes show varying numbers of iron- containing granules which are deep blue in colour, the individual granules can be up to 2 μm in diameter. *(Prussian Blue reaction, May-Grunwald–Giemsa stain)*

Siderocytes (Pappenheimer bodies) in peripheral blood film may be found (Fig.16.15B) in red blood cell after splenectomy and not normally.

Note: Laboratory diagnosis of anaemia resulting from haemoglobinopathies are discussed in chapter 17.

MISCELLANEOUS CHANGES OF RED CELLS

For description of **target cells, elliptocytes** and other morphologically altered red cells — vide Table11.1 (Chapter Blood film).

Irregular contracted cells

Several types of irregularly-contracted red cells can be distinguished. In drug-induced haemolytic anaemia, a proportion of the cells appear contracted with slightly irregular margins (Fig. 16.16). These cells are smaller than normal and usually densely stained. Contracted red cells are also seen in favism and in films of some unstable haemoglobinopathies. These may be red cells from which Heinz bodies have been extracted by the spleen.

Table 16.10 : Distinguishing features of iron deficiency anaemia and thalassaemia major

Features	Iron deficiency anaemia	Thalassaemia major
Peripheral smear		
Anisocytosis and poikilocytosis	Mild	Moderate to severe
Target cells	Occasional	Plenty
Reticulocytes	Normal	10-12%
Abnormal red cells (normoblasts) :		
Early	Nil	2.3 %
Intermediate	Nil	3-5 %
Late	Nil	8-12 %
Abnormal white cells :		
Myelocytes	Nil	5-10%
Metamyelocytes	Nil	2-6 %
Biochemical tests		
Bone marrow iron store	Markedly depleted	Markedly increased
Serum iron content	Markedly diminished	Markedly increased
Blood transferin saturation	< 16 %	> 70 %
Serum bilirubin	Normal	Slightly raised
Serum electrophoresis		
Hb F	Nil	20-70 %
Clinical finding	Pallor	Hepatomegaly with pallor

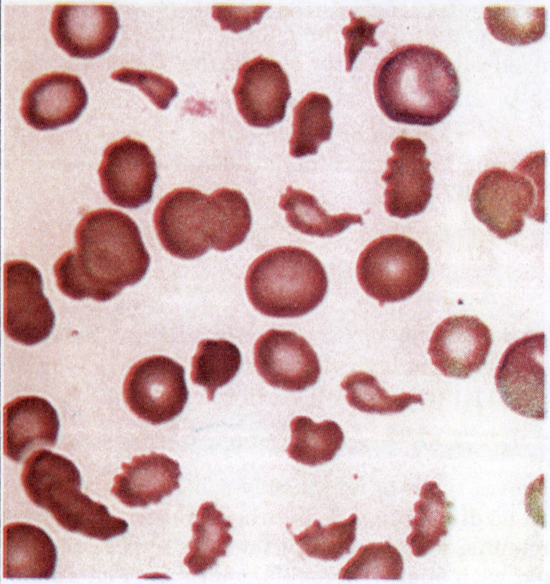

Fig. 16.16. Blood film Microangiopathic haemolytic anaemia : Contracted and distorted cells with irregular and angular shape. Such red cells are known as triangular or helmet cells. Red cell fragments, some with spinous processes and polychromatic cells are also present. *(Wright's stain)*

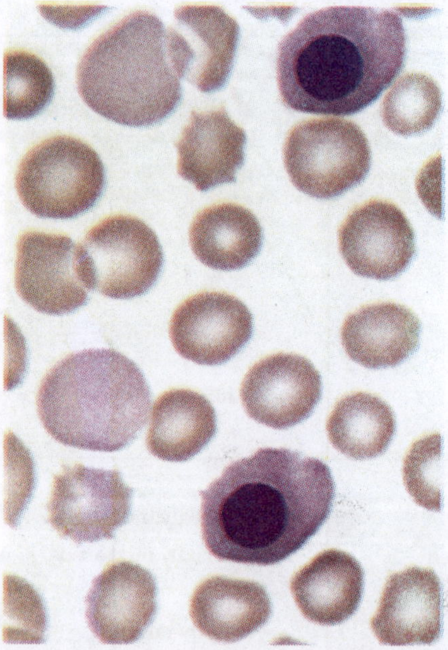

Fig. 16.17. Blood film showing polychromasia and nucleated red blood cells. The large polychromatic cells have stained blue grey and there are nucleated red blood cells. *(May-Grunwald–Giemsa stain)*

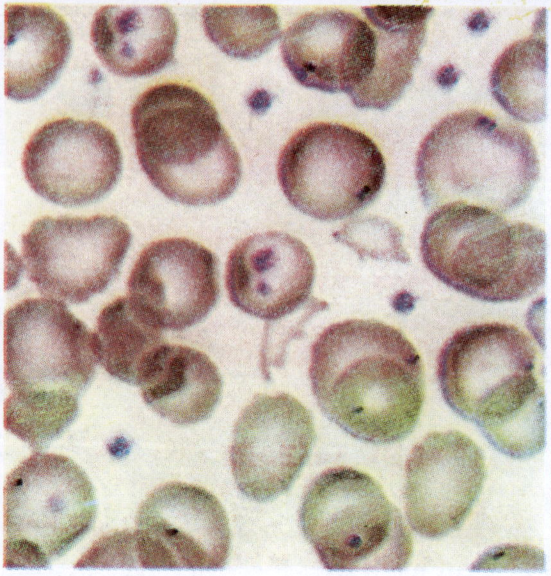

Fig. 16.18. Howell-Jolly bodies in peripheral blood: These are seen near the periphery of the cell (from a post-splenectomy patient who developed megaloblastic anaemia). Macrocytes contain Howell–Jolly bodies. *(Leishman stain)*

Polychromasia

Although the term suggests that the erythrocytes are being stained many colours, but in practice they are found to stain bluish grey — these are reticulocytes (Fig. 16.17). Cells that stain shades of blue, blue polychromasia, are usually young reticulocytes.

Siderocytes

Siderocytes are red cells that contain granules of non-haem iron. These granules are made of a water-insoluble complex of ferric iron, lipid, protein and carbohydrate. Siderotic material (or haemosiderin) reacts with potassium ferrocyanide giving a deep blue colour, i.e., positive *Prussian* blue reaction (Fig. 16.15B). When the granules are stained by Leishman stain (Romanowsky dyes), the granules appear as basophilic and are referred to as *Pappenheimer* bodies.

Significance of siderocytes

1. Siderocytic granules are not normally seen in peripheral blood except after splenectomy. Reticulocytes after delivery from borne-marrow are normally sequestered in the spleen for a time where they complete haem synthesis and utilise the iron stored in the cytoplasm. After splenectomy, ripening of reticulocytes takes place in the blood stream.

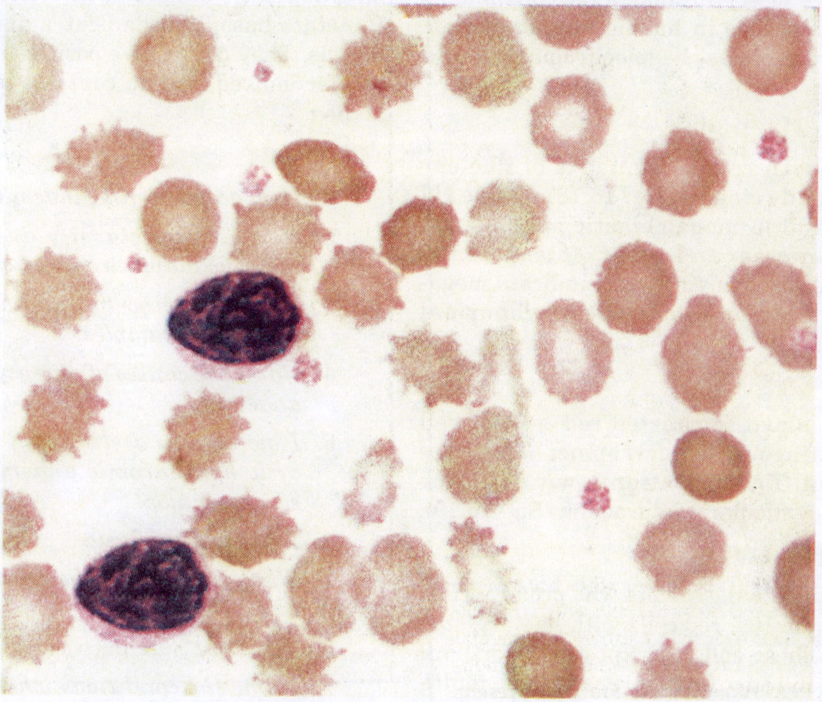

Fig. 16.19. Burr cells in peripheral blood : Blood film shows the contracted red blood cells with spiny surface projections which are often referred to as 'burr' cells because of their resemblance to the burrs from certain plants. Burr cells are deformed poikilocytes. These are commonly seen in chronic renal failure *(Leishman stain)*.

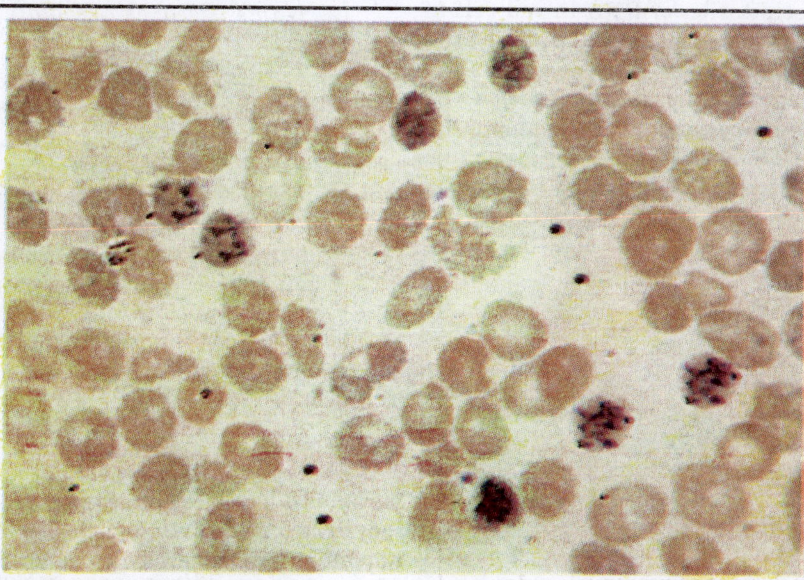

Fig. 16.20. Haemoglobin 'H' inclusions in peripheral blood smear showing small fine inclusions in the red cells that appear after incubation with Brillant Cresyl Blue see the contrast with the more coarse basophilic granules of the reticulocytes. *(Brilliant Cresyl Blue)*

2. Percentage of erythroblasts recognisable as *sideroblasts* increases in haemolytic anaemias, megaloblastic anaemias, haemochromatosis and haemosiderosis.

Howell–Jolly (HJ) bodies

These are smooth round remnants of nuclear chromatin (usually singly) (Fig. 16.18). Single HJ bodies are found in megaloblastic anaemia, in haemolytic anamia and after splenectomy. Multiple HJ bodies in a single cell indicate megaloblastic anaemia or some type of abnormal erythropoiesis.

Burr cells

Burr cells are small contracted red cells or cell fragments bearing one or a few spines. These are found in blood films of patients with various disorders, but particularly in uraemia (Fig. 16.19).

Haemoglobin H inclusions

In patients with α-thalassaemia who produce HbH (β4) contain some 10% red cells with haemoglobin H inclusions. These cells on exposure to brillant cresyl blue, as in reticulocyte preparations, multiple blue green spherical inclusions develop (Fig. 16.20).

Basophilic stippling

Basophilic stippling (or punctate basophilia) results from precipitation of RNA in red cell in which numerous granules are distributed throughout the cell (Fig. 16.21). These cells are associated with a significant increase in the generation of erythrocytes, as in response to haemorrhage or haemolysis, e.g., thalassaemia, megaloblastic anaemia, infection, liver disease. Punctate basophilia indicates disturbed erythropoiesis. They do not give positive reaction in *Perl's test* for ionised iron, in contrast to Pappenheimer bodies.

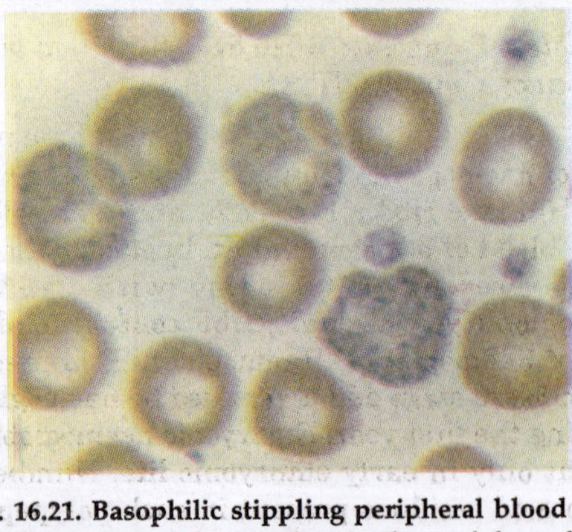

Fig. 16.21. Basophilic stippling peripheral blood film, shows fine basophilic stippling in three of the red cells present in this illustration (prepared from a patient suffering from lead poisoning). *(Leishman)*

QUESTIONS

1. *How do you define anaemia?*
2. *How do you classify anaemia on morphological appearance of red cells?*
3. *What is microcytic hypochromic anaemia, give some examples?*
4. *Name the causes of microcytic hypochromic anaemia.*
5. *How do you distinguish between microcytic hypochromic anaemia from thalassaemia major?*
6. *What is hypoplasia?*
7. *What is acquired haemolytic anaemia and name its causes?*
8. *What are Siderocytes and Burr cells?*
9. *Name the conditions where you get target cell (vide Table 11.1).*
10. *What is the pathogenesis of megaloblastic anaemia?*
11. *What are stomatocytes?*
12. *Name diseases associated with spherocytosis.*
13. *Name the hereditary red cell diseases associated with enzyme defect.*
14. *What is warm antibody?*
15. *What are the bone marrow changes in different anaemias?*
16. *What is osmotic fragility test and its use?*
17. *What are Hb-H inclusions?*
18. *What are siderocytes?*
19. *What is basophilic stipling?*
20. *What are deficiency anaemias?*
21. *Which is the common parasite producing deficiency anaemia?*
22. *How do you distinguish between hereditary spherocytosis and acquired spherocytosis of immunohaemolytic type?*
23. *Why some cells are osmotically fragile?*
24. *What is the cause of haemolysis in G6PD deficiency?*

Chapter 17

Haemoglobinopathies

NORMAL HAEMOGLOBIN MOLECULE

The main constituent of red cell is haemoglobin, nearly 90% of dry weight of red cell. The main function of red cell is to carry oxygen.

Haemoglobin is a globular molecule of conjugated protein (molecular weight 65000) made up of 4 subunits, each consisting of a haem core with a polypeptide chain attached (Fig. 17.1). The haem core is constant while the polypeptide chains occur in pairs. Haemoglobin type is determined by the amino acid sequence in the polypeptide chains. The haem groups transport oxygen.

There are thus 2 pairs of polypeptide chains (called globin) in each haemoglobin molecule, 2 of the sub-units containing one type of polypeptide and 2 containing another. Till now 5 types of polypeptide chains are identified, α, β, γ, δ and ε. On the basis of the nature of polypeptide chain pairs, four types of haemoglobins are described (Fig. 17.2) :

Haemoglobin A – $\alpha_2\ \beta_2$	97% adult Hb
Haemoglobin A2 – $\alpha_2\ \delta_2$	3% adult Hb
Haemoglobin F– $\alpha_2\ \gamma_2$	Foetal Hb
Embryonic haemoglobin $\alpha_2\ \varepsilon_2$	Early embryonic Hb

Note that α chain occurs in all normal haemoglobins. Normal adult haemoglobin is designated as HbA; foetal haemoglobin, HbF and that found in sickle cell anaemia, HbS. Since Hb synthesis is inherited from both parents, these Hb can be depicted as :

Normal adult haemoglobin = AA = (αα/ββ) = $\alpha_2\ \beta_2$

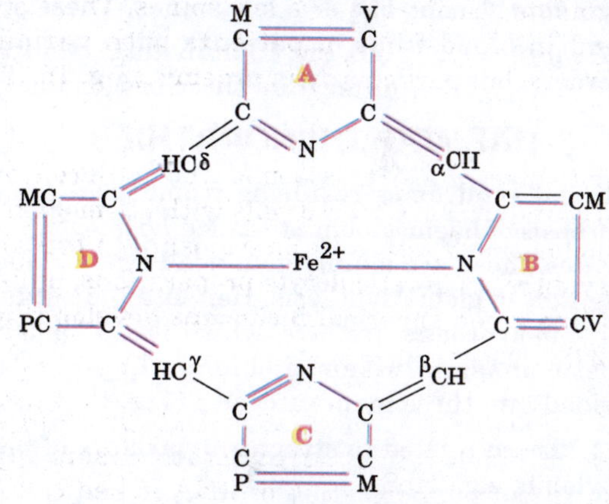

Fig. 17.1. Structure of haem with 4 pyrrole rings (A, B, C, D)

Sickle cell trait = AS = $\alpha_2\ \beta_2^{6\ val}$, differs from HbA in the substitution of valine for glutamine in the 6th position of the β chain amino acid sequence.

Sickle cell anaemia = Hb SS = $\beta_4^{6\ val}$, in which all haemoglobins are HbS.

Normal haemoglobin : There are three main types of haemoglobin found in normal individuals: HbA, HbF and HbA_2 (Fig. 17.2). The haemoglobin in the blood of a normal adult, haemoglobin A is mostly present (97%) along with 2–3% of haemoglobin A_2. In adult, HbF content is about 0.2% of haemoglobin. Haemoglobin F is present only in foetal stage and is replaced by haemoglobin A during the first year. Embryonic haemoglobin is present only in early embryonic life. Number of amino acid residues present in each polypeptide chain :

α chain 141

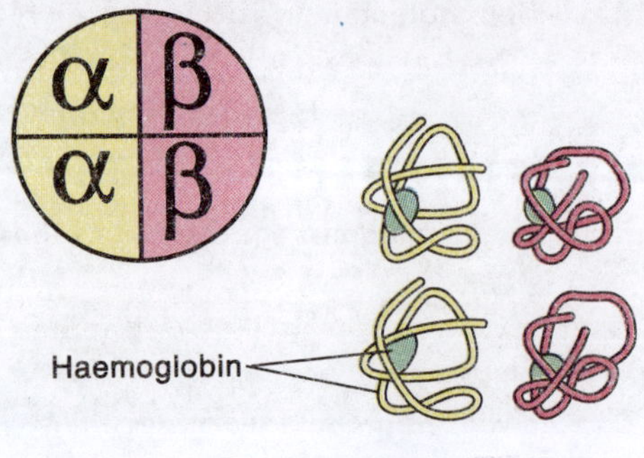

Fig. 17.2. Diagrammatic illustration to show structure of haemoglobin molecule

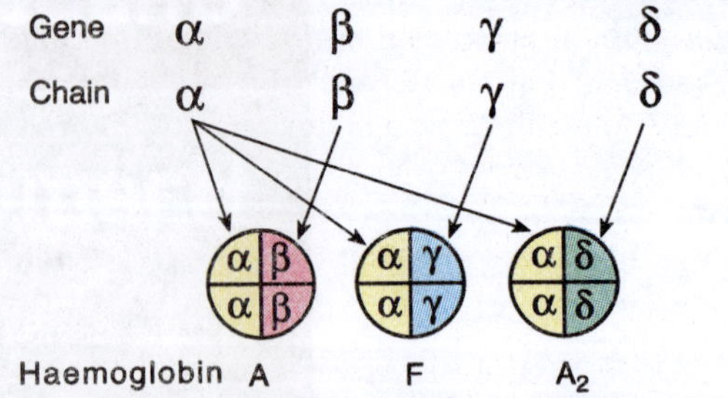

Fig. 17.3. Normal haemoglobin molecules formed by gene determined polypeptide chains which combine as dimers with α-γ β-γ and δ-chains

β chain	....	146
δ chain	....	146, but 10 individual residues differ from those of β chains.

HAEMOGLOBINOPATHIES

Clinical syndromes resulting from disorders of synthesis of haemoglobin are called *haemoglobinopathies.* These are mainly genetically determined disorders of globin synthesis. Hereditary disorders of haem synthesis are rare, which lead to sideroblastic anaemia. Haemoglobinopathies may be divided into three main categoies (Fig. 17.2).

1. Those related to structural variants of haemoglobin, e.g., HbS.

2. Those due to failure to form HbA, e.g., thalassaemia.

3. Those due to *failure to complete the normal neonatal switch* from HbF to adult HbA, which leads to a group of disorders called hereditary persistence of foetal haemoglobin (HPFH).

HAEMOGLOBIN VARIANTS

History : There is chemical difference between fetal (F) and adult (A) haemoglobin which has been known for over 140 years (Von Körber, 1866). Immunologic differences between these two haemoglobins were studied more recently (Darrow *et. al.,* 1940). Herrick in 1910 first described a clinical entity belonging to this group, sickle cell anaemia. Pauling *et al.* (1949) opened a new chapter in introducing fruitful field of investigation of haemoglobinopathy when they reported specific and characteristic properties of sickle cell haemoglobin. The studies initiated by them made a new approach to the study of variants of human haemoglobins, which subsequently led to much information of clinical importance.

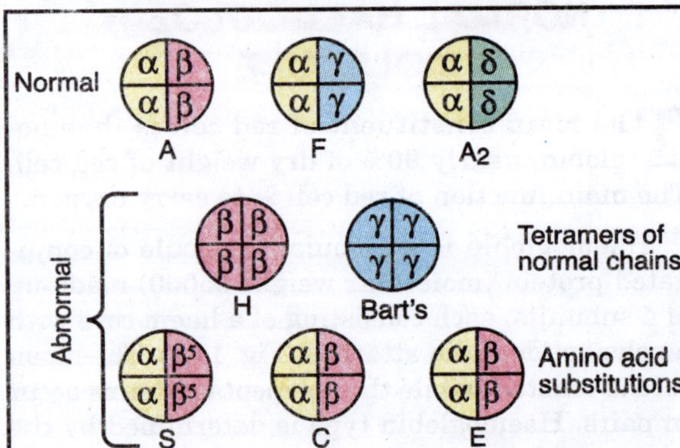

Fig. 17.4. Common types of normal and abnormal haemoglobin molecules

Table 17.1
Functional classification of Hb variants

Hb polymorphism	HbS	$\alpha_2\ \beta_2^{6\ val}$	Sickle cell trait
	HbC	$\alpha_2\ \beta_2^{6\ Lys}$	Mild haemolytic anaemia
	HbD Punjab	$\alpha_2\ \beta_2^{121\ Glut}$	No anaemia
	HbE	$\alpha_2\ \beta_2^{26\ Lys}$	Mild microcytic anaemia
Tetramers of normal chains	Hb Bart's	γ_4	
	HbH	β_4	
	Hb($\alpha^A{}_4$)	α_4	
Other Variants	Hb Lepore	$\alpha_2\ (\beta\ \delta)_2$	Contain two normal α-chains with two abnormal hybrid chains consisting of the β– and δ– chains

Haemoglobin variants in 90% cases, usually result from substitution of a single amino acid by an amino acid of a different type in a single chain, but multiple substitutions do occur and more than one chain may be involved. Over 300 variants are recognised but only a few produce clinical disease, the most common being haemoglobins S, C, D and E.

More than 18 different varieties of haemoglobins are already fully characterised and identified. Other variants of haemoglobin have been announced and await identification, and undoubtedly more will follow.

Nomenclature : By international agreement, capital letters of the alphabet are used for their identification in the order of discovery, except for those that had already been associated with a particular letter at the time when the new nomenclature was agreed upon. When two or more haemoglobins are involved in a haemoglobinopathy syndrome, the major is listed first; the same preference is given to thalassemia.

Biochemistry : The genetically determined haemoglobin differences are located in the globin component of haemoglobin, not in the haeme. Till now, significant biochemical differences have been found in Hb F (fetal haemoglobin), specifically in the total amino acid composition as compared with Hb A.

Modern nomenclature includes the number of amino acid residue in the superscript along with the substituted amino acid residue; e.g.

HbS = $\alpha_2\ \beta_2{}^{6\ val}$ ... i.e., at position 6 glutamine is replaced by valine.

Genetic regulation

Control of haemoglobin synthesis is inherited from both parents.

1. *Genetic defects* inherited as autosomal codominants.
2. *One normal and one abnormal gene* : heterozygous.
3. *Both abnormal genes* : homozygous.

In most haemoglobinopathies there is anaemia of varying degrees. The anaemia is hemolytic for which the haemoglobin abnormality is responsible. Another finding common to most haemoglobinopathies is presence of target cells in the peripheral blood. Their numbers vary. They are characteristic but not specific.

The inherited disorders of haemoglobinopathies may be classified as follows :

I. **Structural haemoglobinopathies**

Synthesis of haemoglobin occurs with altered amino acid sequence resulting in production of defective haemoglobins, e.g., Hb S, haemoglobin sickling.

II. **Thalassaemias**

There is defective biosynthesis of globin chains leading to decreased synthesis of either α– or β–globin chain of Hb A ($\alpha_2\ \beta_2$).

1. α Thalassaemias
2. β Thalassaemias
3. δβ, γδβ, αβ Thalassaemias

III. **Thalassaemic haemoglobin variants**

1. HbE
2. Hb constant spring
3. Hb Lepore

Identification of the Haemoglobins

Alkali Denaturation. Hb F is resistant to denaturation by highly alkaline solutions whereas all other

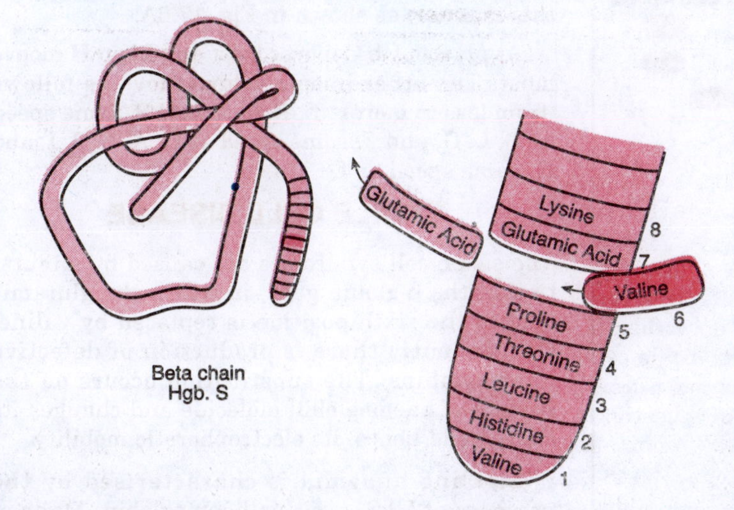

Fig. 17.5. Substitution of valine for glutamic acid in 6th position from amino terminal in β-polypeptide chain, producing sickle cell haemoglobin (Hb S) ($\alpha_2\ \beta_2$ 6 Glu → Val)

Table 17.2 : Result of analysis of blood in different Hereditary Anaemias

	Haemoglobin A	Haemoglobin F	Haemoglobin S	Haemoglobin C	Anaemia	Target Cells	Sickled Cells in Blood Smear	Nucleated Red Cells	Increased Reticulocytes	Stippled Cells	Hypochromia	Hemolytic Jaundice	Splenomegaly
	%	%	%	%									
Normal newborn	10–50	45–90	–	–	–	–	–	±	±	–	–	–	–
Normal adult	97–100	0–2	–	–	–	–	–	–	–	–	–	–	–
Sickle cell trait	50–80	N	20–40	–	–	0–4	–	–	–	–	–	–	–
Sickle cell anaemia (homozygous Hb S)	–	N-25	30–99	–	+++	5–30	++	+	+	–	–	+	±
Hb C trait	55–75	N	–	25-40	–	0–40	–	–	–	–	–	–	–
Homozygous Hb C	–	N–4	–	60–99	+	40-100	–	±	+	–	–	+	+
β–Thalassaemia minor	98–100	N	–	–	+	5–10	–	±	+	+	++	±	+
β–Thalassaemia major	10–90	10–90	–	–	++++	10–40	–	+++	++	+	++	++	+++
Sickle cell-Hb C	–	N–10	35-65	35-65	++	20-80	+	+	+	–	–	+	++
Sickle cell-thalassaemia	0–20	N-20	60-90	–	+++	20-40	+	++	+	+	+	+	++

N = normal; + = presence of condition; – = absence of condition

human haemoglobins are destroyed alkali. This method can detect Hb F when present in excess of 2 per cent of the total haemoglobin.

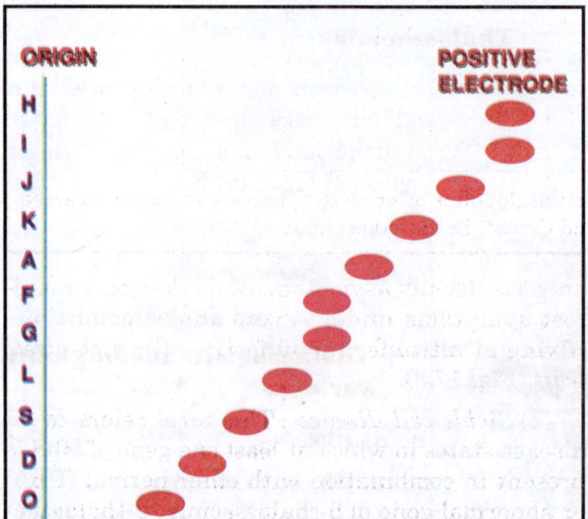

Fig. 17.6A. Relative migrations of the human haemoglobins after electrophoresis on filter paper

Paper Electrophoresis

Proteins are electrically charged molecules. They move at different rates of speed in an electric field. Additional differences are related to the hydrogen ion concentration of the solution employed. Most of the haemoglobins are identified in this manner, as shown in Fig. 17.6A.

At pH 8.6, Hb C moves least and I and H mopve most. The other haemoglobins move as follows (from less to more) : E, Q, D, Q and S, same speed as D; L, G, and F, same speed as G; A, K, J, I, and H, same speed as I.

SICKLE CELL DISEASE

The sickle cell syndromes are caused by a mutation in the β-globin gene, in which the glutamic acid in the sixth position is replaced by valine. Consequently there is production of defective haemoglobins. The substitution occurs on the surface of haemoglobin molecule and changes its charge and hence, its electrophoretic mobility.

Sickling anaemia is characterised by the presence of HbS — sickle haemoglobin. Many of the erythrocytes exhibit a definite sickle shape and stain much more heavily than surrounding erythrocytes.

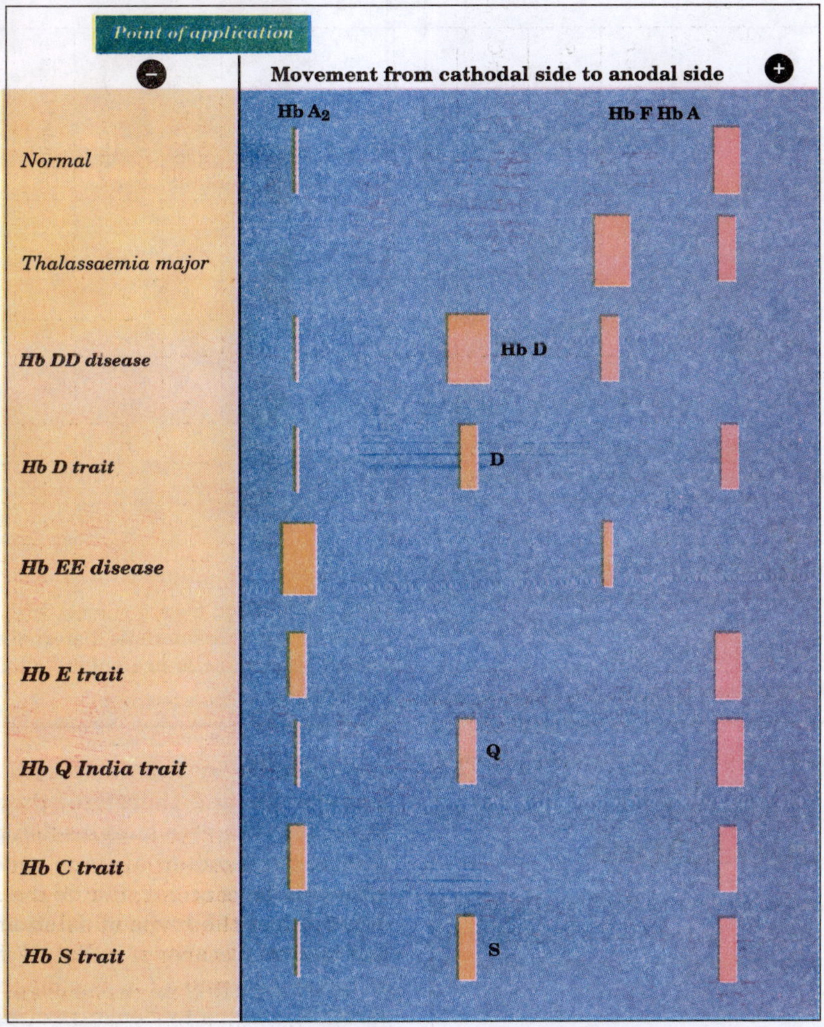

Fig. 17.6B. Figure shows relative migration of human immunoglobulins after electrophoresis on starch Agarose at pH 8.6, Hb S, D, Q move in the same region; Hb A_2, E and C move in the same region

HbS — Substitution of valine for glutamic acid in 6th position of β chain ($\alpha_2\ \beta_2^{6\ val}$). See table 17.2.

Types

(1) *Sickle cell trait* (Hb–AS); heterozygous, symptoms are mild; resistant to falciparum malaria.

(2) *Sickle cell anaemia* (Hb–SS); Homozygous HbS disease (Fig. 17.7).

Homozygous individuals (Hb SS), in whom all the haemoglobin is HbS, always show manifestations of sickle cell disease and this may be fatal in childhood. Heterozygotes (Hb AS) have 40–50% HbS, are carriers of the sickle gene, and most patients are usually asymptomatic as they only manifest symptoms under severe anoxic conditions (flying at altitude, 15000 feet) — the *sickle cell trait* (Fig. 17.8).

(3) *Sickle cell disease* : This term refers to all disease states in which at least one gene of HbS is present in combination with other normal (HbA) or abnormal gene of β-thalassaemia, α-thalassaemia, HbD, HbE, HbC, HbQ or any other haemoglobinopathy (Table 17.2).

HbS/C disease behaves like a mild variety of sickle cell anaemia. HbF reduces the risk of sickling, for this reason clinical symptoms do not develop before the age of six months.

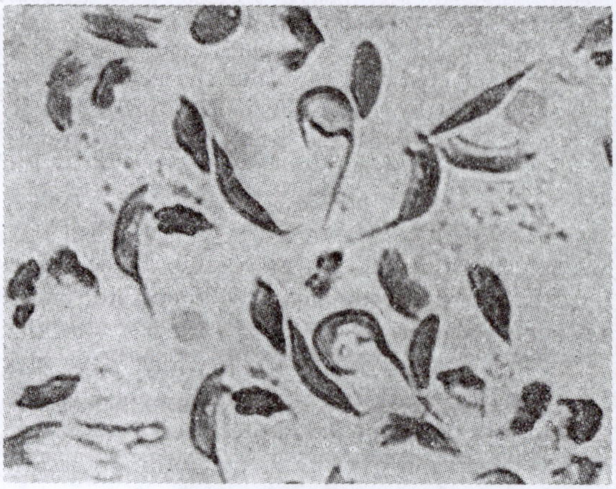

Fig. 17.7. Blood film : HbSS disease showing target cells and sickle cells (metabisulfate preparation)

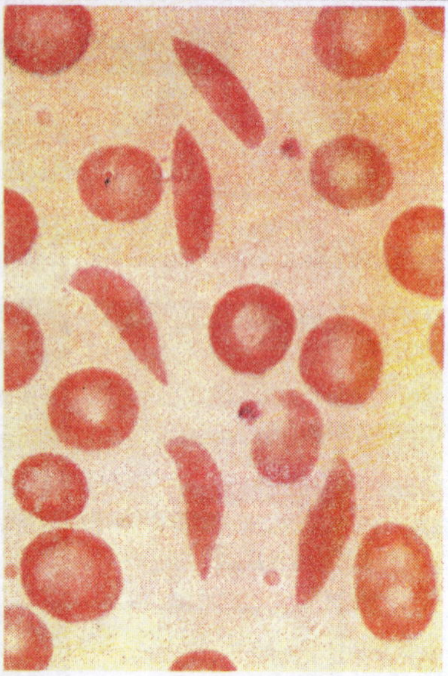

Fig. 17.8. Blood from a subject with sickle cell trait showing the characteristic distorted shapes assumed when the red cells are subjected to a low oxygen tension

Epidemiology : Patients with sickle cell anaemia are frequently found in equatorial Africa. Sickle haemoglobin is named for the fact that red cells on incubation in absence of oxygen acquire the shape of a sickle or half-moon.

Clinical features : HbS molecules stack abnormally and cause sickling in reduced oxygen state producing anaemia, splenomegaly, haemolytic jaundice and poor general resistance. The heterozygous trait is considered as carrier or trait.

THALASSAEMIA

Thalassaemia develops due to lack or diminished level of synthesis of α or β globin chain of HbA. Classification of thalassaemias are given in tables 17.3 and 17.4.

(1) Alpha (α) thalassaemia : The α chains are coded for by two duplicated genes on chromosome 16, and therefore, there are 4 genes. Thus, for complete suppression of α chain synthesis, deletions of all four genes is required. Abnormalities of varying degrees are produced depending on the type of deletion. Classification and clinical features of α-thalassaemia are shown in tables 17.2 and 17.3. The diagnosis of α-thalassaemia is made by demonstrating a reduced α/β chain ratio.

Table 17.3 : Alpha thalassaemia : Classifiction and clinical features

Gene	*Genotype*	*Clinical and laboratory features*	*Hb pattern*	
			Newborn	After first year
One gene deleted	– α/αα	Silent α–thalassaemia	Hb Bart's 1–2%	None
Two genes deleted	– –/αα	α–thalassaemia trait, mild anaemia and hypochromia	Hb Bart's 2–20%	None
Three genes deleted	– –/–α	HbH disease; haemolytic (Hb 7-9 g/dl); red cells severely hypochromic with HbH inclusions, may become folate deficient	Hb Bart's 20–40%	Hb H 5–30% Hb Bart's ± trace
Four genes deleted	– –/– –	Lethal in utero with hydrops foetalis (still-born baby)	Hb Bart's > 80% HbH, Hb Portland	

α-thalassaemia is most common in Asians. The four common classic α-thalassaemias include (see Table 17.3) :

(i) α-thalassaemia–2 trait, in which one of the four α-globin loci (α gene) is deleted;

(ii) α-thalassaemia–1 trait, in which two coci are deleted.

(iii) *HbH disease,* with three loci deleted; and

(iv) *hydrops foetalis,* with all the four loci deleted, with Hb Bart's.

Thalassaemia—2 trait is silent carrier state and asymptomatic.

α-thalassaemia–1 trait resembles β–thalassaemia minor. It produces asymptomatic hypochromia and microcytosis.

Haemoglobin H disease (Fig. 17.12A and B) : HbH is β chain tetramer, Hb (β_4), in which three of the 4α chain genes are absent. Functionally, HbH is useless. A chronic anaemia with the clinical picture of thalassaemia intermedia is usual, though the severity varies. The disease has been described in all racial groups, especially in South-East Asia, Middle-East and Greece. It is rare in Negroes.

Blood picture shows decreased MCV and MCH with hypochromia and target cells. Reticulocyte count ranges between 4 to 5%. Vital staining with brilliant cresyl blue (oxidising dye) induces pale blue inclusion bodies (HbH precipitates) in many red cells, which contrasts with the deep blue precipitates of RNA in reticulocytes. Single large Heinz bodies are seen after splenectomy.

(2) Beta (β) thalassaemia – Table 17.5

The β chains are coded for by a single gene on

Table 17.4
Beta thalassaemia : Classification and clinical features (β^+ = some β chains present)

Genotype	Type	Clinical and laboratory features
β^o/β^o, β^+/β^+ } Homozygous	*Thalassaemia major;* transfusion dependent; 98% HbF; HBA — absent, excess α chains form aggregates in red cells and red cell precursors	Severe hypochromic microcytic anaemia; increased reticulocyte count; target cells and basophilic stippling; increased iron stores; nucleated red cells present, requires blood transfusion.
β^o/β, β^+/β^+	*Thalassaemia intermedia*	Severe, but does not need regular blood transfusion.
β^o/β, β^+/β } Heterozygous	*Thalassaemia minor;* raised HbA_2	Mild to moderate hypochromic microcytic anaemia.

Table 17.5 : β–Thalassaemias

Syndrome	Genotype	Clinical and laboratory features	Hb pattern
Homozygous states :			
β^+ thalassaemia	β^+/β^+	Thalassaemia major: or thalassaemia intermedia	↓ Hb A. ↑ Hb F, variable Hb A_2
β^o thalassaemia	β^o/β^o	Thalassaemia major	0 Hb A, variable Hb A_2 residual Hb F
$\delta\beta^o$ thalassaemia	$\delta\beta^o/\delta\beta^o$	Thalassaemia intermedia	0 Hb A and Hb A_2, 100% Hb F
Hb Lepore	Lepore/Lepore	Thalassaemia major	0 Hb A, Hb A_2; 75% Hb F, 25% Hb Lepore
Heterozygous states :			
β^+ thalassaemia	β^+/β^+	Thalassaemia minor	↑ Hb A_2, slight ↑ Hb F
β^o thalassaemia	β^o/β	Thalassaemia minor	↑ Hb A_2, slight ↑ Hb F
δ/β^o thalassaemia	$\delta\beta^o/\delta\beta$	Thalassaemia minor	5–20% Hb F
Hb Lepore	Hb Lepore/β	Thalassaemia minor	↑ Hb F, ↓ Hb A_2, 5–15% Hb Lepore

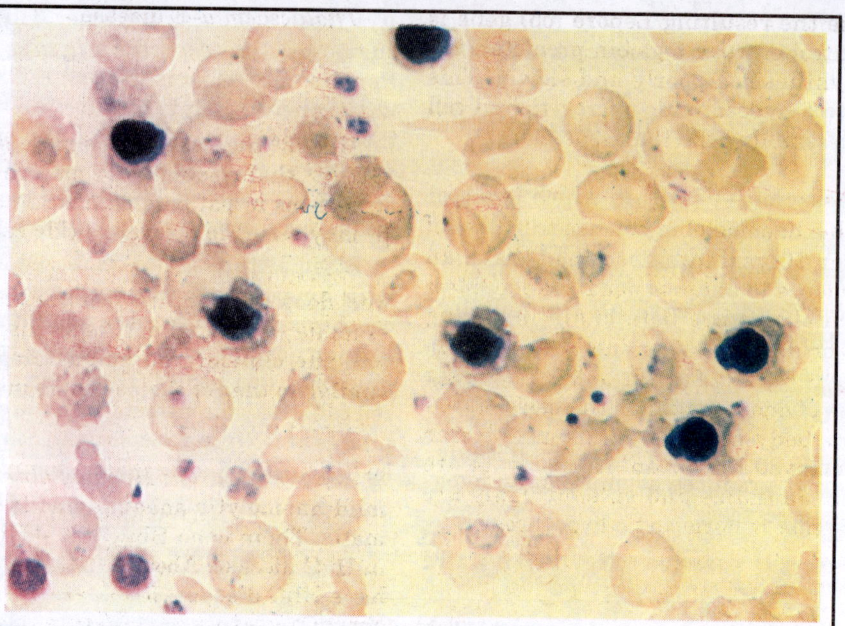

Fig. 17.9. Blood film : β-thalassaemia major showing late normoblasts, few, target cells, hypochromasia, anisochromasia, anisocytosis and numerous poikilocytes

chromosome 11. Mutations in this gene result in a failure to synthesise β chains (β^o) or in reduced synthesis of β chains (β^+). Failure to form β chain (β–chain thalassaemia) is the commonest type and is frequently seen in the Mediterranean area. Failure to synthesise β-chain leads to an excess of α chains within red cells which gets precipitated and damage the erythrocytes. Since the α chains do not form tetramers, there is no abnormal Hb formed. The deficiency of HbA is compensated by an increase in HBA_2 and F.

β–thalassaemia is the commonest type and prevalent throughout the world in large number.

These cells with accumulated free α chains are destroyed in the R.E.S. (extravascular haemolysis).

Types of β-thalassaemia (Table 17.4)

1. *Thalassaemia minor* : Heterozygotes, presents as hypochromic microcytic anaemia with little or no clinical disability (Figs. 17.10, 17.11).

2. *Thalassaemia intermedia* : It is the double heterozygotous state in which there occurs moderately severe anaemia. Such patients grow into adulthood and are not transfusion dependent.

3. *Thalassaemia major* (Cooley's anaemia) (Figs. 17.9, 17.11) : Cooley and Lee (1925) first described the severe and fatal form of anaemia of erythroblastic type which was peculiar to children of Mediterranean origin. Homozygotes develop serious haemolytic anaemia accompanied by splenomegaly and mild jaundice. Repeated blood transfusion is necessary. Demonstration of thalassaemia trait in both parents is usually adequate to establish the diagnosis.

Distribution

About 250 million, 4.5% of world population is affected by thalassaemia and allied disorders (WHO Report, 1995). β-thalassaemia is prevalent throughout running from Mediterranean, North-west Africa through the Middle east, Pakistan, India and South-East Asia. **Higher prevalence is seen Greece, Cyprus, Sardinia, Italy, Thailand and parts of Malaysia**. In India, β-thalassaemia is observed throughout the country and a 35 million people are carriers with a higher incidence in the Punjabis, Sindhis, Bengalis, Gujratis, Parsis and Lohanas.

Haemoglobin Lepore [$\alpha_2\ (\delta\beta)_2$]

Hb Lepore [$\alpha_2\ (\delta\beta)_2$] is an abnormal haemoglobin having a normal α-chain combined with a composite δβ-chain (Table 17.5). This arises as a result of chromosome misalignment by an unequal crossover and recombination event that fuses the proximal end of the δ-gene with the distal end of the closely linked β-gene resulting in a fused δβ gene. Because the resulting Lepore (δβ) gene is under the control of weak δ-globin promoter, the δβ-chain is synthesised poorly and slowly. This fusion leads to a hypochromic microcytic red cell morphology resembling the thalassaemias.

UNSTABLE HAEMOGLOBIN

The unstable haemoglobin belongs to a class of mutants, over 70 variants described, have an increased tendency to undergo denaturation. Most of the abnormalities are beta chain involving substitution or deletion of amino acid, e.g., Hb Bristol $\alpha_2\beta_2{}^{67Asp}$, Hb Zurich $\alpha_2\beta_2{}^{63Arg}$. This increased rate of denaturation is the basis of congenital Heinz body haemolytic disease. Heinz bodies are removed by spleen. All patients are heterozygous. Jaundice and splenomegaly are common. Anaemia is normocytic hypochromic.

(3) THALASSAEMIA IN ASSOCIATION WITH ABNORMAL HAEMOGLOBINS

Thalassaemia is often associated with abnormal haemoglobins, such as HbS, HbC, HbD, HbE, etc. Such thalassaemic states associated with abnormal haemoglobin are manifested as :

Thalassaemia–S disease

Thalassaemia–C disease

Thalassaemia–D disease

Thalassaemia–E disease

Sickle cell thalassaemia (HbS /β° thalassaemia)

HbS /β° thalassaemia is more dangerous than HbS/β⁺ thalassaemia. β⁺ may result in clinical symptoms in patients with sickle cell trait, while β° may result in a severe sickle cell syndrome.

β-thalassaemia with HbC or HbD is mild and does not require treatment. HbE/β thalassaemia, a South-East Asian disorder, is severe and the clinical and haematological picture is similar to that of thalassaemia major.

OTHER HAEMOGLOBIN DISEASES

HAEMOGLOBIN C : *Haemoglobin C disease* is a mild haemolytic anaemia and is often asymptomatic. There is no HbA, 93% – HbC and 7% HbF in HbC disease. About 0.02% Negroes in America have HbC disease. RBCs are normocytic normochromaic with an admixture of microcytes and spherocytes, numerous target cells and a few reticulocytes. *HbC trait* (HbAC), heterozygous asymptomatic state without anaemia and is prevalent in West Africans and in 2–3% American blacks. Mild hypochromia with about 40% targets may be present.

HAEMOGLOBIN D : It is found in India. HbD-

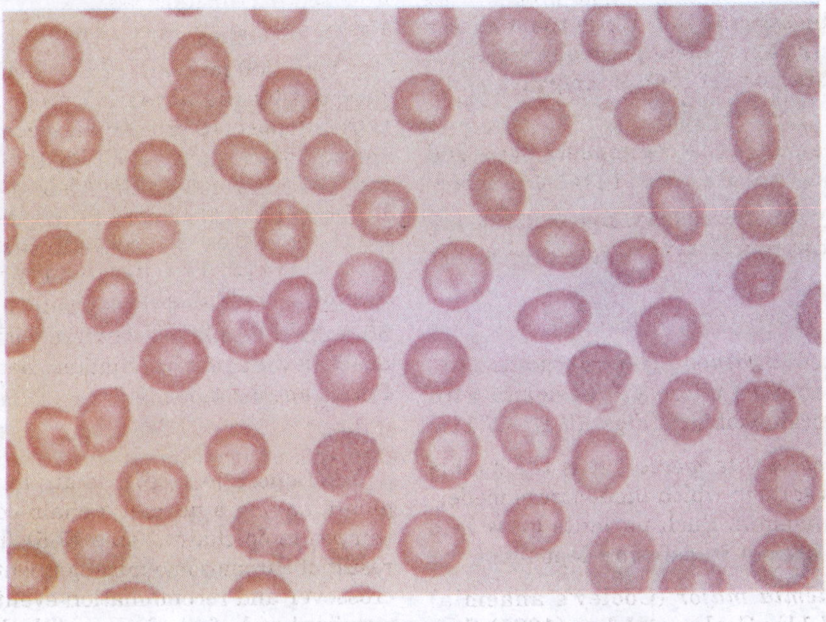

Fig. 17.10. Blood film : β-thalassaemia minor

Punjab and HbD-Los Angles are the same (α_2 $\beta_2^{121\ Gln}$) and constitute the most common D-variant in blacks in America (< 0.02 per cent). The trait shows normal blood smear and is asymptomatic. Incidence of homozygous D disease is rare, and virtually asymptomatic without anaemia. In some persons, a few target cells may be found and osmotic fragility is decreased. In HbD disease, HbD is 95% and HbA_2 is normal.

HAEMOGLOBIN E : HbE is found in South-East Asia including India, but does not occur in blacks. HbE trait (HbAE) is asymptomatic without any haemotologic abnormality. Homozygous HbE disease is a mild anaemia with microcytosis and target cells and a slightly decreased red cell survival.

LABORATORY INVESTIGATIONS

Test employed

1. Blood count and stained film study
2. Osmotic fragility of red cells
3. Sickling phenomenon of red cells (HbS)
4. Alkali denaturation test for estimation of HbF
5. Estimation of HbA_2
6. Bone marrow study
7. Electrophoretic study for haemoglobin by cellulose acetate paper strip at alkaline pH.

A. BLOOD COUNT AND FILM

1. **Blood count** : A full blood count including red cell, white cell, reticulocyte, platelet count, haemoglobin level, MCV and MCH, provides useful information for the diagnosis of thalassemia (α and β).

2. **Peripheral smear** : Peripheral smear shows characteristic red cell changes, such as target cells with HbC and sickle cells with HbS.

Blood picture thalassaemia :

Hb	.....	usually less than 10 gms%
MCV, MCH, MCHC	.....	diminished
Total RBC	.....	3-3.5 million /cu.mm
Total WBC	.....	10,000–30,000/cu.mm shift to left
Total platelets	.....	1-3 lacs/cu. mm
Reticulocytes	.....	10-12%

Different count :

Neutrophils	.....	50-60%
Lymphocytes	.....	15-25%
Monocytes	.....	5-10%
Eosinophils	.....	2-4%
Basophils	.....	0-5%
Abnormal cells		
Myelocytes	.....	5-10%
Metamyelocytes	.....	2-6%
Normoblasts		
Early	.....	2-3%
Intermediate	.....	3-5%
Late	.....	8-12%

Morphologically, the red cells show features of anisocytosis, poikilocytosis, hypochromia, polychromasia and presence of target cells.

3. **Reticulocyte count** : Reticulocytes are moderately increased in haemolytic anaemias (10-15%). Reticulocytosis is a hallmark of haemolytic anaemia that reflects the ability of the bone marrow to respond.

B. OSMOTIC FRAGILITY OF RED CELLS

Osmotic fragility of red cells is moderately decreased in thalassaemia and hereditary elliptocytosis. Reticulocytes and red cells from splenectomised patients are osmotically resistant due to a greater amount of cell membrane compared to normal red cells.

C. SICKLING TEST

Principle

It is a screening test to detect HbS. Sickling can be observed by sealing a drop of blood between a glass slide and a coverslip as wet film and incubating at 37°C for 1 hour. The red cells become distorted, appearing like leaf or sickles when oxygen in the blood has been used up almost completely.

The process of sickling is hastened up by addition of a drop of reducing substance like glucose, sodium metabisulfite or sodium dithionite solution to blood, which enhances deoxygenation of Hb and sickling of HbS.

Method

Two types of screening tests are in current use, both detect presence of HbS in red cells but do not distinguish sickle cell trait from other sickle

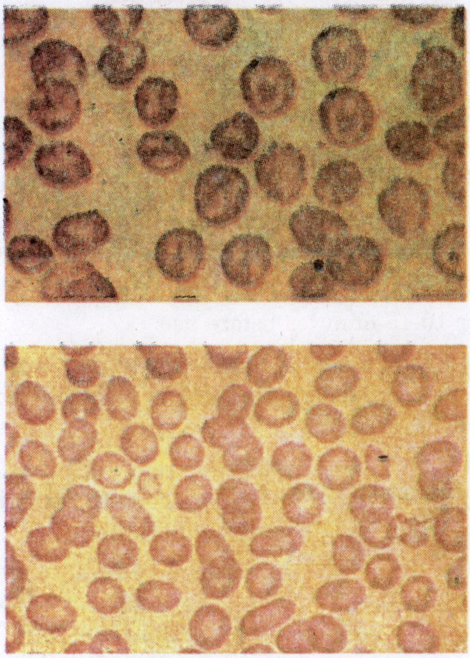

Fig. 17.11.(A) Blood film, **haemoglobin C disease. The numerous target cells and cells with an elongated central density are characteristic. (B)** Blood film, **beta-thalassaemia** trait. Microcytosis; increased number of elliptocytes.

syndromes. However, sickling occurs more rapidly with greater amounts of HbS in the cells. In cases with positive sickling, haemoglobin electrophoresis (Fig. 17.6) should be done for precise diagnosis of sickle syndrome.

1. **Sickling test** — Using metabisulfite : Standard "sickle cell preparation" consists of mixing a drop of blood over a glass slide with a drop of 0.2% sodium metabisulfite solution on which a cover- glass is placed and then the border of the coverslip is sealed with petroleum jelly so that no air can enter the wet film. The film is incubated at 37°C for 30 minutes and examined under microscope (Fig. 17.7). Metabisulfite totally deoxygenates blood and induces sickling.

2. **Solubility test** — Using dithionite : It is a solubility test in which HbS red cells are lysed by a high tonic strength of dithionite solution (sodium hydrosulfite) at pH 6.8 (with phosphate buffer). The reduced HbS is insoluble in the buffer and produces opacity. The test is useful in mass screening for the presence of HbS as there is no need of a microscope.

D. Bone marrow changes

Bone marrow shows features of normoblastic reaction with hypercellularity. The haemosiderin content is highly increased in the marrow.

E. Alkali denaturation test for HbF

Principle

Adult haemoglobin gets denatured in alkali, while foetal haemoglobin resists alkali denaturation. A haemolysate is alkalinised, HbF maintains its pink colour, while HbA turns colourless. This "one-minute alkali-denaturation test" is useful in identification of HbF.

(a) Method of Singer et al., 1951

Reagents

1. *Alkali solution* : 0.12 N KOH or NaOH kept in refrigerator in plastic or paraffin lined bottles.

2. *Precipitating agents*

Hydrochloric acid (sp. gr. 1.18)	....	2.5 ml
50% Saturated ammonium sulphate solution	....	1000 ml

3. *Ammonia solution* : Dilute 0.4 ml of concentrated ammonia (sp. gr. 0.88) to a litre with water.

Technique

Haemolysate preparation

Blood	....	0.5 ml
Sod. citrate solution (3-8%)	....	2.0 ml

Mix well, centrifuge, and then wash the packed cells in normal saline thrice. Then add one volume of distilled water and half volume of chloroform. The mixture is centrifuged for 20 minutes at 1500 r.p.m. The supernatant is decanted off and the haemoglobin solution is adjusted to 10 g% by adding distilled water. Determine haemoglobin concentration (H_1). The haemolysate can be stored for a prolonged period at – 20°C.

Test

1. *Alkali* — 3.2 ml in a test tube in a water bath at 20°C.
2. *Haemolysate* — 0.2 ml added quickly rinsing well and gently shaking the tube for 10 seconds.

Start a stop-watch when the haemoglobin is added. At the end of one minute, add rapidly 6.8 ml precipitating reagent to stop the reaction instantaneously, Mix well by inverting 6 times and filter immediately. The filtrate H_2 is a 1 to 50 dution of the original haemoglobin solution (H_1).

Filtrate

1. Colourless — Normal adult Hb (HbA), when, less than 2% of foetal Hb in initial haemoglobin.

2. Coloured (faintly brown to deep red) – alkali resistant Hb (HbF), if HbF is more than 2%.

Prepare a Hb solution by adding 0.2 ml haemolysate to 200 ml with ammonia solution, extinction of which corresponds to 5% alkali resistant Hb in the test procedure.

Calculation : Read the standard and test in a colorimeter at 415 nm.

$$\frac{\text{Reading of unknown}}{\text{Reading of standard}} \times 5 \text{ g } \%$$

Interpretation of HbF level

1. *Thalassaemia* — 20-60% alkali-resistant Hb (HbF)
2. *Normal adult* — less than 1% HbF
3. *Hb Barts* — is alkali resistant
4. *Insignificant* — if less than 4 g % alkali-resistant Hb.

(b) Modified Betke method

1. *Cyanide solution* :Potassium cyanide 0.2 g, potassium ferricyanide 0.2g, water to 1 litre.
2. *Sodium hydroxide* (1.2 mol/l) : NaOH 48.0 g, water to 1 litre.
3. *Saturated ammonium sulphate* : A 50% saturated ammonium sulphate solution.

All reagents are brought to room temperature for 10-15 minutes before use.

1. Add 0.6 ml of lysate (100 g/l) to 10 ml of cyanide solution. This makes cyanmethaemoglobin (HiCN) solution.

2. To 2.8 ml of HiCN solution, add 0.2 ml NaOH solution. After mixing thoroughly, it is left for exactly 2 min at room temperature.

3. Then 2.0 ml of 50% saturated solution of ammonium sulphate is added and mixed thoroughly and allowed to stand for 10 min. The ammonium sulphate lowers the pH and precipitates the denatured haemoglobin.

4. Filter through a Whatman No. 42 filter paper and collect the filtrate.

5. The remaining HiCN solution is used as standard. Read the absorbance of the standard and the filtrate (test) in a spectrophotometer at either 413 nm or 520 nm.

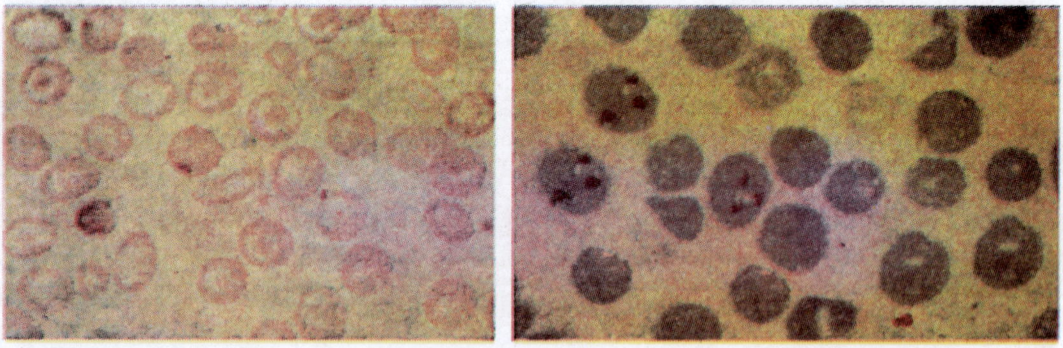

A B

Fig. 17.12. (A) Blood film, haemoglobin H disease. A form of alpha-thalassaemia, this has the combination of microcytic hypochromic red cells and haemolysis. Target cells are numerous. **(B)** Film made after incubation of blood with brilliant cresyl blue, haemoglobin H disease. Two reticulocytes have dark blue precipitates of RNA. Several red cells contain multiple smaller pale blue precipitates of HbH (A and B; by courtesy of Dr. McDonald K. Home).

Calculation :

$$\% \text{ Hb F} = \frac{\text{Reading of filtrate} \times 100}{\text{Reading of standard} \times 20}$$

Interpretation

A normal and a raised HbF control is tested with every batch of samples. Hb F control of 10% Hb F is prepared from a mixture of cord and adult blood.

HbF : 0.2–1.0% — Normal adult.

HbF : 1–5% — In 30 to 50% of β-thalassaemia traits.

HbF : 15–20% — Heterozygous HPFH.

HbF : > 45% — β-thalassaemia major.

F. Demonstration HbH (β4)

HbH preparation : Two parts of fresh blood and one part of 1% brilliant cresyl blue (as for reticulocyte) are mixed in a test tube and incubated at 37 °C for three hours and, therefore, blood films are prepared and dried in air.

Observation

During incubation, the unstable HbH gradually precipitates as multiple small pale blue inclusions uniformly distributed on the red cell membrane, which are distinguished from dark blue precipitates of RNA in reticulocytes (Fig. 17.12A).

G. Haemoglobin electrophoresis

Principle : Electrophoretic separation of haemoglobin is used for the qualitative detection of the presence of abnormal haemoglobins especially for Hbs C, D, E and S. Haemoglobin molecules in alkaline solution have a negative charge and move towards the anode. Haemoglobin solution of the haemolysate prepared from the blood is applied over the strip of cellulose acetate on an electrophoresis apparatus using Tris buffer (pH 8.9). The different types of haemoglobins get separated on the cellulose acetate strip according to their electrophoretic mobility (Fig. 17.6B). Better separation of Hbs occurs on starch gel.

Observation

Separated haemoglobin bands are compared with different controls maintained as stock standard in "haemoglobin bank". HbA remains stationary since its anodic movement balances the endosmotic flow of buffer which carries HbA_2 and HbD towards the cathode. Good separations are obtained with haemoglobins A, C, D, H, S and A_2, but HbE and HbA_2 or HbS and HbD exhibit similar mobilities.

Final characterisation consists of purification of abnormal haemoglobins with starch block electrophoresis and hybridisation to see the abnormality in α or β chain and "finger printing".

QUESTIONS

1. *What is thalassaemia trait?*
2. *What is β thalassaemia major?*
3. *What is the cause of haemolysis in β thalassaemia major?*
4. *What is the diagnostic test for thalassaemia major?*

Chapter 18

Erythrocytosis and Polycythaemia

ERYTHROCYTOSIS

In erythrocytosis and polycythaemia there is a genuine increase in the absolute number of erythrocytes. *Absolute erythrocytosis* may result from :

I. **Polycythaemia (primary)**

When there is a pathological (neoplastic) proliferation of red cells arising out without erythropoietin stimulus, it is called primary proliferative polycythaemia. Here, the disorder is intrinsic to the progenitor cells of the bone marrow, and serum erythropoietin levels are usually reduced. Polycythaemia may be of two types :

(i) *Erythraemia* (pure erythrocytosis). Erythraemia may be familial and sporadic.

(ii) *Polycythaemia vera* (PV).

II. **Secondary polycythaemia of physiological response**

There is an excessive stimulation of an otherwise normal bone marrow in secondary polycythaemia (also known as erythrocytosis) by a pathological stimulus, such as hypoxia, in which erythropoietin production is increased.

Causes

1. *Hypoxia* : Altitude, pulmonary disease or congenital heart disease with cyanosis, abnormal haemoglobins with high oxygen affinity.
2. *Tumours producing erythropoietin or other erythropoietic stimuli* : Certain benign and malignant tumours of kidney, liver, bronchus, uterus and cerebellum (haemangioblastoma) and with renal cysts.

POLYCYTHAEMIA VERA

PV is a myeloproliferative disorder resulting from clonal expansion of a haematopoietic stem cell associated with excessive overproduction of erythrocytes, and, to a lesser extent, elevated peripheral granulocyte and platelet counts.

Pathophysiology

There is excessive proliferation of erythroid, myeloid and megakaryotic elements within the bone marrow (Figs. 18.1 and 18.2). Blood and bone

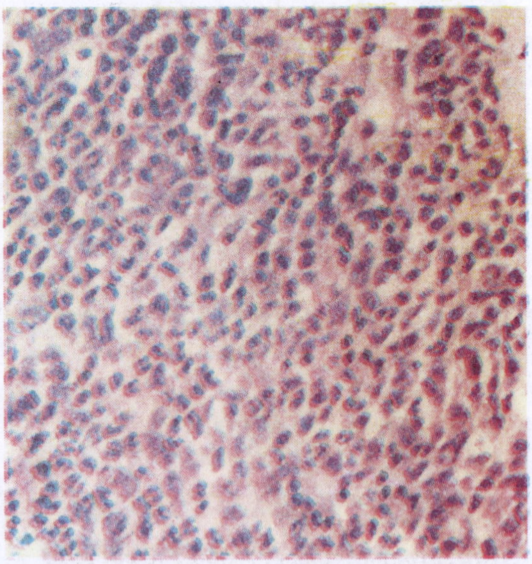

Fig. 18.1. Bone marrow biopsy. Polycythaemia rubra vera showing markedly hyperplastic marrow. Marrow spaces are completely filled with haemopoietic, leucopoietic tissue as well as megakaryocytes. *(Haemalum and Eosin)*

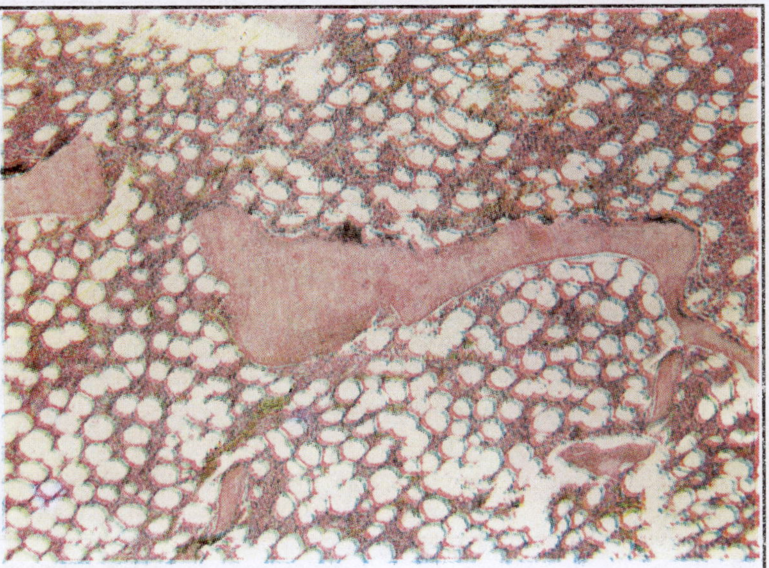

Fig. 18.2. Vertebral marrow section. Normal : Showing bone trabeculae, fat spaces and haemopoietic tissue in normal proportions. *(Haemalum & Eosin)*

marrow contain increased number of pleuripotent colony-forming of stem cells. These cells give rise to mixed colonies granulocytic, erythroid, macrophage and megkaryocytic elements (CFU–GEMM) in culture in the absence of added erythropoietin. This endogeneous erythroid colony formation in PV is abolished with antibodies to erythropoietin, suggesting increased sensitivity to erythropoietin.

Clinical features

Patient usually presents with symptoms referable to blood volume; headache, vertigo, tinitus, or blurred vision. Diagnosis is made most often during routine blood count.

Laboratory diagnosis of PV

(i) Haemoglobin : Usually more than 18 g% in males and 16 g% in females.

(ii) Significant elevation of red cell count (8-10 million/cu. mm).

(iii) Thrombocytosis : > 400,000/cu. mm.

(iv) Leucocytosis : > 12,000/cu. mm.

(v) Leucocyte alkaline phosphatase : Increased.

(vi) Serum vitamin B_{12} : More than 900 pg/ml or vitamin B_{12}-binding capacity greater than 2,200 pg/ml.

Course and prognosis

PV is a chronic disease and affected subjects usually live 10 to 20 years under good control. Phlebotomy, chlorambucil, radioactive phosphorus (^{32}P) and hydroxyurea are useful to control the manifestations of the disease.

(a) Progressive anaemia with more immature granulocyte and with more circulating nucleated red cells occur in 20-40% of patients.

(b) About 25% cases progress to myelofibrosis in 5–25 years and in whom splenomegaly crosses even umbilicus.

(c) Few cases may transform to acute myeloid leukaemia (AML) or myelodysplastic syndrome (MDS).

- Most patients die of vascular complications.

Treatment

1. *Venesection* alone is benificial as it lowers Hb values to 15 g%.
2. *Myelosuppression* by low dose busulphan to reduce platelet count to four lakh per cu. mm.
3. *Alpha-interferon.*

Table 18.1 : Distinguishing features of polycythaemia vera and seconday polycythaemia

Polycythaemia Vera	Secondary Polycythaemia
1. A disorder of stem cell.	1. Secondary to various causes such as hypoxia at high altitude, uterine myomas, renal cell carcinoma, haemangioblastoma of cerebellum and phaeochromocytoma in which there is increased production of erythropoietin.
2. Not related with hypoxia, O_2 saturation > 92%.	2. Associated with hypoxia, O_2 saturation < 92%.
3. Erythropoietin level is decreased.	3. Erythropoietin level is increased.
4. There is splenomegaly.	4. –ve.
5. Bone marrow shows trilineage hyperplasia.	5. Not present Features of underlying disorder are present.
6. Abnormal karyotype is present.	6. Normal karyotype.

SECONDRY POLYCYTHAEMIA

Secondary polycythaemia, also called relative or pseudopolycythaemia, in which the cause is known (Table 18.1). The secondary causes are all associated with increase in erythropoietin level.

QUESTIONS

1. *Define erythrocytosis.*
2. *What is polycythaemia vera?*
3. *How do you diagnose a case of PV?*
4. *How do you distinguish between a primary and a secondary polycythaemia?*
5. *How do you distinguish between a primary and a secondary polycythaemia?*

Chapter 19

Leukaemia

Malignant neoplastic diseases of white cells can be classfied as :

1. Lymphoid neoplasms.

2. Myeloid neoplasms : Myeloid neoplasm arises from haemopoietic stem cells that give rise to cells of the myeloid lineage — erythroid, granulocytic and/or thrombocytic types.

Leukaemia is a malignant state of haemopoietic tissue characterised by widespread proliferation of leucopoietic cells in the bone marrow with or without appearance of abnormal premature leucocytes in peripheral blood.

INTRODUCTION

CLASSIFICATION ON CELL TYPE

Classification of leukaemia is broadly related to the cell of origin (e.g., *lymphoid* or *myeloid*) as well as to the rapidity of the clinical course (e.g., *acute* or *chronic*).

Classification based on rate of progress of disease

1. ***Acute leukaemia*** : It is of sudden onset and life expectancy, without treatment, is short (3-4 months). The bone marrow is usually packed with primitive cells (blast cells) of the series involved and very little evidence of differentiation.

2. ***Chronic leukaemia*** : It is of gradual onset and the patients have usually been unwell for years and survive a much longer time. The neoplastic proliferation consists mostly of more differentiated cells (myelocytes, metamyelocytes, neutrophils in CML, small mature lymphocytes in CLL) and few blast cells.

In both *acute* and *chronic leukaemias* the total count of leucocytes usually exceeds 15,000/cu. mm in blood along with plenty of premature leucocytes. The term *subleukaemic leukaemia* is used when the total leucocyte count is within or below normal limits but abnormal cells are found in the blood. The term *aleukaemic* is applied when there are no abnormal cells in peripheral blood and the leucocyte count is normal or subnormal. All patients presenting with subleukaemic or aleukaemic disease have acute leukaemias and the diagnosis is established by examination of bone marrow which contains more than 30% blast cells. Acute leukaemia may occasionally present as an aplastic anaemia.

In leukaemias, there is a failure of cell maturation. Proliferation of cells which do not mature occupy more marrow space at the expense of normal cells. Eventually the immature cells spill into the blood.

ACUTE LEUKAEMIAS

FAB CLASSIFICATION (Tables 19.1, 19.2, 19.3)

Although the dominant cell in an acute leukaemia is usually an immature blast cell, it is possible to recognise a number of subtypes, within the myeloid and lymphoid categories, on the basis of variability in the morphological features of blast cells. A collaborative *French-American-British* (FAB) group has described a classification system which is generally accepted (FAB classification); and is based on blood and bone marrow morphological features of abnormal cells stained by Romanowsky stain, and by histochemical studies (Table 19.3).

1. Acute myeloid leukaemia (AML)

AML (also called acute non-lymphoblastic

Table 19.1 : FAB classification of acute leukaemias		
Classification	***Cell types***	***Characteristics***
M0 (*Undifferentiated myeloblastic*)	Primitive cells	Undifferentiated stem cell.
M1 (*AML without maturation*)	Myeloblasts	Non-granular myeloblasts usually containing one or more distinct nucleoli.
M2 (*AML with maturation*)	Myeloblasts, promyelocytes	Maturation beyond the promyelocyte stage. Cells containing Auer rods are common.
M3 (*Acute promyelocytic leukaemia*)	Hypergranular promyelocytes	The majority of the cells are promyelocytes with a characteristic pattern of heavy granulation.
M4 (*Acute myelomonocytic leukaemia*)	Monocytoid cells	Immature and mature cells of both myeloid and monocytic lineage.
M5 (*Acute monocytic leukaemia*) Two subtypes	(M5a) – Monoblasts (M5b) – Monoblasts Promonocytes Monocytes	Poorly differentiated monoblastic. Differentiated monoblasts; promonocytes and monocytes.
M6 (*Acute erythroleukaemia*)	Erythroblasts	Bizarre erythroblasts. Erythroblasts with multiple lobation of the nucleus, multiple nuclei, nuclear fragments, giant forms and megaloblastic features.
M7 (*Acute megakaryocytic leukaemia*)	Megakaryocytes	Immature megakaryocytes with abnormal platelets are prominent.

Table 19.2 : FAB classification of acute lymphoblastic leukaemia		
Classification	***Cell types***	***Characteristics***
L1, Childhood – ALL (B – ALL and T – ALL)	Microlymphoblasts	Small lymphoblasts, scanty cytoplasm, regular round nuclei, nucleoli often not present or inconspicuous.
L2, Adult – ALL (Mostly adult T – ALL)	Large undifferentiated lymphoblasts	Pleomorphic larger lymphoblasts. Nucleoli are always present, irregular or cleft nuclei.
L3, ALL (B – ALL)	Burkitt type	Large blast cells with oval to round regular nucleus, basophilic cytoplasm, one or more nucleoli. Majority of cells are undifferentiated type, identical to that described in Burkitt lymphoma cells.

leukaemia, ANLL) is divided into eight types based on the direction of differentiation along one or more cell lines and the degree of maturation (Table 19.1). M0 is an undifferentiated or stem cell leukaemia; M1, M2 and M3 show predominantly granulocytic differentiation. M4 shows both granulocytic and monocytic, M5 predominantly monocytic, M6 predominantly erythroblastic and M7 megakaryocytic differentiation.

2. **Acute lymphoblastic leukaemia (ALL)** : ALL is divided into 3 types, L1, L2, L3, according to the occurrence of individual cytological features and the degree of heterogenecity in the leukaemia cell population (Table 19.2).

CHRONIC LEUKAEMIAS

Chronic leukaemias are also divided basically into myeloid and lymphoid categories and they show predominantly myelocyte and mature lymphocyte, respectively.

1. *Chronic myeloid or myelocytic leukaemia (CML).*
2. *Chronic lymphoid or lymphocytic leukaemia (CLL).*

Table 19.3 : Morphologic subtypes of acute leukaemia (FAB classification)

Sub-type	Common name	Morphology	Histochemistry: Peroxi-dase	Histochemistry: Non-sp. esterase	Histochemistry: PAS	percentage of cases	Typical protein markers
M0	Undifferentiated	Primitive cells	–	–	–	2	CD 34, 33, 13
M1	AML without maturation	Myeloblasts predominate, distinct nucleoli, few granules	+/–	+/–	–	20	CD 34, 33, 13
M2	AML with maturation	Myeloblastic and promyelocytes predominate, Auer rods ±	+++	+/–	–	25	CD 34, 33, 15, 13
M3	Acute promyelocytic leukaemia	Promyelocytes predominate, hypergranular, often with multiple Auer rods per cell	+++	+	+/–	10	CD 33, 13, (HLA–Dr–)
M4	Acute myelomonocytic leukaemia	Monocytoid appearing cells in peripheral blood; M4 with eosinophilia is a subtype	+/–	+++	–	20	CD 34, 33, 15, 14, 13
M5	Acute monocytic leukaemia	Two subtypes identified : (a) undifferentiated; (b) differentiated with 80% promonocytes and monocytes	–	+++	+/–	20	CD 33, 15, 14, 13
M6	Acute erythro-leukaemia	Predominance of erythroblasts and markedly dysplastic erythroid precursors	+/–	–	+++	5	CD 33, glycoprotein
M7	Acute megakaryo-cytic leukaemia	Pleomorphic, undifferentiated blasts react with antiplatelet antibodies and contain platelet peroxidase	–	+/–	++	5	CD 33, 41
L1	Acute lymphoblastic leukaemia (ALL)	Small homogeneous round blasts with scanty cytoplasm, 1–2 nucleoli	–	–	+++	75	CD 10, 19, 34, T dt
L2	ALL	Pleomorphic larger blasts with more cytoplasm and prominent nucleoli (1–2)	–	–	+++	20	CD 10, 19, 34, T dt
L3	ALL	Large blast cells with basophilic vacuolated cytoplasm and vesicular nuclei; undifferentiated cell type	–	–	+++	5	CD 19, 20, sIg

Certain haematological disorders with abnormal cells in blood that do not completely fulfil the criteria of acute or chronic leukaemia are relatively common. These are collectively termed *myelodysplastic syndrome,* and discussed at the end of the chapter.

DIAGNOSIS OF ACUTE LEUKAEMIAS

The morphological features of abnormal leucocytes (myeloblasts, monoblasts, lymphoblasts, etc.) are discussed in chapter 13.

CLINICAL FEATURES

There is failure of cell maturation in acute leukaemias leading to accumulation of immature cells in bone marrow and blood. Although acute leukaemia may occur at any age but in children the highest incidence is in first 6 years and in adult at all ages. Acute myeloid leukaemia is about eight times more common than acute lymphoblastic leukaemia in adults. Acute lymphoblastic leukaemia is more common in young children. The spleen and liver are often enlarged. Enlarged lymph node is a common feature of lymphoblastic leukaemia.

INVESTIGATIONS

A. Blood picture

Typical blood picture of acute leukaemia is of anaemia, thrombocytopenia with a moderate to marked increase of leucocytes, majority of which are *blast cells.*

Total WBC count : Subnormal level to markedly elevated; average 20 to 100,000/cu. mm.

Differential count (Table 19.5)

Immature cells :

Blast cells	30 to 90 per cent
Intermediate type cells	10 to 15 per cent.

Mature cell :

Neutrophils	10 to 15 per cent
Lymphocytes	10 to 15 per cent
Normoblasts	0 to 2 per cent.

Blast cells : Myeloblasts, lymphoblasts and monoblasts are very similar morphologically. They are usually cells with 15–20 μm diameter, with round or oval nucleus and one or more nucleoli (Fig. 19.4; Table 19.6). The type of leukaemia is determined by taking into account their morpho-

Table 19.4: Distinguishing features of myeloblast, monoblast and lymphoblast

	Myeloblast	*Monoblast*	*Lymphoblast*
Leishman / May-Grunwald Giemsa			
Azurophilic granules	Few Auer rods +	—	—
Nucleoli	2–5	2–4	1 or 2
Sudan Black B	> 5% blasts	—	—
Peroxidase	+ or ++	—	—
Nonspecific esterase	+ (+ in M_4 and M_5 AML)	±	—
PAS	+ (diffuse)	+	—

Table 19.5: Differential nucleated cell count in acute leukaemias (%)

Acute myeloblastic leukaemia	*Acute lymphoblastic leukaemia*	*Acute monoblastic leukaemia*
Immature cell		
Myeloblast 40–60	Lymphoblast 40–60	Monoblast 40–60
Myelocyte 8–10	Prolymphocyte 8–10	Promonocyte 8–10
Myelomonocyte 2–5		
Mature cell		
Neutrophil 10–15	Neutrophil 10–15	Neutrophil 10–15
Lymphocyte 10–15	Lymphocyte 12–20	Lymphocyte 10–15
Monocyte 1–3	Monocyte 0–2	Monocyte 4–8
Abnormal red cell		
Intermediate normoblast 0–1	0–1	0–1
Late normoblast 0–2	1–3	0–2

logical features and results of cytochemical staining and immunotype markers. In addition, a small number of nucleated red cells may be seen in peripheral smear. Their distinguishing features are shown in Table 19.4. Only 2% of adult and less than 1% of childhood acute leukaemias fail to be categorised using these methods.

B. Other findings :

Total RBC	3 to 3.5 million/cu. mm
Total platelets	40,000 to 60,000/cu. mm
Haemoglobin	8 to 9 g%
Bleeding time	prolonged due to thrombocytopenia
Clotting time	prolonged due to hypofibrinogenaemia

C. Bone marrow (Figs. 19.2, 19.4, 19.6, 19.7, 19.8, 19.10, 19.11)

Hypercellular marrow and blast cells of the particular type are usually the outstanding feature. Erythroblasts and megakaryocytes are usually reduced.

Differentiation of Acute Leukaemias

The type of acute leukaemia is determined by considering the following factors (Table 19.4).

1. *Morphology* of the abnormal cell in blood film.
2. *Cytochemical* staining.
3. *Cell surface* makers.

(a) Morphological appearance

The principal features of various morphological types of blast cells are discussed in Chapter 13, and also shown in Table 19.3 and Table 19.4.

(b) Cytochemical stains

Cytochemistry is an adjunct to Leishman/May-Grunwald-Giemsa staining for determination of the category of leukaemia.

(a) *Myeloperoxidase* and *Sudan Black B* : Positive in some immature cell of myeloid series and, to a lesser extent, monocytic series.

(b) *Periodic Acid Schiff* (PAS) : Positive in lymphoblasts and sometimes in erythroblasts in erythroleukaemia (M6) (Fig. 19.4).

(c) *Nonspecific esterase* : Positive reaction, inhibited by sodium fluoride, in monocyte series.

(d) *Acid phosphatase* : Reaction is focal positive in T cell acute lymphoblastic leukaemia blast cells, diffuse reaction occurs in monocytic cells.

Serum lysozyme (muramidase) : Lysozyme level in serum rises to a very high level in myelomonocytic (M4) and monocytic (M5) leukaemia.

(c) Cell surface markers

Haematopoietic cells acquire cell surface antigens and receptors at various stages of differentiation, which may also be present on leukaemic blast cells (Table 19.2). Acute leukaemia may thus be classified based on the nature cell markers. This is particularly useful in lymphoblastic leukaemias (Table 19.3).

(d) Surface markers used for classification of ALL (Table 19.6)

(i) *Surface Ig* (sIg), a B lymphoid cell markers.

Table 19.6 : Acute lymphoblastic leukaemia immunophenotypes

Type	*Characteristic features*	*Marker*	*Frequency*
Common (derived from precursors of pre-B lineage)	cALL antigen Pan B antigen	CD 10, 19, 34 T dt	60%
T lineage	E (SRBC) rosette + Pan T antigen and cALL antigen-negative	CD 2, 5, 7, T dt	20%
Pre-T (early thymic T cells)	No rosette formation Pan T antigen	CD 1	5%
B lineage)	Surface Ig+	CD 19/CD 20	5%
Pre-B lineage	Cytoplasmic μ chains only	—	4%
Null cells	No definitive markers	—	10%

(ii) *Sheep erythrocyte (SRBC) rosette* formation, T cell marker.

(iii) *Surface and internal antigens* : It is detected by the help of specific monoclonal antibodies which include : common acute lymphoblastic leukaemia (cALL) antigen, T and B lymphoid cell surface antigens, a cytoplasmic μ chains, whose presence in absence of surface I_g serves as an index of pre-B cell status.

(iv) *Deoxynucleotidyl transferase* estimation by immunofluorescent study shows high level of enzyme in ALL than AML.

(v) *PCR* with probes specific to chromosomal break points are useful.

These tests are usually adequate to divide acute leukaemias of both types into various subtypes.

D. FAB typing

I. Acute myeloid leukaemia

In the FAB classification of *acute leukaemia*, the range of cells found in the peripheral blood mirrors the abnormal population in the bone marrow.

1. In acute myeloid leukaemia M0 category, the great majority of nucleatd cells in the blood are stem cells (undifferentiated cells). The nuclei of these atypical blast cells have fine structure, nucleoli are pale, no thickening of chromatin at the circumference (Fig. 19.1). They have a thin narrower border of basophilic cytoplasm. It is not possible from marrow or blood film to state whether these very primitive cells are lymphoblastic, myeloblastic or monoblastic origin.

2. The immature cells are myeloblasts in MI category (Fig. 19.2), more mature cells are found in addition to myeloblasts in M2 (Fig. 19.3), and hypergranular promyelocytes in M3 (Fig. 19.4).

3. More than 30% blast cells of myeloid and monocytic lineage with granulocytic and monocytic differentiation are seen in M4 (Fig. 19.5); and monoblast, promonocytes and monocytes predominate in M5 (Fig. 19.6).

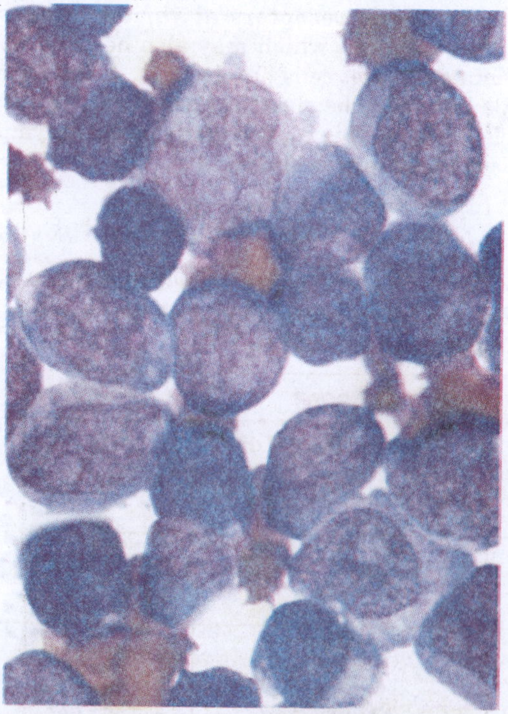

Fig. 19.1. Blood film. Acute undifferentiated leukaemia — M0. All cells are atypical blast cells. Nuclei have fine structure and nucleoli are pale (*Leishman*)

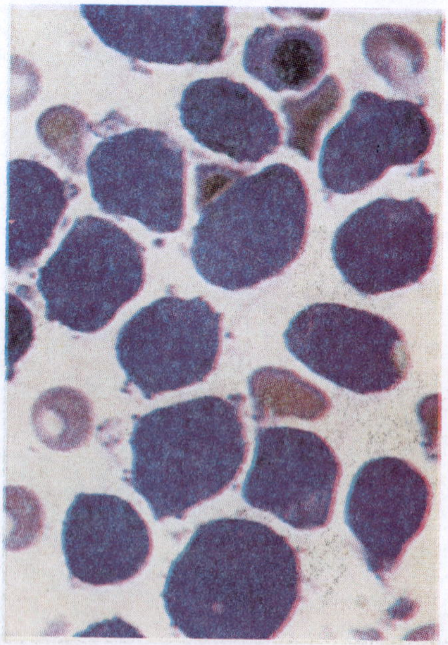

Fig. 19.2. Marrow film. Acute myeloid leukaemia — M1 showing non-granular myeloblasts without any granulocytic differentiation (*Leishman*)

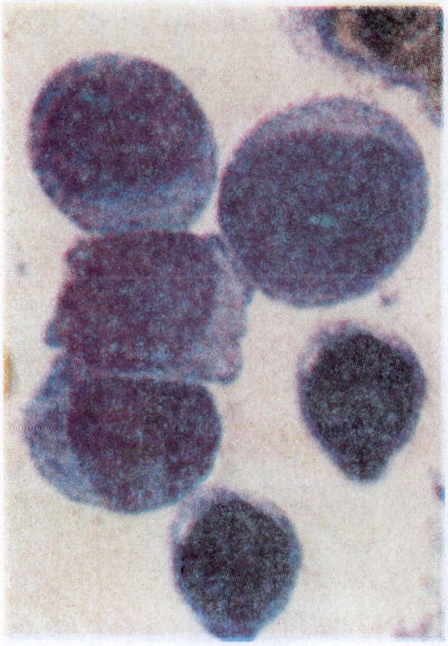

Fig. 19.3. Blood film. Acute myeloid leukaemia – M2, showing some degree of maturation beyond promyelocyte stage with dysplastic cells.

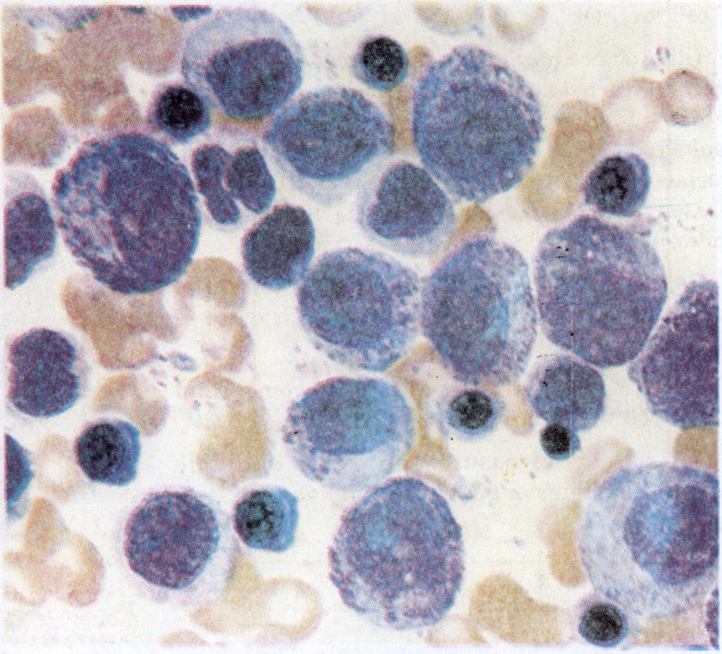

Fig. 19.4. Marrow film. Acute myeloid leukaemia – M3, showing predominantly promyelocytes with coarse granulation.

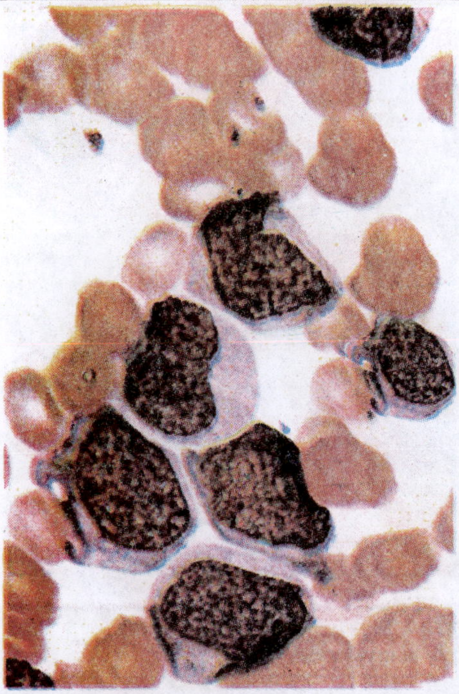

Fig. 19.5. Blood film. Acute myelomonocytic leukaemia – M4, showing primitive cells of monocytic series, monoblast and promonocyte, and primitive cells of myelocyte series promyelocyte and myeloblasts.

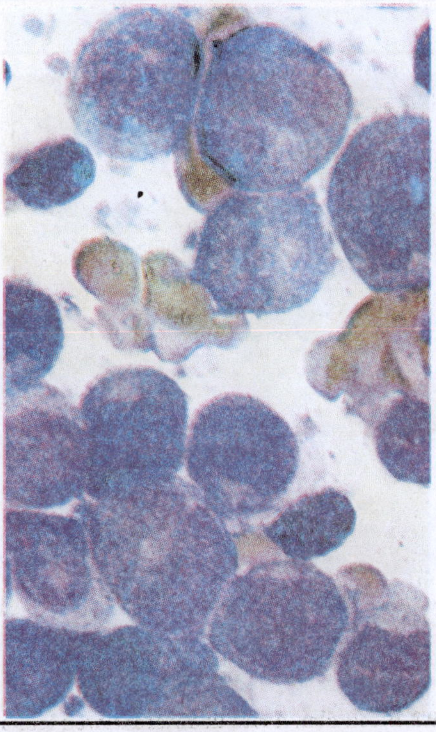

Fig. 19.6. Marrow film. Acute monoblastic leukaemia — M5 (b), showing cells of monocytic series monoblasts and promonocytes.

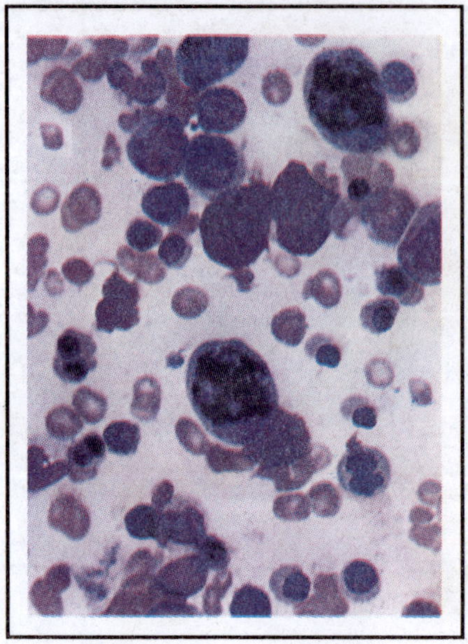

Fig. 19.7. Marrow film. Erythroleukaemia – M6 under low power

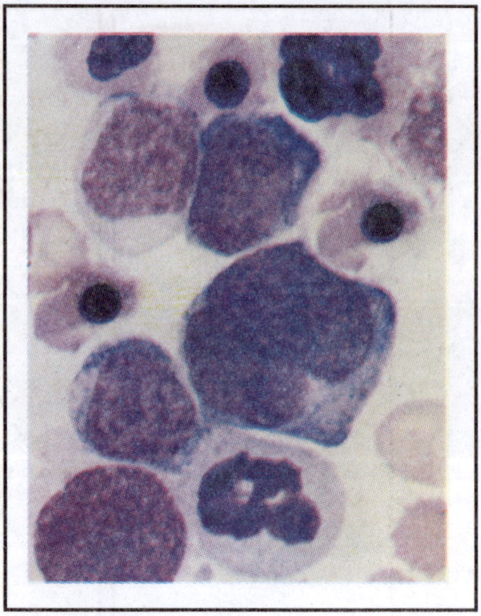

Fig. 19.8. Marrow film. Erythroleukaemia – M6, showing bizarre nature of erythropoiesis. Erythroblasts with multiple lobation of nucleus are present

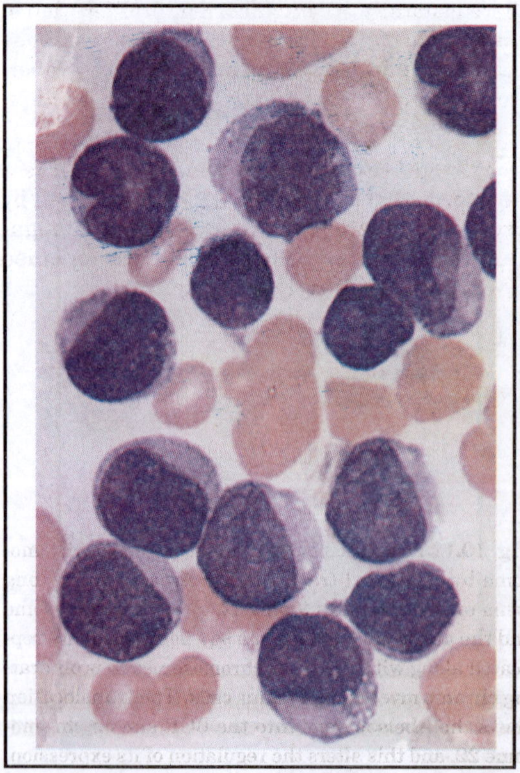

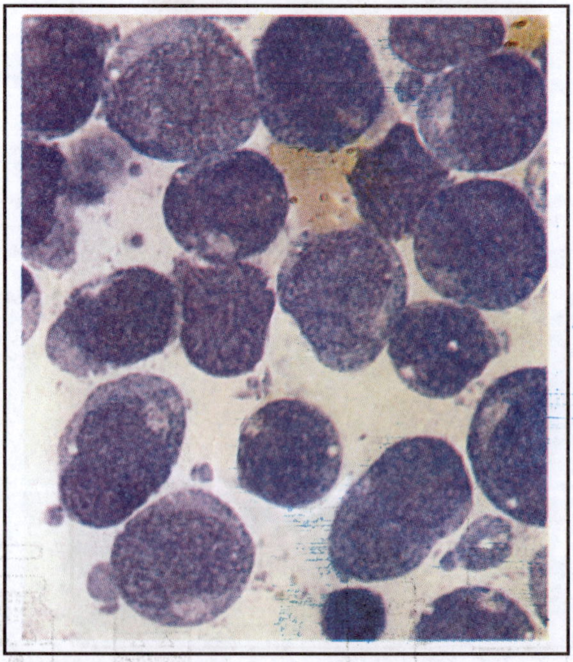

Fig. 19.10. Marrow film. Acute myeloid leukaemia – M1

⇦ **Fig. 19.9.** Blood film. Acute myeloid leukaemia – M1, showing myeloblasts of varying size

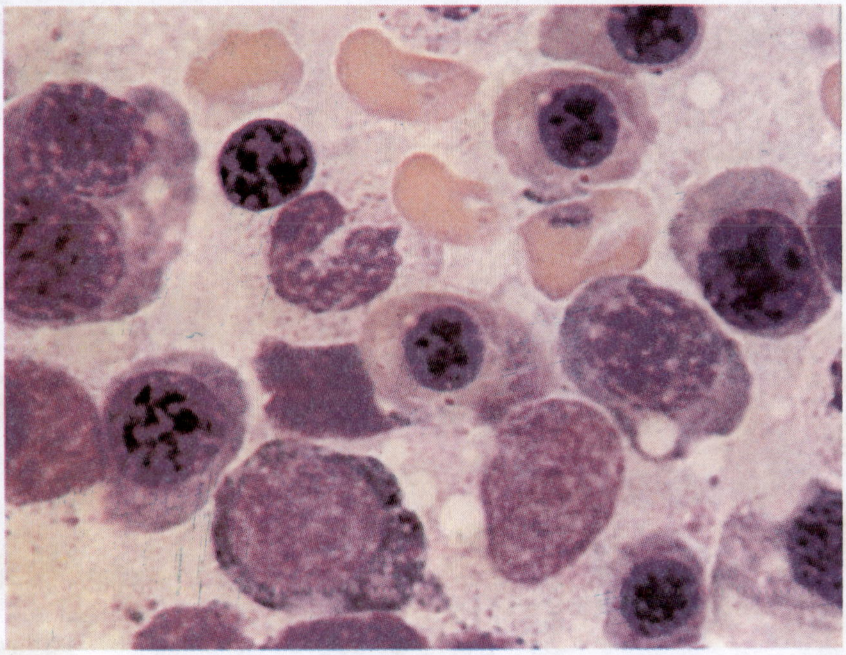

Fig. 19.11. Myelodysplastic syndrome

4. In *erythroleukaemia* M6 (Figs. 19.7; 19.8), there generally occurs abnormal proliferation of both erythroid and myeloid precursors in bone marrow leading to a mixture of variable proportions of *proerythroblasts* and *myeloblasts*. Variations may occur.

5. *Megakaryoblastic leukaemia* (M7), is a rare form of acute leukaemia, characterised by predominance of megakaryocytes or megakaryoblasts in the bone marrow, accompanied by an increase in reticulin fibres.

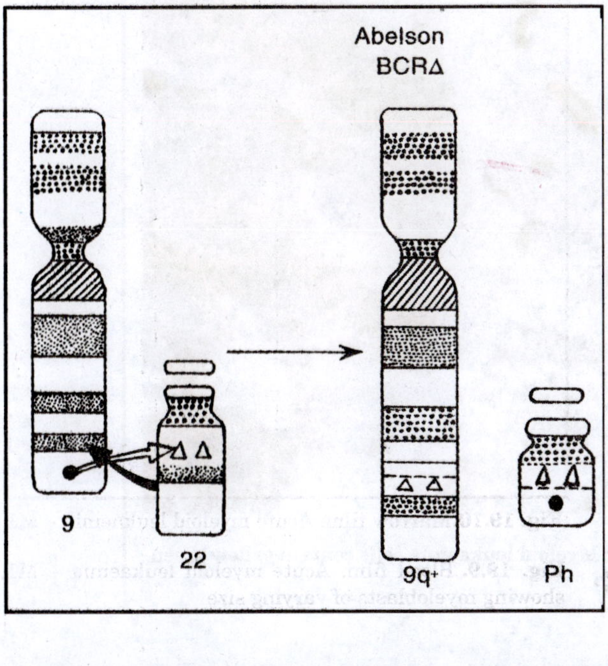

Fig. 19.12. Formation of the Philadelphia (Ph) chromosome by reciprocal translocation of parts of the long arms of chromosomes 9 and 22. The Ph chromosome and the abnormal chromosome 9q+ persist and are replicated along with the other chromosomes in proliferating chronic myeloid leukaemic cells. The translocation shifts the Abelson gene into the BCR site on chromosome 22, and this alters the regulation of its expression.

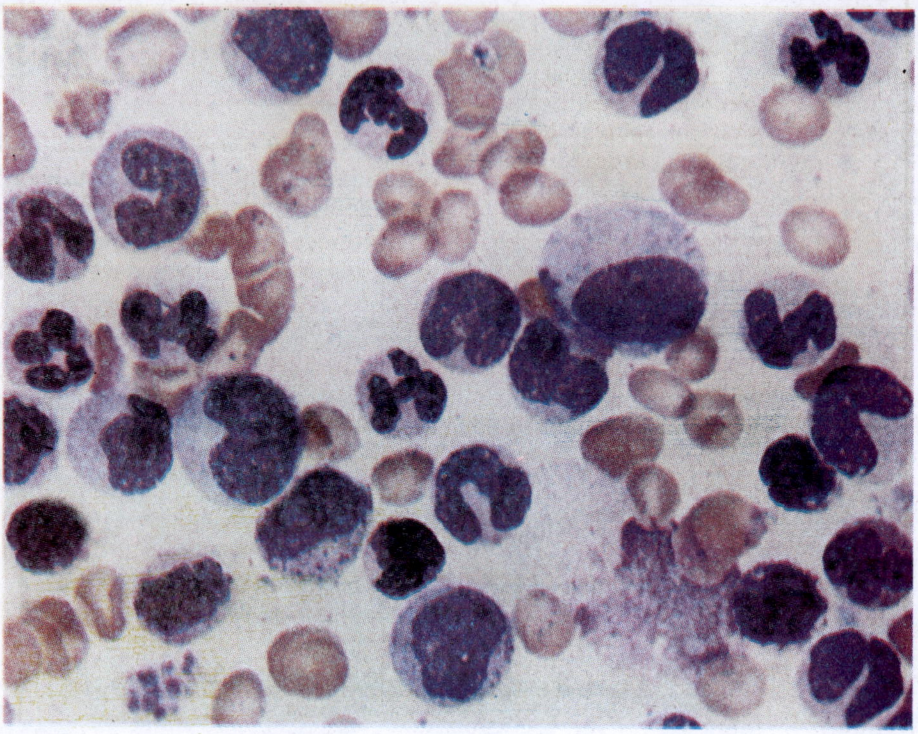

Fig. 19.13. Chronic myeloid leukaemia (blood film) showing many myelocytes, metamyelocytes, band form and segmented neutrophils

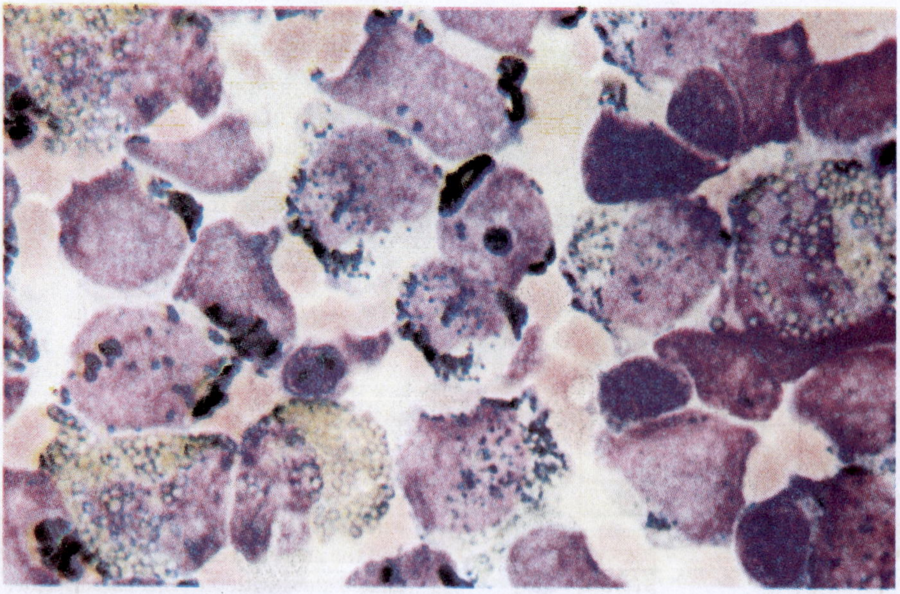

Fig. 19.14. Peroxidase stain (marrow film) : Myeloid leukaemia cells contain yellow green peroxidase positive granules

II. Acute lymphoid leukaemia

Small lymphoblasts with scanty cytoplasm predominate in L1 ALL (Fig. 19.15), the presence of pleomorphic large lymphoblasts with definite nucleoli indicate L2 ALL category (Fig. 19.16). The great majority of immature cells are undifferentiated type in L3 ALL.

CHRONIC MYELOID LEUKAEMIA (CML)

Syn : Chronic granulocytic leukaemia, Chronic myelogenous leukaemia

CLINICL FEATURES

Chronic myeloid leukaemia is a disease of middle age (30-60 years), with a peak incidence at 55 years, onset is insidious, symptoms often having been present for months and the disorder may be diagnosed accidentally on routine blood test. Spleen enlarges progressively and the discomfort associated with splenomegaly may bring the patient to the doctor. Incidence of CML in India is higher than that of CLL.

Although the disease progresses as a chronic process in most patients, but blastic transformation is a frequent termination of the chronic course. In blast crisis, the characteristics of disease usually alters to that of acute leukaemia with a fatal course. Prognosis of chronic myeloid leukaemia is worse than chronic lymphatic leukaemia.

LABORATORY FEATURES

Blood picture (Fig. 19.13)

The typical blood picture includes moderate anaemia, markedly elevated total leucocyte count with 20% or more of myelocytes and with a full spectrum of cells of granulocytic series. Platelet count may be normal but is elevated in one-half of cases.

Total WBC : 100,000 to 500,000/cu. mm

Differential count

Myeloblasts	2–4%
Myelocytes	50–60%
Metamyelocytes	10–15%
Neutrophils	20–25%
Lymphocytes	10–15%
Eosinophils	1–2%
Monocytes	1–3%

Other findings

Total RBC	3 to 4 millions/cu.mm
Platelets	20,000–400,000/cu.mm
Haemoglobin	9–10 g%

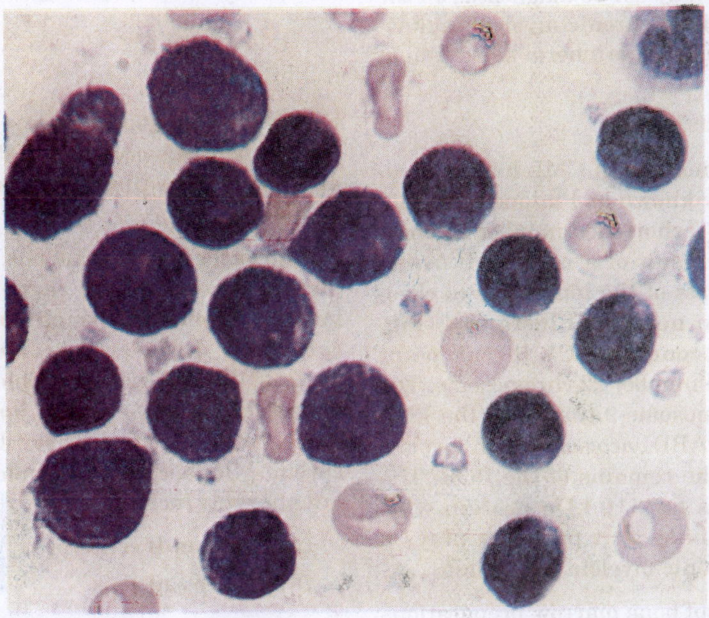

Fig. 19.15. Acute lymphoblastic leukaemia (marrow film) – L1. Small lymphoblasts with indistinct nucleoli

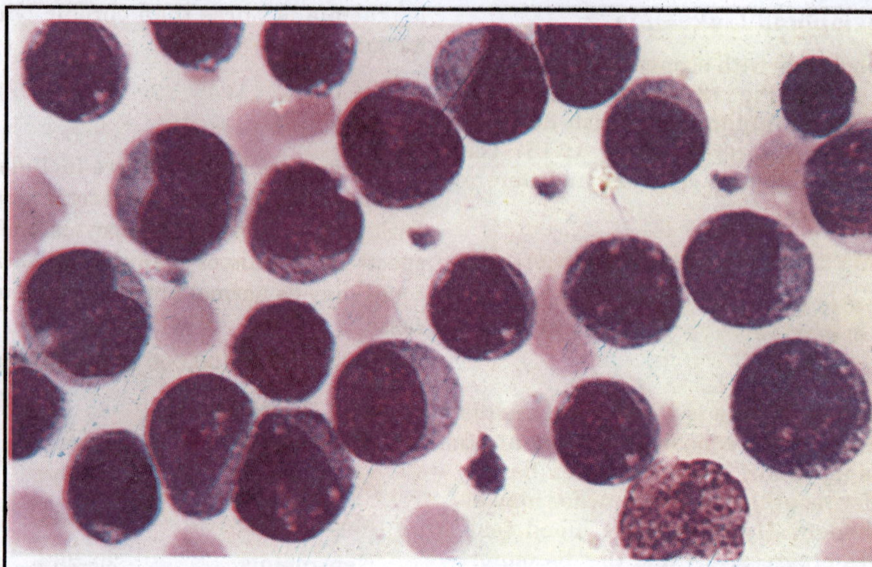

Fig. 19.16 Acute lymphoblastic leukaemia – L2. (Marrow film), showing large lymphoblasts with prominent nucleoli

Bone marrow

Bone marrow aspirate yields hypercellular fragments with complete or partial replacement of fat spaces. It is markedly hypercellular due primarily to granulocytic proliferation, with all stages represented. It should be remembered that even a typical bone marrow may not be diagnostic; on the other hand, diagnosis of chronic myeloid leukaemia can be made from the peripheral blood film in most cases.

Chromosomal findings

About 90% of patients with CML have a chromosome abnormality known as Philadelphia (Ph) chromosome. This is a shortened number 22 chromosome and is the result of a reciprocal *translocation* between parts of the long arms of chromosome 22 and 9 in nearly all instances (Fig. 19.12). The break occurs in BCR (break point cluster region) on the number 22 chromosome. The fragment from chromosome 9 that joins the BCR carries the Abelson (ABI) *oncogene* which forms a *chimeric* gene wih the remains of the BCR. The chimeric gene codes for 210 kDa protein with tyrosine kinase activity that probably plays a causative role in chronic myeloid luekaemia.

Cytogenetic study of bone marrow preparations at metaphases of cultured peripheral granulocytes reveal the association of Ph-22 chromosome of neoplastic cells. After treatment, Ph chromosome persists in the immature bone marrow cells but not in mature blood cells. With the onset of *blastic crisis,* additional chromosomal changes may develop.

CHRONIC LYMPHOCYTIC LEUKAEMIA (CLL) Figs. 19.17 and 19.18

Clinical features

CLL is the commonest variety of leukaemia, majority of the cases occur after 45 years with a peak at 65. It is more than twice as common in men as in women.

The onset is very insidious. Most patients complain of tiredness and vague illness or enlargement of superficial lymph nodes. The disease is commonly discovered accidentally during the investigation of another problem. Enlarged lymph nodes are usually evident. Spleen is usually palpable. Anaemia develops slowly. Common types of chronic lymphocytic leukaemia based on nature of lymphocytes incldue :

(a) Common B cell type

(b) Rare T cell type

(c) Hairy cell leukaemia (B cell type)

(d) Prolymphocytic leukaemia

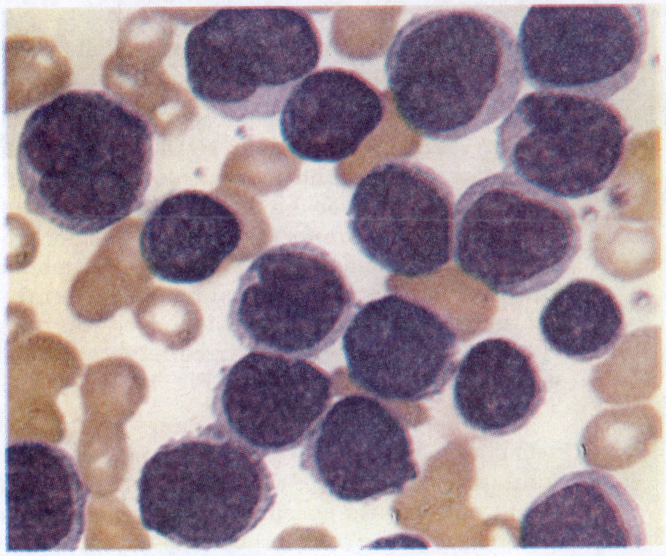

Fig.19.17. Pro-lymphocytic leukaemia (blood film) showing prolymphocytes with indented nuclei and lymphoblasts with large nucleoli

LABORATORY FEATURES

Blood picture

Total WBC : 200,000 to 400,000/cu. mm

Differential count (Fig. 19.18)

Lymphoblasts	rare
Lymphocyte	85–90%
Neutrophils	4–8%
Monocytes	1–2%.

The lymphocytes are predominantly of small variety and they are monotonously similar (Fig. 19.18). Lymphoblasts are rare but undifferentiated lymphocytes may increase in number in the terminal stages.

Other findings

Total RBC	3 to 4 million/cu. mm
Total platelets	1 to 1.5 lac/cu mm
Haemoglobin	8 to 10 g %

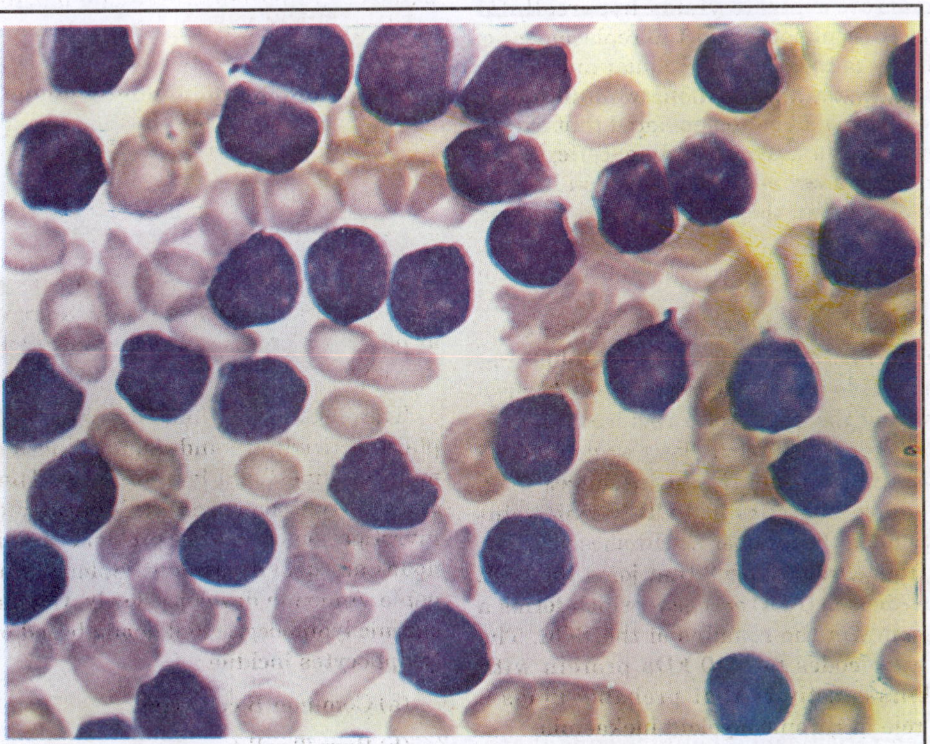

Fig. 19.18. Chronic lymphocytic leukaemia (blood film). There are medium sized lymphocytes with uniformity, few smaller lymphocytes and several larger cells are also present

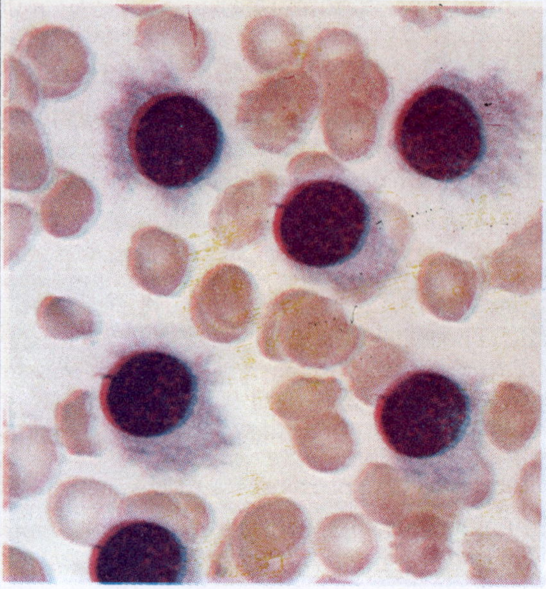

Fig. 19.19. Hairy cell leukaemia (leukaemic reticulo-endotheliosis) (blood film). Grey blue cytoplasm of hairy cell exhibits irregular villi giving rise to irregular serrated hairy edge and pseudopodial extension.

Bone marrow

Increase in lymphocytes with a corresponding reduction of megakaryocytes, myeloid precursors and erythroid precursor. Since the lymphocytes in bone marrow are morphologically normal, examination of marrow films may be equivocal to blood picture. Bone marrow examination is not usually necessary since the diagnosis is established by examination of peripheral blood.

Cell surface markers

Most cases of CLL, lymphosarcoma cell leukaemia and prolymphocytic leukaemia (Fig. 19.17) are of B cell lineage and only a small per cent of cases are derived from T cells. A human T cell virus (HTLV) has been isolated from T cell of CLL and other cutaneous T cell lymphomas.

HAIRY CELL LEUKAEMIA

Hairy cell leukaemia, first described by Bouroncle (1958), is a rare disorder of middle and late adult life, characterised by proliferation of abnormal mononuclear cells with hairy cytoplasmic projections in the reticuloendothelial organs (bone marrow, spleen) and peripheral blood (Figs. 19.19 and 19.20). Most patients have marked splenomegaly.

LABORATORY FEATURES

Pancytopenia or depression of only two cell lines is the usual findings, with variable numbers of hairy cells.

Hairy cell : It is a medium sized cell, 10-20 μm diameter, with round to oval nucleus, though many are notched or dumbell shaped. The chromatin pattern is uniformly reticular. The chromatin is more condensed in some cells resembling that of lymphocytes. Cytoplasm is moderate, stains grey blue and exhibits irregular villi resulting in an irregular scarred hairy edge and also pseudopodial extensions (Fig. 19.20).

Cytochemical examination shows presence of acid phosphatase in hairy cell which is resistant to inhibition by tartrate; this is in contrast to the isoenzymes of acid phosphatase present in other haemic cells. The cells are usually subtypes of B lymphocytes, although others say that the cells have both phagocytic and B cell properties.

Blood picture

Total WBC : 3,000 to 4,000/cu. mm.

Differential count

Neutrophils	— 30–50%
Lymphocytes	— 35-55%
Monocytes	— 2–3%
Eosinophils	— 1–2%
Abnormal cells (hairy cell)	— 10–50%

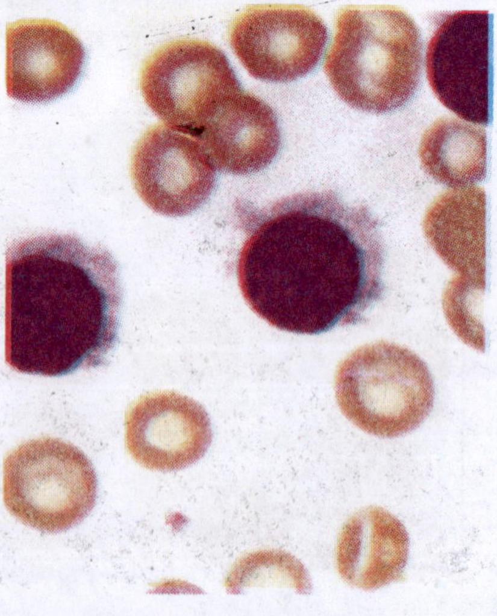

Fig. 19.20. Hairy cell leukaemia showing irregular cytoplasmic villi of the lymphocyte

Other findings

Total RBC	3 to 3.5 million/cu. mm
Total platelets	60,000 to 100,000/cu. mm
Haemoglobin	8.5 to 9.5 g%.

Bone marrow

It varies in cellularity, both hypercellular and hypocellular areas are present with reticular fibrosis. There is usually proliferation of abnormal mononuclear cells with hairy cytoplasmic projections.

MYELOPROLIFERATIVE DISORDERS

Myeloproliferative diseases are a family of disorders characterised by increased blood cell production which arise in a clonal manner from abnormalities of a single pluripotential stem cell (Fig. 19.21). The disorders in this family include :

1. Chronic myelogenous leukaemia (CML),
2. Agnogenic myeloid metaplasia with myelofibrosis (MF, also called idiopathic myelofibrosis),
3. Polycythaemia rubra vera (PV) and
4. Essential thrombocythaemia.

In each disorder, erythroid, myeloid and megakaryocytic elements proliferate excessively, but to varying degrees, in the bone marrow; and in addition there is extramedullary haematopoiesis (often resulting in splenomegaly). In these disorders, it has been experimentally shown that one precursor cell gives rise to abnormal erythrocytes, granulocytes and megakaryocytes but not to lymphocytes.

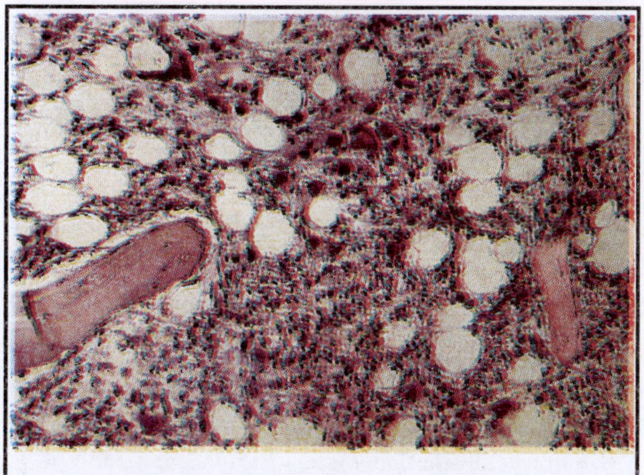

Fig. 19.21. Bone-trephine needle biopsy : Acute myelofibrosis. Haematopoietic tissue is reduced grossly

The erythroid, granulocytic-monocytic and megakaryocytic cell lines are derived from a common cell line which supports the concept that myeloproliferative disorders are clonal in nature which has arisen from a single haematopoietic cell. The new clone gradually replaces the normal cells due to proliferative advance over normal cell.

Despite difference in the predominant cell line released into the periphery in four disorders, the features of bone marrow, at the time of presentation, show many similarities which may be indistinguishable. The presence of sheets of abnormal macrophages is common to all. Other common features include : (i) hyperuricaemia secondary to increased cell turnover, (ii) abnormal levels of serum B12 and its binding capacity, (iii) increased leucocyte alkaline phosphatase activity.

Pluripotent stem cells, although, are constantly present normally in circulation in a very small number; but in these disorders, they appear in much increased number and take up residence in liver and spleen to produce extramedullary haematopoiesis. The primary pathogenic event is thought to be a mutation leading to a malignant haematopoietic clone at the level of a pluripotent stem cell.

CML, PV and essential thrombocythaemia are discussed in relevant chapters. A brief outline on agnogenic myeloid metaplasia will be presented here.

Agnogenic Myeloid Metaplasia with Myelofibrosis

(*Syn : Idiopathic myelofibrosis, myelosclerosis with myeloid metaplasia*)

DEFINITION

It is a chronic, progressive panmyelosis of clonal disorder of haematopoietic stem cell characterised by a triad of findings :

(a) varying degree of fibrosis of the marrow,
(b) massive splenomegaly due to extramedullary haematopoiesis, and a
(c) leucoerythroblastic anaemia with marked red cell abnormalities, circulating normoblasts, immature granulocytes, and atypical platelets.

CLINICAL FEATURES

Idiopathic MF typically occurs above the age of 50, and has an insidious onset, weight loss, anaemia and abdominal discomfort due to splenic enlargement. Hepatomegaly is seen in 50–70% cases. X-ray of bone shows diffuse or patchy osteosclerosis in about 30–50% patients.

Pathophysiology

Fibroblastic proliferation is believed to be due to platelet derived growth factor or tumour growth factor from platelets and megakaryocytes. Type III collagen is usually the cause of myelofibrosis. Anaemia is due to several factors : marrow failure, ineffective erythropoiesis and haemolysis.

Laboratory features

Blood picture

Total count :

RBC : 3.5 to 4.5 million /cu. mm

WBC : 15,000 to 30,000/cu. mm

Platelet : 200,000 to 450,000/cu. mm (increased in 50% cases initially but later falls below normal leading to thrombocytopenia).

Reticulocyte count : Increased (3–5%).

Haemoglobin : 8 to 10 g%.

Differential count

Neutrophils	50-65%
Lymphocytes	20–30%
Monocytes	0–2%
Eosinophils	1–3%
Abnormal cells :	
Myeloblasts, Promyelocytes, Myelocytes, Metamyelocytes	10–12%
Normoblasts	3–8%
Megakaryocytes	1–2%

Peripheral "smear" study

Anaemia : Normocytic normochromic anaemia, frequently with some hypochromic red cells and basophilic stipling. There is moderate degree of anisocytosis and marked degree of poikilocytosis with tear drop forms (dacrocytes) and elliptocytes.

Normoblasts : These are often present in blood out of proportion of anaemia.

Abnormal leucocytes : Myeloblasts, promyelocytes, myelocytes and metamyelocytes are present in significant number, the number of myeloblasts may reach 10% or more. Neutrophils exhibit basophilia and 'Pelger-Huet' anomaly (failure of normal segmentation of granulocyte nuclei) are typical features.

Bone marrow : Aspiration of marrow is usually impossible, especially later in the course of the disease. Marrow material is collected by a needle or surgical biopsy.

(i) *Early stage* : Hypercellular with panmyelosis and increased megakaryocytes which are often abnormal.

(ii) *Late stage* : Bone marrow is fibrotic with residual islands of atypical megakaryocytes, erythroid and granulocytic precursors. Fibrosis is of loose connective tissue with abundant reticulin fibres but scanty collagen. The bony trabeculae are sometimes irregularly thickened (myelosclerosis).

Course : Patient develops progressive anaemia and enlargement of spleen, haemolysis turns out to be an important cause of anaemia. Infectious episode is common. Portal hypertension occurs in 10–20% cases. Median survival is about 3 years. In patients with longer survival, the terminal event is often an acute leukaemia.

MYELODYSPLASTIC SYNDROMES (MDS) Figs. 19.22 and 19.23

The myelodysplastic disorders are a heterogeneous group of leukaemia–related conditions characterised by an anaemia refractory to haematinics, with or without neutropenia and thrombocytopenia. The bone marrow may be normocellular or hypercellular. The FAB Cooperative Group (Bennel 1992) has described and classified these disorders into five categories employing the basic criteria which is summarised in Table 19.7. Agranular blast cells and blast cells with a few azurophilic granules are included as blasts, promyelocytes are excluded.

Table 19.7
Myelodysplastic syndrome : FAB classification

Type	Bone marrow
1. Refractory anaemia (RA)	Blasts < 5%
2. Refractory anaemia with ring sideroblasts (RARs)	Blasts < 5% Ring sideroblasts > 15%
3. Refractory anaemia with excess of blasts (RAEB)	Blasts 5–20%
4. Refractory anaemia with excess of blasts in transformation (RAEB)	Blasts 20–30%
5. Chronic myelomonocytic leukaemia (CMML)	Peripheral blood monocytes > 1000/cu mm

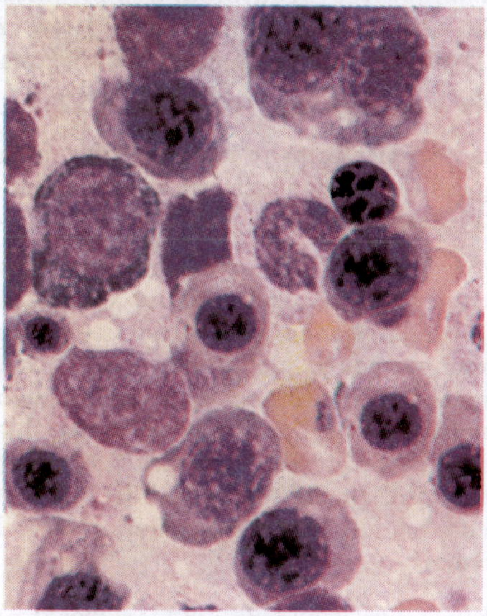

Fig. 19.22. Myelodysplastic syndrome (marrow film), showing erythroid hyperplasia with dyserythropoiesis and megaloplastic features

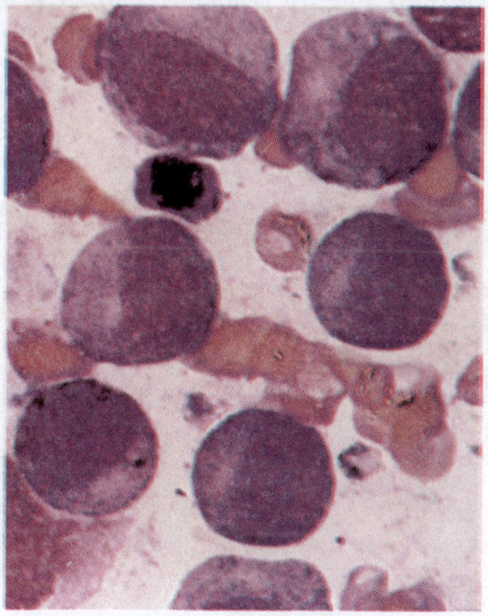

Fig. 19.23. Myelodysplastic syndrome with hypogranularity of myelocytes

Although the aetiology of MDS is not clear, some patients of any age occasionally develop a secondary form of the disease who have had treatment with radiotherapy, chemotherapy or a combination of both. The most common cytogenic abnormalities observed include deletion of long arm of chromosome 5 and 7 or trisomy 8.

CLINICL FEATURES

MDS occur primarily in persons over 50, and usually present with anaemia refractory to haematinics, recurrent infections and haemorrhagic manifestations. MDS have several features in common with acute leukaemia but differs from AML in their chronic course of illness and lesser degree of blast cell infiltration of the bone marow (less than 30%). Since transformation to overt acute myeloid leukaemia of the high proportion of cases take place, Sarrni (1977) termed *pre-leukaemic leukemia* to this group of disorders. Transformation is seen more frequently in refractory anaemia with excess blasts.

LABORATORY DIAGNOSIS

Blood picture

Total count :

Total WBC : Neutropenia of variable degree; average 2500–3500/cu. mm.

Total RBC : 3.5–4.0 million/cu. mm.

Total platelets : Usually reduced, very low count in some cases, average 50,000 to 100,000/cu. mm.

Haemoglobin : Markedly diminished; average 5–7 g%.

Differential count

Neutrophils	15–30%
Lymphocytes	40–60%
Monocytes	Increased in CMML
Abnormal cells :	
Myeloblasts	1–3%
Promyelocytes	0–10%
Myelocytes	0–5%
Metamyelocytes	0–5%
Normoblasts	1–2%

PERIPHERAL SMEAR

Red cells : Mild to severe normocytic, or mildly macrocytic anaemia. Red cells may be dimorphic, simultaneous presence of hypochromic and normochromic RBCs, particularly in refractory anaemia with ring sideroblasts. Nucleated red cells often with dyserythropoietic changes may be present. Basophilic stippling of RBC is often seen.

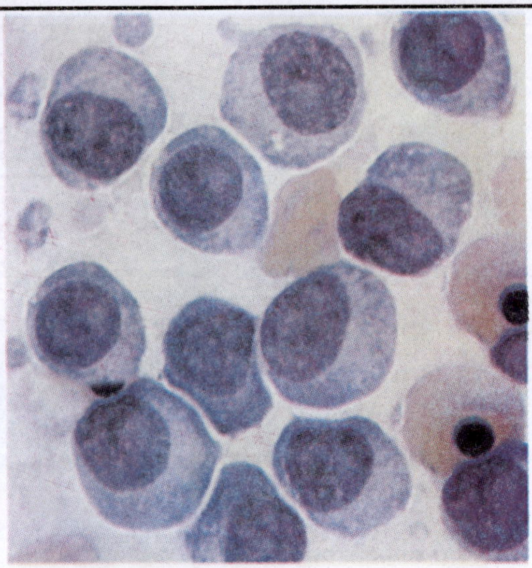

Fig. 19.24. Marrow film : Plasma cell myeloma

White cells : Variable degree of neutropenia, often a shift to the left in the neutrophil series is present; myeloblast is occasionally seen. Pelger-Huet nuclear configuration of neutrophil with bilobed nucleus and agranular granulocytes are commonly encountered.

Monocytes are characteristically increased in chronic myelomonocytic leukaemia.

Thrombocytes : Platelets are significantly reduced and in some cases at a very low critical level. Dysfunctional large platelets are present.

Bone marrow (Figs. 19.22 and 19.23)

It is normocellular to hypercellular with morphological evidence of disordered development of all cell lineages.

Red cell series : The proportion of erythroid precursors show considerable variation but dyserythropoietic features of red cell precursors are common, which include asynchrony between maturation of cytoplasm and nucleus, nuclear fragmentation, multinuclearity, megaloblastoid changes, cytoplasmic vacuolation, basophilic stippling and Howell-Jolly bodies. Marrow iron stores are usually increased and often sideroblasts are present.

White cell series : There is evidence of dysgranulopoiesis including aberrant staining of primary granules of myeloid precursors, hypogranular granulocytes, Pelger-Huet type cells, variably increased proportion of blast cells.

Thrombocyte series : Megakaryocytes and large monolobular megakaryocytes and abnormal large platelets are also seen.

Course of MDS

Behaviour of MDS vary widely between the

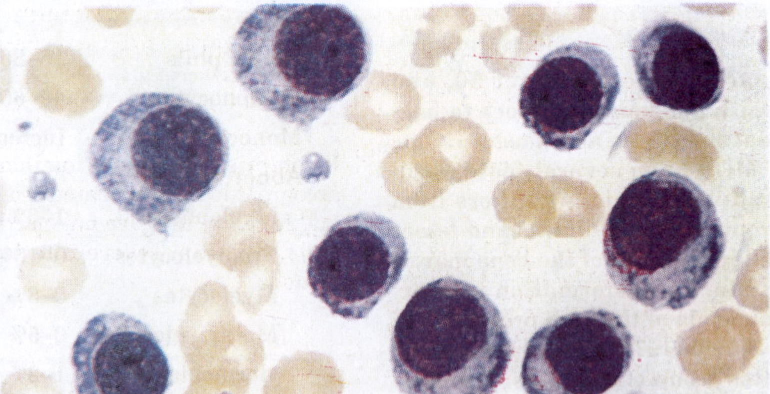

Fig. 19.25. Blood film : Plasma cell leukaemia

Table 19.8
Distinguishing features of chronic myeloid leukaemia and leukaemoid reaction

	Chronic myeloid leukaemia	Leukaemoid reaction
Total WBC/cu. mm	50,000 – 450,000	20,000 – 100,000
Immature cells	About 5% myeloblasts and large number of mylocytes	Some band forms and myelocytes
Neutrophil alkaline phosphatase score	Decreased (0-40)	Increased (150-350)
Philadelphia chromosome	Positive	Negative
Splenomegaly	Moderate to massive	No
Eosinophilia	–ve	+ve
Basophilia	–ve	+ve
Cause	No cause	Present

groups and also within particular category. The first two are relatively chronic disorders. In mild cases, active therapy is not required. Where anaemia is a sole problem, blood transfusion provides good quality of life for many years. The last 3 categories show a more aggressive course with a tendency to terminate as acute myeloid leukaemia. Mostly elderly persons are affected.

PLASMA CELL DYSCRASIAS AND RELATED DISORDERS

Plasma cell dyscrasias are a group of disorders that have in common :

(i) the proliferation of a single clone of immunoglobin producing plasma cells (Fig. 19.24) and (ii) a resultant increase in serum levels of one specific class, subclass and type of immunoglobulin or its fragments.

The group is divided into six major variants which include : (1) *multiple myeloma,* (2) localised *plasmacytoma* (solitary myeloma), (3) *Waldenstrom's macroglobulinaemia,* (4) *heavy-chain disease,* (5) primary or immuno-associated *amyloidosis* and (6) *monoclonal gammopathy.*

PLASMA CELL LEUKAEMIA (Fig. 19.25)

A few plasma cells are sometimes found in peripheral blood in multiple myeloma. Only in rare instances of myeloma in which large numbers of plasma cells circulate (> 20% of blood leucocytes), the term plasma cell leukaemia is applied. Plasma cell leukaemia is an advanced stage of the disease with tissue invasion, and prognosis is poor.

LEUKAEMOID REACTION

Leucocytosis (neutrophilia) is a common feature of inflammations, especially that caused by bacteria. Sometimes an extremely high leucocyte counts (40000 to 100000/cu. mm) similar to that found in leukaemia are obtained. These are called leukaemoid reactions. Leucocytosis results from accelerated release of cells from bone marrow reserve pool triggered by IL–1 and TNF. Peripheral blood contains some immature forms (band forms, myelocytes) in addition to mature neutrophils. Neutrophil alkaline phosphatase score is high in contrast to chronic granulocytic leukaemia (Table 19.8).

LEUCOERYTHROBLASTIC REACTION

It comprises of circulating immature granulocytes accompanied by nucleated red cells (erythroblasts) and found in massive haemorrhage, severe haemolysis, hypoxia, severe infection, and metastatic tumour.

QUESTIONS

1. *How do you classify leukaemia?*
2. *What is the Fab classification of acute leukaemia?*
3. *Mention the different nucleated cell counts in acute leukaemias.*
4. *How do you distinguish myeloblast from monoblast?*

5. *How does cytochemical studies help to determine the category of acute myeloid, acute lymphoid leukaemia?*
6. *How to distinguish myeloblast from lymphoblast?*
7. *How is aleukaemic leukaemia diagnosed?*
8. *Which of the acute leukaemias has got better prognosis?*
9. *Which is the type lymphoid cell from which most acute lymphoblastic leukaemias arise?*
10. *Which is the cell type of origin in majority of cases of chronic lymphocytic leukaemia?*
11. *Which chronic leukaemia has got a worst prognosis?*
12. *Which leukaemia is more frequent in India?*
13. *What are the common age incidences of CMC and CLL?*
14. *What is a hairy cell leukaemia and its laboratory features?*
15. *What is myeloproliferative syndrome (MDS)?*
16. *Name the diseases included in MDS.*
17. *What is plasma cell leukaemia?*
18. *What is leukaemoid reaction? How do you distinguish between leukaemia and leukaemoid reaction?*
19. *Name the causes of leukaemoid reaction.*
20. *What is leucoerythroblastic reaction?*

Chapter 20

Haemorrhagic Disorders and Investigation of Haemostasis

NORMAL HAEMOSTASIS

Haemostasis is the mechanism by which bleeding from an injured blood vessel is arrested by formation of a thrombus which seals the injured vessel.

The normal haemostatic mechanisms have two primary functions : to maintain the blood in a fluid state and to prevent blood clots from developing in intact blood vessels and to arrest bleeding from injured vessels. This is achieved by a balance between many complex, interrelated systems which include *blood vessels, platelets, plasma coagulation proteins, inhibitors* and *fibrinolytic system.*

Injury to the wall of blood vessel is immediately followed by constriction of the vessel resulting in slowing of blood flow; activated platelets adhere to the damaged wall and subsequently aggregate to form a platelet plug which arrests haemorrhage. This is followed by conversion of the platelet plug into the definitive clot (Fig. 20.1).

Platelet and Vessel wall interaction

Injury leads to vasoconstriction due to serotonin and other vasoconstrictors liberated from plate-

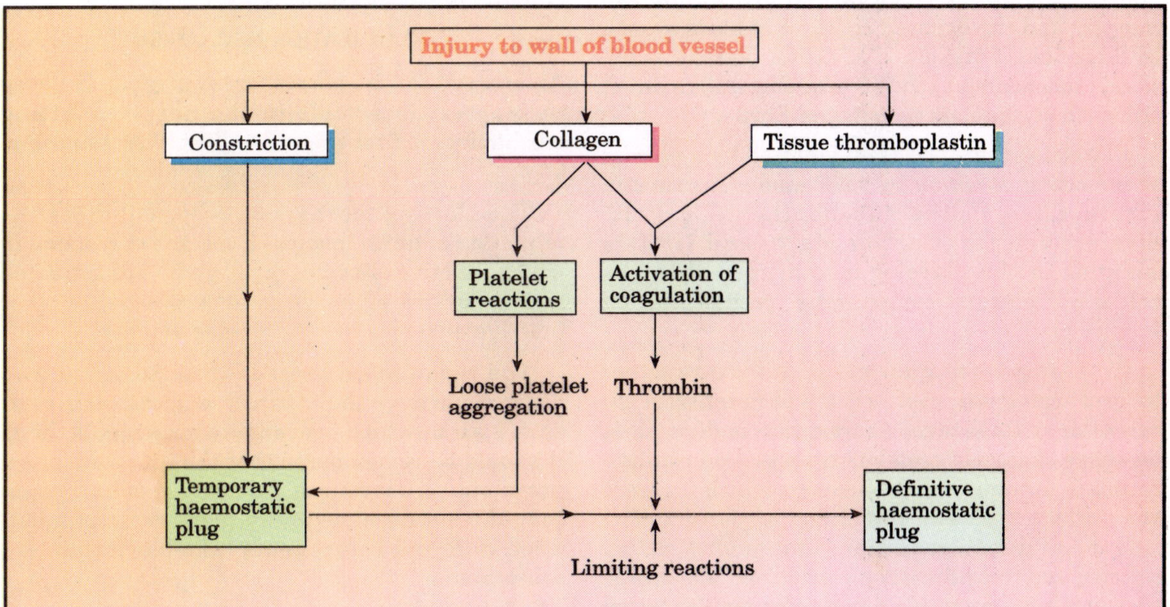

Fig. 20.1. Normal haemostasis

lets. The platelets leave the blood flow immediately after vessel injury to reach to the subendothelium which may be measured in milliseconds.

Endothelial cell possesses proteoglycan coat which contains heparin sulphate and other glycosaminoglycans. Heparin sulphate and glycosaminoglycans can activate *antithrombin III,* an inhibitor of coagulation enzymes. Endothelial cell can also generate *angiotensin II,* a local vasoconstrictor. Thus constriction occurs following injury even in microcirculation in vessels without smooth muscle cells. Endothelial cell also produces *von Willebrand Factor* (vWF), essential for adhesion of platelet to the subendothelium. vWF is secreted both in circulation and towards the subendothelial matrix.

Platelets are not activated with healthy endothelial cells due to *non-thrombogenecity* of endothelium.

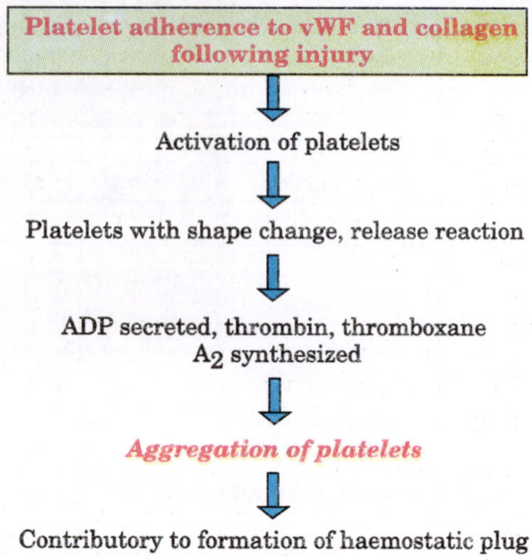

Fig. 20.2. Role of platelets in coagulation

Formation of haemostatic plug (Fig. 20.2)

Platelet adhesion to subendothelium has two components :

(i) *Adhesion* : When blood vessel is damaged, circulating platelets react with collagen fibrils of subendothelial surface. Platelet adhesion at high speed flow of blood in the capillary bed depends on plasma protein, vWF which forms a bridge to the platelet membrane receptor and glycoprotein Ib complex and the exposed collagen of blood vessel. In larger blood vessels, e.g., aorta, platelet adhesion is independent of vWF probably due to direct adhesion of platelets to collagen fibrils.

Platelet contact is closely followed by a process of *spreading adhesion* by vWF and/or fibronectin incorporated in the subendothelial matrix, divalent cations (Ca^{++} or Mg^{++}) and IIb/IIIa complex in the platelet membrane. With the release of platelet components, recruitment of further platelets occur simultaneously.

(ii) *Aggregation* : Platelets stick to one another to form aggregates. Fibrinogen and fibronectin are essential at this stage. Aggregation is dependent on shape change of platelets from discoid configuration to formation of pseudopods which increase the surface area and likelihood of contact. The release of dense granular components, *ADP, calcium* and free *arachidonic* acid from membrane phospholipids provides a powerful amplification feedback to aggregate platelets in the vicinity (Fig. 20.2). Thus, a larger, firmer aggregates of platelets is formed.

Fate of the haemostatic plug

Autolysis of the platelets in haemostatic plug gradually takes place and is replaced by fibrin, and the haemostatic plug is transformed into a dense fibrin mass in 24–28 hours. The fibrin mass is then gradually digested by fibrinolytic enzyme system and the vessel wall defect is covered by endothelial cells (Fig. 20.4).

COAGULATION MECHANISM

An overview of the participants currently believed to play critical roles in the normal clotting mechanism is first presented (Table 20.1 and Fig. 20.3).

The clotting mechanism responsible for the formation of fibrin involves a cascade of reaction in which inactive enzymes (zymogens) are activated and the activated enzymes in turn activate other inactive enzymes by its protease activity.

The coagulation cascade (Fig. 20.3) has two distinct parts — the *intrinsic* and *extrinsic* systems, both of which converge to activate factor X. It should be remembered that the illustration is a gross simplification of intricate mechanism of coagulation because many more reactions between different components take place than are illustrated.

I. Intrinsic pathways

The initial reaction in the intrinsic pathway is activation of inactive factor XII (Hageman factor)

Table 20.1 : Plasma coagulatiuon factors

Factor	*Synonym (probable)*	*Synthesis site dependent*	*Vit. K*	*Functions*
I	Fibrinogen	Liver	No	Clot structural protein
II	Prothrombin	Liver	Yes	Serine protease
III	Thromboplastin	Tissue factor	—	—
IV	Calcium	—	—	—
V	Proaccelerin	Liver	No	Cofactor
VI	*Nonexistent*	—	—	—
VII	Proconvertin	Liver	Yes	Serine protease
VIII–C	Antihaemophilic globulin (AHC)	Liver	No	Cofactor
VIII–R	von Willebrand factor	Endothelium	No	Cofactor for platelets
IX	Christmas factor	Liver	Yes	Serine protease
X	Stuart-Power factor	Liver	Yes	Serine protease
XI	Plasma-thromboplastin antecedent ((PTA)	Liver	No	Serine protease
XII	Hageman factor, glass contact factor	? Liver	No	Serine protease
XIII	Fibrin stabilising factor	Liver	No	Transamidase
Fletcher factor, PreKallikrein		? Liver	No	Serine
Fitzgerald factor, HMW Kininogen		? Liver	No	Cofactor

to active factor XIIa. This occurs when blood is exposed to the collagen fibres of the subendothelial tissue of blood vessels. This reaction is greatly enhanced by the negative charges of subintima of injured vessel wall. Active factor XIIa then activates factor XI (plasma thromboplastin) and active factor XI (XIa) in turn activates factor IX (Christmas factor). Activated factor IX (IXa) forms a complex with phospholipid of aggregated platelets and activates factor VIII. The activated factor VIII (VIIIa) activates factor X in the presence of calcium. Recent studies suggest that the formation of Xa by this indirect path may proceed at a rate equal to or greater than that of activation of X by VIIa /tissue factor (the classic "extrinsic pathway"). The intrinsic pathway is assessed *in vitro* by the *activated partial thromboplastin time* (APTT).

Vitamin K dependent factors include factor II (prothrombin), X, IX, and protein C and S.

II. Extrinsic pathways

The extrinsic pathway is triggered by the release of tissue factor (tissue thromboplastin) which is a protein-phospholipid mixture that activates factor VII. The tissue thromboplastin and factor VIIa activate factors IX and X (classical pathway). Tissue factor is produced by many tissues, e.g., human endothelial cells, smooth muscle cells and fibroblasts. Extrinsic pathway is measured by the *prothrombin time* (PT).

Common pathway

Once formed, activated factor Xa in turn activates prothrombin (factor II) leading to conversion of prothrombin to the active enzyme thrombin. Thrombin cleaves peptide fragments from the α and β chains of fibrinogen to fibrin monomers, that subsequently assemble into polymetric fibrin clot. Further strengthening of these fibrin polymers is done by the action of activated XIIIa, a transamidase which cross-links adjacent molecules of polymerised fibrin. Factor XIII is converted to its active form by the action of thrombin in presence of calcium ions. Thrombin, therefore, plays two vital roles in coagulation : (i) conversion of fibrinogen to fibrin and (ii) the activation of factor XIII so that the fibrin cross-links can be stabilised.

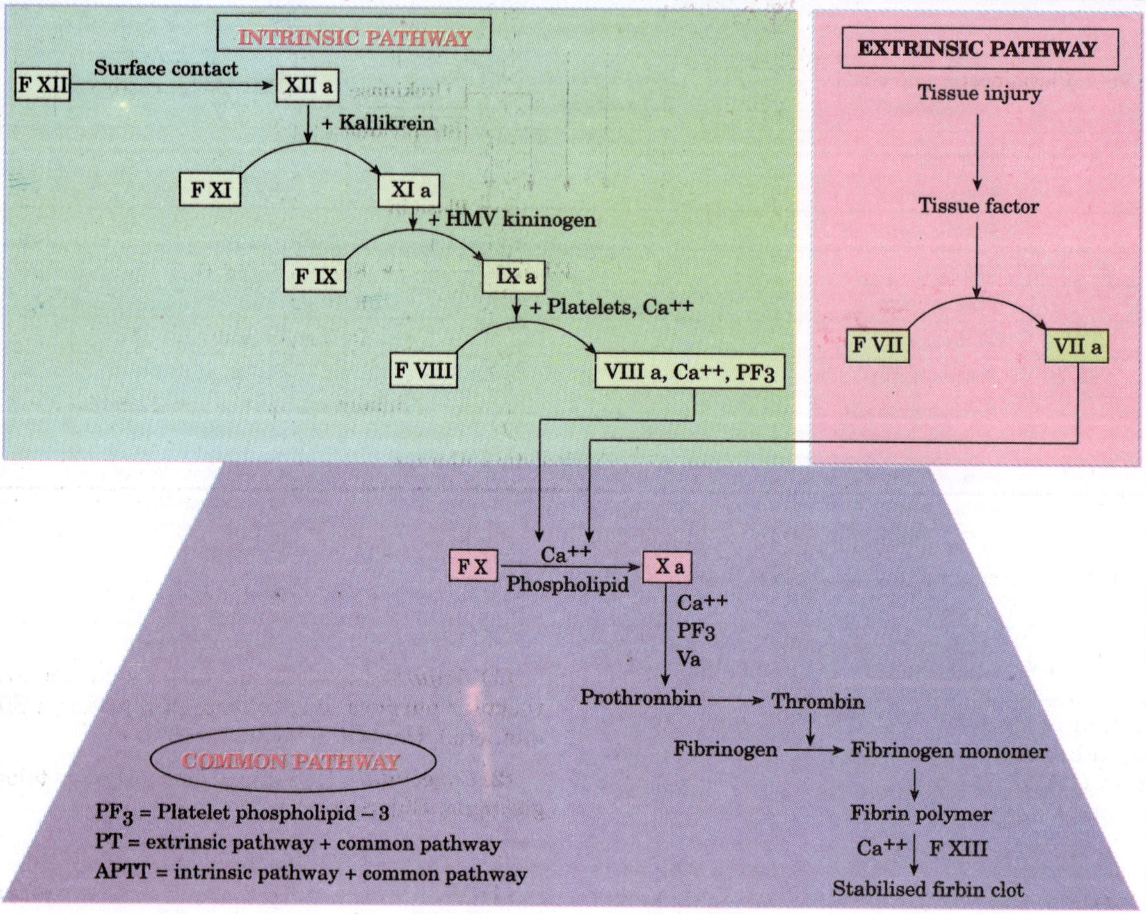

Fig. 20.3. Coagulation pathways

Congenital or acquired deficiencies of single or multiple components of the clotting system lead to a bleeding diathesis characterised by joint and muscle haemorrhage and prolonged bleeding after trauma or surgery, e.g., haemophilia.

REGULATION OF COGULATION

The coagulation process, once activated, would continue until all the fibrinogen in the plasma was converted to fibrin in absence of strict regulatory mechanisms. This process is controlled by two important physiological inhibitors of coagulation which include *anti-thrombin* III (AT III) and *protein C/protein S system.*

(i) AT III neutralises thrombin and several other activated clotting factors (Xa, IXa, XIa, XIIa). Heparin accelerates the speed of action.

(ii) Protein C and protein S are synthesised in liver and are vitamin K dependent. Protein C is also synthesised by endothelial cells. Protein C is converted by thrombin to an activated form. The activated protein C, in conjunction with its cofactor protein S, inhibits factor Va and factor VIIIa.

Other coagulation inhibitors include C1 inhibitor (an inhibitor of classical complement pathway), α macroglobulin and α_1–antitrypsin.

Fibrinolysis

Thrombi prevent loss of blood from vessel but they must be removed as healing occurs. This removal occurs through fibrinolytic system. This consists of an inactive proenzyme *plasminogen* which is activated to proteolytic enzyme *plasmin* by several plasminogen activators (Fig. 20.4). Although, the main physiological substrate for plasmin is fibrin, it also digests fibrinogen and factors V and VIII.

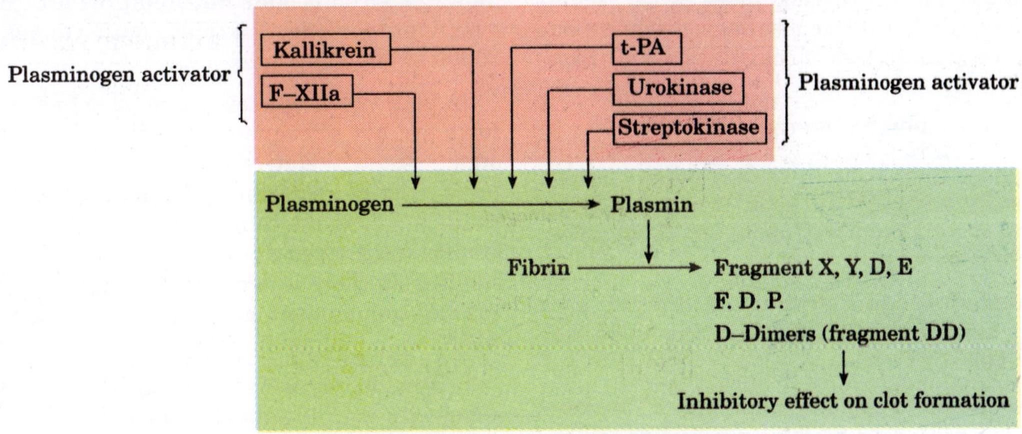

Fig. 20.4. Fibrinolytic pathways

There are several types of plasminogen activator : (i) *tissue plasminogen activator* (t-Pa) and (ii) *urokinase plasminogen activator* (u-Pa) secreted by endothelial cells are most important. They convert plasminogen to the active enzyme *plasmin* which degrades fibrin to fibrin degradation products (FDPs). The system is regulated by inhibitors — plasminogen activator inhibitors (PAIs) and by α_2 plasmin (α_2–P1) and C_1 inhibitor.

Hypercoagulability state

Hypercoagulability may be defined as an alteration of blood or, specially, the clotting mechanism with increased tendency to thrombosis. The hypercoagulable state, also called thrombophilia, is not a common cause of thrombogenesis.

(i) The best-understood and prototype of hypercoagulable state is one with inherited deficiency of anticoagulants *antithrombin II*, protein C, or protein S. Affected persons suffer from various thrombosis and recurrent thromboembolism in adolescence or early adult life. It is easy to understand the cause of these thrombotic tendencies in these patients. However, these hereditary diseases are quite uncommon.

(ii) There is another group of patients with hypercoagulable state in which there is no hereditary cause and where it is difficult to do unravel the cause of pathogenic thrombotic diathesis, eg., nephrotic syndrome, following severe trauma or burns, in later pregnancy, with cardiac failure, in disseminated cancer, and in females having used oral contraceptives (both arterial and venous thrombosis).

HAEMORRHAGIC DISORDERS

Causes of bleeding disorder

I. Disorders due to capillary defects

(1) *Acquired* : Senile purpura, symptomatic vascular purpura (due to drugs, infections, uraemia, etc.), Henoch Schonlein purpura.

(2) *Congenital* : Hereditary haemorrhagic telengiectasia, Ehlers–Danlos disease.

II. Disorders due to platelet abnormalities

(1) ***Qualitative abnormalities*** : Congenital abnormalities (disorders of membrane glycoproteins, e.g., thrombasthenia, Burner-Soulier syndrome; presence of defective platelet granules, e.g. storage pool disorders); drugs (aspirin, thromboxane A, indomethacin, dextran).

(2) ***Quantitative abnormalities***

(a) *Thrombocytopenia* : (i) Primary or idiopathic thrombocytopenia. (ii) *Secondary thrombocytopenia* : Secondary to other causes, e.g., drug, infiltration, DIC, chemicals, infections and hypersplenism.

(b) *Thrombocytosis* : Thrombocytosis as nonspecific reactive response to chronic bleeding or inflammation. *Essential thrombocythaemia,* a malignant condition of megakaryocytes.

III. Coagulation disorders

(1) ***Congenital*** : Haemophilia A and B, von Willebrand's disease, other congenital deficiency disorders of fibrinogen, prothrombin, factors V, XII, XIII, Fletcher and Fitzgerald.

(2) ***Acquired*** : (i) Disseminated intravascular coagulation (DIC). (ii) Haemorrhagic disorders due to circulating inhibitors of coagulation. (iii) Excessive fibrinolysis.

THROMBOCYTOPENIC PURPURA

The term purpura is used for disorders involving bleeding from capillaries with the production of petechial spots. Thrombocytopenia is the commonest cause of purpura.

Thrombocytopenic purpura is defined as a platelet count below 100000/cu. mm blood (see chapter 10).

There are three basic mechanisms of thrombocytopenia : decreased platelet production, shortened platelet survival time and splenic sequestration.

Types

Thrombocytopenic purpura may be :

(1) Primary, known as essential or idiopathic.

(2) Secondary to some known causes (chapter 9).

IDIOPATHIC THROMBOCYTOPENIC PURPURA (ITP)

(Syn : Primary or essential ITP)

ITP is a disorder characterised by thrombocytopenia in almost all cases, caused by auto-antibodies, often directed against membrane glycoprotein of platelets. The antiplatelet antibody binds to platelets and agglutination of platelets results in premature splenic removal of these platelets. There are two forms of ITP, acute and chronic. Both types show normal or increased megakaryocytes in the marrow, shortened platelet survival and absence of splenomegaly.

1. ***Acute ITP***

It is a self-limiting disease, occurs most commonly in children between 2-6 years of age and accounts for most cases in children. It is characterised by acute onset with haemorrhage into skin and mucous membrane with an average platelet count of 20000/cu. mm blood. In about 80% of cases there is a previous history of viral respiratory tract infection 1-3 weeks prior to onset of petechiae. Eighty per cent cases recover spontaneously in 2-6 months and recurrence is rare.

2. ***Chronic ITP***

Chronic ITP is usually a disease of young to middle aged females. Onset is less abrupt and undergoes remissions and relapses alternating over long periods. Platelet count ranges from 30000 to 80000/cu. mm.

In both types, epistaxis, gum bleeding, haematuria are not infrequent. Bleeding from internal organs, though relatively uncommon, may occur in brain, uterus, intestine and lungs. Thrombocytopenia is a common complication of HIV infection. Unlike antiplatelet antibody (IgG) bound to platelets in ITP, there is deposition of immune complexes and complement on the surface of platelets in AIDS.

3. ***Senile purpura*** : The subcutaneous tissue along with dermis undergoes atrophy in advanced age. As a result small capillaries at some sites become supportless which bleed on trivial trauma usually in the form of ecchymosis. In such cases capillary resistance test is positive.

Investigations

1. Reduction in platelet count ranges from just below normal to 20000/cu mm (20000 to 80000). Sometimes platelets look morphologically abnormal.
2. Bleeding time prolonged (30 minutes or longer).
3. Demonstration of antiplatelet antibody.
4. Demonstration of shortened platelet survival time by compensated thrombocytolytic test.

ESSENTIAL THROMBOCYTHAEMIA

It is a malignant condition of megakaryocytes in which increased platelet production is sustained, in addition platelets have aberrant function. Patients present with excessive bruising and bleeding or with venous or arterial thrombosis.

Diagnosis

Blood film reveals platelet aggregates, giant forms and fragments of megakaryocytic cytoplasm. Bone marrow smear shows hypercellular marrow with a background of platelet aggregates.

HAEMOPHILIA

Until 1952 it was thought that coagulation abnormality in haemophilics was always caused by deficiency of factor VIII (AHF), it was then found that blood of some patients was deficient in a previously unrecognised clotting factor which was termed Christmas factor (factor IX). The term haemophilia A is now used to describe congenital deficiency of factor VIII (now called VIII–C) and haemophilia B to describe the congenital disorder when factor IX is deficient.

Haemophilia A is five times more common than haemophilia B.

Haemophilia A (classic haemophilia)

Haemophilia A, the classical haemophilia, is the commonest of all congenital disorders of coagulation (one in 10000 males) and is due to reduced amount and activity of factor VIII–C. Some patients lack plasma factor VIII–C, whereas others have a nonfunctional factor VIII–C molecule present in normal concentrations.

Classification

(i) *Severe haemophilia* A : Overt clinical symptoms develop when factor VIII activity is less than 1% of normal.

(ii) *Moderate haemophilia* A : When activity of factor VIII is 1-5% of normal. APTT is prolonged in both severe and mid forms.

(iii) *Mild haemophilia* A : When activity of factor VIII is 6-25% of normal. These patients are usually asymptomatic, but post-traumatic bleeding, e.g., following surgery or trauma, may be somewhat excessive. This may show a normal APTT.

Majority (75%) of haemophilic patients have family history with an X-linked inheritance pattern. In the remainder (25% cases), the mutation of the factor VIII–C gene may be new. A haemophilic patient's daughters will all be carriers and all his sons will be normal. Since factor VIII-C (AHF) is determined by a defect on the the X-chromosome, with the result that hemizygous males are primarily affected. Male inheriting a gene of haemophilia shows deficiency of factor VIII–C and the plasma concentration of same varies from complete deficiency to 30% of normal.

Clinical features

Severe haemophilics are usually diagnosed shortly after birth as they develop extensive cephalhaematoma or bleeds profusely after circumcision. Normal level of factor VIII–C in plasma is 0.5 to 1.5 i.u./ml. The degree of bleeding is related to the plasma factor VIII–C level; patients with less than 0.02 i.u./ml are classified as having severe haemophilia; 0.02-0.10 i.u./ml as moderate and those with greater than 0.10 i.u./ml as mild form of the disease.

Mild haemophilics typically bleed excessively only in association with trauma or surgery. Patients with severe haemophilia experience haemarthrosis in large joints and muscles.

Haemophilia B (*Christmas disease*)

Congenital deficiency of factor IX, or *haemophilia B,* is inherited as an X-linked disorder that presents with the historical and clinical features of classic haemophilia (haemophilia A). The aberration most often results in a reduction of the plasma factor IX-level, but can be due to qualitative defects of factor IX structure. The severity of bleeding is similar to that of haemophilia A.

Laboratory findings

1. *Haemophilia A* : Clotting time greately increased; prothrombin time is normal, deficiency of factor VIII-C and prolonged APTT.

2. *Haemophilia B* : When prothrombin time and factor VIII-C levels are normal and APTT is prolonged, assay of factor IX activity should be performed.

Female carrier of haemophilia A tend to have reduced activity of factor VIII-C levels because of random inactivation of the X chromosome in the developing foetus (*Lyonisation*). The measurement of factor VIII-C : von Willebrand factor (vWF) ratio is reduced in carriers in comparison with normal individuals.

In carrier women of haemophilia the levels of factor VIII appear normal by immunoassay but the coagulant activity of factor is only half of the antigen levels. The ratio of factor VIII activity : factor VIII antigen levels are determined and the ratio is than 0.5 in carriers.

The recent development of recombinant factor VIII-C has increased the safety of factor VIII-C therapy. The normal factor VIII gene has been cloned.

VON WILLEBRAND DISEASE

The von Willebrand factor (vWF) is a protein synthesised by endothelial cells and megakaryocytes. It is an autosomal hereditary disease. It performs two important functions.

1. *Carrier protein* : vWF acts as carrier protein (stabilisation factor) of factor VIII in the circulation. Consequently, a deficiency of vWF results in a secondary reduction in AHG in circulation.

2. *Adhesion of platelets* : The other function of vWF is to form bridges between platelets and

subendothelial components allowing adherence of platelets to damaged vessel walls. A deficiency of vWF, therefore, also results in prolonged primary haemorrhage after trauma.

Clinical features

Clinical features resemble that of thrombocytopenia due to reduced platelet function. Such patients characteristically bleed from mucous membrane and cutaneous sites, such as bruising, epistaxis, menorrhagia, gastrointestinal haemorrhage.

Investigations

1. Prolonged bleeding time (VIII–C)
2. Low level of factors VIII and vWF (VIII R) — responsible for prolonged BT.
3. Associated factors deficiency lead to prolongation of APTT.

Disseminated Intravascular Coagulation (DIC)

It is an acquired haemorrhagic disorder characterised by diffuse intravascular clotting, caused by the release of thromboplastic material into the circulation.

Pathogenesis

DIC is caused by — (i) entry of tissue factors that act as pro-coagulants into circulation and (ii) extensive endothelial damage.

Naturally occurring circulating inhibitors normally inactivate the coagulants and macrophages clear them. Thus, the process of DIC is augmented by stasis and reticuloendothelial blockade. The natural inhibitors and macrophages cannot reach the site of stasis.

Causes : A wide variety of underlying causes can initiate DIC (Table 20.2).

Table 20.2 : Causes of disseminated intravascular coagulation

Types	Causes
Infections	Septicaemia, specially gram negative *(E. coli, Klebsiella)* and meningococcal; streptococcus pneumonia; malaria.
Obstetric	Abruptio placentae, retained dead foetus, pre-eclampsia, amniotic fluid embolism.
Surgical	Specially of the heart and lung.
Cancers	Cancers of lung, pancreas, prostate.

Mechanism and clinical features

Extensive endothelial damage occurs by a wide variety of causes, for example endotoxin liberated during gram negative septicaemia may activate platelets, leucocytes and Hageman factor (XII) leading to initiation and promotion of coagulation cascade. Similarly, tumours and traumatised or necrotic tissue factor into the circulation act as triggering agents on endothelial cells leading to initiation of coagulation cascade. Bacterial endotoxin, in addition, induces the expression of tissue factor on the surface of monocytes and endothelial cells which accelerate coagulation reaction. Intravascular coagulation occurs with consumption of platelets, factors V and VII and fibrinogen throughout the microvasculature in the form of small thrombi. This early thrombotic phase of DIC is followed by a procoagulant consumption and secondary fibrinolysis by activation of fibrinolytic system. Continued fibrin formation and fibrinolysis causes depletion of haemostatic components (coagulation protein and platelets) leading to generalised bleeding, e.g., purpura fulminans in meningococcaemia. Most patients develop extensive skin and mucous membrane bleeding on surgical incision or venepuncture and catheter sites.

Fibrin degrading products (FDP) are increased in DIC as well as in primary fibrinolytic conditions.

Test for FDP

Commercially latex kit are available which contains latex particles coated with specific antibodies to purified FDP. Patient's sera or plasma are tested at different dilutions with latex kit of anti-FDP serum/ plasma.

Investigations

1. Thrombocytopenia.
2. Prolonged prothrombin time.
3. Activated partial thromboplastin time prolonged.
4. Prolonged thrombin time.
5. Low fibrinogen and increased level of D dimer (evidence of fibrinolysis).

LABORATORY INVESTIGATION OF BLEEDING DISORDERS

It is essential to record a careful history of all bleeding episodes which will suggest whether the

Table 20.3 : Investigation of haemostatic function

	Investigation	Information obtained
1.	**Blood film**	*Underlying* disease : aplastic anaemia, leukaemia *Platelet* : morphology and number *RBC* : morphology, e.g., target cells, RBC fragments (microangiopathic haemolysis).
2.	**Platelet count**	*Thrombocytopenia*
3.	**Bleeding time**	*Platelet dysfunction, thrombocytopenia, von Willebrand's disease.*
4.	**Coagulation time**	*Haemophilia A, B, von Willebrand's* disease, *disorders of clotting factors.*
5.	**Prothrombin time (PT)** (extrinsic pathway)	*Warfarin therapy, liver disease, DIC.*
6.	**Activated partial thromboplastin time (APTT)** (intrinsic pathway)	*Heparin therapy, haemophilia A and B, DIC.*
7.	**Fibrinogen consumption**	*Congenital hypofibrinogenaemia, DIC.*
8.	**D dimers**	*Fibrinolysis, DIC.*

Table 20.4 : First-line screening tests in patients with acute bleeding disorder

	PT	APTT (PTTK)	TT	Platelet count	Condition
1.	N	N	N	N	Disorder of platelet function, factor XIII deficiency, disorder of vascular haemostasis, normal haemostasis.
2.	Long	N	N	N	Factor VII deficiency, early oral anticoagulant.
3.	N	Long	N	N	Factors VIII-C, IX, XI, XII, prekallikrein, HMWK deficiency. von Willebrand's disease, circulating anticoagulant.
4.	Long	Long	N	N	Vitamin K deficiency, oral anticoagulants, factors V, VII, X, II deficiency.
5.	Long	Long	Long	N	Heparin, liver disease, fibrinogen deficiency, hyperfibrinolysis.
6.	N	N	N	Low	Thrombocytopenia.
7.	Long	Long	N	Low	Massive transfusion liver disease.
8.	Long	Long	Long	Low	DIC, acute liver disease.

Table 20.5 : Result of screening tests in patients with chronic bleeding disorder (N = normal, L = long)

	PT	APTT (PTTK)	TT	Bleeding time	Condition
1.	N	N	N	L	Platelet dysfunction, disorders of vascular haemostasis.
2.	N	L	N	L	von Willebrand's disease.
3.	L	N	N	N	Factors VII deficiency.
4.	N	L	N	N	Factors VIII-C, IX, XI, XII, PK or HMWK deficiency circulating anticoagulants.
5.	L	L	N	N	Factors V, X or prothrombin deficiency, liver disease.
6.	L	L	L	N	Deficiency or defect of fibrinogen.

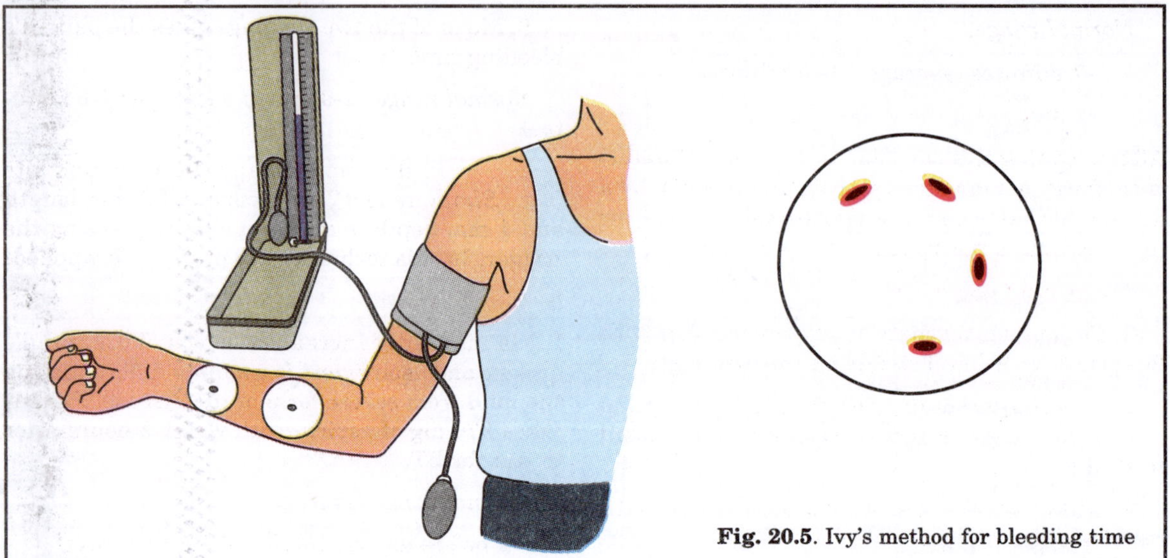

Fig. 20.5. Ivy's method for bleeding time

bleeding tendency is due to disorders of blood platelets or coagulation system and fibrinolytic system. An approach to such evaluation is outlined in Table 20.3. The first-line laboratory tests done in acute bleeding disorder is shown in Table 20.4 and the common pattern of results obtained on chronic bleeding disorders are shown in Table 20.5.

I. Complete Blood Count and Blood Film Study

A complete blood cell count and examination of the blood smear screen for abnormalities in bone marrow with evidence of underlying disease, such as aplastic anaemia and leukaemia.

Visualisation of the formed elements is helpful in patient evaluation.

RBC : Schistocytes (fragments of red cells) suggest microangiopathic haemolytic anaemias as seen in disseminated intravascular coagulation. Target cells are found in liver disease and in thalassaemia.

Platelet : The presence of large platelets in blood film indicates increased platelet turnover as seen in immune thrombocytopenia or platelet destruction by artificial cardiac prostheses. There is an inverse relation between platelet count and bleeding time.

II. Bleeding Time (BT)

It is a screening test used for the detection of abnormalities of blood vessels and platelets.

Principle : A standardised cut is made on the skin and the time during which the cut/incision bleeds is measured. Cessation of bleeding indicates formation of haemostatic plugs.

The time old *Duke's* and *Ivy's* methods for measurement of BT is still in practice in some centres. Nowadays the *Template method* is preferred.

A. Ivy's method (Fig. 20.5)

1. A sphygmomanometer cuff is wrapped around the patient's arm above the elbow and inflated to 40 mm Hg and the same pressure is maintained throughout the test.

2. Volar surface of forearm is cleansed with rectified spirit and an area of skin devoid of superficial veins is selected. The skin is stretched laterally by thumb between thumb and forefinger of left hand, and two separate punctures, 5–10 cm apart, are made in quick succession by free hand, using a disposable lancet or No. 11 surgical blade. Any microlance with about one man width with a cutting depth of 2.5 mm is suitable.

3. Timing is begun as soon as the punctures are made and bleeding starts.

4. Blood extruding from the cut is blotted off gently but completely with filter paper at 15/30 seconds interval till the bleeding stops. The time is noted.

When the bleeding has ceased, a sterile adhesive strip is placed on the wounds.

Normal range

2.0–7 minutes (average 1.0–6 minutes).

B. Duke method

After cleaning the ear lobe (or heel of an infant) with spirit, a 3 mm deep stab wound is made by a disposable lancet in the margin of ear lobe (or heel). Result is recorded as in Ivy method.

C. BT by template method

1. Patient sits on chair having an arm rest with forearm exposed and steady on the arm rest.

2. A sphygmomanometer cuff is wrapped around the patient's arm above elbow and inflated to 40 mm Hg.

3. Volar surface of forearm is cleaned with rectified spirit and an area of skin devoid of superficial veins is selected. A template is placed 5-6 cm distal to the antecubital crease.

4. The template is made of plastic having a slit of 9 mm length and the thickness is that of the plastic. The angle of the blade is fitted in the plastic in such a manner that the incision made through the slit is nine mm in length and one mm in depth.

After placing the template on the forearm, it is pressed against the skin to flatten the skin surface and the slit remaining parallel to the antecubital fossa. Incision is made parallel to the crease to avoid retraction of skin. If incision is made at right angle to crease, stem gets retracted producing a bigger spindle-shaped wound.

5. The skin is penetrated by the blade through the slit and an incision is made along the entire length of the slit. The whole process is carried carefully with a smooth and rapid movement. A stop watch is started as soon as the puncture is made and bleeding starts.

6. At a distance of 1.5 cm to 2 cm from the site of first incision, a second incision is made and a second stop watch is started.

7. Blood extruding from the incisions is blotted off gently but completely with filter paper (Whatman No.1), without touching the wound edges or skin, every 15/30 seconds interval till the bleeding stops. Time is noted.

When the bleeding stops, the edges of the incisions are carefully opposed and sterile adhesive strip is placed on the wounds.

8. Mean of the two readings gives the patient's bleeding time.

Normal range : 2-9 minutes (average 1-6 minutes).

Note : In the commercially available test kits (e.g., *Simplate test* , an incision of 5 mm length and 1 mm depth is made on simply pressing the trigger. In this technique, no pressure is applied.

D. Aspirin test

BT is markedly increased in von Willebrand's disease and aspirin test is useful in differentiating the mild from severe form of the disease. Patient takes 970 mg of aspirin with water 2 hours prior to test for BT.

Normal range (average)

BT before aspirin intake — 1-6 minutes

BT after aspirin intake — 4-10 minutes

In mild form of von Willebrand's, BT is normal while severe form of the disease it is markedly prolonged after aspirin intake.

Principle : Aspirin irreversibly blocks the action of platelet cyclooxygenase and thereby it prevents conversion of arachidonic acid into endoperoxides and prostaglandins leading to failure of platelet aggregation. Hence coronary artery disease patients are treated with aspirin to prevent thrombus formation. However, aspirin therapy may cause increased bleeding after injury.

Prolonged bleeding time

1. Thrombocytopenia – essential and secondary types.
2. Qualitative platelet defects.
3. von Willebrand's disease.
4. Vascular defects.
5. Others : Uraemia, antiplatelet medication (e.g. aspirin).

III. Platelet aggregation test

The test can only be performed in a reference laboratory. Platelet aggregometry provides additional information on qualitative defect of platelet. When citrated platelet-rich plasma is continuously stirred in a platelet aggregometer and light beam passed through the suspension, platelet aggregation in response to an added chemical stimulus can be monitored by changes in light transmittance. Increased degree of aggre-

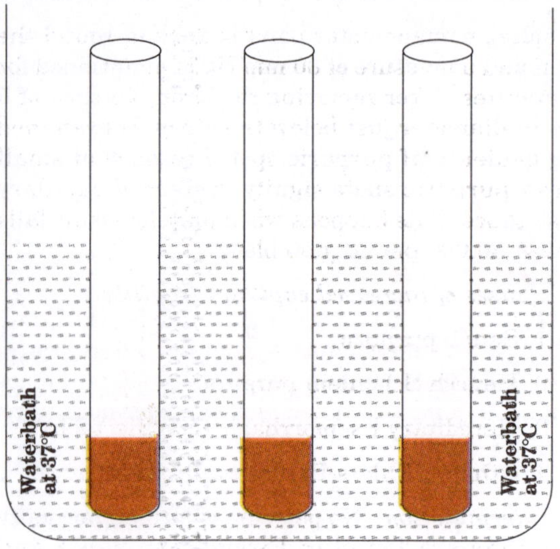

Fig. 20.6. Lee and White method for clotting time

gation of platelets is measured as an increase in light transmission.

Platelet-rich plasma (PRP) : It is obtained by centrifuging citrated blood for 10-15 minutes. Then PRP is carefully removed by a Pasteur pipette without disturbing red cell layer.

Test substances : These include ADP, collagen, epinephrine, sodium arachidonate and the agglutinating agent ristocetin.

Interpretation

A normal platelet aggegation curve with percentage transmittance and time is prepared. In *von Willebrand's (vWB) disease,* platelet aggregation test is unresponsive to the agglutinating agent ristocetin, whereas it is responsive in *thrombasthaenia*.

IV. Coagulation time (CT)

Principle : It is the time required by whole blood (venous) for clot formation *in vitro*. Although CT test measures all 3 stages of coagulation, but it is more sensitive to deficiencies in substances necessary for intrinsic pathway of coagulation. It is most important that care must be taken not to allow entry of any tissue thromboplastin into the sample of blood since a very small amount of the same can shorten the coagulation time. CT is usually not affected by a mild to moderate deficiency of platelets as only a very small number of platelets are required for normal coagulation.

1. Lee and White method (Fig. 20.6)

(i) Make a clean venepuncture with as little trauma as possible to the connective tissue between skin and vein.

(ii) Withdraw 4-5 ml blood by a siliconised dry glass syringe or disposable plastic syringe. After detaching the needle, deliver one ml of blood in each of the three 8 × 75 mm test tubes.

(iii) The 3 tubes with blood are allowed to stand in upright position at room temperature. Where facilities are available, a 37°C water bath or incubator may be used.

(iv) Coagulation in the tube can be ascertained by tilting the tube or by gentle tipping. The first tube is gently tilted every minute and the remaining tubes are examined every half minute. The average of the clotting time in 3 tubes gives the result.

Since the speed of coagulation increases with temperature, the test should be done at a particular temperature.

Normal range : 4-9 minutes at 37°C.

2. Capillary tube method of Wrights

Blood is collected from a clean finger prick in 3-4 fine capillary tubes. The tubes are sealed at both ends by flame and left in a water bath at 37°C. After one minute, one end of the tube is broken gently, and breakage of tube is repeated every 15/30 seconds until a thin line of unbroken coagulum is stretched between the two broken ends.

Normal range : 6-10 minutes and longer if done at room temp. This method is not recommended.

Prolonged coagulation time

CT gives a rough indication of intrinsic pathway of coagulation mechanism. it is prolonged under the following conditions. The sensitive indicator of efficiency of intrinsic pathway of coagulation is activated partial thromboplastin time (APTT/PTTK). CT is prolonged only when in severe deficiency of factor (VIII 98% deficiency), IX or fibrinogen (e.g., afibrinogenaemia).

1. Haemophilia A and B;
2. von Willebrand's disease;
3. Liver disease when liver is unable to synthesise factors II, V, VII and X;
4. Hereditary hypoprothrombinaemias;

5. Hereditary hypofibrinogenaemias.

6. Heparin therapy.

V. Clot retraction study (Fig. 20.7)

Collect 5 ml blood into a 10 ml graduated centrifuge tube of glass. A dry glass rod is placed inside the tube with its upper end passing through a perforated cork. The tube is then incubated at 37 °C in a water bath for one hour.

The glass rod along with the clot is gently lifted up and the clot is drained. Then the volume of expressed serum-cell suspension is read.

$$\text{Percentage of clot retraction} = \frac{\text{Vol. serum cell}}{\text{Vol. of blood}} \times 100$$

Normal range : 48-64%.

Interpretation : Since retraction of blood clot is directly related to the total number and functional capability of platelets, clot retraction study is useful in assessment of platelet function.

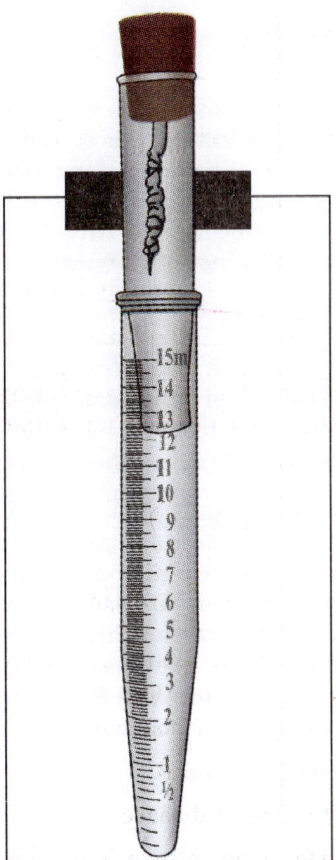

Fig. 20.7. Glass-ware for clot retraction test

VI. Capillary fragility test (Hess's test)

A sphygmomanometer band is applied round the arm and a pressure of 80 mm Hg is maintained for 5 minutes. After removing the band, an area of 5 cm in diameter just below the elbow is examined for evidence of purpuric spot. Presence of small fresh purpuric spots signify decreased capillary resistance. This happens when platelet count falls below 50,000 per cu. mm blood.

Causes of increased capillary fragility

1. Senile purpura
2. Henoch Schonlein purpura
3. Hereditary haemorrhagic telangiectasia
4. Others : Ehlers-Danlos syndrome scurvy.

Interpretation : No petechia is formed normally but they are found in thrombocytopenia and decreased capillary resistance (von Willebrand's disease).

VII. Prothrombin time (quick one-stage test)

Principle : The test measures the time plasma takes to clot in the presence of an optimal concentration of tissue factor, i.e., thromboplastin (usually an extract of brain). The reaction in the test depends on factors V, VII, X and I, II (Table 20.4) which are synthesised by liver. Hence PT must be tested before performing liver biopsy.

Materials

A. *Reagents*

1. Commercial thromboplastins : Majority of thromboplastins now in use are extracts of brain or lung or rabbit, available in powder as well as in liquid form.

2. Diluent ($CaCl_2$, 0.025 mol/L) : The test reagent is prepared fresh before use.

B. *Plasma* : Patient's and control (normal) plasma samples are obtained as follows (9 volumes of blood and 1 volume of 3.8% sodium citrate) :

Anticoagulant, 3.8% sodium citrate soln.	=	0.5 ml
Whole blood	=	4.5 ml

Blood and citrate mixture is mixed well gently. Less amount of anticoagulant is added to avoid excessive dilution of coagulation factors.

Method

1. Deliver 0.1 ml of plasma in a small test tube placed in a water bath (37°C).

2. Add 0.1 ml of calcium chloride to 0.1 ml thromboplastin in a test tube. Place the container or tube of calcium chloride-thromboplastin solution in the water bath.

3. Wait for 2-4 minutes for allowing to warm to 37°C.

4. Then add 0.2 ml of warmed $CaCl_2$ thromboplastin solution to the plasma and mix the contents of the tube and start the stopwatch.

5. The tube is continuously tilted within the water bath and watched for clot formation. As soon as the fibrin clot is developed, the watch is stopped and the time is recorded.

The test is carried out in duplicate on the patient and control plasma and their mean values are recorded.

Let the prothrombin time of control plasma be 12 seconds and that of patient is 20 seconds, then the results are reported as follows.

Results :

1. Prothrombin Time (PT)
   - of control plasma ..... 12 seconds
   - of patient's plasma ...... 20 seconds
2. Prothrombin Index $= \dfrac{\text{PT of control plasma}}{\text{PT of patient's plasma}} \times 100$

$$= \frac{12}{20} \times 100 = 60\%$$

Normal range

Normal range varies between 12 to 15.5 seconds. The variation is due to particular tissue factor used. If possible, a preparation calibrated against the International Reference Thromboplastin should be used.

Normal control value should be obtained from 20 normal men and 20 women (non-pregnant and not on oral contraceptives). The upper limit of normal control is 1.2 (i.e., 1.2 times higher value).

Interpretation

PT provides an assessment of extrinsic coagulation system. The common causes of prolonged prothrombin time one stage test include :

1. For monitoring anticoagulant therapy.
2. Liver disease, particularly obstructive jaundice, cirrhosis.
3. Vitamin K deficiency.
4. Disseminated intravascular coagulation.
5. Deficiency of factors mainly comprising of the classical "extrinsic pathway" factors V, VII, X, fibrinogen (II), prothrombin (I), and the presence of some inhibitors.

Note : PT is not prolonged in haemophilia A and haemophilia B (Christmas disease).

Monitoring anticoagulant therapy

1. *Prothrombin time* (PT) : It provides an assessment of extrinsic coagulation system (Table 20.4 and Table 20.5).

Liver synthesises factors V, VII and X. These factors are essential for PT. Therefore, prothrombin time must be tested before doing liver biopsy.

2. *APTT* : It provides an assessment of intrinsic coagulation system (Table 20.4, 20.5). Deficiency of any factors XII, XI, IX and VIII prolongs APTT (Table 20.4). For monitoring heparin therapy APTT is done.

VIII. Activated Partial Thromboplastin Time (APTT)

(*Syn* : Partial thromboplastin time with Kaolin, PTTK)

Principle : The test measures the clotting time of plasma after the activation of contact factors (Kaolin or other surface acting agents which activate the surface clotting factors XII and XI) but without added tissue thromboplastin. It indicates the efficiency of "intrinsic pathway".

The activation of contact factors is to be standardised first, for which the plasma is first preincubated with Kaolin. A standardised phospholipid preparation called partial thromboplastin is added as a platelet substitute following the addition of an excess of calcium, to allow the test to be carried out on platelet poor plasma. Phospholipid is obtained from soyabean.

APTT depends not only on the contact factors XII and XI, and on factors VIII and IX, but also on reactions with factors X, V, prothrombin (factor) and fibrinogen (factor). The test is also sensitive to the presence of circulating anticoagulants (inhibitors) and heparin.

Reagents

1. *Plasma* : Platelet-poor blood of patient and control normal are collected in 3.8% sodium citrate (9 vols. solution + 1 vol. blood). Platelet-poor plasma (PPP) is prepared by centrifuging at 4000 RPM for 15 minutes.

2. *Kaolin* : Suspension of Kaolin (0.5 g%) in barbitone buffered saline (pH 7.4) is prepared, to which a few glass beads are added to aid resuspension. The suspension is stable at room temperature for an indefinite period. Other insoluble surface acting agents include cellic or ellagic acid which can also be used in place of Kaolin.

3. *Phospholipid* : Many lyophilised phospholipid reagents are available from commercial house and the working solution is prepared at their direction.

Method

1. Mix 0.5 ml of phospholipid reagent with equal volume of Kaolin suspension in a test tube and keep in a water bath at 37°C.

2. Place 0.1 ml of control and test (patient's) plasma in tubes marked 'C' and 'T' respectively and add 0.2 ml of Kaolin phospholipid solution in tube marked "C", mix the contents and start the stopwatch immediately. Keep in the water bath at 37°C for exactly 10 minutes with occasional shaking. Then 0.1 ml of pre-warmed $CaCl_2$ solution is added and stopwatch is started. The time taken by the mixture to clot is recorded.

Same procedure is repeated with the tube marked 'T' and the time required for clotting is recorded. The test should be repeated with control and patient's plasma at least once. The mean value is taken into account in both the cases.

Normal range : 35 to 43 seconds. An abnormal result is indicated when the clotting time of patient is 10 or more seconds more than the control time.

Interpretation (Table 20.4, 20.5)

The result is interpreted in conjunction with the results obtained in quick one stage prothrombin time test. It provides an assessment of intrinsic coagulation system.

1. It is prolonged in deficiencies of factors XII, XI, IX and VIII. Factor VII deficient plasma provides a normal result.

Factor VIII consists of two fractions : (i) VIIIC (the precoagulant protein or AHG) and its activity is measured by APTT, and (ii) VIII vWF fraction that helps in attachment of platelet to subendothelial collagen (Table 20.1).

2. When one stage prothrombin test is normal, APTT is prolonged in either factor VIII or factor IX and rare deficiencies of factors XII and XI, prekallikrein or HMW Kininogen and also the presence of inhibitors.

3. APTT is prolonged in certain diseases, e.g., DIC, liver disease, massive transfusion with stored blood, administration of heparin and circulating anticoagulant.

4. Generally APTT is a very sensitive test. It is very useful in diagnosis of haemophilia A and B.

5. Normal result indicates that there is no significant deficiency of the above mentioned factors.

6. APTT is done for monitoring heparin therapy.

Precaution : (1) The test does not measure platelet factor 3 activity, as a substitute for platelet is used. (2) False normal result may be obtained when blood is contaminated with tissue juice. Hence blood by clean venipuncture is to be collected.

IX. Thrombin Time Test

Principle : The test measures the time plasma takes to clot after the addition of a solution of exogenous thrombin. Thrombin time is influenced by the concentration and activity of fibrinogen and also by the presence of inhibitory substances.

Reagents

1. *Plasma* : Platelet-poor plasma of patient and normal control.

2. *Thrombin solution* : A commercial bovine thrombin is available (Ortho Lab; Parke Davis & Co.), stored frozen (–20°C) in a strength of 50 NIH unit solution. Working solution is prepared freshly by diluting the stock in barbitone buffered saline in a plastic tube.

Method

1. Take 0.1 ml of barbitone buffered saline and 0.1 ml of citrated plasma in a test tube in water bath at 37°C.

2. Add 0.1 ml of working thrombin solution and start the stop watch immediately and note the time required for clot formation. Test is repeated at least once.

Expression of results

Results are expressed in seconds as mean of the two readings for the control and the test plasma. In addition to noting clotting time, the quality of clot should be observed and compared with normal clot.

Normal range : 13 to 15 seconds, result above 20 seconds is regarded as abnormal.

Interpretation

Prolongation of thrombin time may occur due to :

1. Hypofibrinogenaemia, e.g., DIC.
2. Increased concentration of fibrin degrading products (FDP) as in DIC.
3. Presence of heparin interferes in thrombin-fibrinogen reaction.
4. Transparent bulky clot is formed in abnormal fibrin polymerisation, e.g., liver disease and some congenital dysfibrinogenaemias.

Sometimes significant increase of fibrinogen in plasma also prolongs thrombin time.

QUESTIONS

1. *What are the plasma coagulation factors?*
2. *What is intrinsic pathway of coagulation?*
3. *Name the receptors on platelets mediating adhesion and aggregation.*
4. *Name the different techniques for BT. Which is preferable method of test for BT and why incision is made parallel to anticubital vein in template method?*
5. *What is the fate of haemostatic plug?*
6. *What is fibrinolytic pathway and its utility?*
7. *Name the factors involved in common coagulation pathway.*
8. *What is haemophilia and what are its types?*
9. *In which condition capillary fragility is increased?*
10. *What is the usefulness of Hess's test?*
11. *By which test oral anticoagulant therapy is monitored?*
12. *Name the test done for monitoring oral anticoagulant therapy and that for heparin therapy.*
13. *What is prothrombin index?*
14. *Why the proportion of blood to citrate is 9 : 1 for determining PT?*
15. *Name the contact factors and other factors on which APTT is dependent.*
16. *Name the fractions of factor VIII. How are these measured? Which fraction is measured by APTT?*
17. *What is thromboplastin?*
18. *What is the role of senile purpura?*
19. *Name the role of kaolin in APTT.*
20. *What is partial thromboplastin in APTT?*
21. *What is the source of thromboplastin in PT?*
22. *Name the causes of DIC.*
23. *What are the causes of prolonged CT?*
24. *What are Vit K dependent coagulation factors?*
25. *What is hypercoagulable state? Give some examples.*
26. *Which cells synthesise factor VIII?*
27. *How is haemophilia A classified?*
28. *How do you diagnose different types of haemophilia?*
29. *How to detect carriers of haemophilia?*
30. *How do you diagnose von Willebrand's disease?*
31. *Name the causes and pathogenesis of DIC.*
32. *What is clot retraction study?*

Chapter 21

Blood Group. Rh System and Blood Transfusion

Significant progress has been achieved in the understanding of red cell surface antigens in relation to various diseases.

BLOOD GROUPS AND ANTIGENS

Red blood cells of human being contain glycoproteins and glycolipids on their surface which constitute the blood group antigens. About 200 red cell antigens are described. After Landsteiner's discovery of ABO system in 1901, 15 well-defined blood group systems have been identified, some of which are shown in Table 21.1. Of these only two blood group systems, **ABO** and **Rh** are of major clinical importance and constitute major antigens. The other blood group systems are of less importance because the red cell antigen is weak and naturally occurring antibodies are encountered only occasionally or rarely.

Table 21.1
Some major blood group system in historical order of discovery

Year	*System*	*Main antigens*	*Chromosome location*
1901	ABO	A, B	9
1927	MNS	M, N, S, s	4
1927	P	P_1, P, p^k, p	22 (?)
1939	Rhesus	C, c, D, (d), E, e	1
1945	Lutheran	Lu^a, Lu^b	19
1946	Kell	K, k, Kp^a, Kp^b, Js^a, Js^b	—
1946	Lewis	Le^a, Le^b	19
1950	Duffy	Fy^a, Fy^b	1
1951	Kidd	Jk^a, Jk^b	2

Genotype refers to the genes present on the chromosome, whereas phenotype is the red cell antigen on the surface of the cell.

Antibodies

There are mainly two types of antibodies to the red cell antigens : naturally occurring and immune.

1. *Naturally occurring antibodies* : These are formed in the blood without any obvious antigenic stimulus and found in the serum of individuals lacking it, e.g., isoagglutinins of ABO system. They are either wholly or partially IgM and react better with corresponding antigen at a temperature below 37°C. Naturally occurring antibodies are rarely or occasionally seen in other blood group systems.

It appears that antigens very similar to A and B of red cell are common in the environment, such as the intestinal bacteria and possibly foods to which newborns are exposed and the infants rapidly develop antibodies to those foreign antigens not present in their own cells. Thus, type A persons develop anti-B antibodies, type B persons develop anti-A antibodies, type O persons develop both, and type AB persons develop none (Table 21.2).

2. *Immune or acquired antibodies* : These are produced in persons in response to stimulation by a red cell antigen which is not present on their own red cells or in their body fluids, e.g., Rh antibodies, which are not naturally occurring and are formed only as an acquired immunologic phenomenon either after mismatched blood transfusion or after pregnancy. Most of the immune antibodies react best at 37°C and may be either IgG or IgM, usually the former.

ABO SYSTEM

The ABO blood group system discovered by Landsteiner in 1901 contains four main groups A, B, AB and O which are determined on the basis of presence or absence of 2 antigens A and B on the red cell membrane (Table 21.2). These antigens are glycosphingolipids.

Table 21.2
ABO blood groups and frequency in India

Pheno-type	*Genotype*	*Red cell antigens*	*Antibodies*	*Prevalence in India*
O	OO	(H)	anti A, anti B	33%
A	AA or OA	A	anti B	25%
B	BB or OB	B	anti A	37%
AB	AB	A + B	None	5%

ANTIGENS

The presence or absence of A, B or O antigens on red cells is under the control of three allelic genes, A, B and O situated in a single locus on the long arm of chromosome 9, which are inherited in pairs. The A and B genes are co-dominant, and the O gene is amorph (silent), i.e., it has no effect on antigenic structure.

The cellular expression of A and B antigens is determined by a further gene, the H gene, which is inherited independently of ABO system. The H gene is located on chromosome 19. The alleles H and h are inherited independently of ABO genes. Most individuals are homozygous for H gene (HH). The H gene codes for an enzyyme fucosyl transferase which converts the carbohydrate precursor into H substance (L-fucose), on which the A and B gene products act. The A and B genes code for specific enzymes (glycosyl transferases) which convert H substances into A and B antigens (Fig. 21.1). A and B antigens are formed by terminal addition of N-acetyl-D-galactosamine and D-galactose, respectively, to H substance.

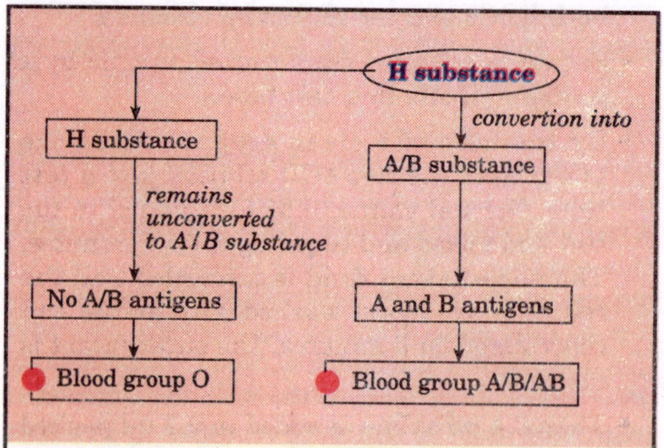

Fig. 21.1. Action of A and B gene on H substance

Bombay phenotype : Since O gene is a 'silent' allele, it does not produce any active transferase and hence the H substance persists unchanged in group O. In the absence of H genes (designated as *hh*), the precursor substance remains unconverted, and therefore, A and B genes, if present, cannot be expressed, and Oh or Bombay type results. Individuals of this extremely rare **Oh** or **Bombay phenotype** (Bhende *et al*, 1956) have anti-A_2, anti-B and anti-H in blood, all active at 37°C. These persons can only be safely transfused with same Oh group blood.

Subgroups of A

Several subgroups of A exist, most important are A_1 and A_2. Group AB has similar subgroups A_1B and A_2B. Thus, the frequency of occurrence of ABO system in Caucasians increases to six : A_1, A_2, B, A_1B, A_2B and O. About 80% of group 'A' and group AB belong to group A_1 and A_1B respectively, the remainder belong to group A_2 and A_2B. The distinction can be made conveniently by the use of anti-A_1 lectin, a potent anti-A agglutinin which has been extracted from the seeds of *Dolichos biflorus*. It agglutinates only A_1 red cells.

Antigens weaker than anti-A are occasionally encountered—called A_3, A_x etc. These variations in A antigen of erythrocytes are due to mutant forms of the glycosyl transferases produced by the A gene, which are less efficient at transferring N-acetyl-D-galactosamine to H substance.

Appearance of A, B, H antigens

The A, B and H antigens appear on red cells early in foetal life and remains unchanged for life. At about one year of age the number of antigen sites reaches the adult levels. The antibodies appear in blood of infants at detectable level by about 6 months of age.

Secretors and nonsecretors

The ability to secrete ABH substances in water-soluble form of glycoprotein (secretory status) is controlled by a dominant secretor gene *Se* (allele *se*). About 80% of Caucasian population are secretors (genotype *Se Se* or *Se se*) and the rest are nonsecretors (*se se*). Saliva and other body fluids of the secretors contain H substance together with A and/or B substances depending on their blood group.

ANTIBODIES

1. Naturally occurring antibodies

Naturally occurring anti-A and anti-B antibodies (agglutinins) are usually of the IgM class and they cannot cross the placenta from mother to foetus. They are most active at 20°C, but can also react at 37°C. These are complete antibodies and cause agglutination of corresponding antigens on red cells in saline suspension. Natural "anti-A_2B" in O group persons is usually of IgG class which is less readily agglutinated by A and B cells.

Serum of group O person contains both anti-A and anti-B antibodies, that of group A contains anti-B, group B contains anti-A and group AB contains neither anti-A nor anti-B antibodies (Table 21.2).

The subgroups of A, A_1 and A_2 are of some practical importance, in that A_2 cells react less strongly with anti-A sera. Thus, group A_2 is liable to be interpreted as O and A_2B as B. Hence an anti-A serum should be so selected that it should give strong reactions with A_2 cells as well as A_1 cells. To avoid the wrong interpretation of blood group, red cells of patients are mixed with good quality anti-AB serum and mixed well and allowed to stand for 3-5 minutes, the serum will agglutinate all Ags except O. Thus A_2 antigen can be detected.

Anti-A_1 and anti-H antibodies : Further, anti-A_1 may occasionally be encountered in the group-A_2 subjects (1-2%), active at 37°C, which can destroy transfused A_1 cells.

Anti-H antibody reacts strongly with O and A_2 cells; and sometimes found in the serum of group A_1, A_1B or B persons. The anti-H lectin of *Ulex europaeus* plant seed strongly agglutinates O red cells. These antibodies react at low temperature (20°C) as cold agglutinins. They rarely react with appropriate red cell antigens at a temperature above 30°C. However, the anti-H antibody found in serum of subjects with Oh (Bombay) phenotype normally reacts with O red cells and sometimes causes lysis at 37°C.

2. Immune antibodies

Immune anti-A or anti-B is of the IgG class, and is usually the result of immunisation due to

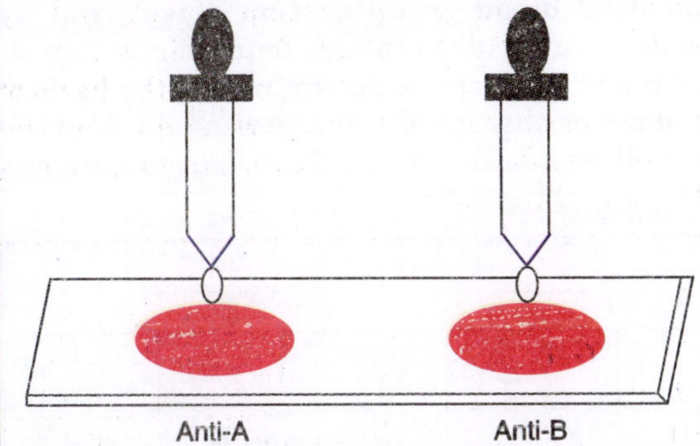

Fig. 21.2. Anti-A anti-B Blood grouping : slide test

foetal maternal haemorrhage, TAB vaccine and incompatible transfusion with ABO blood. These are incomplete antibodies and do not cause agglutination of corresponding red cells in saline suspension, hence they are demonstrated by Coombs' test.

METHOD OF BLOOD GROUPING

ABO grouping may be performed by tube or slide methods or in microplates. Monoclonal anti-A and anti-B reagents are used. The slide method is satisfactory in an emergency, but less sensitive than tube tests in detection of weak anti-A or anti-B in reverse serum grouping.

Preparation of red cell suspension

- A volume of 4 to 5 ml venous blood is collected in a plain vial and allowed to clot. Alternatively, the blood is collected in ACD solution in the proportion of 1 part of ACD solution and 3 parts of blood.
- Clotted sample of blood is preferable since both RBCs and serum can be obtained.
- Serum is collected from clotted sample by a pasteur pipette in a test tube.
- By the help of a clean dropper RBCs are taken from the clot/ACD solution into a test tube. Normal saline (0.85%) is added to the test and mixed and centrifuged for 5 minutes. The supernatant fluid is discarded and the red cells are again washed with saline and centrifuged for 5 minutes. The supernatant is discarded.
- Then 0.4 ml saline is added to 0.1 ml packed red cell to get a 20% saline suspension.

1. Slide method (Fig. 21.2)

Specimen : A 20% saline or citrated cell suspen-

Table 21.3 : Interpretation of ABO grouping and its prevalence

Antibody added	*Anti–A*	*Anti–B*	*Anti–AB*	*Result Group*	**Prevalence in** *India %*	*Europe*
Agglutination	–	–	–	O	33	46
	+	–	+	A	25	42
	–	+	+	B	37	9
	+	+	+	AB	5	3

sion is used. Alternatively, fresh blood by finger prick or cells from clotted sample of blood may be used.

Reagent : (a) Monoclonal anti-A and anti-B reagents. (b) Vial of anti-AB antibody.

Test :

1. Take a clean glass slide and label on both corners; Anti-A on left and Anti-B on right. Another clean glass slide is taken and labelled on one side (left) Anti-AB.

2. Two drops of blood are placed by a Pasteur pipette at each corner. Two separate slides are also sometimes used — one for Anti-A and other for Anti-B. Two drops of blood are also placed on the slide with marking Anti-AB.

3. Using a commercial reagent dropper, one drop of Anti-A is added on the cell suspension in left side and similarly one drop of Anti-B serum on the right side separately. Likewise, 1 drop of Anti-AB serum is added on the Anti-AB labelled slide with cell suspension.

4. Mix the serum-cell suspension separately in each corner by a glass rod or wooden swab-stick breaking off the used portion after each mixing. It is then tilted carefully with hands for 2-3 minutes.

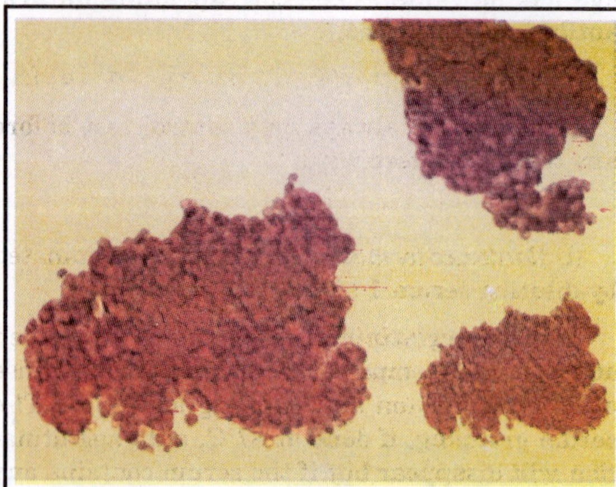

Fig. 21.3. Tube test : Agglutination of red cells

Result : Results are read within 2 to 5 minutes which is based on positive or negative agglutination (Fig. 21.3 and Table 21.3).

(i) *Group* A : Agglutination with anti-A serum (left corner) but not with anti-B serum (right corner).

(ii) *Group* B : Agglutination with anti-B (right side) but not with anti-A (left side).

(iii) *Group* AB : Agglutination on both sides.

(iv) *Group* O : No agglutination on any side. Slide with AB antiserum will agglutinate Ags except O.

2. **Tube Method (Fig. 21.3)**

Specimen : 20% saline or citrated cell suspension.

Test :

(i) Take 3 plastic or glass tubes (75 × 12 mm) and add one drop of each of grouping serum to the tubes labelled anti-A, anti-B and anti-AB, respectively.

(ii) Add one volume of 2% red cell suspension to each tube.

(iii) Mix the suspension by tapping the tubes and leave them undisturbed at room temperature or at 37°C for $1–1^1/_2$ hour and examine for agglutination.

Reading :

Using a Pasteur pipette take supernatant up to 0.5 mm and 1–2 mm red cells. Expel the supernatant and cells on a slide, place a cover glass and examine microscopically (Fig. 21.3) for agglutination and the result is interpreted as given in Table 21.3.

Result : Blood group A, B, AB or O is defined.

Controls : Control should be set up with each grouping serum using red cells of known group (Table 21.3).

Advantage

Tube method of blood grouping is better than that of slide test because the reaction between the red cells and corresponding antibodies in serum is enhanced as a result of centrifugation, consequently weaker antigens like A_2 are also detected. Tube technique is recommended for both ABO and Rh grouping.

Serum grouping (*Reverse grouping*)

Reverse grouping preferably by tube method is necessary to confirm the result of red cell grouping by tube/slide method.

In the serum grouping, normally cells of groups A (A_1), B and O are mixed with patient's serum and examined. O cells serve as a control for unexpected antibodies. A_2 cells also should be used when there is suspected presence of anti–A_1. Any discrepancy between the results of red cell grouping and serum grouping should be investigated further.

Cross-matching

Once donor's group of the same ABO and Rh D type as that of the recipient is found, donor's cells are to be cross-matched with the serum of the patient. Cross-matching must be done before a blood transfusion is given. It is done to prevent transfusion reactions by detecting antibodies in the recipient's serum that may react with donor's red cells. During cross-matching recipient's serum and donor's red cells are taken and the following tests can be done :

(a) **Saline cross match** detects IgM antibodies.

(b) **Albumin technique** detects IgG antibodies.

(c) **Enzyme technique** detects IgG and some IgM antibodies.

(d) **Antiglobulin test** or **Coombs' test** detects IgG antibodies.

Routine cross-matching

Slide test :

(1) Take a drop of recipient's serum on a slide.

(2) Add a drop of 5% saline suspension of donor's red cells to the recipient's serum.

(3) Mix the two.

(4) Examine macroscopically and microscopically for agglutination or lysis.

Tube test :

The test may also be done on a tube using 2 drops of donor's serum and 2 drops of 5% saline suspension of recipient's cells. Incubate at 37°C for 30 minutes.

Centrifuge at 3000 rpm for 1 minute. Observe macroscopically and microscopically for agglutination or lysis (Fig. 21.3).

Result

No agglutination or haemolysis is observed in a matched recipient's and donor's samples.

In case *mismatching* of blood of donor and recipient, haemolysis/agglutination occurs. As both red cell and serum grouping is done, tube method is more accurate.

Differentiation of group A_1 from A_2

This is done by using extracts of certain plant seeds, *lectins*, that agglutinate red cells.

1. A saline extract of seeds of *Dolichos biflorus* is now routinely used in subtyping A cells. It agglutinates A_1 and A_1B cells preferentially.

2. Saline extract of seeds of *Ulex europaeus* is an anti-H lectin. It agglutinates A_2, A_2B and O cells more strongly than A_1, A_1B and B cells.

Serum grouping in infants below 4 months of age has no value as the corresponding natural antibodies are absent.

Causes of discrepancies in ABO grouping

There should always be a control test before any tests are interpreted.

1. **False positive results**

(i) *Rouleaux formation* which can be eliminated by diluting serum 1 : 2 or 1 : 4 in saline.

(ii) *Cold agglutinin in serum of patient* : When active at room temperature, cold agglutinins cause autoagglutination and pan agglutination. The serum grouping, if done at 37°C, auto-agglutination will disappear but if the serum contains any anti-A and/or anti-B, it will still react. Blood grouping should then be repeated after washing the patient's red cells in warm (37°C) saline. It is useful to test red cells of patients with group-AB serum that contains no antibody.

(iii) *Warm antibodies absorbed to red cells of patient* : Such cells undergo auto-agglutination in normal serum as seen in autoimmune haemolytic anaemia. They give a positive direct Coombs' test.

(iv) *Infected red cells* : Infection of red cells by bacteria both *in vivo* and *in vitro* may cause polyagglutinisation in normal sera. Bacterial enzymes expose T receptors on red cell surface. Since most human sera contain anti-T antibodies, such infected cells get agglutinated in normal serum. As a result, group O cells may appear as AB.

Universal donor and recipient

Under normal circumstances, transfusion of donor's blood of the same ABO type as that of the recipient is done. But in an urgent situation when ABO identical red cells are not available, transfusion of ABO compatible red cells may be made. For example, group O individual (having no antigen) can donate red cells to a recipient of any ABO type, and the type AB recipient (having both A and B antigens) can receive red cells of any ABO type. Hence, group O individual is considered as *universal donor* and group AB subject as *universal recipient.*

Anti-A and/or anti-B of the donor plasma get diluted in recipient's serum and usually does not produce any significant immunological reaction when one or two bottles of blood are transfused. However, red cells should be transfused in these circumstances instead of whole blood, least the antibodies present in donor's serum may destroy recipient red cells.

THE Rh SYSTEM

The rhesus (Rh) system was so named because Landsteiner and Wiener (1940) produced the original antibody in rabbits by injection of red cells from Rhesus monkey, which agglutinated about 83% human red cells.

ANTIGENS

Fisher postulated that Rh antigens (C, c, D, d, E, e) are determined by three pairs of closely linked allellomorphic genes located on chromosome 1, C or c, D or d and E or e. Every individual carries one member of each pair of these genes derived from each parent. Each gene is responsible for production of a specific antigen. The antigen controlled by D locus is the strongest immunogen, called the Rh D antigen. The six Rh genes give rise to 8 allellomorphs and eight antigenic patterns of Rh system (Table 21.4). Fisher's nomenclature has been accepted by WHO Expert Committee (1977).

Table 21.4
The Rh genes in order of frequency (Fisher)

	Genes	Antigenes	Approx. frequency (%)		
			Caucasian	*Black*	*Chinese*
Rh positive	CDe	CDe	41	18	73
	cDE	cDE	14	11	19
	cDe	cDe	3	29	Rare
	CDE	CDE	Rare	Rare	Rare
Rh negative	Cde	Cde	1	1	2
	cdE	cdE	1	Rare	–
	cde	cde	39	26	0.02
	CdE	CdE	Rare	Rare	0.04

THE Rh(D) SYSTEM

Rh D is a strong antigen and other antigens of Rh system are much less antigenic than D and are of less clinical importance. In practice, therefore, Rh positive or Rh negative depends on the presence of D antigen on surface of red cells which can be detected by a strong anti-D serum. Rh D antigens are present in about 95% of Indians, 85% Caucasians and 90% of Chinese. About 5-6% Indians are Rh D negative. However, occasionally, other antibodies, such as anti-E, anti-C, anti-c, and rarely anti-e develop as a result of pregnancy or transfusion; they may develop also in D positive subjects. During blood transfusion Rh D negative donors should preferably be tested with anti-C and anti-E serum and only those giving negative results (cde) should be selected as donors.

ANTIBODIES

The six sera containing antibodies corresponding to the Rh antigens are denoted by the terms anti-C, anti-c, anti-D, anti-d, anti-E and anti-e. Five of the six antisera have been detected in human but no serum containing anti-d has yet been found. The counterpart of D is probably not antigenic or amorphic.

In contrast to ABO system, there are no naturally occurring antibodies against Rh system (exception anti-E, rare). They are immune in origin and arise in serum only in consequence of Rh incompatible pregnancy or transfusion. Rh antibodies are usually IgG in nature and can cross the placenta and is of great clinical significance since D negative individuals are relatively easily stimulated to produce anti-D antibody when exposed to Rh D positive cells.

Rh D^u

A variant of D named D^u appears in weak forms on red cell membrane and complicate Rh typing. The D^u differs from 'normal' D by its smaller number of antigenic binding sites. The Du cells are not generally agglutinated by anti-D sera. It can be detected by strong anti-D serum and by Coombs' test. As donors, Du individuals should be considered as Rh positive and as recipients they should be transfused with Rh negative blood.

Rh D GROUPING

Rh D typing is usually done at the same time as ABO grouping. It is advisable to use two different anti-D reagents as a check against errors.

High titre monoclonal anti-D reagent has now made it possible to use the same technique in Rh grouping as for ABO grouping. Both slide and tube tests may be performed but tube tests give better result.

Slide method

Test cells : Clotted blood is used. A 2–5 per cent suspension of red cells is prepared in the patient's own serum after the clot has been broken by a glass rod.

Test :

1. Place one drop of anti-D on a slide.
2. Add one drop of test cells suspended in their own serum.
3. Mix well and tilt for a few minutes.

Result : Clumping of cells (macroscopic or microscopic) indicate Rh D positive, and no clumps indicate Rh D negative.

Tube test

1. Add 1 drop of anti-D serum in test tube.
2. Then add 1 drop of 2% red cell suspension in saline.

The serum and cell suspensions are mixed, incubated at 37°C for 1-2 hours and examined macroscopically and microscopically as in ABO grouping.

Result

Presence of agglutination indicates RhD positive blood group.

Controls

Known Rh D positive and Rh D negative red cells should be tested with each set of test cases.

HAEMOLYTIC DISEASE OF THE NEWBORN (HDN)

HDN may be due to (a) Rh disease and (b) ABO disease.

Rh Haemolytic disease

This disorder, previously known as erythroblastosis foetalis, is a haemolytic disease of the newborn due to attack in the Rh positive foetal red cells by maternal antibodies of IgG type which can cross the placental barrier. It is an isoimmune disorder as the antigen and antibody come from different persons, although of the same species.

In HDN, the mother is Rh-negative while father and foetus are Rh-positive. The incidence of HDN in Rh negative mother is about 1 in 500 births, although in about 25 pregnancies in 500, the mother is Rh-D negative. Sensitisation of mother does not occur as often as might be anticipated, becuase a significant number of foetal red cells are required to enter the maternal circulation which may occur during placental separation at the time of delivery or abortion. This induces antibody response in the mother. The first pregnancy usually escapes provided the woman has not been previously sensitised by transfusion with Rh positive blood. During a subsequent pregnancy, the maternal anti Rh antibodies, usually IgG class, cross the placenta and damage the foetal red cells producing HDN. The clinical features of HDN include anaemia, jaundice, hepatomegaly, splenomegaly and often kernicterus. Clinical jaundice may be absent for first 24 hours after birth and thereafter deep unconjugated hyperbilirubinaemia leading to kernicterus occurs. Severe cases show cardiac failure and generalised oedema (hydrops foetalis).

Laboratory investigations

1. Isoimmune anti-D are mostly IgG type and do not agglutinate Rh-D positive red cells in

saline. *Direct Coombs' test* with foetal red cells from cord blood becomes positive.

2. Estimation of *serum bilirubin* of cord blood shows mainly unconjugated bilirubin.

3. Peripheral blood smear shows a large number of *nucleated red cells* with 10-15% reticulocytes.

Diagnosis of isoimmunisation of mother

When the mother is Rh-negative and the father is Rh-positive, the maternal serum must be tested for antibodies by **Indirect Coombs' test** on 32nd and 36th week of each pregnancy.

ABO Haemolytic disease

Haemolytic disease may also occur in the newborn due to maternofoetal ABO incompatibility, particularly when the mother is group O and the foetus is either group A or group B. Individuals of group A or group B possess IgM natural antibodies which cannot cross the placental barrier. But persons with O group contain predominantly IgG class anti-A and anti-B which can cross the placenta.

Immunisation also occurs due to foetal-maternal haemorrhage when anti-A or anti-B antibodies are developed in mother by stimulation with foetal cells.

Although ABO haemolytic disease is more common than Rh haemolytic disease, but generally the infants are mildly affected. This is probably due to fewer antigenic sites of A or B group erythrocytes. The first born does not usually escape as with Rh immunisation. The **Direct Coombs'** test with foetal red cells is often negative but **Indirect Coombs'** test with neonatal serum (cord blood) is more commonly positive.

Coombs' (Antiglobulin) Test (Fig. 21.4)

This test is used for demonstrating the presence of IgG antibodies directed against the RBCs. As IgG antibodies (incomplete antibodies) do not cause agglutination of RBCs when red cells and serum are mixed in saline, antiglobulin (Coombs) serum is added that combines with IgG antibodies on the surface of RBCs leading to agglutination of RBCs. The RBCs should be washed with saline to remove free gamma globulin, so that when antiglobulin is added, it is not neutralized by other globulins. Coombs' test is of two types : direct and indirect.

Direct Coombs' Test

The test detects antibodies coated on the surface of red blood cells, when the sensitisation red cells has taken place in vivo.

Method

(1) RBCs of patient are taken from the clot/ EDTA blood/citrated blood in a test tube. Normal saline is added to RBCs and mixed. Centrifuge the tube at 2,500 rpm for 5 minutes and the saline is decanted.

(2) RBCs are washed twice again in the same way.

(3) After washing for three times, a 5% saline suspension of RBCs is prepared.

(4) To 2 drops of saline red cell suspension add 2 drops of antiglobulin serum. Mix well and incubate at 37°C for 5 minutes.

(5) The content in the tube is centrifuged at 1,000 rpm for 1 minute. The cell button is dislodged. Then gently resuspend the cells and look for agglutination both microscopically and macroscopically. One positive control and one negative control is set up with each test.

(6) For positive control, 1 ml Rh +ve EDTA blood is taken in a test tube and washed with N-saline thrice. To 2 drops of 5% saline suspension, add 2 drops of anti-Rh (anti-D) IgG antibody. Incubate at 37°C for 10 minutes for antibody to get coated on the surface of RBCs.

(7) Wash with saline thrice to remove the excess of Ab. Now these RBCs are coated with antibody (control). Take 2 drops of coated RBCs and add 2 drops of antiglobulin serum and incubate at 37°C. Agglutination should be positive.

(8) Negative control : RBCs of normal individual's serve as a negative control.

Result : Agglutination of the test sample indicates the presence of antibody on the surface of red cells, i.e., giving positive Direct Coombs' Test.

Indications for direct antiglobulin test

(i) Haemolytic disease of newborn (baby's red cells in cord blood are subjected to direct Coombs' test).

(ii) Autoimmune haemolytic anaemia.

Direct test demonstrates in vivo attachment of antibodies to red cells.

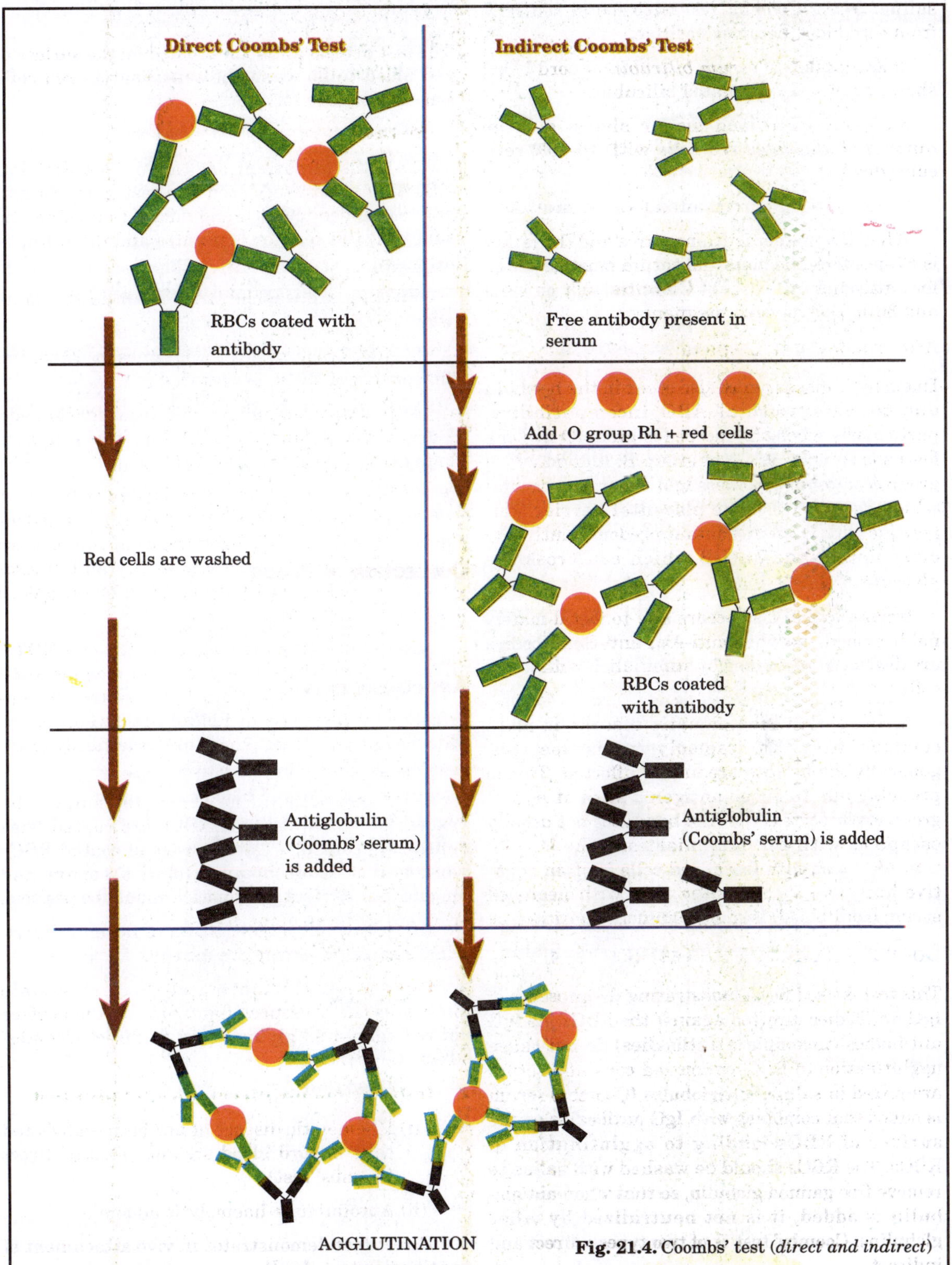

Fig. 21.4. Coombs' test (*direct and indirect*)

INDIRECT COOMBS' TEST

It is employed to detect antibodies that are present in the serum.

(1) Put 2 drops of patient's serum in a test tube.

(2) Two drops of 5% "O" red cell suspension made from any Rh D positive "O" group person.

(3) The mixture is incubated at 37°C for 8-10 minutes.

(4) Red cells are washed with normal saline thrice to remove the excess of antibodies.

(5) The supernatant is removed. The "O" RBCs thus treated with test serum becomes coated with (IgG) anti-Rh antibodies of the patient (if antibodies are present).

(6) Two drops of Coombs' serum (antiglobulin) are added and incubated at 37°C for 10 minutes. Then it is centrifuged at 2,000 rpm for 1 minute. The red cells are resuspended by gentle agitation and examined macroscopically and microscopically for agglutination.

Result : Positive indirect Coombs' test shows agglutination of RBCs due to the presence of antibodies in the test serum.

Indications

(i) In haemolytic disease of newborn — serum of mother is tested to detect anti-Rh antibody, and (ii) in cross-matching to detect incompatibility of recipient's serum with donor's cells.

BLOOD TRANSFUSION

Transfusion medicine is a multi-disciplinary speciality comprising of selection and utilisation of blood and blood components in the treatment on prevention of disease. The old term blood banking has been replaced by the term transfusion medicine to stress the importance of patient care and evaluation of the clinical results in this speciality by Klein in 1987.

DONOR SELECTION

(1) Individual in apparent good health.

(2) *Age* : At least 18 years of old (age of maturity); no upper limit, may be upto 70 years.

(3) *Body weight* : 50 kgs for collection of 450 ml; of blood in 63 ml anticoagulant (CPD or CPDA-1) plus upto 30 ml of additional blood for purpose of testing.

(4) BP, pulse rate and temperature within normal limit.

(5) Minimum haemoglobin 12.5 gm% and PCV – 38%.

(6) *Check up of infectious diseases* : High risk history for AIDS, temporary active disease under treatment such as tuberculosis, syphilis, influenza and other infections.

(7) *For one year* : after hepatitis B immunoglobulin administration, after therapeutic rabies vaccination (after animal-bite), sexual contact with a prostitute.

(8) *For two months* : after recent transfusion of blood.

(9) *For six weeks* : after recent delivery of a baby.

(10) *For one month* : after treatment for benign prostatic hyperplasia, German measles vaccination, vaccination with oral polio, measles, mumps and yellow fever.

COLLECTION OF BLOOD

Blood is collected in a blood bank in aseptic conditions after proper grouping and cross-matching in a bottle containing anticoagulant.

ANTICOAGULANTS

Citrate was first used as a blood anticoagulant in 1914 (*Hustin*). Then it was further improved, dextrose was added to citrate in 1916 (Rous) that provides energy to red blood cells, and citric acid was added to citrate-dextrose solution in 1943 (Loutit) to bring down pH of the solution. This new solution, acid citrate dextrose (ACD) has a lowered pH and can be heat sterilised. This is the standard blood anticoagulant.

Subsequently citrate phosphate dextrose (CPD) was developed by adding phosphate buffer to ACD to increase adenosine triphosphate (ATP) production that increases red blood cell viability (*Gibson, 1957*).

1. *CPD solution*

   Sod. citrate
   Phosphate buffer
   Dextrose

   or

   CPDA-1 : It contains CPD + Adenine (improves survival of stored red blood cells, from 21 days to 35 days).

Table 21.5 : Blood components and their uses

Blood Component	*Characteristics or derivative*	*Volume Shelf-life*	*Indications*
Whole blood	RBC and plasma, WBCs and platelets not viable after storage of 24 hours. Blood 450 ml + ACD or CPD 63 ml.	Store at 1°C–6°C 520 ml ACD/CPD — 21 days CPDA–1 — 35 days	Where massive transfusion is needed.
Packed red cells	Packed RBC with reduced volume of plasma	Store at 1°C-6°C 260 ml same as whole blood	Thalassaemia major, Sickle cell anaemia, severe anaemia of any cause, aplastic anaemia.
Platelet concentrate (single-donor) by apheresis*	Platelets (3×10^{11}), some WBC (lymphocytes), 250 ml plasma, few red cells.	250–300 ml store at room temperature (20°C-24°C). Constant, gentle agitation — 5 days.	Thrombocytopenia
Granulocyte concentrate (single-donor) by apheresis*	Granulocytes (1.0×10^{10}), some WBC (i.e., lymphocytes) 250 ml plasma, few red cells.	Store at 20°C – 24°C temp, constant, no agitation 12-24 hours.	Severe granulo cytopenia.
Fresh frozen plasma (FFP)	Plasma proteins, all coagulation factors, complement	200-260 ml. 1 year at –18°C or colder	DIC, treatment of factors V or IX deficiency, bleeding in liver disease.
Cryoprecipitate (obtained by thawing FFP at 4°C)	Rich in factors VIII, IX, XIII, fibrinogen and other plasma proteins.	10-15 ml 1 year at –18°C or colder	Most useful in von Willebrand disease, factor VIII deficiency (haemophitea A, B), or hypofibrinogenaemia).
Factor VIII concentrate	Factor VIII	25 ml, 2 years at 2-8°C storage as per manufacturer's instructions	Used in deficiency of Factor VIII
Rh immune globulin	Ig G anti-D (Rho)	1 ml. $1^1/_2$ year at 2-8°C	To Rh negative women in HDN

* **Apheresis donation** : Haemapheresis is a procedure in which blood is removed from a donor anticoagulated and separated into components. After retaining the desired components, the unwanted portions remaining are returned to the donor. There are cell/plasma separators which separate different blood components by centrifugal force, and plasmapheresis are now available that use special membrane allowing cellular elements to pass through the membrane and plasma.

2. *ACD solution*

Citric acid Sod. citrate
Dextrose

Both the anticoagulants are stored at 2-6°C in refrigerator.

PRE-DONATION CHECK UP

(i) ABO grouping
(ii) Hepatitis BsAg
(iii) Test for syphilis
(iv) Rh-D typing
(v) HIV testing
(vi) Hepatitis C antigen

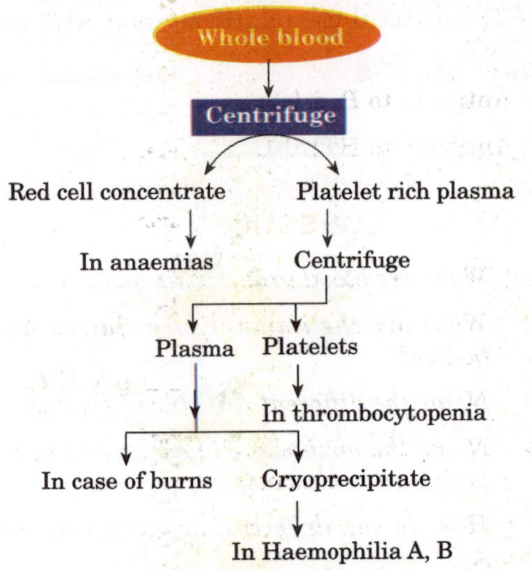

Fig. 21.5. Chart of blood components

BLOOD COMPONENTS

The various blood components include :

(a) Whole blood

(b) Red cell components (packed red cells)

(c) Plasma, fresh frozen plasma — FFP

(d) Platelet concentrates

(e) Cryoprecipitate

Table 21.5 and Fig. 21.5 show the common blood components and derivatives used in haemotherapy. These are prepared from whole blood by means of refrigerated centrifuges.

Preparation by centrifugation

(i) For packed RBC or platelet component, blood is centrifuged at high spin at 5000 g for 5 minutes.

(ii) For preparation of cryoprecipitate or cell-free plasma, blood is centrifuged at high spin at 5000 g for 7 minutes.

(iii) For preparation of platelet concentrate, blood is centrifuged at low spin at 2000 g for 3 minutes.

The centrifugation is done at room temperature (20°C to 24°C) for preparation of a platelet concentrate. For preparation of all other blood components, centrifugation is performed between 1°C to 6°C.

RED CELL COMPONENTS

The red cells are obtained by centrifuging the blood. Haematocrit is 55-75% in the packed cell unit.

These can be stored in a refrigerator at 4°C and shelf life is 1 month. From the packed cell, white cells are withdrawn as buffy coat and such red cell preparation is preferred.

Indications

(1) Thalassaemia major

(2) Aplastic anaemia

(3) Sickle cell anaemia

(4) Hypovolaemia due to haemorrhage

(5) Severe anaemia of any cause

SELECTION OF BLOOD COMPONENTS

Whole Blood : Whole blood (vide Table 21.5) is a product containing all the red cells and most of the plasma. The platelets and WBCS in whole blood are not active as they require separation from whole blood and special storage conditions are required for maintaining their viability and function. Whole blood should not be infused in persons with chronic anaemia and normal blood volume.

Red blood cells : Red blood cells or packed cells (Table 21.5) are obtained from whole blood by overnight sedimentation under refrigerated storage or by refrigerated centrifugation.

Leucocyte-reduced red blood cells : It can be obtained by using 3-log leucoreduction filters. Another simple method is to prepare packed cells using cold centrifuge and the packed cells are washed twice with 300-400 ml of saline, using centrifugation and removal of the buffy coat.

Plasma : Fresh frozen plasma (PFP) is prepared by centrifuging whole blood and then 200 to 260 ml of the upper liquid plasma is removed.

Other blood products : Platelet concentrate, granulocyte concentration etc., are mentioned in Table 21.5.

HAZARDS OF BLOOD TRANSFUSION

A. Immediate complications

1. *Haemolytic reactions* : Mostly caused by ABO mismatches.

2. *Chill-fever reactioins* : Predominantly due to reaction of recipient alloantibodies to donor's white cells.

3. *Contaminated blood* : It contains gram negative rods, particularly some enteric bacteria that grow preferentially at 4°C and produce endotoxin. Transfusion of endotoxin contaminated blood may cause shock, generalised bleeding and death. However, such contamination is rare.

4. *Allergic reactions* : Urticaria and anaphylaxis.

5. *Circulatory overload* : This is a common side effect of transfusion which may lead to congestive cardic failure. The risk can be minimised by using packed cells.

6. *Air embolism* : A rare side effect.

B. Delayed complications

1. *Infections* : Hepatitis, malaria, syphilis, cytomegalovirus, HIV, HTLV-I, II, HSV, *T. gondii*, EBV.

2. *Post transfusion thrombocytopenic purpura* is caused by recipient antibodies to donor platelets.

3. Thrombophlebitis.

SCREENING TESTS FOR DONATED BLOOD UNITS (Mandatory)

1. Hepatitis B surface antigen (HBS Ag)
2. Antibody to HIV-1 and HIV-2.
3. Antibody to *Treponema pallidum* (syphilis)
4. Malarial parasite

Other optional tests

1. Antibody to *Hepatitis C virus*
2. Antibody to *Cytomegalovirus*
3. Surrogate tests for Non-A, Non-B hepatitis (Hepatitis B core antibody and ALT activity).
4. Antibody to *P. falciparum.*
5. Antibody to HTLV-I.

QUESTIONS

1. *What are blood group antigens?*
2. *What are the immune or acquired antibodies?*
3. *Name the different ABO blood groups.*
4. *Name the methods of blood grouping and which method is better.*
5. *How do you differentiate group A_1 from A_2?*
6. *Name the causes of discrepancy in ABO blood groupings.*
7. *What is the utility of cross matching?*
8. *What is Bombay phenotype of blood group?*
9. *What are the sub-groups of blood group A?*
10. *Name the differences between complete and incomplete ABO antibodies.*
11. *How do you store blood and its components?*
12. *What are the hazards of blood transfusion?*
13. *Name the causes of haemolytic disease of newborn (HDN).*
14. *What is HND due to Rh disease?*
15. *What is called one unit of blood?*
16. *Name the different blood components.*

Section II

MICROSCOPIC PATHOLOGY (General Pathology)

Section II contains

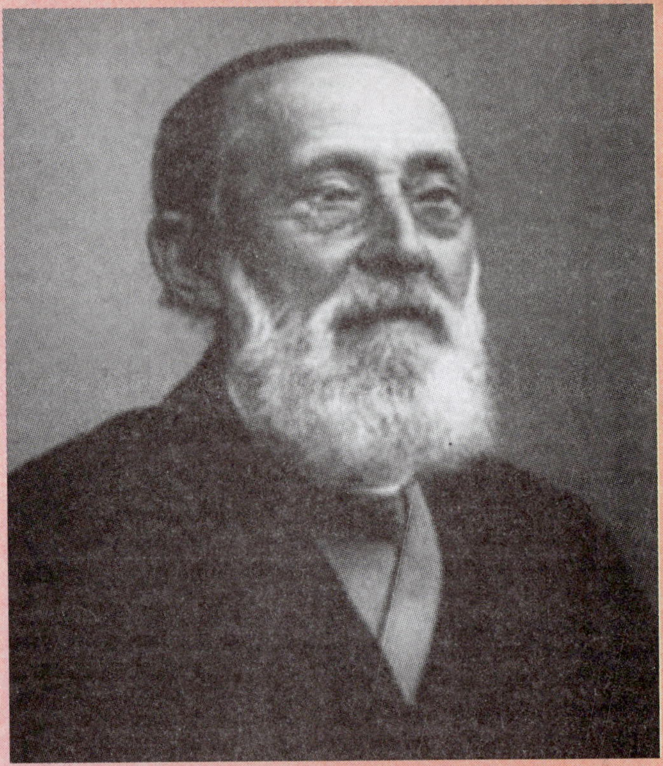

Rudolf Virchow (1821–1902)

Father of Modern Pathology — *Rudolf Virchow was a German physician and described cellular basis of disease. He introduced histopathology as a diagnostic branch. His important discoveries include : Virchow cells (Lepra cell), Virchow node (enlarged left supra-clavicular lymph node in cancer of the stomach), Virchow space in brain tissue, and Virchow's triad in pathogenesis of thrombosis.*

Chapter 22

Inflammation and Repair

Inflammation is defined as the dynamic process by which living tissues react to injury. Depending upon the clinical course and tissue reaction, it is categorised as acute or chronic. The initial stages are called *acute inflammatory* reaction but when the process is prolonged, the inflammation may be *subacute* or *chronic.*

The inflammatory reaction occurs in the surviving adjacent vascular and connective tisues. The specialised parenchymal cells do not participate.

The essential features of acute inflammation are :

(1) *Hyperaemia* : Vascular dilation involving both capillary and arteriole.

(2) *Exudation of fluid* : Increased passage of protein-rich fluid occurs through the wall of the blood vessels into the interstitial tissue leading to local oedema and dilution of toxin.

(3) *Emigration of leucocytes* : Neutrophils (mainly) and few mononuclear cells pass through intracellular space of the venule into tissue spaces.

Morphological types of acute inflammation

1. **Suppurative (purulent) inflammation :** It is an acute inflammation in which the exudate is rich in neutrophil leucocytes. Suppurative inflammation most commonly results from bacterial infection where both viable and dead neutrophils are present. Necrotic tissue and tissue fluid in acute inflammatory exudate form a semiliquid material known as pus, from which the term *purulent inflammation* is derived.

2. **Fibrinous inflammation :** It is a type of acute inflammation where the acute inflammatory exudase possesses high plasma protein content. Fibrinogen derived from plasma gets converted to fibrin and is deposited in tissues. This type of inflammation is observed in membrane-lined cavities, e.g., pleura, pericardium and peritoneum. The fibrin strands form a mat-like sheet causing adhesion between adjacent surfaces.

3. **Serous inflammation :** In this type of acute inflammation, the principal tissue response is an outpouring of fluid with a low plasma protein and cell content, e.g., skin in response to burns.

ACUTE INFLAMMATION

The type of acute inflammatory exudate depends on the nature of injured tissue and the offending agent.

M.E. Section shows :

(i) Hyperaemia with marked dilatation of small blood vessels.

(ii) Large number of neutrophils and excess of fibrin (pink-stained).

(iii) There are several degenerated neutrophils (pyknotic nucleus) and small numbers of macrophages (Fig. 22.1).

OUTCOME OF ACUTE INFLAMMATION

Factors involved

Three factors determine the outcome of infection which include :

(1) Severity of tissue damage,

(2) capacity of specialised cells within the damaged tissue to replicate and regrow which is called regeneration, and

(3) type of agent that caused tissue damage.

Types of cells involved

Three broad groups of cells exist in the context of cell cycle.

(1) ***Labile cells*** : These cells include covering epithelium, bone marrow, lung parenchyma which normally shows continuous turnover, hence regeneration is excellent.

(2) ***Permanent cells*** : Such as adult neurones, that are incapable of proliferation, heal by scarring.

(3) ***Stable cells*** : Such as liver cells and renal tubular epithelium, that show normally little proliferation but remain capable of rapid cell division following injury. Chances of regeneration are good here.

RESOLUTION

It involves complete restitution of normal architecture and function. Here tissue damage is slight and tissue involved is capable of making good any loss of specialised tissue (regeneration), e.g., restitution of normal structure and function of lung following lobar pneumonia.

REGENERATION

Regeneration refers to growth of cells and tissues to replace the lost structures. It involves the capacity of proliferation of surviving cells and migration of surviving cells into the vacant space, e.g., regeneration of epithelia of skin and GIT, alveolar lining cells (following pneumonia) and regeneration of axonal process of peripheral nerve (regeneration of one part of cell and not formation of new cell, i.e., cell body of the neurone).

In cases of partial hepatectomy and unilateral nephrectomy, there is compensatory growth rather than true regeneration.

HEALING

Healing consists of variable proportion of two distinct processes : regeneration and laying down of fibrous tissue, e.g.,

(a) Healing of a cutaneus wound demonstrates both regeneration of epithelium of skin and healing of the epidermis repair by scarring.

(b) In inflammation of pleura, pericardium and peritoneum, healing occurs by scar (fibrous) tissue and there is no regeneration.

REPAIR AND HEALING

GRANULATION TISSUE (Figs. 22.1 and 22.2)

Process of repair begins early in inflammation, sometimes as early as 24 hours after injury. Repair of the site of tissue damaged by scar formation is a common type of healing. It begins as a proliferation of young connective tissue cells (fibroblasts) and proliferation of small blood vessels (capillaries) by mitotic division of connective tissue and endothelial cells respectively (by 3 to 5 days). The elongated fibroblasts and buds of capillary endothelial cells grow into and permeate the exudate, producing a highly vascularised, reddish, interconnected network of granular (because of granular appearance) mass called *granulation tissue.*

(a) Early form (vascular) granulation tissue (Fig. 22.1)

Histology

(i) Section shows plenty of newly formed dilated thin-walled capillaries with evidence of budding.

(ii) The capillary loops are lined by a single layer of endothelial cells.

(iii) Spaces between the capillaries are occupied by plenty of young fibroblasts, macrophages, lymphocytes and neutrophils.

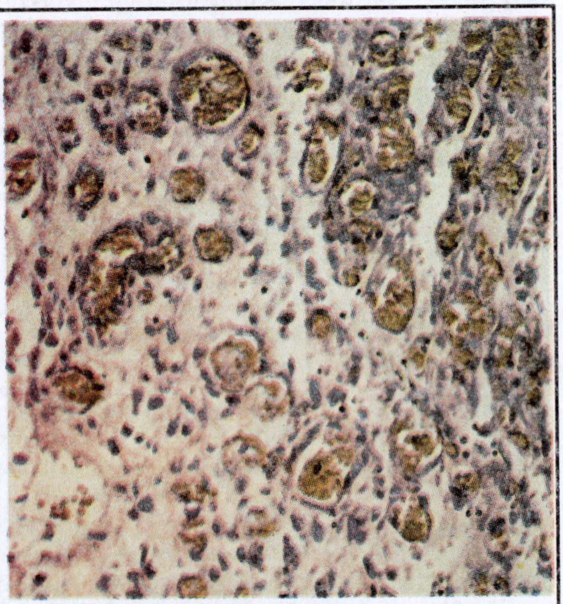

Fig. 22.1. Granulation tissue : Early stage of vascular granulation tissue, HE × 300

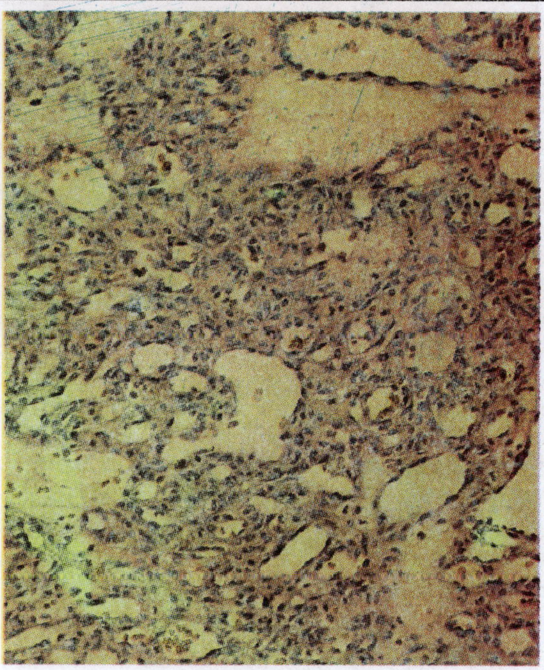

Fig. 22.2. Pyogenic granuloma : skin, showing granulation tissue, HE × 100

(b) Late form granulation tissue (Fig. 22.2)

There is a gradual laying down of collagen by proliferating fibroblasts, and eventually a dense fibrous scar is produced.

Histology : Section shows — (i) Numerous plump fibroblasts with few lingering lymphocytes. (ii) Capillary vessels are relatively small.

CHRONIC INFLAMMATION

Chronic inflammation may result :

(a) following acute inflammation when the causal agent is persisting or,

(b) primary where there is no pre-existing acute cause.

Types

1. **Non-specific chronic inflammation** : Here the damaging stimulus persists despite the presence of acute inflammation. Granulation tissue formation and attempts at fibrous repair go on concurrently instead of sequentially, e.g., chronic ulceration of stomach, chronic inflammation of bronchi and chronic inflammation of colonic mucosa. Histological appearance is dominated by lymphocytes and fibroblasts.

2. **Primary chronic inflammation** : Common causes include :

(a) *Persistent specific infections,* e.g., tuberculosis (Fig. 25.9), leprosy (Figs. 25.14, 25.15, 25.16) where the microorganisms are resistant to attack of neutrophil and the offending bacteria survive intra-cellularly within the macrophage. There is a strong cytotoxic response (Type IV hypersensitivity) mediated by T lymphocytes that produce lymphokines which attract and activate macrophages. These are called histiocytic granuloma or chronic granuloma.

(b) Granuloma resulting from foreign material, such as silicates, including asbestos (Fig. 25.12).

(c) *Auto-immune diseases*, e.g., auto-immune thyroiditis.

(d) *Granuloma* of unknown aetiology, e.g., sarcoidosis, Crohn's disease. These two conditions histologically show features of histiocytic granuloma and are also referred to as chronic granuloma.

Chapter 23

Degeneration, Amyloidosis and Necrosis

CELLULAR RESPONSE TO INJURY

The normal cellular metabolism is maintained by plasma membrane, mitochondria and nucleus. A variety of injurious agents may be involved in cellular injury, such as hypoxia, physical and chemical agents, toxins (bacterial, plants, of snake, etc), viruses, abnormal immunological reactions, nutritional deficiencies and genetic abnormalities. The outcome depends upon severity of the injury and status of cell (Fig. 23.1).

Failure of cellular adaptation

Cells that are intrinsically unable to adapt to injury exhibit several characteristic morphological changes, at first seen ultrastructurally and later on visible to light microscope (Fig. 23.1).

Cells that are unable to adapt metabolic stress, e.g., hypoxia, cease to synthesize structural proteins and begin to face difficulties in supplying energy to sustain electrolyte gradients and support other membrane functions.

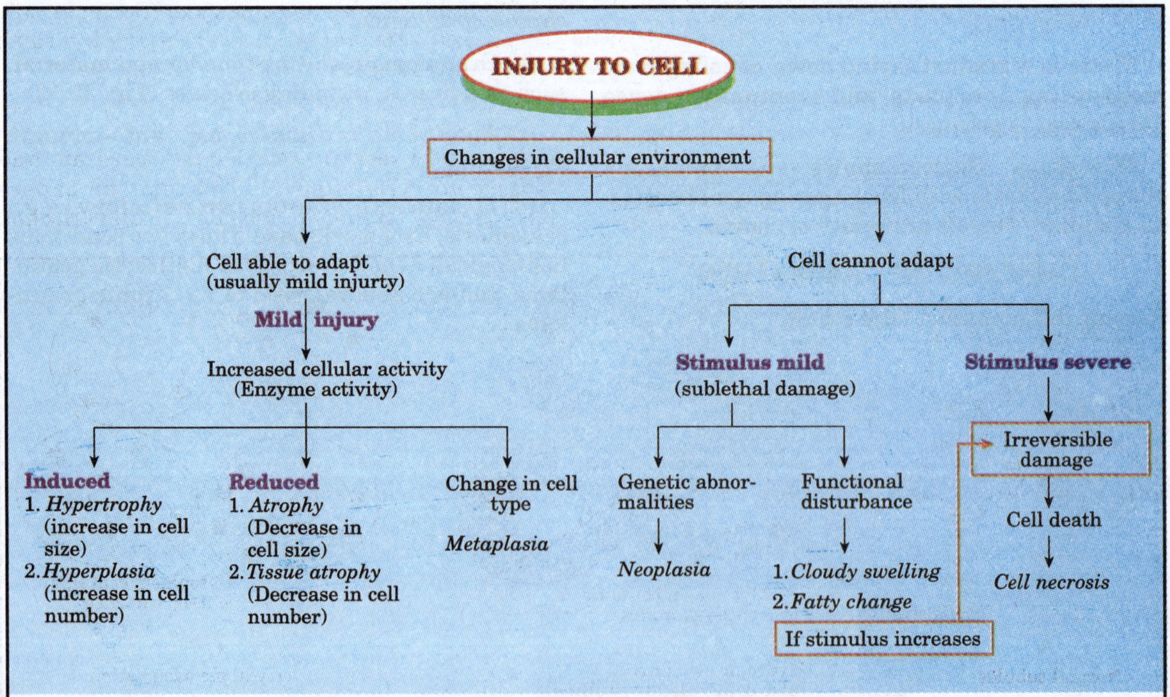

Fig. 23.1. Severity of the injury and status of cell

In *sublethal damage*, the first ultrastructural evidence of cell shows swelling of membrane-bound organelles, particularly endoplasmic reticulum and mitochondria. This change of cell probably results from accumulation of electrolytes and water due to the early damage to the enzymes of the membrane sodium pump. This alteration of cell is potentially reversible if the noxious stimulus is insufficient to cause cell death. The term **degeneration** is in applied such alteration of cells.

DEGENERATION

The term degeneration refers to the state of a living cell with altered biochemical, functional and morphological state resulting from a mild (sublethal) stimulus of injury. Light microscopic study shows fluid accumulation in such cells which makes them pale staining or vacuolated known as *hydropic degeneration* (formerly known as cloudy swelling) — see Figs. 23.2 and 23.3. In special situation, certain cell types (e.g., hepatic cells) respond to metabolic stress by failing to metabolise fatty acids, thus there is accumulation of lipid within the cytoplasmic vacuoles giving rise to so-called *fatty change* (Fig. 23.4). When the causative metabolic stress is removed, such early manifestations of cell change is reversible.

HYDROPIC DEGENERATION

This change may be observed in any tissue with minor injury especially renal tubular epithelium.

Histology (Figs. 23.2 and 23.3)

(i) Structure of kidney

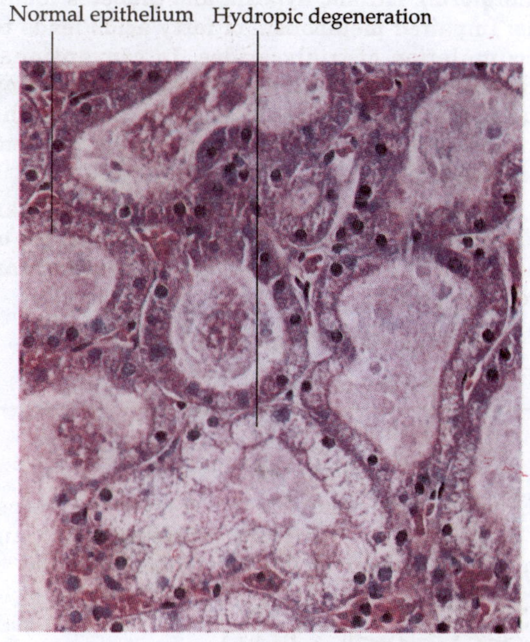

Fig. 23.3. Hydropic degeneration : Kidney (HP × 300)

(ii) some tubules show normal looking epithelial cells, and

(iii) some tubules are damaged : Cells are pale and vacuolated and exhibiting hydropic degeneration.

FATTY CHANGE : LIVER

It is usually seen in liver but myocardium and kidney are also affected. The common causes fatty change (steatosis) include : toxins (alcohol,

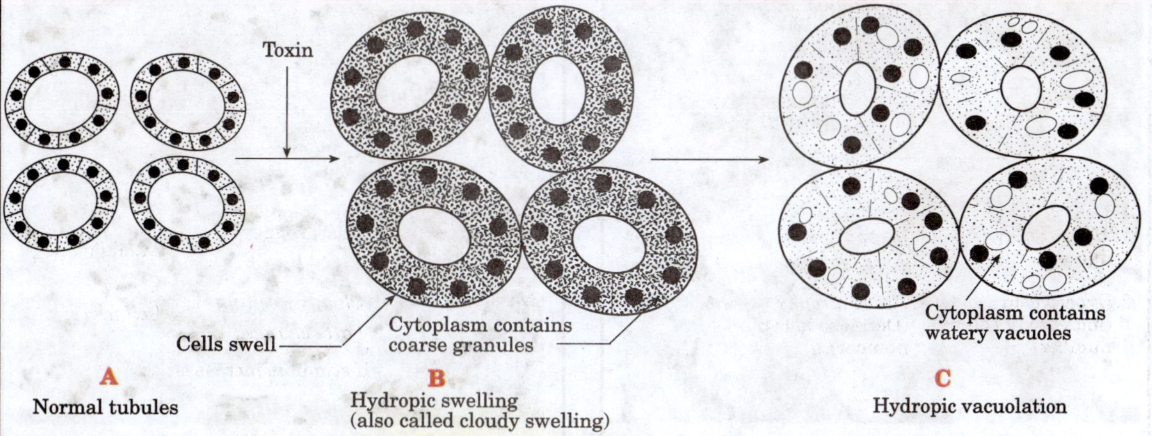

Fig. 23.2. Microscopic appearances of—(A) normal tubules, (B) tubules in hydropic swelling and (C) tubules in hydropic vacuolation

chloroform), chronic hypoxia and diabetes mellitus. Impaired metabolism of fatty acids leads to accumulation of triglycerides. In conventional preparation of section, e.g., paraffin embedding and HE staining, organic solvents used in the processing dissolve the fat leaving an empty, non-staining hole.

For demonstrating fat in *frozen section,* Sudan IV, Oil red O, etc. are to be used. The example of the liver section is a wedge biopsy of liver from an alcoholic person.

Histology (HP) (Figs. 23.4A & B)

(i) Structure of liver.

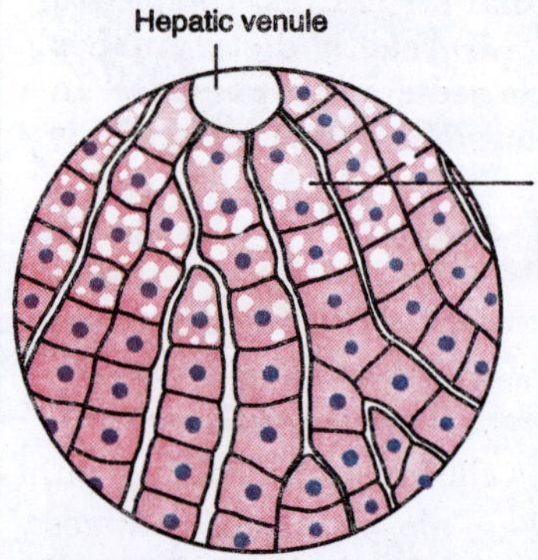

Fig. 23.4A. ME : Fatty liver (diagrammatic)

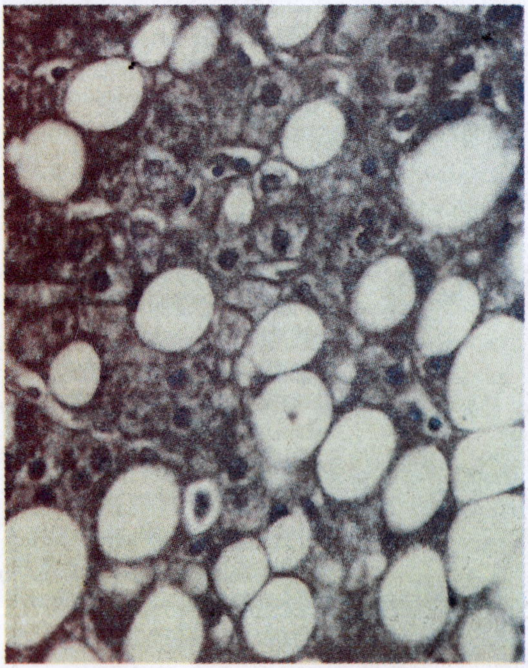

Fig. 23.4B. HE Section : Diffuse fatty change of liver (HP × 350)

(ii) Architecture of hepatic lobule is normal.

(iii) Hepatocytes contain large vacuole pushing the nucleus to periphery and also some fat cysts due to fusion of some lipid-layden cells (Fig. 23.4B).

AMYLOIDOSIS

Amyloidosis is a condition characterised by the extracellular deposition of an abnormal fibrillar protein (waxy substance, termed amyloid).

Nature of amyloid

Chemically amyloid fibrils are made up of :

(a) A major variable component — more than 90%.

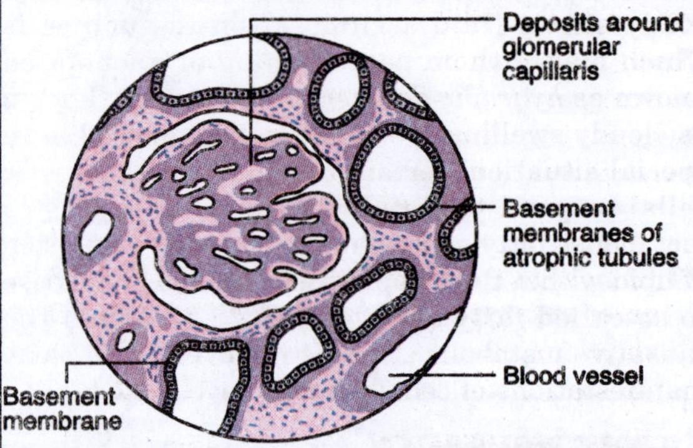

Fig. 23.5A. ME : Amyloid deposition in kidney (diagrammatic)

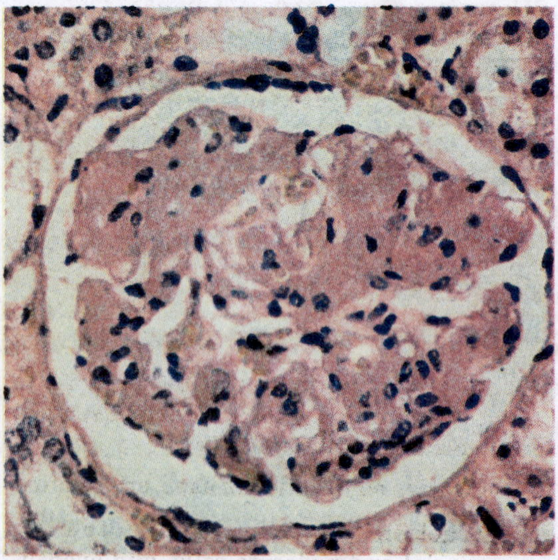

Fig. 23.5B. HE Section : Homogeneous eosinophilic deposit of amyloid in the glomerulus (HP × 300)

(b) A minor constituent of amyloid protein — a glyceroprotein normally present in serum.

Distribution : Amyloid is a homogeneous eosinophilic substance deposited in the extracellular compartment (interstitium) of the tissues. In section stained by HE, amyloid is seen as uniformly eosinophilic (pink-staining) homogeneous material. It may occur in many tissues but kidneys, spleen, adrenals and heart are more frequently affected.

Pathogenesis : The amyloid has a particular predilection for deposition in the walls of blood vessels and basement membranes. Progressive accumulation of amyloid results in cellular dysfunction either preventing normal diffusion through extracellular tissues or by physical compression of the parenchymal cells.

Amyloidosis may be systemic process affecting many organs simultaneously (*systemic amyloidosis*) or it may affect one organ or tissue (*localised amyloidosis*).

Macroscopy

(i) At *post-mortem,* the affected organs look pale, enlarged and possesses a firm waxy structure.

(ii) *Staining with Lugol's iodine* : Amyloid material looks brown whereas normal tissue appears yellow.

Light microscopy

(i) *Congo red stain* : Amyloid shows red staining, apple green birefringence in polarised light. Normal tissue looks pale pink and there is no birefringence.

(ii) *Immuno-staining* : useful for specific constituents, e.g., protein.

Electron microscopy

Amyloids appear as closely packed interlacing fibrils, 70–100 nm in diameter.

AMYLOID KIDNEY

Deposition of amyloid usually begins in the glomerular mesangium and capillary basement membrane leading sequentially to :

(i) progressive obliteration of capillary lumina,

(ii) destruction of glomerular endothelial, mesangial and podocyte cells, and eventually complete replacement of the glomerulus by confluent mass of amyloid occurs.

(iii) Walls of renal arteries and arterioles may concurrently show infiltration by amyloid causing impairment of blood supply to the glomeruli.

(iv) Interstitial spaces of renal tubules are often infiltrated by amyloid further compromising tubular function.

Histology (Figs. 23.5B, 23.6)

(i) HE section of kidney (Fig. 23.5) shows homogeneous eosinophilic material in the mesangium and along basement membrane of glomerulus tuft.

(ii) The amyloid material is difficult to distinguish from normal structures. Congo red staining (Fig. 23.6) readily distinguishes amyloid which is red-stained material. In this picture glomerulus and an arteriole is affected.

NECROSIS

When a cell or a group of cell in a living body sustains irreversible damage, a succession of histological changes take place. These cellular changes, indicative of cell death, constitute necrosis.

Although there are no morphological changes initially, but sooner (within a few hours) the cell membrane and intracellular organelles are disrupted which can be demonstrated by electron microscopy.

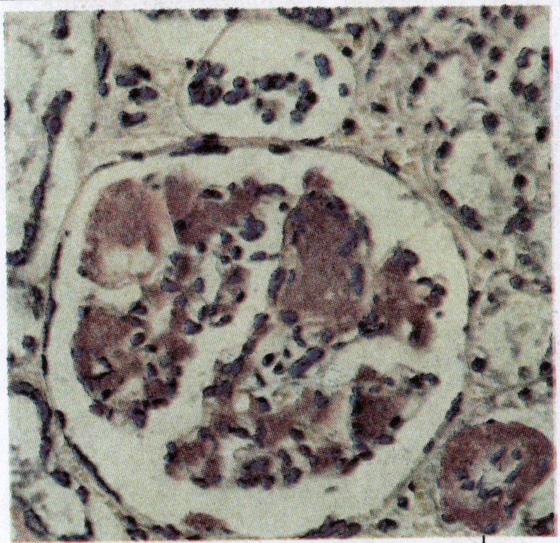

Fig. 23.6. Amyloid kidney and amyloidosis of arteriole (Congo red stain) (H × 250)

Types of Necrosis

Morphologically, patterns of tissue necrosis, are of four types (based on macroscopic appearance) : coagulative, liquefactive, caseous and enzymatic necrosis.

1. Coagulative necrosis

This type of necrosis is usually caused by lack of blood supply and common in infarcts of solid organs, e.g., heart, spleen and kidney.

Macroscopically

Area is swollen, firm and pale.

Microscopically (Fig. 23.7A and B)

(i) Architecture of tissue is maintained in the infarcted area with loss of cellular details.

(ii) Nucleus shows either karyorrhexis (fragmentation into tiny bits) or karyolysis (total dissolution and disappearance). Nuclei show pyknosis (condensed intensely basophilic and dot-like).

(iii) Cytoplasm is opaque, strongly eosinophitic (strong affinity for red dye eosin) and granular.

2. Liquefactive necrosis

In the brain consistently, and in other tissues where there is a large amount of fluid and enzyme activity is marked, the necrotic areas undergo softening and are filled with turbid fluid.

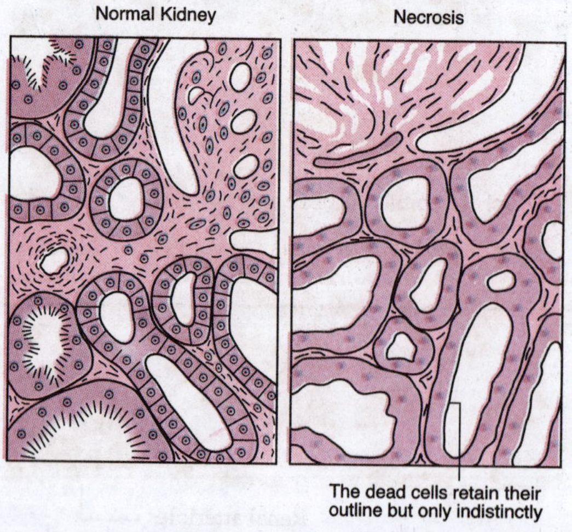

Fig. 23.7A. ME : Coagulative necrosis of kidney (diagrammatic)

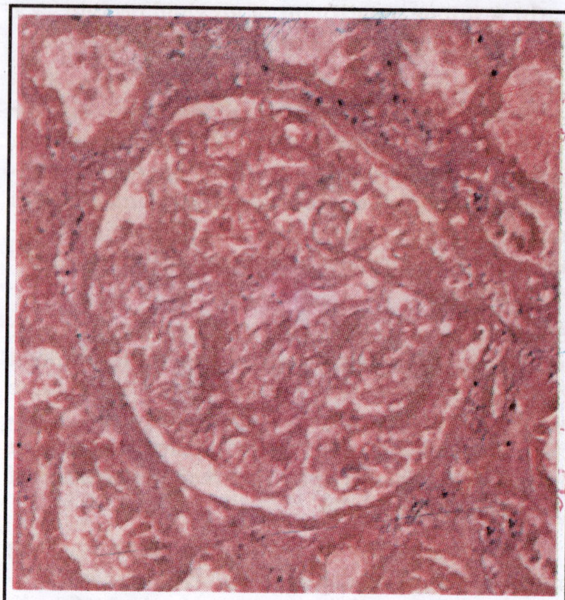

Fig. 23.7B. Coagulative necrosis : Kidney (HE × 150)

The term colliquative necrosis was originally used to describe the microscopic appearance of infarct brain due to arterial occlusion. Since this appearance is not a specific form of necrosis but results from dissolution of the tissue following an initial phase of coagulative-like necrosis, the term is replaced by liquefactive necrosis.

Microscopy

(i) Because of relative lack of extracellular structural proteins, such as reticulin and collagen in brain, hypoxia leads to rapid loss of tissue architecture as autolysis occurs. This results in the early formation of semiliquid mass of dead cells.

(ii) Liquefactive necrosis is often associated with infection caused by pyogenic bacteria such as in abscess.

3. Caseous necrosis

Caseous necrosis is characteristic of tuberculosis. The necrotic tissue has a cream-cheesy appearance, slightly greasy to touch. *Microscopically*, there is a granular eosinophilic material without any architectural details of (mother) tissue or nuclear debris. Surrounding tissue shows chronic granuloma. There are also Langhan's type giant cells in caseous necrosis (vide tuberculous granuloma).

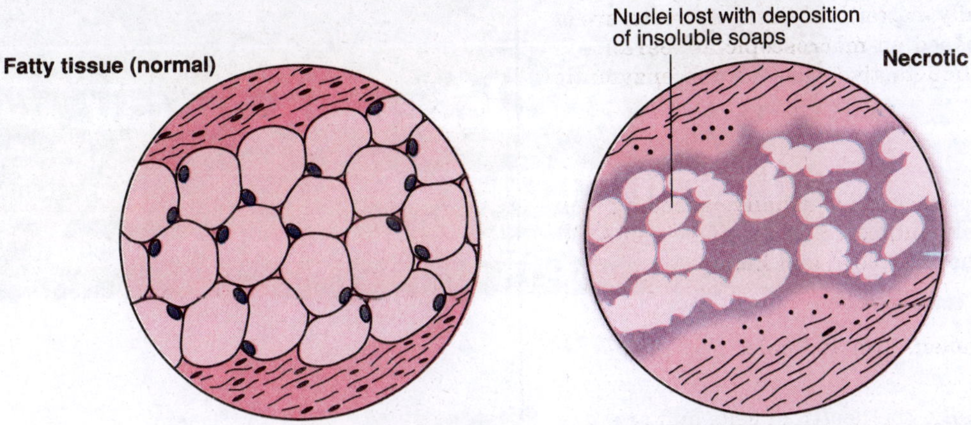

Fig. 23.8A. ME : Fat necrosis (schematic)

4. Fat necrosis

The enzymatic fat necrosis is the term used to denote focal areas of necrosis of fat in the peritoneal cavity, classically seen in omentum, resulting from liberation of activated pancreatic lipases in cases of acute pancreatitis. Enzymes released by the damaged pancreatic acini break up the inert neutral fats into reactive fatty acids that elicit inflammation.

Macroscopic examination (Figs. 23.8A and 23.8B)

Extensive haemorrhagic necrosis of pancreas and surrounding tissues occur. Numerous chalky white spots are often seen in peripancreatic and omental fat.

Histology

(i) Foci of necrotic tissue are surrounded by a dark staining rim of inflammatory cells.

(ii) Foci of calcium soaps seen as amorphous, granular and basophilic material.

(iii) Surrounding zone shows inflammatory reaction.

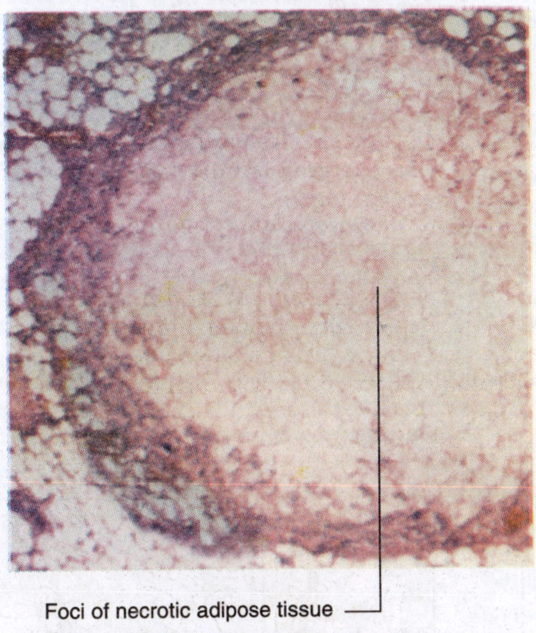

Fig. 23.8B. Fat necrosis in acute pancreatitis (HP × 200)

Chapter 24

Fluid and Haemodynamic Derangements

(Oedema, Congestion, Thrombosis, Infarction)

Physiologically, the health of cells and organs depends on an unbroken circulation to supply oxygen, nutrients and to remove waste products. Abnormalities in vascular permeability or haemostasis can lead to cell injury even when there is intact blood supply.

OEDEMA

Oedema is an accumulation of excess fluid in extravascular (interstitial) tissues. Oedema may be of two categories :

(i) Oedema resulting from local increase in *vascular permeability*, where the oedema is local and the accumulated fluid is a protein-rich exudate with a specific gravity usully over 1020, conversely,

(ii) oedema fluid resulting from *hydrodynamic* derangement, is typically a protein-poor transudate with a specific gravity less than 1012.

PULMONARY OEDEMA

Pulmonary oedema results from increased hydrostatic pressure in the pulmonary circulation. Any condition in which left ventricle and atrium fail to empty adequately, there is an increased pressure in the affected chamber which is transmitted back to pulmonary venous system and pulmonary capillaries. This leads to congestion of pulmonary capillaries and then dilatation of capillaries with erythrocytes, causing increased hydrostatic pressure and transudation of plasma fluid. Fluid accumulates in the alveolar septae, which along with the congested vessels leads to septal widening. The fluid then escapes into the alveolar spaces leading to pulmonary oedema (Fig. 24.1A & B).

Histology

(i) Pulmonary alveoli are filled with eosinophilic coagulated material (that has leaked from the congested capillaries).

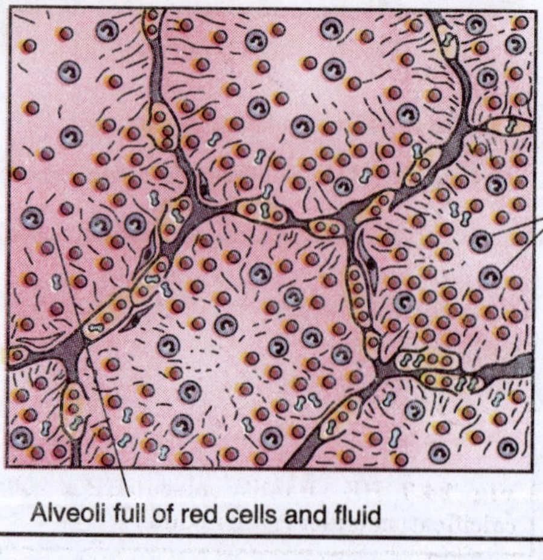

Fig. 24.1A. Pulmonary congestion and oedema (ME)

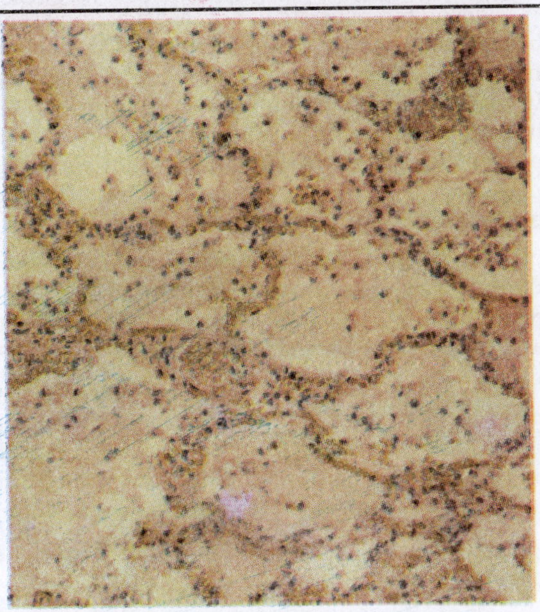

Fig. 24.1B. Pulmonary congestion and oedema (× 140)

(ii) Such transudate is usually cell-free but in this picture few polymorphonuclear leucocytes are present, suggesting that bronchopneumonia was starting to develop.

Cerebral oedema (Fig. 24.2)

Cerebral oedema is encountered in clinical disorders like encephalitis, meningitis and also close to certain focal lesions including abscess, tumour etc.

Histology : There is an accumulation of fluid around the cells and in perivascular Virchow-Robin spaces which leads to formation of clear wide space around the cells and blood vessels. The fibrillar matrix also becomes loose as a result of accumulation of fluid in the interfibrillar spaces.

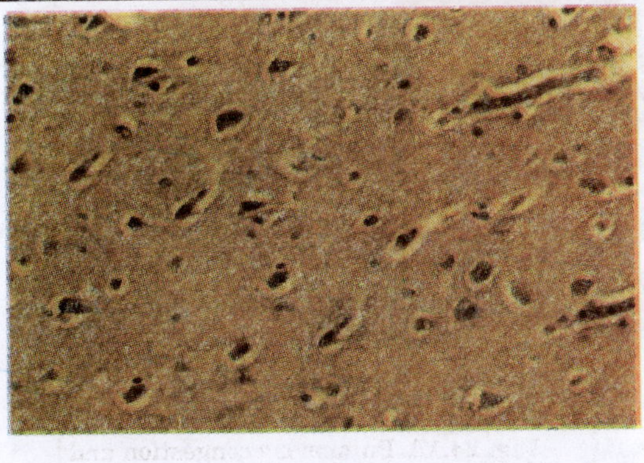

Fig. 24.2. HE Cerebral edema, HP × 250 : Section shows clear space around blood vessels and cerebral cells

CONGESTION

Congestion is a passive process resulting from impaired outflow of blood from a tissue or organ. In right sided cardiac failure when raised pressure is transmitted to the central veins, it leads to congestion of sinusoids of liver with blood and often the hepatocytes in the centrilobular zones undergo atrophy. This is known as chronic venous congestion (CVC). Similar chronic venous congestion is also observed in spleen and lung.

CVC Liver : CVC liver is grossly also known as nutmeg liver. Normal architecture of liver is maintained. There is zonal alterations of each lobule.

Microscopy (vide Fig. 26.46)

Section shows : (i) Dilatation and congestion of central veins and surrounding sinusoids. (ii) There may be associated micro haemorrhages and pressure atrophy of centrilobular hepatocytes. (iii) Midzonal hepatocytes show fatty change resulting from sublethal hypoxia. (iv) Periportal zone contains normal hepatocytes.

CVC Spleen (Fig. 24.3)

In CVC spleen (Banti's spleen) the spleen is enlarged due to marked expansion of the red pulp. The lymphoid follicles of the white pulp have become widely separated as a result of marked expansion of the red pulp.

Microscopy

(1) Sinusoids show dilatation and congestion, with fibrosis of the septae.

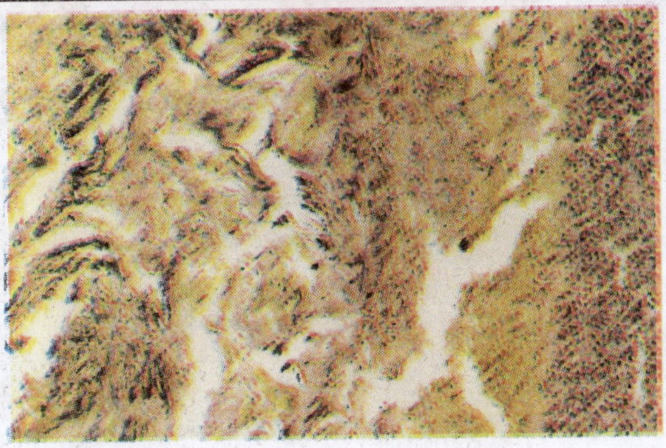

Fig. 24.3. HE : Banti's spleen (HP × 200) showing calcification (siderocytic nodule)

(2) Perivascular haemorrhages have occurred which has lead to organisation with hemosiderin laden macrophages and fibrosis (siderotic nodule, Gamma Gandi bodies).

(3) There may occur giant cell reaction and calcification.

CVC Lung (Fig. 24.4)

Microscopy

CVC lung is also called brown induration.

(i) Edema in the alveoli.

(ii) Septal vessels show congestion, micro-haemorrhages, haemosiderin laden alveolar macrophages (heart failure cells)

(iii) There is septal fibrosis.

Note : The congestion and edema of CVC of lung is to be distinguished from pneumonia. There are plenty of acute inflammatory cells in pneumonic consolidation whereas there is no inflammatory cells in CVC of lung. However, in most cases, CVC lung is a favourable soil for bronchopneumonia to set in.

THROMBOSIS

Thrombosis is an intravascular mass formed from the constituents of blood within a blood vessel or the heart during life.

A thrombus consists of aggregation of platelets bound together by fibrin strands with variable number of red blood cells and white cells trapped in the tangled mass which contribute to the bulk of the thrombus. The main effect is to bring platelets in contact with the vessel wall. The main factors leading to thrombosis are mentioned below.

1. ***Damage to vessel wall,*** particularly endothelium, is the main factor of arterial and intracardiac thrombosis, e.g., atheroma in blood vessel and endocardial damage in case of heart.

2. ***Disorder of blood flow*** in which stasis plays an important role in initiating formation of thrombus in slow-flowing blood, e.g., in veins. In cases of turbulent flow, the arterial vessels and heart are predisposed to thrombus formation.

3. ***Changes in composition of blood*** : It includes :

(i) Increase in platelets, fibrinogen and prothrombin after operation and childbirth, usually after a week (5-10 days).

(ii) Decrease in platelet adhesiveness — after surgery.

(iii) Rarely congenital abnormalities of thrombin inhibitors, e.g., deficiency of antithrombin-II and protein C.

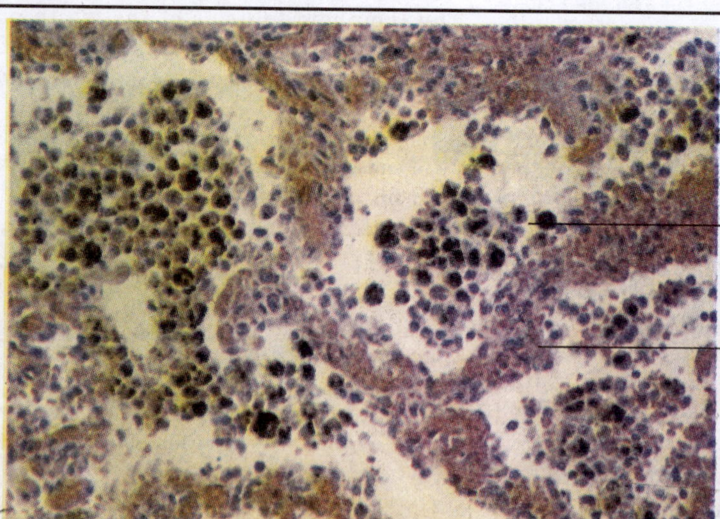

Fig. 24.4. Chronic Venous Congestion Lung — edematous septae and alveoli with hemosiderin laden macrophages

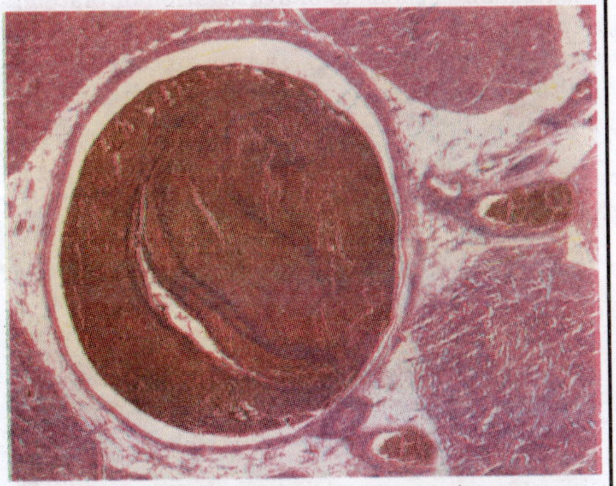

Fig. 24.5. Recent thrombosis in a vein (LP)

(iv) Miscellaneous causes like oral contraceptives, smoking and some cancers.

1. Recent thrombus (Fig. 24.5)

Histology

(i) Thrombus inside a vein of leg.

(ii) It has completely occluded the vessel.

2. Organised canalised thrombus (Fig. 24.6)

Following occlusion of a vessel wall by thrombus, there is an initial inflammatory response in the vessel wall leading to organisation of the thrombus by the ingrowth of granulation tissue from the intima of the wall of blood vessel.

Histology (Fig. 24.6)

An artery is occluded by thrombus and the picture is taken at a later stage of organisation.

(i) Thrombus — occluded the artery.

(ii) Granulation tissue in the lumen showing numerous small blood vessels. These blood vessels may conduct passage of blood across the thrombosed area and some will enlarge later on and acquire smooth muscle walls.

INFARCTION

An infarct is an area of ischaemic necrosis. Infarct is often seen in the periphery of the organ.

Infarction may result either from occlusion of arterial supply (common in myocardium, kidney and spleen), or from obstruction of venous drainage (torsion of bowel loop, testis, ovary).

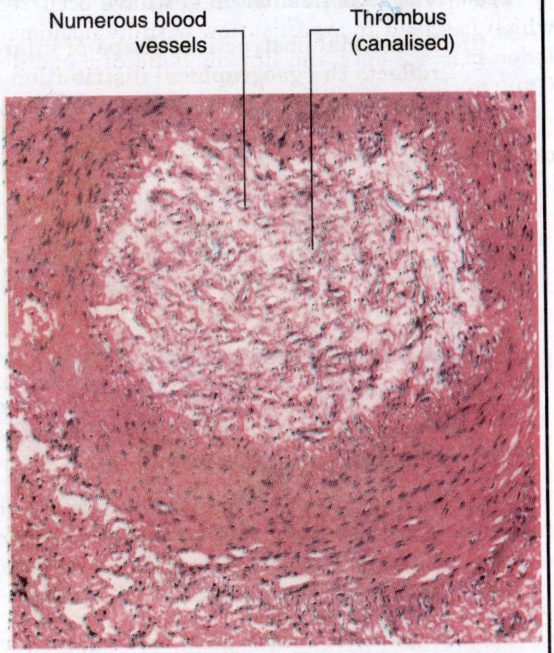

Fig. 24.6. Thrombus with recanalisation (× 140)

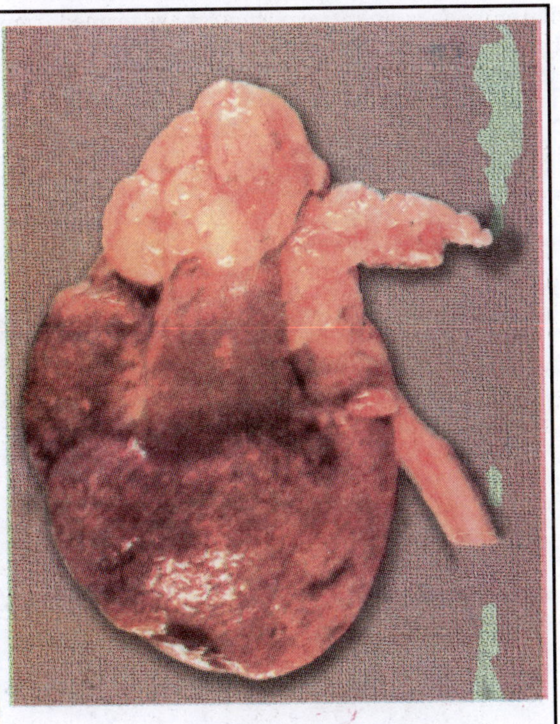

Fig. 24.7. Renal infarct— polar distribution in atherosclerosis

Macrosopic appearance (Fig. 24.7)

(i) In arterial obstruction, shape of infarct reflects the geographical distribution of artery involved.

(ii) Infarct appears wedge-shaped on cut section in most organs.

(iii) Earliest stages are dark red in colour due to congestion and becomes pale in late stages as organisation by granulation tissue occurs resulting in a scar.

Histology (Fig. 24.8)

(i) Infarcted area shows coagulative necrosis (architecture maintained with loss of cellular and nuclear details).

(ii) Cells lining the tubules are necrotic, there is no nuclear staining and cytoplasm is deeply eosinophilic (left side of figure).

(iii) Capillaries of boundary zone (centre) are greatly distended and stroma is oedematous.

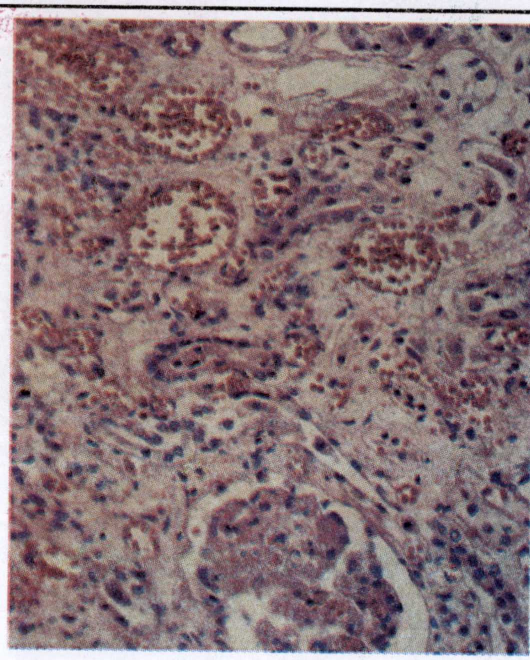

Fig. 24.8. Infarct kidney–edge of a recent infarct (× 150)

Chapter 25

Infectious Diseases

ACUTE INFECTION

Acute appendicitis

Aetiology

Inflammation of appendix is associated with obstruction in 50–80% cases, mostly by faecolith and sometimes by worms (*Enterobius vermicularis*) and others. However, no demonstrable luminal obstruction is detectable in 15-30% cases, where anaerobes (*B. fragilis*) or aerobes (*E. coli, Klebsiella* spp.) or both may be the aetiological agent (Fig. 25.1).

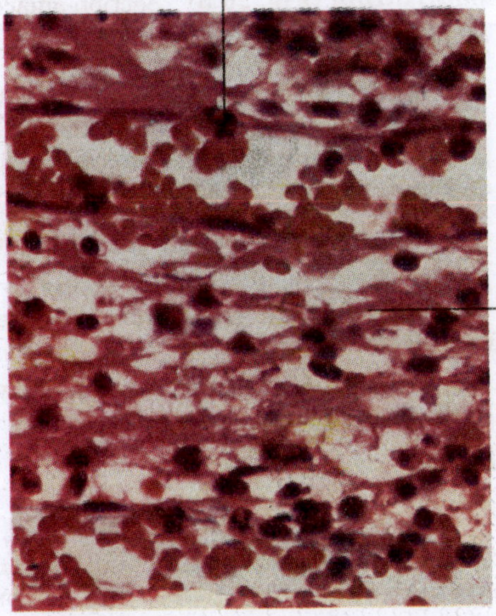

Fig. 25.1. Acute inflammation (early formation of exudate), HE × 150

Morphology

Acute appendicitis is often graded as *early acute* (earliest stage), *acute suppurative* or *acute gangrenous* appendicitis. The beginning of acute appendicitis is usually a superficial ulceration of mucosa. Spread occurs from mucosa to serosa and then rapidly travels lengthwise in the muscular and serous coats.

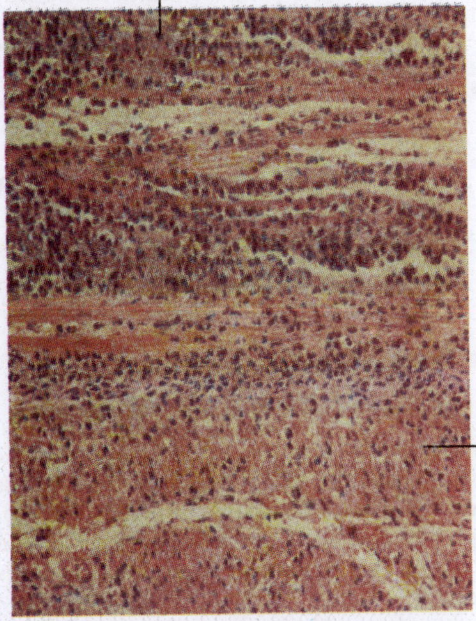

Fig. 25.2. Acute appendicits : Muscle fibres are separated by a pus-like inflammatory exudate consisting predominantly of polymorphonuclear leucocytes, HE × 150

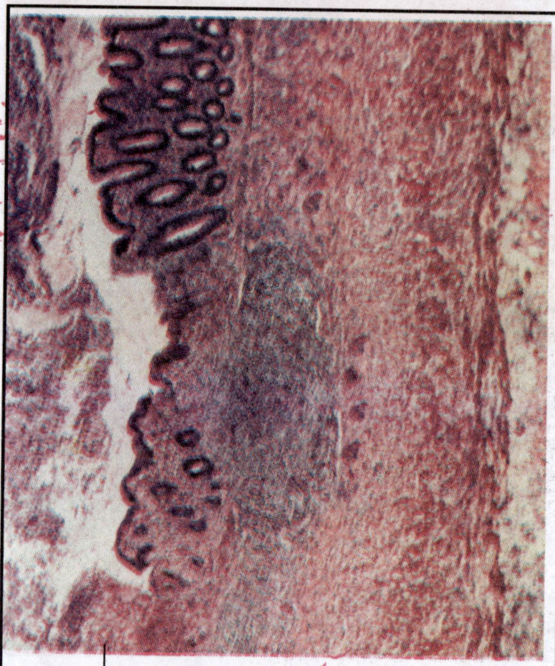

Fig. 25.3. Acute appendicitis : Section shows focal lesion of mucosa infiltrated by polymorphonuclear leucocytes and eosinophils. Base of a gland shows ulceration, HE × 150

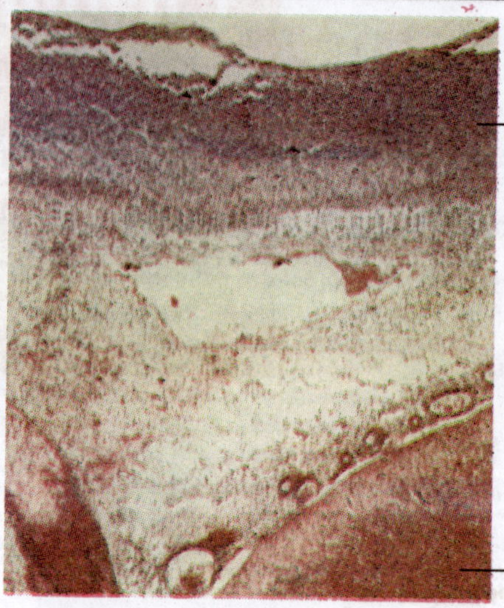

Fig. 25.4. Acute purulent meningitis, HE × 60

Histology (Fig. 25.2, 25.3)

(i) Section shows the picture of appendix.

(ii) Lumen contains exudate and denuded epithelium.

(iii) Lining mucosa is broken and all the coats (mucosa, submucous and muscle coats) are infiltrated with neutrophilic leucocytes.

Diag. Acute suppurtive appendicitis.

ACUTE PURULENT MENINGITIS

Acute purulent meningitis is caused by pyogenic organisms (*Neisseria meningitidis, Streptococcus pneumoniae)*. Acute inflammation of the leptomeninges occur and inflammatory fluid collects in the subarachnoid space, in which neutrophils predominate.

Histology (Fig. 25.4)

(i) The subarachnoid space lying between pia (brain) and arachnoid is distended with inflammatory exudate rich in fibrin and polymorph leucocytes.

(ii) Polymorphs have infiltrated the arachnoid membrane.

(iii) Small blood vessels on the surface of brain are congested.

LOBAR PNEUMONIA

Aetiology and Stages— See Chapter 28 (p. 246).

Microscopic examination

***Red hepatisation* (Fig. 25.5)** : Section shows :

(i) Structure of alveoli of lung.

(ii) Alveoli are filled with inflammatory exudate consisting of large number of polymorphonuclear leucocytes, red cells, degenerated macrophages and fibrin.

(iii) Alveolar wall capillaries are engorged with blood.

Note : (i) The affected lobe would appear red and solid macroscopically.

(ii) A gram stain of aspirate/sputum shows large number of microorganisms.

***Grey hepatisation* (Fig. 25.6)**

(i) Section shows structure of lung.

(ii) Some alveoli contain fibrin, while others contain exudate and plenty of polymorphonuclear leucocytes and scanty red cells.

(iii) A clear zone exists between the exudate and alveolar wall.

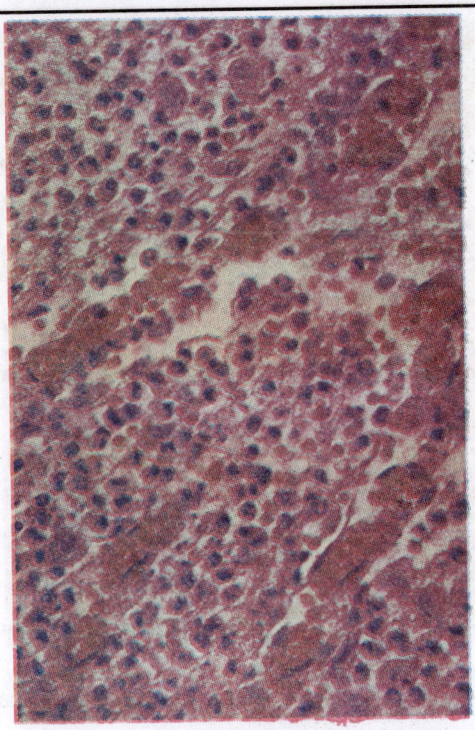

Fig. 25.5. Lobar pneumonia (red hepatisation), HE × 340

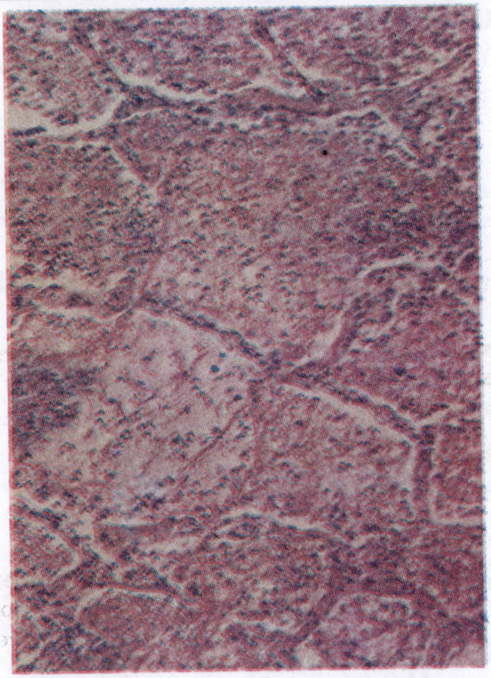

Fig. 25.6. Lobar pneumonia (grey hepatisation), HE × 140

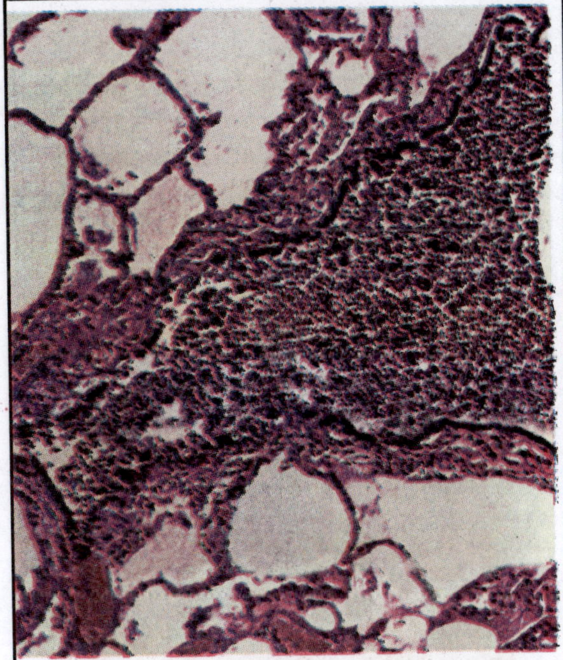

Fig. 25.7. Acute purulent bronchitis, HE × 96

Note : The affected lobe appears grey due to reduced vascularity of the consolidated lung. *S. pneumoniae* are still numerous in the exudate.

ACUTE PURULENT BRONCHITIS

Acute purulent tracheobronchitis and bronchiolitis are probably initiated in most cases by viruses or mycoplasmas, which is followed by bacterial invasion (*S. aureus, H. influenzae).*

Histology (Fig. 25.7)

(i) Mucosa of the airways is acutely inflammed and congested.

(ii) Smaller lobular bronchi and bronchioles are filled by pus-like secretion consisting largely of neutrophil polymorphs.

(iii) Polymorphs are also present within the epithelium of bronchiole, and the blood vessels in the submucosa are greatly dilated.

(iv) Lung parenchyma is usually unaffected in early stages, but alveolar spaces adjacent to the affected bronchioles are often filled with oedema fluid, which may proceed to development of bronchopneumonia.

BRONCHOPNEUMONIA

Aetiology and Pathogenesis : See Chapter 28.

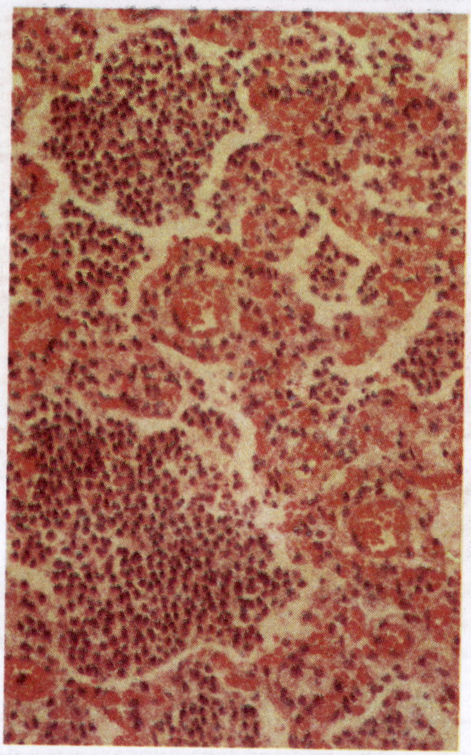

Fig. 25.8. Bronchopneumonia : lung, HE × 150

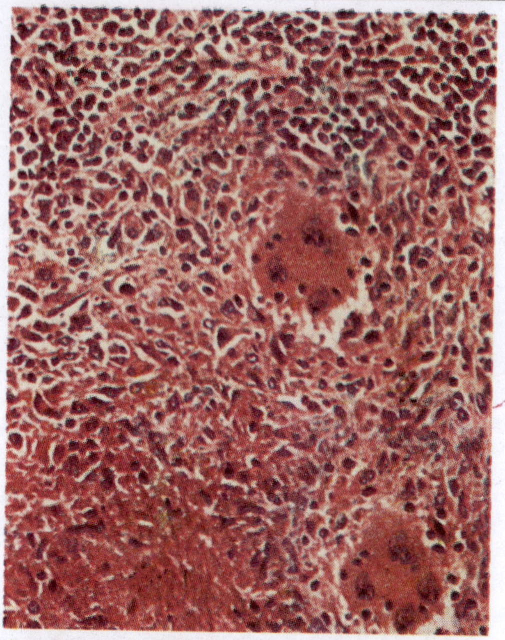

Fig. 25.9. Tuberculous lymph node (LP), HE × 150

Histology (Fig. 25.8)

(i) Section shows structure of lung.

(ii) Bronchioles contain exudate in their lumina and leucocytic infiltration in their walls.

(iii) Peribronchial alveoli are filled up with neutrophils, fibrin and organisms, and are consolidated.

(iv) Consolidated alveoli are surrounded by a zone of compensatory emphysema.

Note :

(i) Inflammatory exudate in the airspace solidifies the lung, hence called, *consolidation*.

(ii) Gram's staining will show fibrin and bacteria in the exudate.

CHRONIC SPECIFIC GRNULOMA

TUBERCULOUS LYMPH NODE

Lymph nodes are focal collections of lymphoid and reticuloendothelial cells. Tuberculous lymphadenitis is common in children and young subjects. Affected lymph nodes are enlarged and matted. Cut section shows presence of many tubercles.

Histology of tubercle (Fig. 25.9)

(i) Section shows the structure of lymph node.

(ii) A granulomatous lesion with —

(a) Central area of caseous necrosis,

(b) surrounded by lymphocytes, histiocytes, epitheloid cells and Langhans' giant cells, and

(c) peripheral zone of fibrous tissue consisting of fibroblasts.

Note : Tubercule bacilli are present in area of caseous necrosis which can be detected by acid-fast staining (Z.N. smear) and culture.

TUBERCULOSIS LUNG (Fig. 25.10)

Histology

(i) Section shows the structure of lung,

(ii) Central granular caseation is surrounded by epitheloid cells and Langhans' giant cells.

(iii) The tubercle is surrounded by fibroblasts and lymphocytes.

Macroscopy : Vide specimen (Chapter 28).

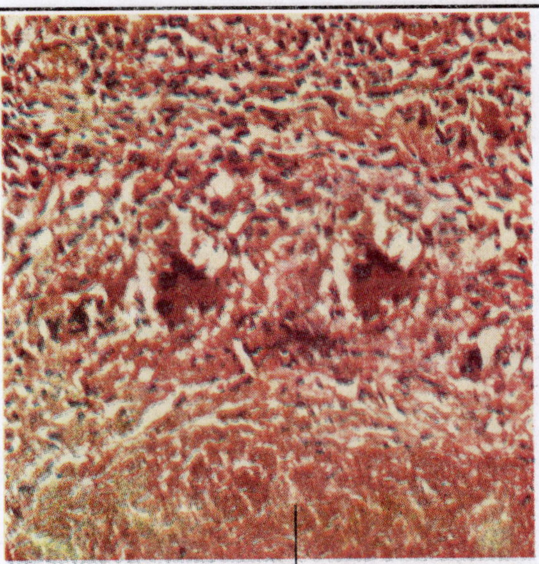

Fig. 25.10. Pulmonary tuberculosis, HE × 100

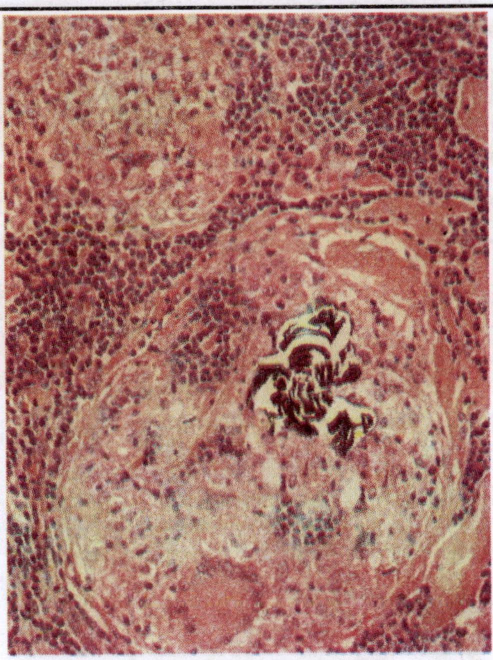

Fig. 25.11. Sarcoidosis in lymph node (HP)

SARCOIDOSIS

It is a chronic granuloma of unknown aetiology characterised by the presence of rounded collections (follicles) of epitheloid cells. It differs from tuberculosis in that there is no central caseation, although small foci of necrosis may be seen in large granuloma. Mediastinal and cervical lymph nodes are more often affected. Cytoplasm of sarcoid giant cells may contain inclusion bodies of 2 types : star-shaped *Asteroid bodies* or small laminated calcified concretions called *Schwamann's bodies*. Although these are characteristics of sarcoid giant cells, they are occasionally found in other chronic granuloma.

Histology (Fig. 25.11)

(i) Architecture of lymph node is lost.

(ii) Lymphoid tissue is largely replaced by several follicles that are composed of epitheloid cells (large cells with eosinophilic cytoplasm and vesicular nuclei).

(iii) Several Langhan's type giant cells are seen.

(iv) Presence of Schwamann body in the larger follicle.

(v) Fibrous tissue at the periphery of the follicle.

Note : No caseation is there.

FOREIGN BODY GRANULOMA

It usually results from a particulate crystalline matter, which may be immunologically inert. The nature of foreign body may be suture, vegetable matter, crystals, fungus, etc. which can be identified, or it may be dissolved during processing of tissue leaving cleft-like spaces as seen in Fig. 25.12. In foreign body granuloma, the giant cells (foreign body type) are formed by fusion of histiocytes which may contain numerous uniform nuclei, scattered in a correspondingly large amount of cytoplasm.

Histology (Fig. 25.12)

(i) Foreign material is enclosed by foreign body giant cells.

(ii) Background shows infiltration of lymphocytes, plasma cells and histiocytes.

(iii) Foreign body is dissolved during the processing of tissue which are represented by cleft-like spaces.

RHINOSPORIDIOSIS

It is a granulomatous disease of man and animal characterised by development of polyp or wart-like lesions primarily affecting the nasal and nasopharyngeal mucosa and less often the conjunctiva

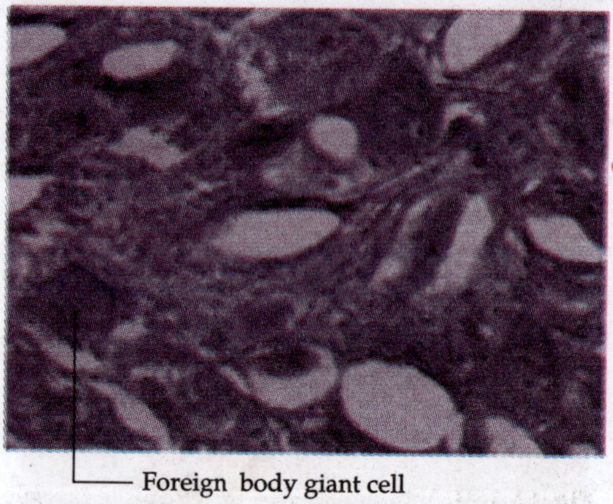

Fig. 25.12. Foreign body granuloma showing cholesterol clefts and foreign body giant cells

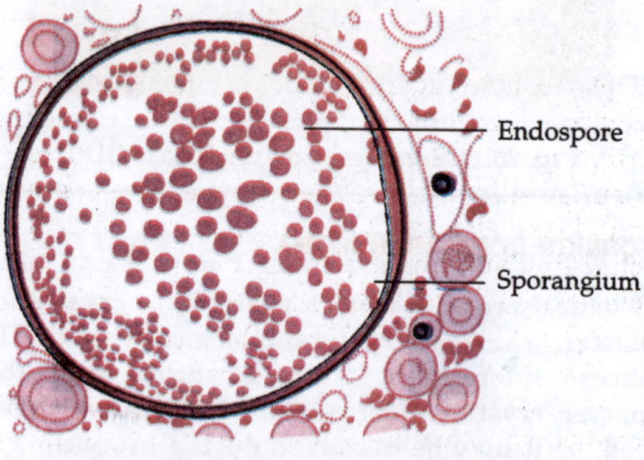

Fig. 25.13. Rhinosporidiosis nose sporangia containing spores lying in nasal mucosa

of the eye. The causative agent is a fungus named *Rhinosporidum seeberi.*

Mode of infection and transmissions are not known. Most cases are found in India and Sri Lanka (80%). Fungus has not been cultivated. Diagnosis is made by demonstration of sporangia in tissue seen on Fig. 25.13.

Histology (Fig. 25.13)

(i) Subepithelial loose connective tissue of nasal mucosa shows mucous glands and varying number of chronic inflammatory cells like lymphocytes, plasma cells and eosinophils.

(ii) Organisms (*R. seeberi)* of the size of red cells with chitinous wall are found in the thick walled sporangia. Spores are also seen in submucosa and surface of mucosa.

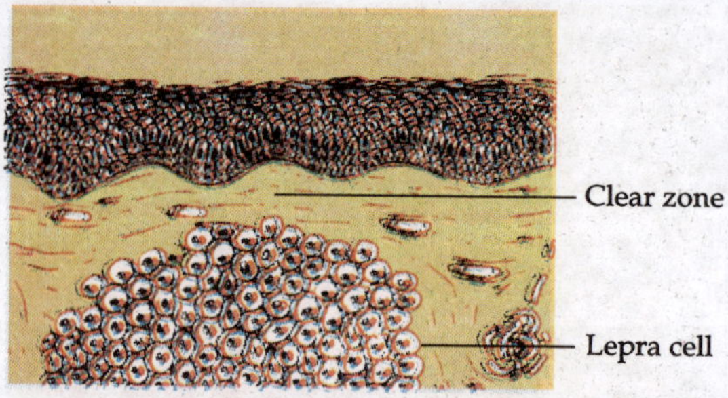

Fig. 25.14A. Lepromatous leprosy

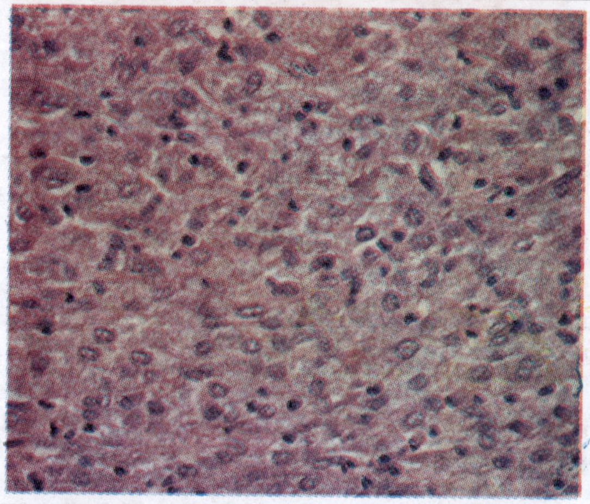

Fig. 25.14B. Lepromatous leprosy skin. Dermis is packed with lepra cell [(large macrophage with vacuole in cytoplasm) (× 300)]

Leprosy

Leprosy or Hansen's disease is caused by *Mycobacterium leprae.* It is less acid-fast than the tubercle bacillus (decolourising agent 5% H_2SO_4 instead of 20% H_2SO_4). Leprosy manifests as two polar forms — tuberculoid and lepromatous.

1. Lepromatous leprosy : In lepromatous leprosy, cell-mediated immune response is impaired because of low host resistance (Figs. 25.14A and 25.14B).

Histology (Figs. 25.14A and B)

(i) Section from lepromatous dermis is packed with nodule of leprosy — lipid-laden foamy macrophages known as *Lepra cells.* Some small lymphocytes and several polymorphs are also seen.

(ii) The dermal aggregates of lepra cells characteristically do not encroach upon the basal layer of epidermis leaving uninvolved (*clear zone*) subepidermal dermis.

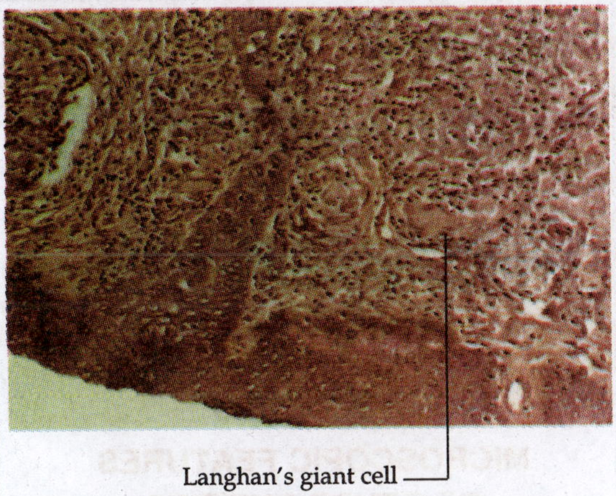

Fig. 25.15. Tuberculoid leprosy : Epitheloid cell granuloma eroding the basal layer of epidermis (× 150)

(iii) Overlying epidermis has become thin and flat.

Note : Stain for AFB (skin scraping) shows numerous bacilli inside cells — often as stacks or globi.

2. Tuberculoid leprosy (Fig. 25.15): Tuberculoid leprosy shows good degree of cell-mediated immune response and has good prognosis.

Histology (Fig. 25.15)

(i) Dermis shows epitheloid cell granulomas that closely resemble *hard tubercles*. They consist of epitheloid cells, Langhans' giant cells, a few lymphocytes at the periphery but no caseation.

(ii) Granuloma erode the basal layer of the epidermis (*Grenz zone*) and dermal nerve twigs.

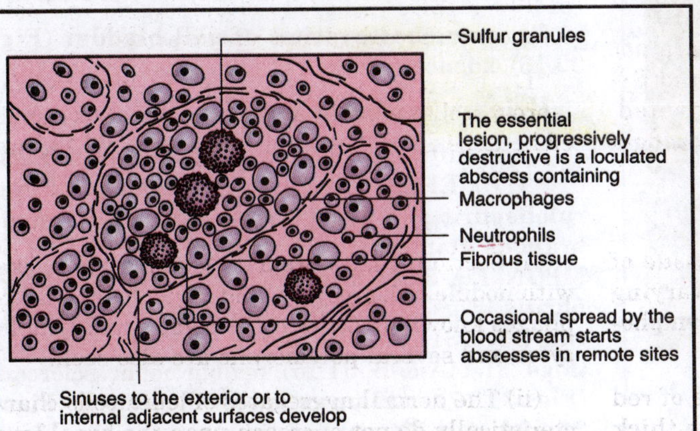

Fig. 25.16A. Actinomycotic abscess

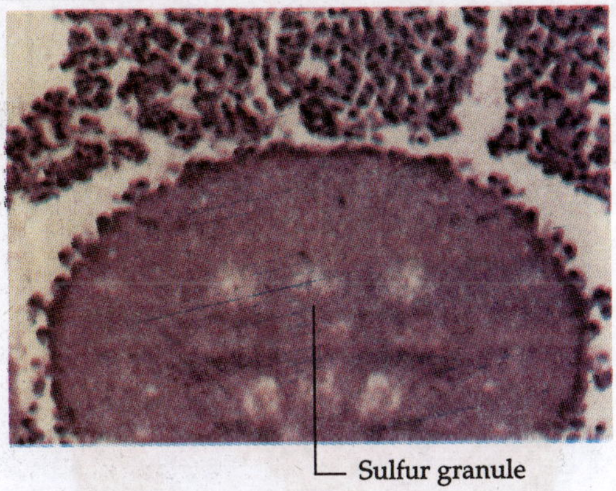

Fig. 25.16B. Actinomycosis — ME : Sulfur granule is surrounded by polymorphs (× 250)

Note : Lepra bacilli are few or absent in acid-fast stain.

Actinomycosis Skin

The causative agent is most commonly *Actinomyces israeli* and head and neck region is commonly affected. These are anaerobic bacteria. There is firm swelling on the lower jaw at the beginning but later abscess with sinuses are formed discharging sulphur granules. Pus contains characteristic yellow sulphur granules.

Histology (Figs. 25.16A and B)

(i) Section shows reaction of granuloma with central suppuration. There are chronic inflammatory cells, giant cells and fibroblasts surrounding the central area of absccess.

(ii) Bacterial colony (sulphur granule) shows basophilic radiating filaments with hyaline eosinophilic club-like ends in the centre of suppuration.

FUNGAL DISEASES

Rhinosporidiosis

Rhinosporidiosis — causative agent is a fungus called *Rhinosporidium seeberi*.

Other important fungal diseases include aspergillosis lung.

Filariasis Lymph Node

Both adult female filarial worm and microfilaria are seen in lymphatic channels near the lymph node. If dead, it may calcify or lead to intense inflammatory reaction characterised predominantly by eosinophils around the parasite. The affected lymph node shows reactive hyperplasia, inflammation and fibrosis around the worm (Fig. 25.17).

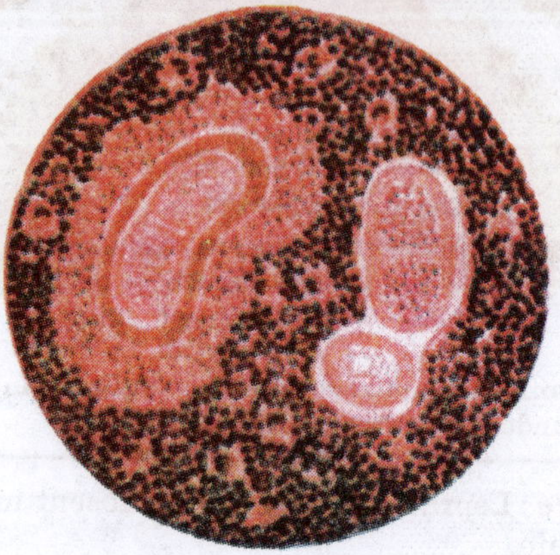

Fig. 25.17. Microfilaria in lymph node with surrounding inflammation and fibrosis

Hydatid disease of liver (Fig. 25.18)

Hydatid cyst is the larval form *Echinococcus granulosus.* These occur most commonly in liver and sometimes in lungs, brain and other deep viscera.

The cyst may be over 10 cm in diameter and shows laminated membrane and the cyst contains clear fluid containing infective scolex (head) of the parasite.

Histology : Cyst wall is pearly white in colour and composed of three distinguished layers :

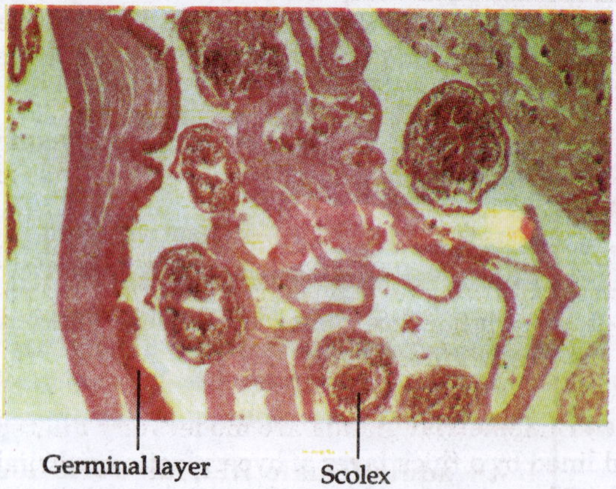

Fig. 25.18. Hydatid cyst liver showing laminated membrane and brood capsule with scolices

(i) ***Endocyst*** : Innermost layer lining the cyst wall is germinal epithelium which gives rise to brood capsules with scolices. Section shows several brood capsules.

(ii) ***Ectocyst*** : It is the characteristic intermediate layer that supports the germinal layer. It is composed of a cellular, chitinous, laminated, hyaline material.

(iii) ***Pericyst*** : This is the outer fibrous layer that results from cellular reaction of the host and consists of mononuclear cells, eosinophils and surrounded peripherally by fibroblasts.

MICROSCOPIC FEATURES OF OTHER ENTITIES

Microscopic (histological) features of some systemic diseases and neoplasms are discussed in Section III (Systemic Pathology) along with description of the specimens, the numbers of relevant figures are mentioned below :

Cardiovascular system (Ch. 27)

Aschoff body (Fig. 27.1).

Respiratory system (Ch. 28)

Nasal polyp (Fig. 28.1), squamous cell carcinoma of lung (Fig. 28.14).

Alimentary system (Ch. 29)

Benign pleomorphic adenoma of salivary gland (Fig. 29.1), peptic gastric ulcer (Fig. 29.6), carcinoid tumour (Fig. 29.13), salmonella enteritis (Fig. 29.15), tuberculosis granuloma of ileum (Fig. 29.17), adenocarcinoma of colon (Fig. 29.24).

Liver, Gall bladder and Pancreas (Ch. 30)

Chronic cholecystitis of gall bladder (Fig. 30.16), adenocarcinoma of pancreas (Fig. 30.18).

Urinary system (Ch. 31)

Acute diffuse proliferative glomerulitis (Figs. 31.3A, B), RPGN (Fig. 31.4), membranous glomerulonephritis — EM features (Fig. 31.5), membranous glomerulonephritis (Fig. 31.7), EM of MPGN (Fig. 31.8), mesangiocapillary glomerulonephritis (Figs. 31.9A, B), chronic glomerulonephritis (Figs. 31.12A &B), diabetic glomerulosclerosis (Figs. 31.14A & B, 31.15), benign nephrosclerosis (Fig. 31.17), malignant nephrosclerosis (Figs. 31.19A and B), chronic pyelonephritis (Figs. 31.21A and B), transitional cell carcinoma bladder (Fig. 31.27).

Chapter 26

Disorders of Growth, Neoplasia, Lymphoma and Systemic Diseases

Cells respond to the environmental changes in several ways. The cells undergo degeneration or cell death when the stimulus is overwhelming (see chapter 23) but when the stimulus is less noxious, cells adapt to new environment by altering their pattern of growth. This may occur in three ways.

Cellular alteration

1. ***Change in size of cells***, e.g., cell size is increased in hypertrophy and cell size is decreased in atrophy.

2. ***Change in the differentiation*** of cells, e.g., metaplasia.

3. ***Change in the rate of cell division***, such as in liver, where proliferation rate is very slow but is increased rapidly following injury.

4. ***Increase in cell number***, e.g., hyperplasia.

Cell types

Intrinsically cells may be grouped into three types for their capacity for cell division :

1. ***Labile cells*** : Cells that divide and *replicate continuously*, e.g., squamous cells in the epidermis.

2. ***Stable cells*** : Cells which normally do not replicate or show little proliferation but which are capable of cell division in response to certain stimulus, e.g., hepatic cells and renal tubular epithelium (*facultative dividers*).

3. ***Permanent cells*** : Cells which are not capable of proliferation (*non-replicatory*), e.g., neurones and cardiac muscle cells. Hence the heart and brain have no capacity of *regeneration*.

GROWTH DISORDERS

Hyperplasia

Hyperplasia is an increase in the number of cells in an organ or tissue resulting in increased volume of tissue or organ.

Hyperplasia occurs in response to a stimulus and the process is reversible.

Types of hyperplasia

(i) *Physiological hyperplasia* may be again — *hormonal hyperplasia* that increases the functional capacity of an organ or tissue when needed (e.g., endometrial glands in adults).

(ii) *Compensatory hyperplasia* (e.g. bone marrow, gut epithelium, skin). In bone marrow there is both hyperplasia and development of new cells from stem cells.

(iii) *Pathological hyperplasia* are mostly caused by excessive hormonal stimulus (e.g., hyperplasia of endometrium) or growth factors (e.g., papilloma viruses producing skin warts).

Hyperplasia plays an important role in wound healing where proliferating fibroblasts and blood vessels aid in repair.

Endometrial hyperplasia : Endometrial hyperplasia occurs when there is abnormal oestrogenic stimulation.

Histology (Figs. 26.1A and 26.1B)

(i) Endometrial glands are moderately dilated and lined by a thick layer of hyperplastic epithelial cells. There is no evidence of secretory activity.

(ii) Stroma is intensely cellular.

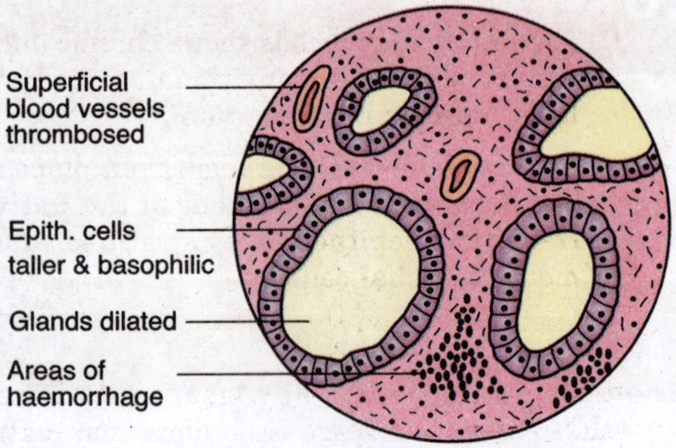

Fig. 26.1A. M.E : Endometrial hyperplasia (due to excess oestrogenic stimulation — anovulatory cycle)

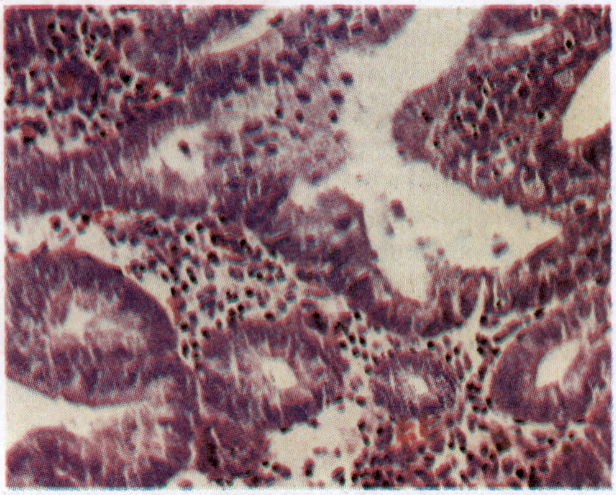

Fig. 26.1B. Endometrial hyperplasia (× 150)

(iii) Numerous mitoses are present in both epithelial and stromal cells.

Note : The lady was on prolonged oestrogen therapy (Fig. 26.1B). Such picture is also seen in oestrogen-secreting ovarian tumours.

Hypertrophy

Hypertrophy is defined as an increase in the size of cells resulting in increase in tissue mass or organ. So the hypertrophied organ has not got any new cell and the cells are just larger. Hypertrophy is seen in *stable cells* of muscle tissue (skeletal, etc.) which normally do not replicate or have little proliferative activity. It occurs in response to a (physical) stimulus (e.g., pregnant uterus), and reversible.

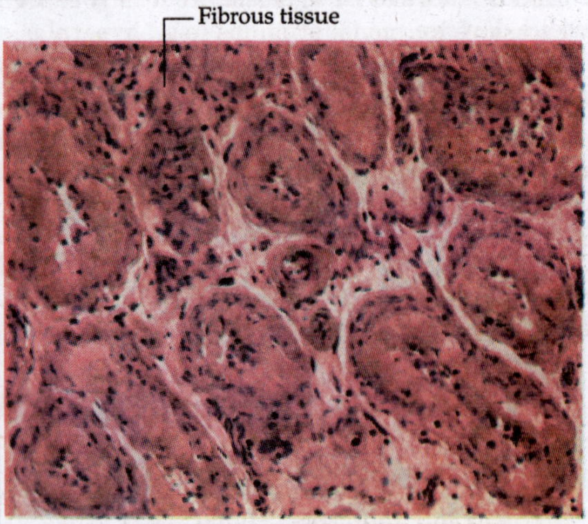

Fig. 26.2. Atrophic testis (× 200)

Atrophy

Reduction in the size of the cell by loss of cell substance is known as atrophy.

Atrophy occurs due to various reasons including disuse atrophy, loss of nerve supply and blood supply, loss of endocrine stimulation, ageing, etc. Atrophy must be distinguished from *hypoplasia* where there is incomplete growth of an *organ* and *agenesis* where complete failure of growth of an organ occurs during embryological development.

Testicular atrophy : Reduced secretion of trophic hormones plays an important role in atrophy of testis and that is the cause in this person of 80 years old (Fig. 26.2).

Histology

(i) *Seminiferous tubules* show thickened wall and pink-stained, a process of *hyalinization*. There is minimal spermatogenic activity.

(ii) *Interstitial tissue* shows increased deposition of fibrous tissue.

Metaplasia

This is a replacement of one type of differentiated (mature) tissue to another by altering their morphological appearance. Altered differentiation of cells takes place from primitive or basal cells.

Metaplasia is a reversible change, commonly seen in lining epithelia but may be found in connective tissue. Metaplasia is considered to be an adaptive process which produces cells better equipped to withstand a new environment.

(a) **Epithelial metaplasia** : Bronchi — the respiratory cuboidal epithelium may be replaced by squamous epithelium under the influence of chronic irritation due to smoking (called *squamous metaplasia*). Similarly, chronic irritation may lead to *squamous metaplasia* of normal transitional epithelium of bladder and columnar epithelium of endocervix (see exfoliative cytopathology).

(b) **Connective tissue metaplasia** : Metaplasia sometimes may be seen in mesodermal tissue. When an area of fibrous tissue is exposed to chronic trauma, it may form bone (*osseus metaplasia*).

Squamous metaplasia

The patient (Fig. 26.3B) had been suffering from chronic bronchiectasis and that caused chronic irritation of the bronchial mucosa leading to squamous metaplasia. Normally lining cuboidal epithelium was replaced by stratified squamous epithelium.

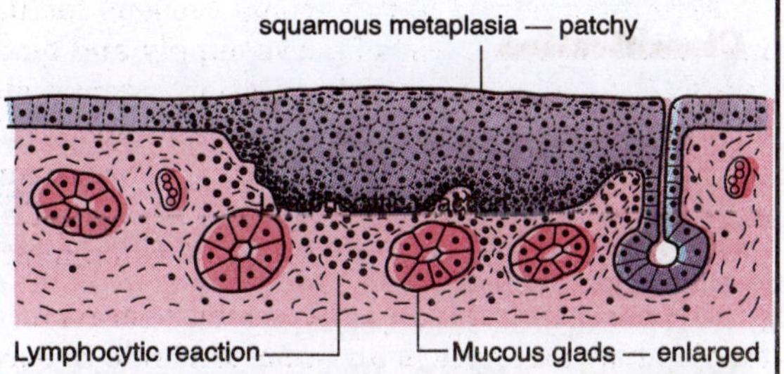

Fig. 26.3A. ME : Squamous metaplasia of larynx

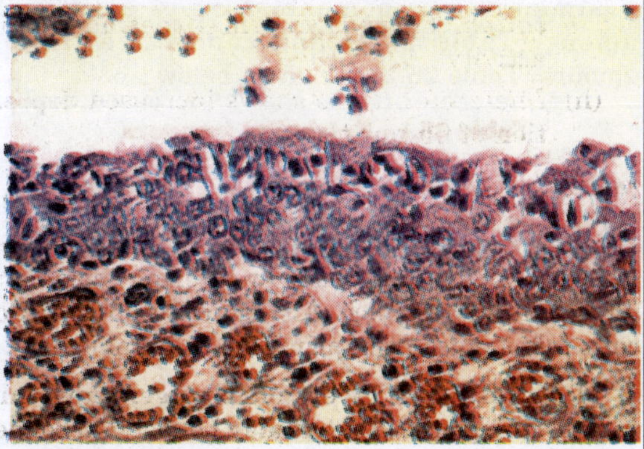

Fig. 26.3B. Microscopic view of squamous metaplasia of bronchial epithelium (× 100)

Histology (Figs. 26.3A and 26.3B)

(i) HE section of bronchus shows chronic inflammatory cells in transitional epithelium layer (chronic inflammation).

(ii) Squamous metaplasia has taken place in one area with replacement of the native transitional epithelium by stratified squamous epithelial cells.

DYSPLASIA

The term dysplasia literally means disordered growth. In dysplasia there is an abnormal maturation of cells and all cytological features of malignancy are present but the cells have not invaded the surrounding tissues. It is frequently encountered in the cervix uteri at the junction of ecto and endocervix. It may occasionally be found in gladular epithelia.

Dysplasia is characterised by the constellation of changes which include (Figs. 26.4A and 26.4B) :

1. loss of uniformity of cells,
2. loss of architectural orientation (polarity),
3. exhibit considerable pleomorphism,
4. nuclear enlargement,
5. hyperchromasia and
6. abnormal mitotic activity even in maturing superficial layers of epithelium.

Like metaplasia, dysplasia is often observed in epithelia subjected to chronic irritation where there are associated inflammatory and repairatory changes, e.g., as seen in cervical and bronchial epithelia. However, it may also occur in absence of tissue damage.

The squamo-columnar junction of cervix is the transformation zone from where squamous metaplasia occurs. Cervical carcinoma and their precursor **cervical intraepithelial neoplasia** (CIN) begins at this site. Dysplastic changes are graded as CIN I, CIN II and CIN III (Figs. 26.4A, 26.4B). Later on, invasive squamous cell carcinoma develops in some cases (vide chapter on exfoliative cytopathology).

Dysplasia of cervix (CIN II moderate dysp) (Fig. 26.4B)

Histology

(i) HE section shows disruption of the normal orderly maturation sequence of squamous cells.

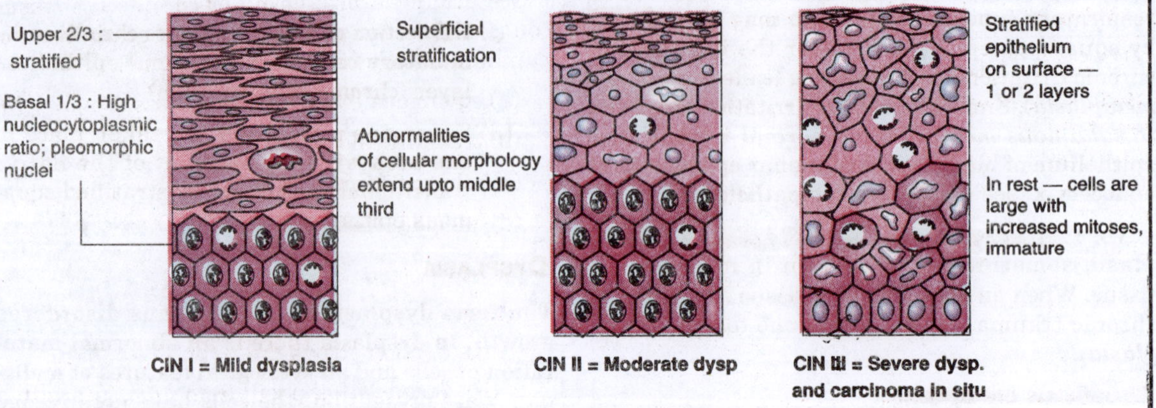

Fig. 26.4A. ME : Based on cellular morphology, cervical dysplasia is graded into CIN I, CIN II and CIN III

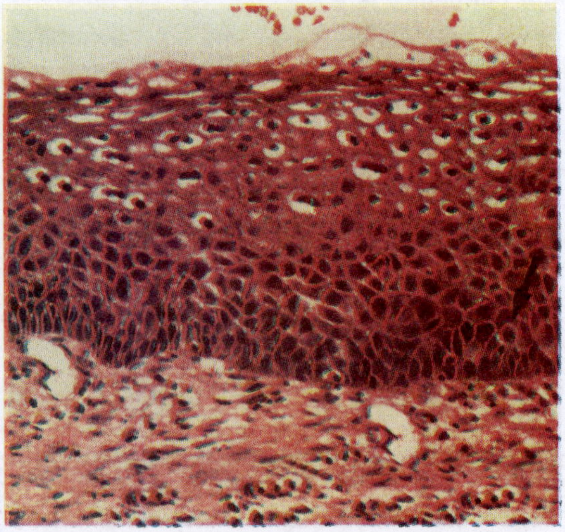

Fig. 26.4B. Cervical dysplasia — CIN II (× 250)

(ii) Cell in mid-strata show very large nuclei with prominent nucleoli.

(iii) Mitotic figures are present above the basal layer.

(iv) Cells show increased nuclear–cytoplasmic ratio (higher ratio of nucleus to cytoplasm).

NEOPLASIA

Neoplasia literally means process of new growth and a new growth is referred to as neoplasia. The term tumour was originally applied to the swelling caused by inflammatory reaction but now it is synonymously used with neoplasm and it has no relevance with inflammation.

Neoplasia (for new growth) describes a state of an abnormal mass of tissue whose growth exceeds and is uncoordinated with normal growth, and continues irrespective of its causative stimulus being withdrawn.

Classification

Neoplasia may be classified based on — (a) cell or tissue of origin, or (b) as benign and malignant according to their behaviour.

Benign tumour : When the margins of the neoplasm are well-defined and cellular growth is entirely local, it is called *benign*.

Malignant tumour : When the margins of the neoplasm are poorly defined and the neoplastic cells infiltrate into and destroy surrounding tissues, it is called malignant neoplasm.

Nomenclature of tumours

Summaries of nomenclature of epithelial tumour (Table 26.1) and connective tissue tumours (Table 26.2) are given below :

Table 26.1 : Epithelial tumours

Tissue of origin	*Benign*	*Malignant*
Surface epithelium	Papilloma	Carcinoma
Examples :		
Squamous	Squamous cell papilloma	Squamous cell carcinoma
Glandular (columnar)	Adenoma (villous or tubular)	Adenocarcinoma
Transitional	Transitional cell papilloma	Transitional cell carcinoma

Table contd. next page

Table 26.1 contd. from previous page

Tissue of origin	*Benign*	*Malignant*
Solid glandular epithelium	Adenoma	Adenocarcinoma
Examples :		
Thyroid	Thyroid adenoma	Thyroid adenocarcinoma
Kidney	Renal adenoma	Renal adenocarcinoma
Liver	Hepatic adenoma	Hepatic adenocarcinoma

Table 26.2 : Connective tissue tumours

Tissue of origin	*Benign*	*Malignant*
Fibrous	Fibroma	Fibrosarcoma
Bone	Oesteoma	Osteosarcoma
Cartilage	Chondroma	Chondrosarcoma
Adipose	Lipoma	Liposarcoma
Smooth muscle	Leiomyoma	Leiomyosarcoma
Skeletal muscle	Rhabdomyoma	Rhabdomyosarcoma

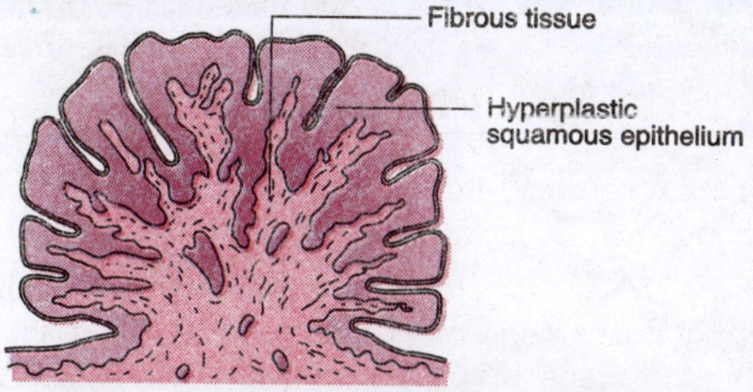

Fig. 26.5A. ME : Squamous cell papilloma *(common wart)*

BENIGN TUMOURS

Epithelial Tumours

There are two main types of benign epithelial tumours, *papilloma* that grow outward from an epithelial surface (e.g., cutaneous or mucosal papilloma) and *adenoma,* which arises from and imitates glandular epithelium.

Papilloma

It is a pedunculated or sessile tumour growing outward from a surface, consisting macroscopically or microscopically visible finger-like or warty projections. Microscopically, neoplastic epithelial cells lie externally around a branching of connective tissue containing blood vessels. Type of epithelium of papilloma is that of surface origin, i.e.,

(a) squamous (skin, palate, larynx, tonsil);

(b) transitional (urinary tract);

(c) columnar (intestinal tract) or

(d) cuboidal (lining of a cyst).

Squamous papilloma of skin

Microscopic examination (Figs. 26.5A & B)

(i) Section shows the structure of skin.

(ii) It consists of papilliform processes with a central core of connective tissue stroma containing blood vessels covered by a thick layer of stratified squamous epithelium.

(iii) The epithelial cells show *hyperkeratosis* (thickening of stratum corneum) and *acanthosis* (increase in thickness of prickle cell layer) and *parakeratosis* (retention of nuclei within the keratinised cell layer).

(iv) The epithelial cells are regular with little evidence of mitosis and basement membrane is intact.

(v) Infiltration of lymphocytes in connective tissue core is frequent.

Fibroadenoma of breast

Fibroadenomas are compound epithelial and connective tissue tumours in which hyperplasia of glandular cells is associated with growth of fibrous tissue. This benign breast tumour is common in

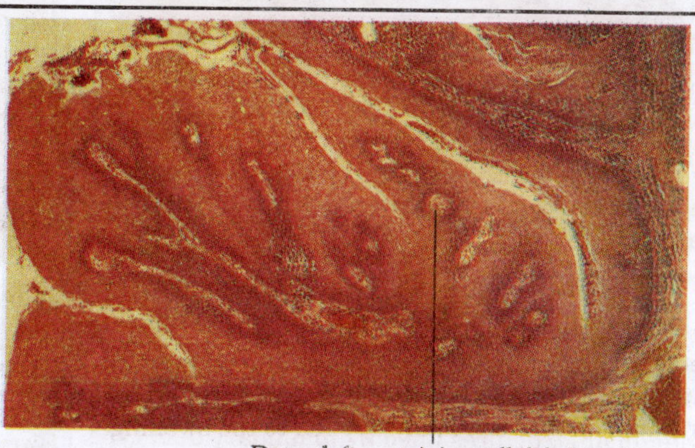

Fig. 26.5B. Squamous cell papilloma of tonsil, HE × 40 arrow indicates blood vessels

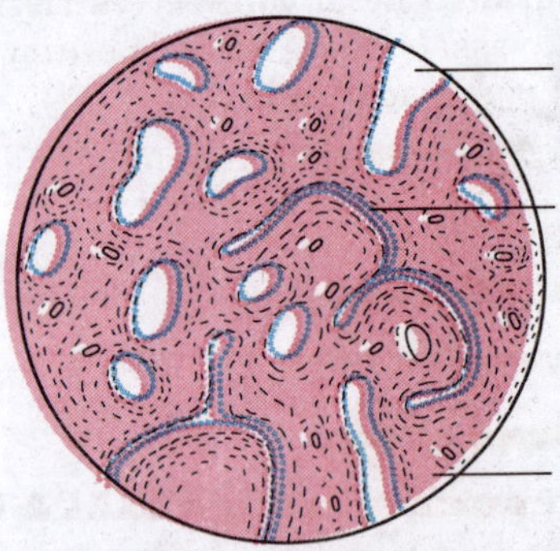

Fig. 26.6A. ME : Fibroadenoma of breast *(pericanalicular)*

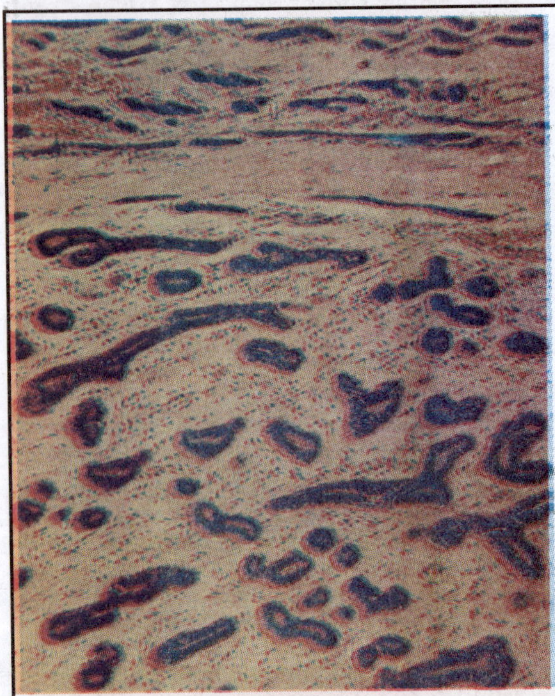

Fig. 26.6B. Fibroadenoma of breast *(pericanalicular type)*. HE × 80

younger women (20-35 years). *Histologically,* fibroadenomas are of two types : pericanalicular and intracanalicular.

Histology

(i) Section shows both epithelial and fibrous stromal components.

(ii) The epithelial components have formed glandular structures lined by mammary duct type single or multiple layers of cuboidal epithelial cells that are regular and have a well-defined, intact basement membrane.

(iii) The stromal component is a loose cellular form of fibrous tissue. The stroma may be myxomatous in very large masses.

Two patterns of growth occur in fibroadenoma, often in the same lesion :

(a) *Pericanalicular type* (Figs. 26.6A & 26.6B)

The epithelial component takes the form of rounded to oval ducts which remain small and undistorted, surrounded by fibrous stroma in a regular manner. Ducts are usually larger, and some are open.

(b) *Intracanalicular type* (Fig. 26.7)

Here connective tissue element proliferates more actively than the epithelial component. The ductal spaces are compressed by extensive proliferation of the stroma and consequently the ducts appear as slits or irregular structures. The nodules of intracanalicular fibroadenoma are surrounded by bands of dense fibrous tissue.

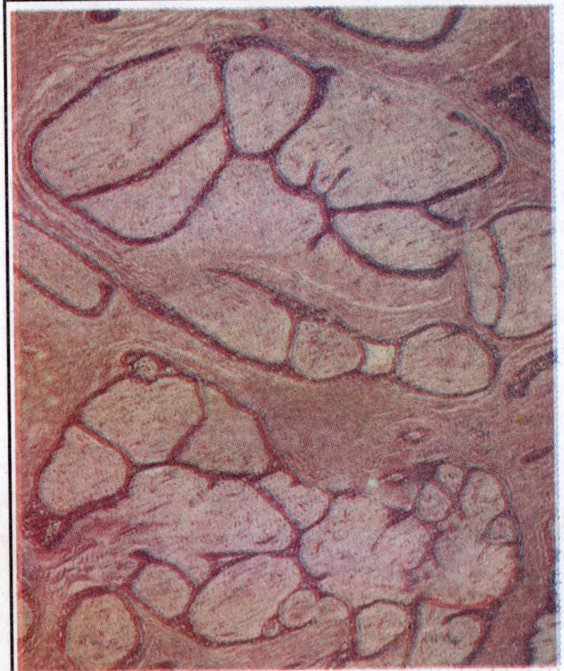

Fig. 26.7. Fibroadenoma of breast *(intracanalicular pattern),* HE × 60

HAMARTOMAS

HAMARTOMA

Hamartoma is thought to be a tumour like malformation or inborn errors of tissue development characterised by focal overgrowth of cells and tissues native to the organ in which it occurs. Hamartoma differs from neoplasm by its inability for limitless proliferation. Examples include *haemangiomas, lymphangiomas, moles* and *developmental cysts* within kidney, etc.

Hamartomas are thought to be present at birth and they grow in step with other tissues of the body, and ceases growth when body growth is complete.

HAEMANGIOMA

Haemangiomas may be composed of masses of cavernous or capillary-like channels filled with blood.

These are common lesions, particularly in infants and children. It is yet unknown whether haemangiomas are true neoplasm or hamartomas. There are several histological variants, e.g., *capillary, cavernous* and *sclerosing haemangioma*. Capillary haemangiomas most commonly occur in skin, subcutaneous tissue and mucous membranes and may also be found in viscera (liver, spleen, kidney). Cavernous haemangiomas occur in skin of head and neck but more frequently seen in viscera (liver, spleen, pancreas).

Note : Haemangioendothelioma and haemangiosarcoma are true tumours and represent the malignant counterparts of the benign angiomatous lesions. Haemangioendothelioma is locally invasive and constitutes an intermediate grade between benign haemangioma and frank anaplastic haemangiosarcoma.

Microscopic examination

Capillary haemangioma (Fig. 26.8A)

It is common in skin.

(i) Section shows plenty of closely packed capillaries forming a lace work.

(ii) The vascular channels are lined by relatively thin endothelial cells.

(iii) Supporting tissue is formed by a few pericyte and fibroblast.

Cavernous haemangioma (Fig. 26.8B)

(i) Section shows plenty of large inter-communicating blood vessels, resembling a cavern.

(ii) Supporting tissue is formed of fibrous septa.

Frequently, both forms are present in the same lesion. Section of liver (Fig. 26.8A) is showing both forms of capillary and cavernous haemangioma.

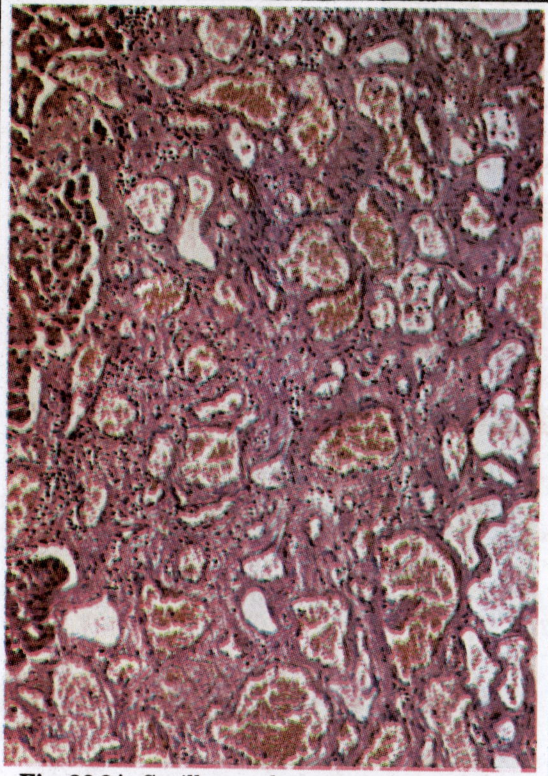

Fig. 26.8A. Capillary and cavernous haemangioma (combined type), HE × 150

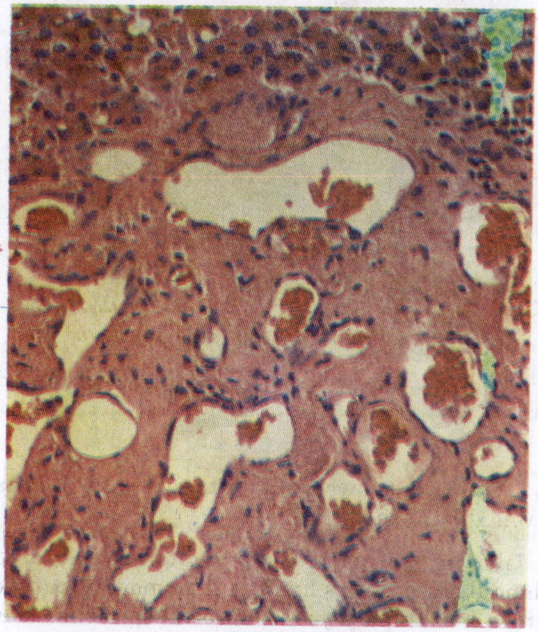

Fig. 26.8B. Cavernous haemangioma, HE × 200

Lymphangioma

It is often congenital (e.g., cystic hygroma in the neck). These are made up of small and large lymphatic channels, containing eosinophilic plasma cells with lymphocytes but there is no RBC. Some authorities consider lymphangioma as angioma.

COMMON MESENCHYMAL TUMOURS

The incidence of benign mesenchymal tumours are much commoner than their malignant counterparts. Mesenchymal tumours may arise in any organ but are most frequently observed in the soft tissue.

BENIGN

Lipomas

Lipomas are benign circumscribed masses of an adult (mature) type of fat tissue. Lipomas are subclassified based on morphological features as *conventional lipoma, fibrolipoma, angiolipoma, myolipoma* and *pleomorphic lipoma.*

Microscopy (Fig. 26.9)

(i) Section shows network of polyhedral clear cells of adipose tissue and the nuclei at the peripheral position.

(ii) Fat cells separated by irregular fibrous septa.

(iii) Blood vessels are within the fibrous septa.

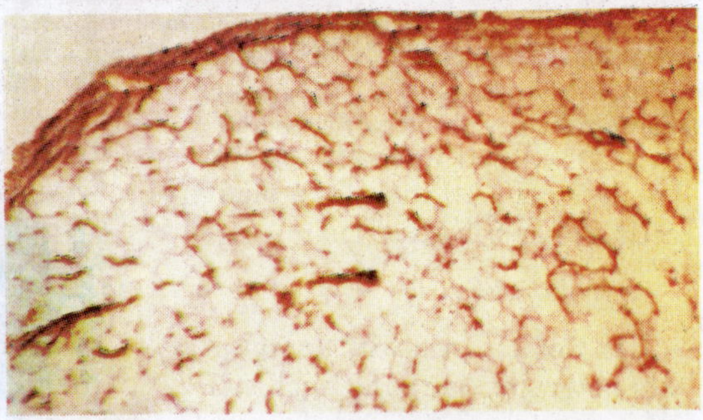

Fig. 26.9. Lipoma (conventional type), HE × 300

LEIOMYOMA UTERUS (Fig. 26.10A)

Leiomyoma is commoner in muscular visceral organs (like uterus, GIT etc.) than in the soft tissues.

Histology

(i) The tumour is composed of mature smooth muscle cells which form bundles that run in all directions producing the whorled pattern, so that some are seen in cross section and others in longitudinal section.

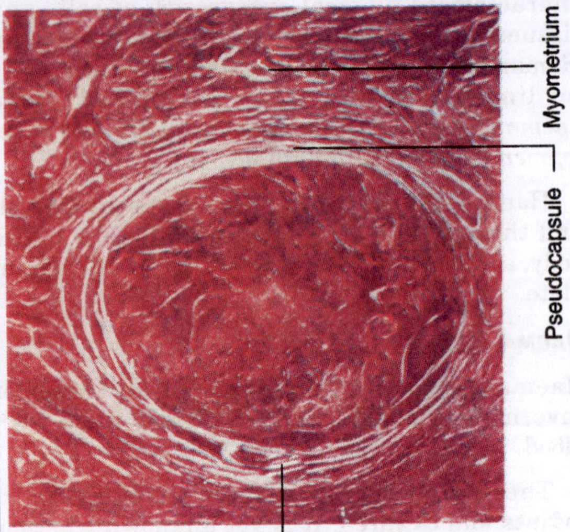

Fig. 26.10A. Leiomyoma uterus, HE × 200

(ii) There is some fibrous tissue between the muscle fibrils and this fibrous component is usually increased resulting in hard and fibrous tumour (*fibromyoma* or *'fibroid'*).

(iii) Blood vessels are within the stroma which may be partially hyalinised.

Macroscopy : Vide specimen (Fig. 33.2).

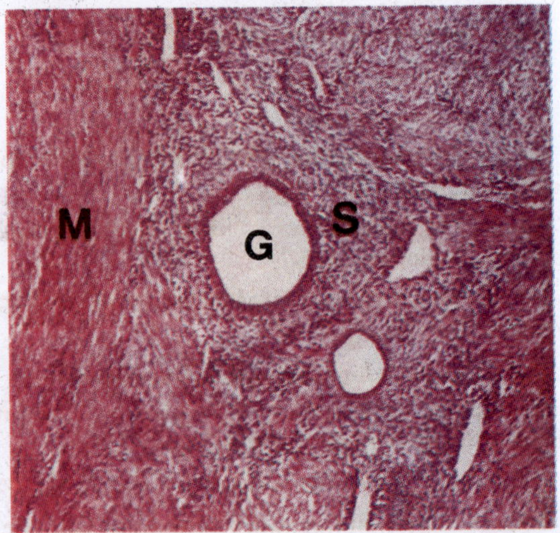

Fig. 26.10B. Adenomyosis uterus, M = muscle, G = gland, S = stroma; HE × 200

ADENOMYOSIS OF UTERUS

In this condition islands of endometrial glands and stroma are present deep within the myometrium.

Microscopical examination (Fig. 26.10B)

(i) Section shows smooth muscle cells.

(ii) Several endometrial glands with stroma are seen in the deeper part of the muscle.

TUMOURS OF SOFT TISSUE

Neurofibroma and Neurilemmoma

Neurofibroma and neurilemmoma are commonly seen in superficial soft tissues. ***Microscopy*** : They consist of elongated spindle cells containing elongated nuclei that are set in a fibrillary background. When the cells and their nuclei exhibit a wavy configuration, it is referred to as neurofibroma, whereas in neurilemmoma there is palisading arrangement of nuclei into regimented rows.

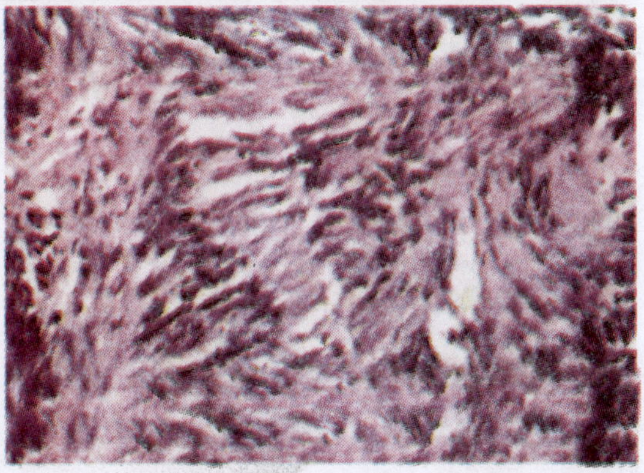

Fig. 26.11A. Neurilemmoma with nuclear palisading

MALIGNANT TUMOURS

I. Malignant mesenchymal tumours *(sarcomas)*

The malignant mesenchymal tumours (or sarcomas) are basically composed of spindle cells with anaplastic features. It is difficult to classify poorly differential sarcomas by means of cell type but in case of some well differentiated sarcomas, they can be typed as fibrosarcoma (collagen fibrils formation), leiomyosarcoma (predominance of myofibrils), liposarcoma (predominance of lipoblasts with fat vacuoles in cytoplasm), chondrosarcoma (preponderance of hyaline cartilaginous matrix), osteosarcoma (predominance of osteoid laid down by tumour cells) etc.

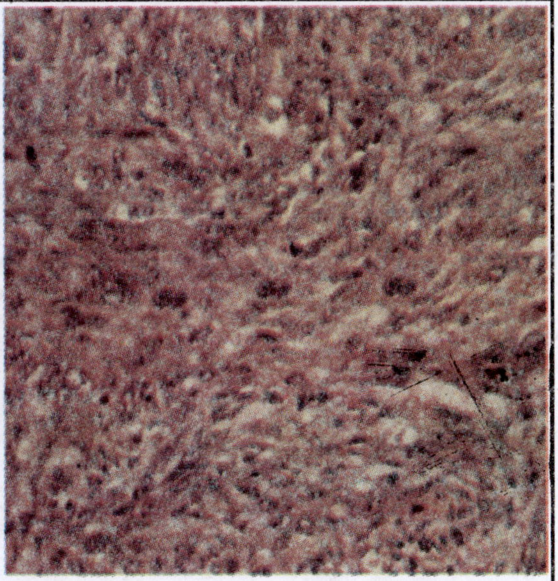

Fig. 26.11B. Sarcoma D spindle cell tumour with features of anaplasia (× 250)

Microscopy (HE section)

(a) *Well differentiated fibrosarcoma shows* :

(i) Tumour consists of spindle-shaped well-differentiated fibroblasts.

(ii) Turn over cells are arranged in fascicles that intersect each other at acute angles exhibiting a herring bone appearance.

(b) *Undifferentiated tumours*

It is difficult to recognise fibroblastic nature of tumour cells as there are plenty of mitoses and cells are anaplastic.

Special staining

(i) Reticulin stain demonstrates abnormal fibres wrapped around each cell.

(ii) Phosphotungstic acid haematoxylin stain demonstrates abundant cytoplasmic fibrils.

Note : (i) It should be kept in mind that many other soft tissue tumours, particularly liposarcoma, synovial sarcoma, malignant and fibrous histiocytoma, retroperitoneal sarcoma, and malignant schwannoma, frequently contains areas closely resembling fibrosarcoma. Only careful study of different blocks will provide correct diagnosis.

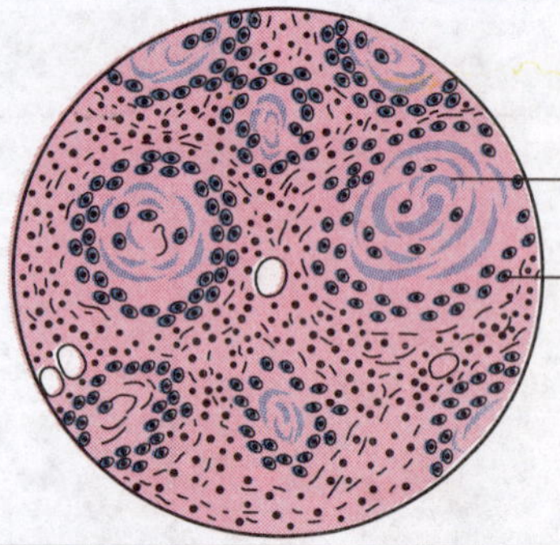

Fig. 26.12. Squamous cell carcinoma skin with a surface ulcer (diagrammatic). The tumour shows numerous keratin pearls and invasion of dermis.

(ii) Presence of giant tumour cells usually means that it is not a fibrosarcoma but more likely to be liposarcoma or malignant fibrous histiocytoma.

II. Malignant epithelial tumours

Skin

The main types of carcinoma of skin arise from basal cell (basal cell carcinoma) and spinous cell (squamous cell carcinoma).

Squamous cell carcinoma

Squamous cell carcinoma occurs not only in skin but also wherever squamous epithelium is found. Hence it may occur in skin, mouth, tongue, larynx, cervix uteri and oesophagus. It may also arise from squamous epithelium formed by metaplasia, e.g., bronchus or urinary bladder. However, squamous cell carcinoma of skin are usually very well differentiated, highly keratinising, containing numerous keratin pearls, slow growing and maintains epidermal structure (hence called epidermoid). In contrast, cervical carcinomas are poorly differentiated and spread early to draining lymph nodes.

Microscopical examination (Figs. 26.12, 26.13)

(i) Section shows the structure of skin.

(ii) Prickle cell layer has broken down the basement membrane and has invaded the dermal layer.

(iii) The cells show following features of malignancy :

(a) great variation in cell and nuclear size.

(b) hyperchromatic nuclei.

(c) large nucleus with increased mitosis.

(d) cells with loss of polarity and infiltration.

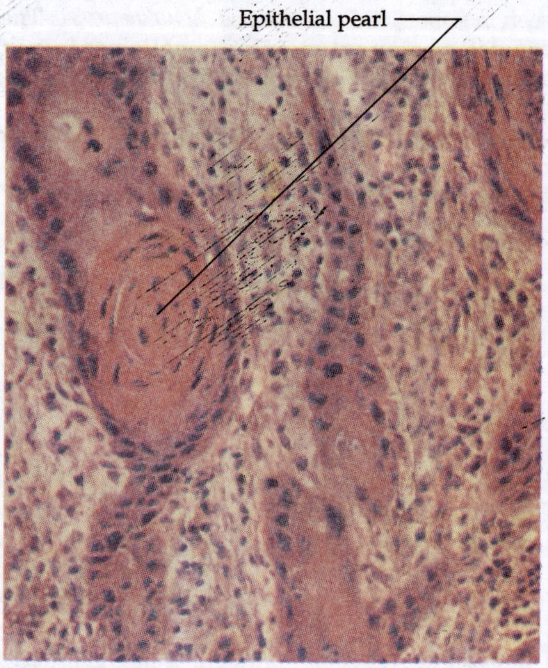

Fig. 26.13. Squamous cell carcinoma of skin, HE × 200

(iv) Formation of cell nest : Keratinised malignant cells are seen in concentric nests (epithelial pearl), the periphery of which is occupied by basal cells (Fig. 26.12).

(v) Stroma is infiltrated by lymphocytes and plasma cells.

Diagnosis : Well-differentiated squamous cell carcinoma.

Basal cell carcinoma (Figs. 26.14A & B)

Basal cell carcinoma (rodent ulcer) is the most frequent type of skin cancer. The tumour arises from the basal cells of the epidermis or epidermal appendages. It occurs most frequently on the light-

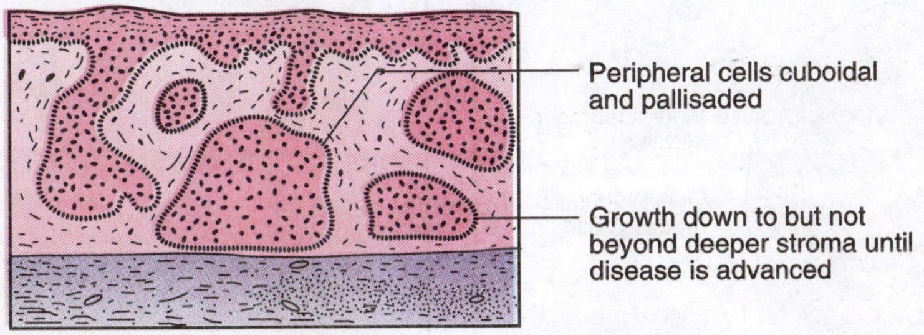

Fig. 26.14A. Basal cell carcinoma

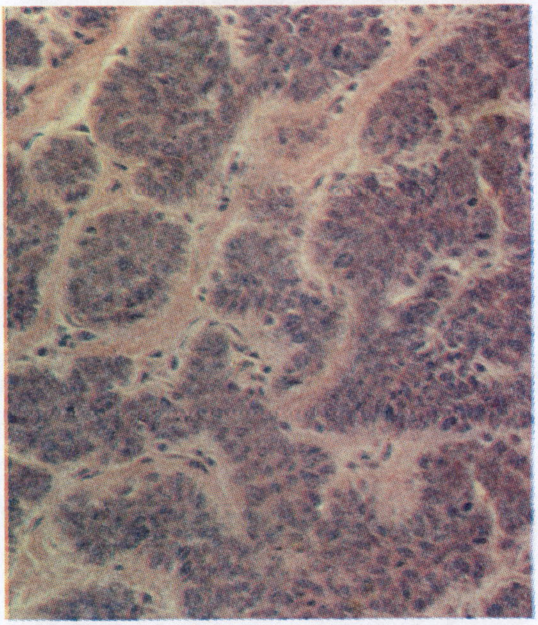

Fig. 26.14B. Basal cell carcinoma of skin, HE × 220

exposed areas of skin, particularly on upper two-thirds of face and about the nose and eyelids. It is a malignant tumour and invades the dermis and any deeper underlying structures, but almost never metastasises.

***Microscopic features* (Figs. 26.14A & B)**

(i) Section shows the structure of skin.

(ii) Proliferated basal cells have produced club-shaped masses of cells that have projected downwards into the dermis.

(iii) The outer layer of clumps of cells are formed by a single layer of columnar cells arranged in a palisading pattern.

(iv) The palisaded columnar cells at the margin stain deeply with haematoxylin, whereas the tumour cells in the centre of the mass are small, basophilic and fusiform in appearance; arranged haphazardly and show considerable mitotic activity.

Note : There is ordinarily no keratinisation or prickle cell formation here.

ADENOCARCINOMA GIT

These are malignant tumours, arising from the secreting surface epithelia as well as from the acinar lining cells of the glands. Common sites of origin include : breast, stomach, large intestine, kidneys, uterus, thyroid and pancreas.

***Microscopy* (Figs. 26.15A & B)**

(i) Section shows the structure of intestine.

(ii) Some submucosal glands show features of malignancy :

(a) hyperchromatic large nucleus with increased mitotic activity.

(b) acinar cells are multilayered with loss of polarity and with evidence of infiltration in the surrounding tissue including muscle layer.

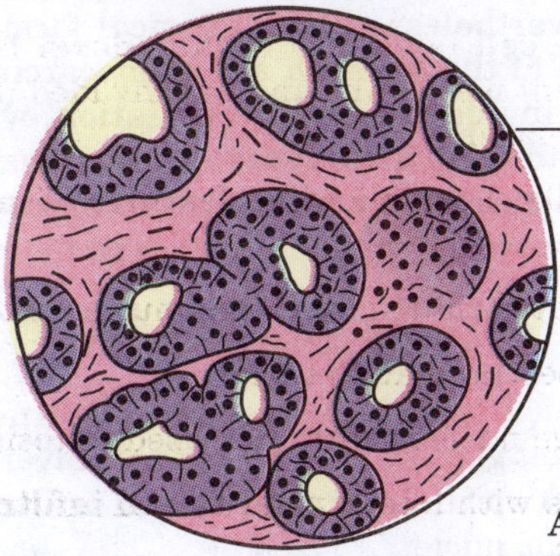

Fig. 26.15A. Adenocarcinoma

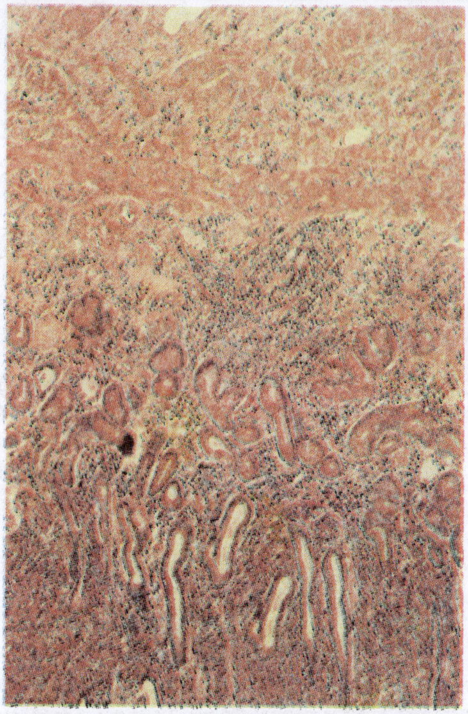

Fig. 26.15B. Adenocarcinoma of stomach, HE × 100

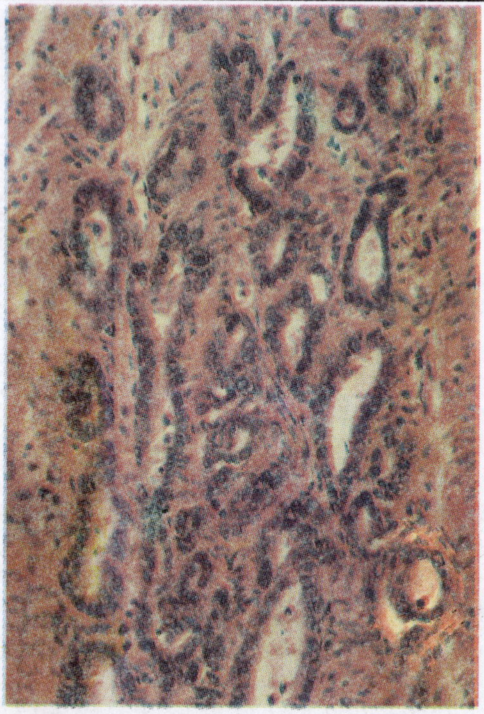

Fig. 26.16. Adenocarcinoma of stomach, HE × 165

Diagnosis

Adenocarcinoma of stomach.

Adenocarcinoma of stomach (Fig. 26.16)

Malignant tumours of stomach cause about 5% of all cancer deaths. Gastric cancer arises from mucus-secreting cells of gastric crypts. They may arise from any part of stomach, but majority develop from antrum and pylorus, more particularly along lesser curvature. Several gross forms of gastric carcinoma are recognised, *fungating polypoid tumour, ulcerative, mucinous, diffuse spreading or infiltrating (linitis plastica)* and *superficial spreading*. Nevertheless, the histological form of all carcinomas of the stomach are adenocarcinomas with varying degree of differentiation, well differentiated to anaplastic types. A metaplastic squamous cell carcinoma *(adenoacanthoma)* or squamous cell carcinoma rarely occurs in pyloric area.

Microscopic features (Fig. 26.16)

(i) The muscle layer is invaded by well formed malignant glands, lined by a single layer of cuboidal epithelium with round or ovoid basophilic nuclei.

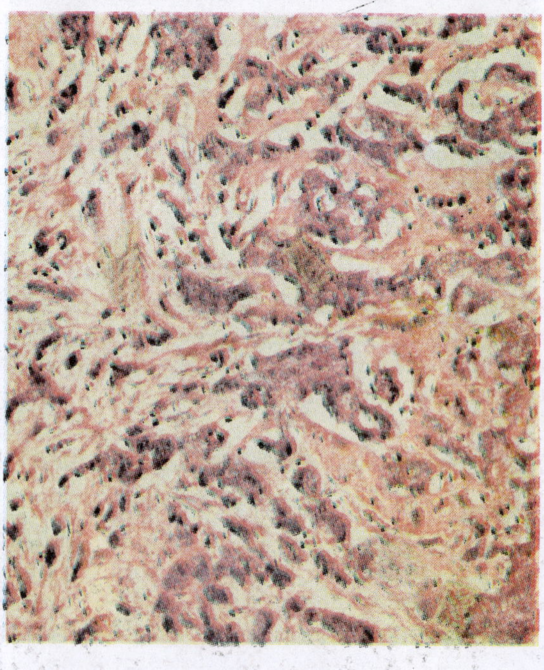

Fig. 26.17. Invasive ductal (scirrhous) carcinoma of breast, HE × 200

(ii) The tumour cells contain relatively scanty cytoplasm and there is no obvious mucin secretion.

(iii) There is considerable mitotic activity.

BREAST : Scirrhous carcinoma of breast

Microscopy (Fig. 26.17)

(i) Section shows islets and cords of cells with hyperchromatic large nucleus and increased mitotic activity.

(ii) Surrounded by abundant dense, productive fibrosis.

(iii) Few islets of malignant cells show glandular pattern.

KIDNEY : Renal cell adenocarcinoma

The most common malignant tumour of kidney is renal adenocarcinoma (formerly called hypernephroma) which arises from the renal tubular epithelium.

Microscopic features (Fig. 26.18)

(i) Section may show the structure of kidney with a zone of normal and tumourous area separated by a fibrous septa (not seen here).

(ii) Tumourous area shows clumps of polyhedral cells with pyknotic nucleus. The cells are arranged in cords or sheets or in the form of tubules.

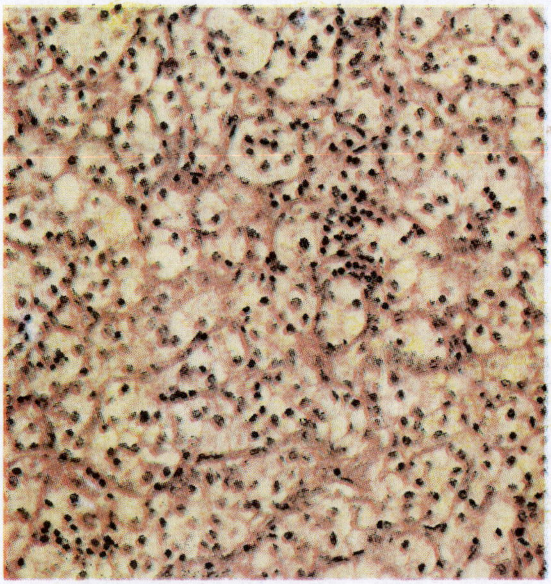

Fig. 26.18. Renal adenocarcinoma, HE × 250

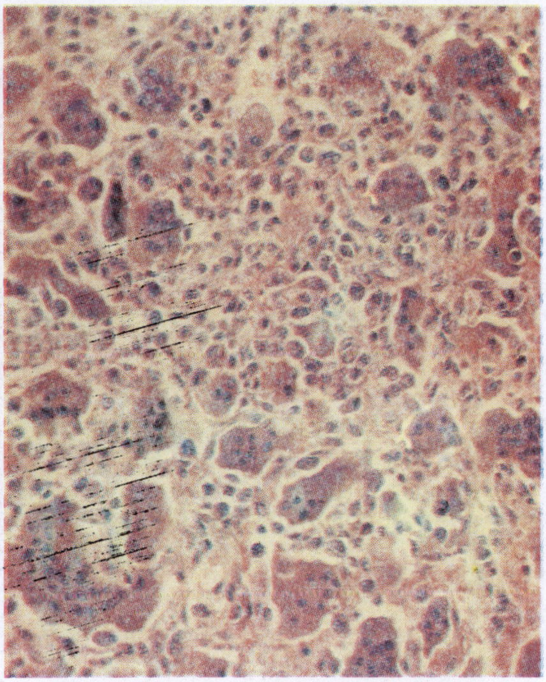

Fig. 26.19. Giant cell tumour of bone, HE × 165

(iii) The cells are vacuolated (due to cytoplasmic glycogen and lipid accumulation).

(iv) Area of haemorrhage and necrosis.

III. Giant cell tumour

BONE

Giant cell tumour of bone

Microscopy (Fig. 26.19)

(i) Section shows highly vascularised stroma consisting of spindle-shaped cells.

(ii) Plenty of osteoclastic type giant cells in the stroma.

(iii) Areas of haemorrhage and deposition of haemosiderin pigment.

(iv) Some blood vessels are surrounded by giant cells.

Diagnosis : Giant cell tumour of bone (osteoclastoma).

PIGMENTED NAEVUS AND MALIGNANT MELANOMA

Pigmented naevi are very common, virtually every person is having at least one. In normal skin, melanocytes are situated among the cells of basal

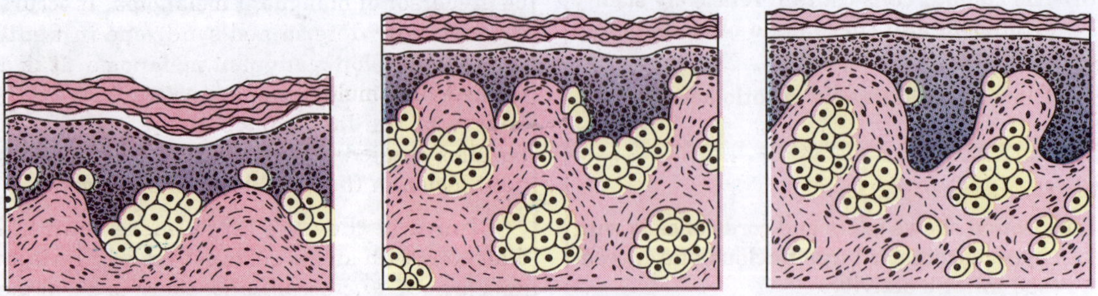

Fig. 26.20A. ME : 3 types pigmented naevus — junctional, compound and intradermal, HE × 200 (diagrammatic)

layers of epidermis in a ratio of one melanocyte per 5-10 basal cells. In early embryonic development, melanoblasts are derived from the neural crest (neuroectoderm) and migrate to the primitive epidermis where they mature into melanocytes. Melanocyte is a rounded cell with clear or pale cytoplasm and contain numerous fine branching processes (dendrites).

Melanocytes synthesise melanin which is then transferred to adjacent keratinocytes. In addition to epidermis, melanocytes are also found in skin adnexa, and some mucosal membranes. Melanocytes may give rise to benign and malignant tumours.

Benign pigmented naevus (Fig. 26.20A)

Every person has a variable number of naevi, also called moles (*L. moles,* a shapeless mass). It is a localised benign abnormality of the melanocytic system, which is usually acquired, and becomes manifest clinically after the first year of life. *Histologically,* they fall between malformation and neoplasia.

Three different patterns of common pigmented naevi are recognised according to the location of melanocytes (Fig. 26.20) :

(a) ***Junctional naevus* (Fig. 26.20A)** : It is the one in which melanocytic proliferation is restricted to basal layers of epidermis (in dermo-epidermal junction). This type of naevus has the potential, although very low, to undergo transformation to malignant melanoma. *Histologically,* cluster of clear cells (melanocytes) is present at the site. It is a brown macule often found in soles, palms and genitalia.

(b) ***Intradermal naevus* (Figs. 26.20A & B)** :

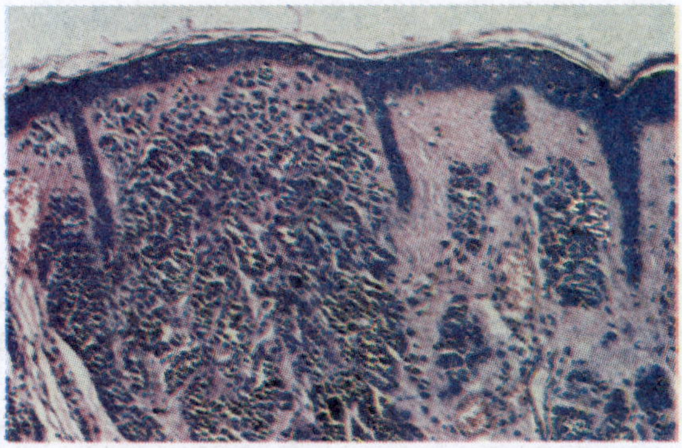

Fig. 26.20B. Intradermal naevus, HE × 200

The melanocytes form clumps in the upper dermis and are not present in epidermis. This type is more common in adults. It may be flat, or slightly elevated or warty, and is often hairy. These naevus cells are more compact and may also contain melanin pigment.

(c) ***Compound naevus* (Fig. 26.20A)** : It combines the features of the junctional and intradermal naevus, and with passage of time, junctional component becomes less prominent and less active.

Blue and cellular naevi

Blue naevus is small and located in head, neck or upper extremity. *Microscopically,* the lesion is characterised by ill-defined dermal proliferation of elongated dermal melanocytes.

Cellular blue naevus is a distinctive variety of blue naevus. Because of its size and intense pigmentation, it is often suspected as malignant.

Microscopically, blue naevus is extremely cellular. They differ from malignant melanoma by the

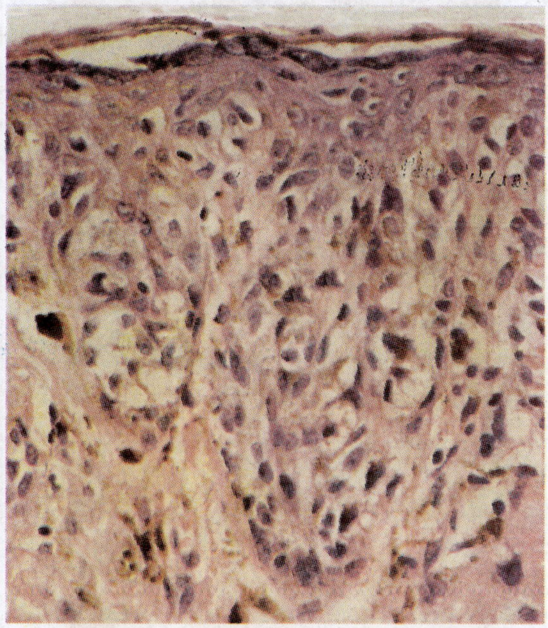

Fig. 26.21. Lentigo maligna skin. It is a premalignant lesion in basal layer of epidermis, the pilosebaceous follicle is replaced by large melanocytes, HE × 220

absence of junctional activity, epidermal invasion and other points. The behaviour of cellular naevus is usually benign but a few cases show recurrence.

Spitz naevus

Spitz naevus (spindle and epithelioid cell naevus). It is a red, pink or brown nodule in the skin of face and characteristically occurs before puberty. *Microscopically,* most of them are compound naevi with a prominent intradermal component. They are composed of spindle cells, epithelioid cells or both.

Dysplastic naevus

Dysplastic naevus (Fig. 26.21) is a recently introduced and controversial concept and is believed to be precursor of malignant melanoma. It occurs as a genetically determined syndrome in families prone to develop malignant melanoma. It is also termed B.K. mole (a name derived from the first letters of the last names of the initial of two families studied). *Lentigo maligna* is a premalignant lesion in the basal layer of epidermis.

Clinically they are large (more than 5 mm diameter) with an irregular outline and variegated appearance. *Microscopically,* there is basal melanocytic hyperplasia with some degree of atypia. Melanocytes may be spindle-shaped or epithelioid. The dermis shows lymphocytic infiltrate.

Malignant melanoma (Melanocarcinoma)

This highly malignant tumour of melanocytes are associated with sunlight exposure and occurs most commonly in the skin, and rarely in eye and other sites. Malignant melanomas occur most frequently in the head, neck area and on lower extremities. Palms and soles are well known locations of cutaneous melanoma. The tumour appears as a pigmented nodular lesion in the skin which may be ulcerated. The tumour presumably arises in the naevus cells in the region of dermoepidermal junction and invades downward into the dermis. The tumour may arise in an existing naevus (junctional or compound but not intradermal) or may arise *de novo.*

Microscopic features (Figs. 26.22A and 26.22B)

(i) Junctional activity of melanocytes has involved the whole of epidermis particularly rete ridges. The melanocytes in the nests in the epidermis exhibit hyperchromatic nuclei with nuclear and cytoplasmic pleomorphism and frequent mitosis. Majority of the cells are spindle-shaped and some are epithelioid-cell-shaped.

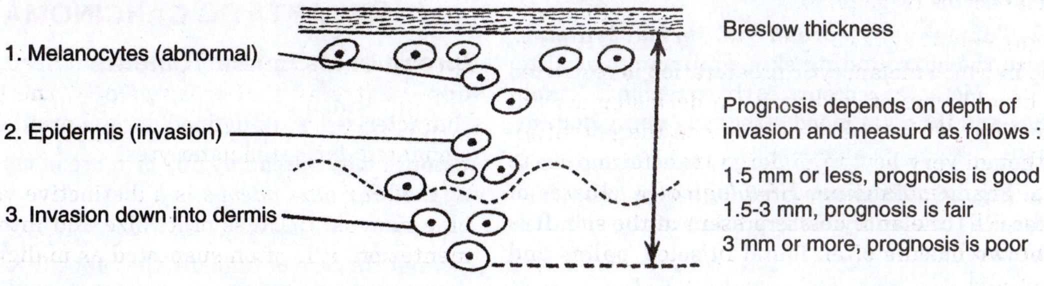

Fig. 26.22A. Assessment of prognostic value of melanoma on the basis of features of malignant melanocytes

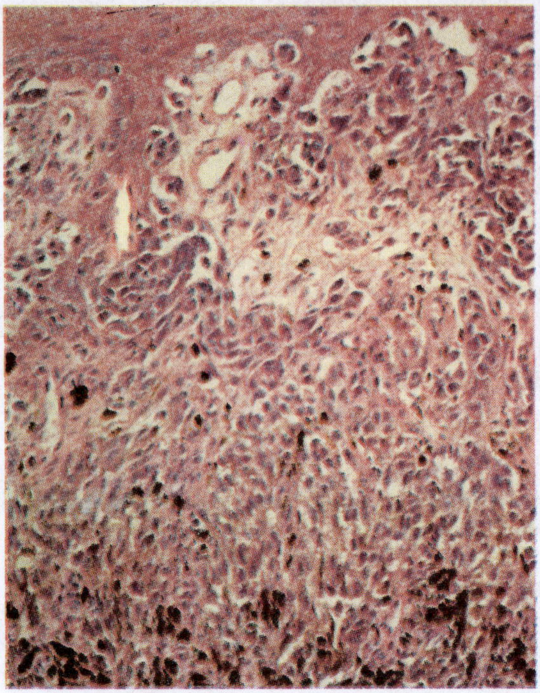

Fig. 26.22B. Malignant melanoma, HE × 100

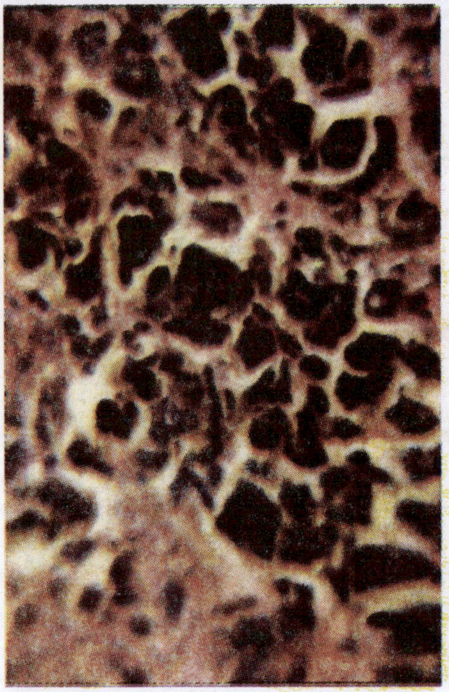

Fig. 26.23. Malignant melanoma, HE × 265

(ii) The tumour cells have invaded downward into the dermis, where there is formation of closely packed masses of cells, mostly spindle-shaped.

(iii) Many cells contain melanin pigment (sometimes amelanotic melanoma are also found).

(iv) Many macrophages laden with melanin (melanophages) are present in the deeper parts of the tumour.

(v) There is a chronic inflammatory cell infiltrate around the margins of the tumour.

Note : 1. Incipient surface ulceration of the tumour is common.

2. Tumour may spread via dermal lymphatics to the surrounding skin producing satellite lesions. Metastasis occurs early to regional lymph nodes and then via blood stream to many distant organs.

3. Fig. 26.22B shows predominance of epitheloid cells that form clusters and scanty spindle-shaped cells.

4. Prognosis of melanoma depends on invasion of dermis by malignant melanocytes (Fig. 26.22A).

5. Clinical types of malignant melanoma include : *superficial spreading melanoma* (most common form), and *nodular melanoma.*

Malignant melanoma (Figs. 26.22B and 26.33)

Microscopy

(i) Section shows clumps of spindle cells with hyperchromatic large nucleus and increased mitotic activity.

(ii) Presence of brownish pigment within the cells and also in the stroma.

(iii) Many macrophages laden with melanin are also present.

METASTATIC CARCINOMA

Spread of Malignant Tumours

Spread and metastasis are the behavioural hallmarks of malignant tumours. Malignant tumours may spread by any or more of the following modes :

(1) **Local infiltration into surrounding tissues** : In case of tumours that appear to possess a capsule, a microscopic examination often may show capsular infiltration by the malignant cells.

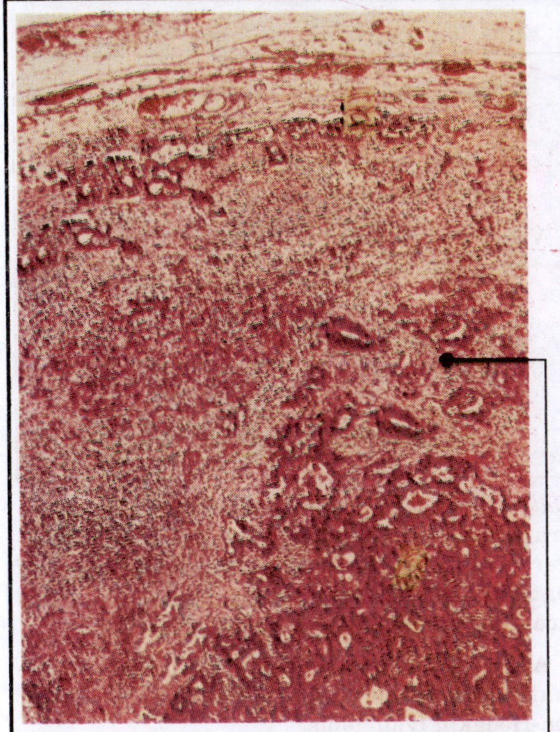

Fig. 26.24. Secondary carcinoma lymph node, HE × 100

(2) **Lymphatic spread** : This route is more often encountered in carcinomas in the form of tumour embroil within lymphatic channels. The lymphatic channels have flattened epithelial cells with thin wall devoid of muscle coat. This type of spread leads to metastasis in draining lymph nodes. Deposits first occur in subcapsular sinuses and may later replace the entire lymph node.

(3) **Hematogenous spread** : This type of spread is more often observed in sarcomas. The venous channels are the portal of entry for malignant cells to form tumour emboli. Certain organs like lungs, liver (and bones and brain) constitute the frequent sites of metastatic deposits.

(4) **Seeding of body cavities** : Disseminated spreads of malignant cells may occur in peritoneum by malignant tumours of ovary and GIT. Primary cancers of pleura may occur (by lung as well as by metastatic tumours to the lung). Malignant cells can be detected cytologically in the peritoneal fluid and pleural effusion fluid by cytological examination of cellular deposit with Papanicolau's staining.

Metastatic carcinoma lymph node

Microscopic features (Fig. 26.24)

HE section is made from a mesenteric lymph node draining adenocarcinoma of colon, and following microscopic features are observed :

(i) Section shows structure of lymph node with distorted follicular architecture. The fibrous capsule is on the right.

(ii) There are a large number of round carcinoma cells impacted in the subcapsular sinus and also have passed down to medullary sinus. Tumour cells have proliferated to a certain extent within the medullary sinus.

LYMPHOMA

Traditionally, the term *lymphoma* was applied to describe proliferation of lymphoid cells arising as discrete tissue masses, while the term lymphocytic leukaemia is used to describe lymphoid neoplasms presenting with widespread involvement of the bone marrow, usually accompanied by the presence of large number of tumour (immature) cells in the peripheral blood. However, the distinguishing line between lymphocytic leukaemia and lymphoma often blurs. Many types of lymphoma occasionally involve bone marrow and produce a leukaemic blood picture. Conversely, tumours identical to lymphocytic leukaemia arise as soft tissue masses without evidence of bone marrow disease.

Another important group of lymphoid neoplasm is *plasma cell* tumour composed of terminally differentiated B lymphocytes. Such tumours most commonly arise in bone marrow and rarely involve lymph nodes or produce leukaemic blood picture.

In view of above, the classification of lymphoid neoplasms has evoked much controversy and confusion. Traditional classification on morphology alone is not satisfactory. A working classification of lymphoid tumours was made by the experts in 1994 known as Revised European-American Classification of lymphoid Neoplasm (REAL). This classification scheme incorporated several objective criteria such as : (i) *immunophenotype,* (ii) *genetic aberrations,* (iii) *morphologic features,* (iv) *clinical features* and (v) *pathologic entities.* More recently, World Health Organisation (WHO) reviewed and updated the REAL classification. The WHO classification (2001) which includes immunochemistry and genetic data is now generally accepted.

Lymphomas are divided into broad groups : *Hodgkin's Lymphoma* (HL) or Hodgkin's disease and non-Hodgkin lymphoma (NHL). Hodgkin's lymphoma is clinically and histologically distinct from NHLs. Moreover, its unique fashion of response to therapy makes it easier for differentiating Hodgkin lymphoma from non-Hodgkin lymphoma which is clinically important.

Non-Hodgkin's Lymphoma (NHL) : Most of the lymphoid neoplasms (80-90%) are of B lymphocyte origin and the remainder are other T cell tumours (9.5%) and rarely of NK cell origin (0.5%).

Classification of lymphoma of all types are given in Table 26.1 below :

Table 26.1
WHO classification of lymphoid neoplasms

I. **Precursor B-Cell Neoplasms**
- Precursor–B-Cell lymphoblastic leukaemia/lymphoma

II. **Peripheral B-Cell Neoplasms**
- Chronic lymphocytic leukaemia/small lymphocytic lymphoma
- B-cell prolymphocytic leukemia
- Lymphoplasmacytic lymphoma
- Splenic and nodal marginal zone lymphomas
- Extranodal marginal zone lymphoma
- Mantle cell lymphoma
- Follicular lymphoma
- Marginal zone lymphoma
- Hairy cell leukaemia
- Plasmacytoma/plasma cell myeloma
- Diffuse large B-cell lymphoma
- Burkitt lymphoma

III. **Precursor T-Cell Neoplasms**
- Precursor T-cell lymphoblastic leukaemia/lymphoma

IV. **Peripheral T-Cell and NK-Cell Neoplasms**
- T-Cell prolymphocytic leukaemia
- Large granular lymphocytic leukaemia
- Mycosis fungoides/Sezary syndrome
- Peripheral T-cell lymphoma, unspecified
- Anaplastic large cell lymphoma
- Angioimmunoblastic T-cell lymphoma
- Panniculitis-like T-cell lymphoma

Table contd. to next column

Table 26.1 contd. from previous column

- Hepatosplenic γδ T-cell lymphoma
- Adult T-cell leukaemia/lymphoma
- NK/T-cell lymphoma, nasal type
- NK-cell leukaemia

V. **Hodgkin-Lymphoma**
- *Classical subtypes* :
- Nodular sclerosis
- Mixed cellularity
- Lymphocyte-rich
- Lymphocyte depletion
- Lymphocyte predominance

Hodgkin's disease : It is characterised by proliferation of large lymphoid cells in which *Reed-Sternberg* cells are present in a background of reactive inflammatory cells of various types accompanied by fibrosis to a variable extent.

After discussing the Hodgkin's lymphoma we shall discuss the more complicated types of non-Hodgkin lymphoma.

Hodgkin's Disease

Hodgkin's lymphoma (HL) previously called Hodgkin's disease (HD) differs from NHL in that :

(i) HD often occurs at extranodal site.

(ii) Classical RS cell is present in most cases.

(iii) RS cells induce accumulation of inflammatory cells.

(iv) Unusual tumours of B-cell type.

Hodgkin's disease usually first becomes clinically manifest by lymph node enlargement, but later by splenomegaly, hepatomegaly and bone-marrow involvement.

The diagnosis of Hodgkin's disease is made based on the distinctive large tumour cells. This neoplastic cell is morphologically distinctive and eponymously termed *"Reed-Sternberg"* (RS) cells (Fig. 26.25). *Classical Reed-Sternberg cell* is large, binucleate with two mirror image nuclei, and contains large pink staining nucleoli giving owl's eyes appearance. These RS cells constitute only a small proportion of cell population of lymph node in Hodgkin's disease. Multinuclear and mono-nuclear variants of RS cell are also found.

In addition to typical RS cell, there are two variants of RS cell : (i) the lacunar cell and (ii) the mononuclear Hodgkin's cell (Fig. 26.25). RS cells are derived from germinal centre or post-germinal centre B-cells indicating that most HDs are unusual tumours of B-cell origin.

Variants RS cell

(i) *Lacunar cell* : There is shrinkage of cell cytoplasm towards cell walll and nucleus leaving a clear zone.

(ii) *Mononuclear Hodgkin's cell* : Nucleus is similar to that of typical RS cell but smaller. These cells are not diagnostic of Hodgkin's lymphoma.

Classification:

Classification based on morphology, immunophenotype and clinical features is given in Table 26.2.

There are five histological sub-forms which correlate with prognosis and response to therapy :

(i) *Lymphocyte-predominant*—slowly progressive.

(ii) *Lymphocyte*—rich.

(iii) *Mixed cellularity*—intermediate progression.

(iv) *Lymphocyte-depleted*—aggressive disease.

(v) *Nodular sclerosis*—slowly progressive.

These five forms of Hodgkin's disease fall under two main groups as follows :

A. Classical Hodgkin's disease (HD):

The classical HD is caused by CD30 B-cells. These are probably caused by EBV. There are three main forms :

1. *Nodular sclerosis* — 70%
2. *Mixed cellularity* — 20%
3. *Lymphocyte depleted* — < 2%
4. *Lymphocyte rich* — < 0.5%

B. Nodular lymphocyte predominant HD (6%):

This form of HD affects young males and prognosis is good. The 'popcorn cells' express B-cell markers and not CD 30 of classical HD. About 3-5% cases of this form transform to diffuse large B-cell lymphoma. EBV is not associated with this form of HD.

Typing is based on the number of RS cells relative to reactive cells in the node. Nodular sclerosis exhibits fibroblastic response with production of collagen.

Prognosis and treatment of Hodgkin's disease depend on histological type and the extent of lymphoreticular involvement.

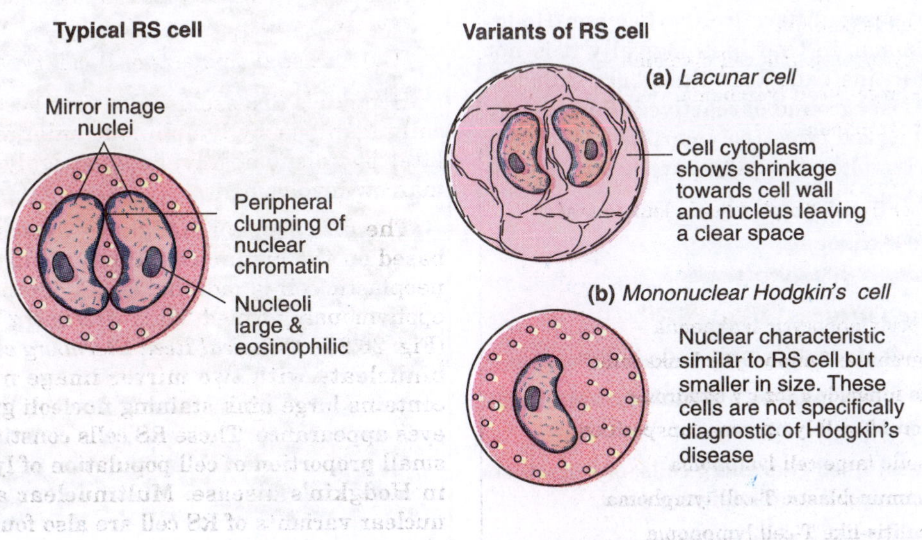

Fig. 26.25. Diagrammatic representation of RS cell

Table 26.2

Classification of Hodgkin's lymphoma

Subtype	Morphology and Immunophenotype	Typical Clinical Features
Nodular sclerosis	There are many lacunar cells and occasional diagnostic RS cells; background infiltrate consists of *T lymphocytes*, eosinophils, macrophages and plasma cells. There are fibrous bands dividing cellular areas into nodules. RS cells include CD15+, CD30+; EBV–.	Stage 1 or 2 disease most common. Mediastinal involvement is frequent. F = M, most patients young adults.
Mixed cellularity	There are good number of mononuclear and diagnostic RS cells. The background infiltrate is rich in T lymphocytes, eosinophils, macrophages, plasma cells. RS cells include CD15+, CD30+; 70% EBV+.	About 50% present as stage 3 or 4, M > F. Biphasic incidence, peaking in young adults and again in adults, older than 55.
Lymphocyte-rich	There are frequent mononuclear and diagnostic RS cells; background infiltrate is rich in T lymphocytes. RS cells CD15+, CD30+; 40% EBV+.	Uncommon. M > F. More common in older adults.
Lymphocyte depletion	Reticular variant : There are frequent diagnostic RS cells and variants with a paucity of background reactive cells; diffuse fibrosis variant; background is hypocellular fibrillar with scattered diagnostic RS cells and variants and few reactive cells. RS cells CD15+, CD30+; most EBV+.	This type is uncommon. More common in older males, HIV-infected individuals, and in developing countries. It often presents with advanced disease.
Lymphocyte predominance	There are many popcorn cell variants in a background of follicular dendritic cells and reactive B-cells. RS cells CD20+, CD15–, C30–; EBV–.	It is uncommon. Young males with cervical or axillary lymphadenopathy. Mediastinal.

Microscopic characteristics

Hodgkin's disease differs from other non-Hodgkin's lymphomas in that histologically it is not monomorphic, instead, Reed-Sternberg cells are present in a background of reactive inflammatory cells of various cell types (polymorphic), including histiocytes, lymphocytes, plasma cells and eosinophil leucocytes.

1. Hodgkin's disease (Lymphocyte-predominant)

Microscopic features (Fig. 26.26)

(i) Architecture of lymph node is lost.

(ii) There are masses of small lymphocytes (B-cells).

(iii) Several Reed-Sternberg cells, one of which containing four nuclei, are seen.

(iv) A few plasma cells are present.

This type has a favourable prognosis.

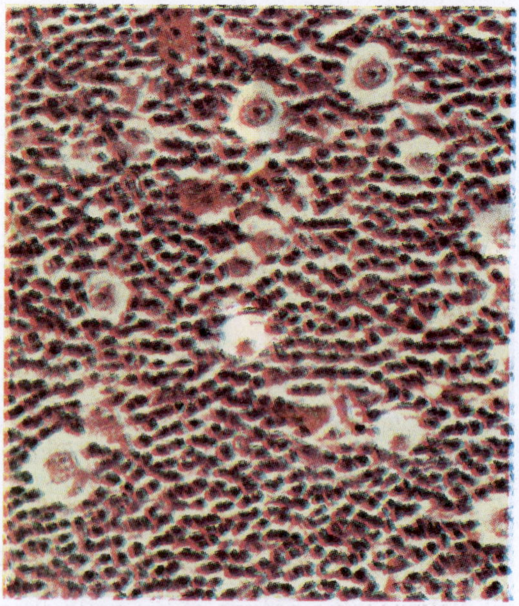

Fig. 26.26. Hodgkin's disease (lymphocyte-predominant pattern), HE × 100

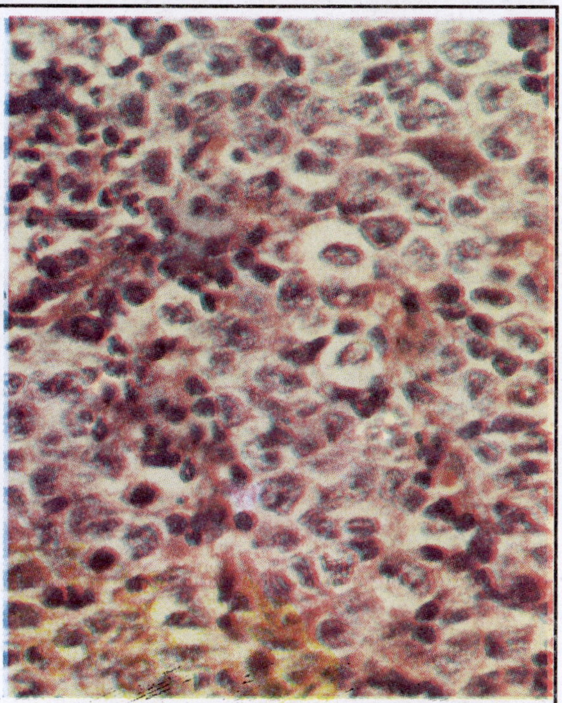

Fig. 26.27. Hodgkin's disease lymph node (mixed cellularity pattern), HE × 100

2. Hodgkin's disease (Lymphocyte-rich type)

This is an uncommon form of HD. The reactive lymphocytes make up the vast majority of the cellular infiltrate. Lymph nodes are diffusely effaced in most cases but sometimes residual B-cell follicles can be seen. This form is differentiated from lymphocyte predominance type HD by the presence of frequent mononuclear and diagnostic RS cells with the characteristic CD45–, CD20–, CD15+, CD30+. It is associated with EBV in approximately 40% cases.

3. Hodgkin's disease (Mixed cellularity pattern)

Next to lymphocyte-predominant pattern is the mixed cellularity type which has also got favourable prognosis.

Microscopic features (Fig. 26.27)

(i) Follicular structure of lymph node is lost.

(ii) Polymorphic nature of the cells show numerical even distribution of lymphocytes, histiocytic-like cells, occasional eosinophils, neutrophils and fibroblasts.

(iii) There are several Reed-Sternberg (RS) cells, lacunar cells (L) and one giant cell.

4. Hodgkin's disease (Lymphocyte-depleted type)

Morphologically this has got two subtypes : *"diffuse fibrosis"* and *"reticular"*. In diffuse fibrosis subtype, a number of lymphocytes and other cells progressively decrease due to deposition of collagen fibres. Reticular type is characterised by a large number of RS cells. The lymphocyte-depleted type has got worst prognosis.

Microscopic features (Fig. 26.28)

HE section shows :

(i) Lymphoid architecture is lost.

(ii) Reed-Sternberg (RS) cells are much more numerous.

(iii) Histiocytes (H), neutrophils (N) and fibroblasts (F) are found (Fig. 26.28).

(iv) Lymphocytes (L) and eosinophils are scanty but still seen.

(v) Areas of necrosis are more common in this type than other types.

5. Hodgkin's disease (Nodular sclerosis)

This pattern of Hodgkin's disease is associated with good prognosis when diagnosed at early stage.

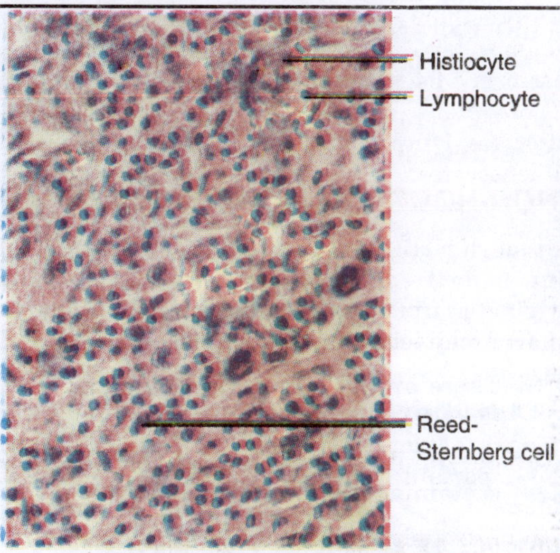

Fig. 26.28. Hodgkin's disease lymph node (lymphocyte-depleted pattern), HE × 100

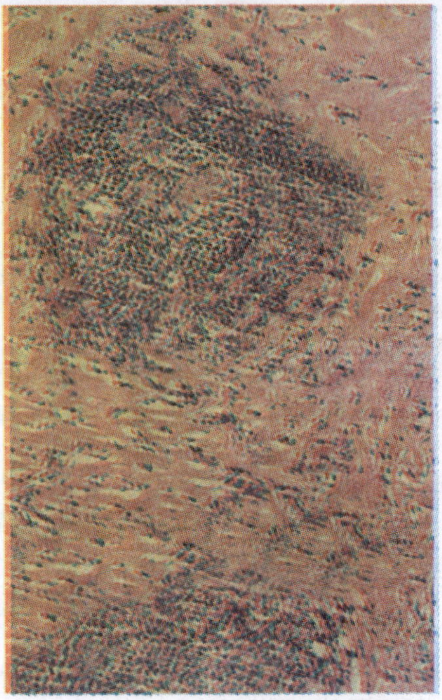

Fig. 26.29. Hodgkin's disease lymph node (nodular sclerosis), HE × 50

Microscopic features (Fig. 26.29)

(i) Lymphoid architecture is lost.

(ii) Broad well defined bands of collagen have separated the cellular Hodgkin's tumour mass into islands, imparting a nodular appearance to the cut surface of the node.

(iii) Cell type within nodule may be lymphocyte-predominance, lymphocyte-depletion or mixed type. Here in this picture, there are a large number of lymphocytes with RS cell.

NON-HODGKIN'S LYMPHOMA (NHL)

Although NHL may be derived from T- or B-cells, but majority are B-cell in type. Tumor rarely originates from true histiocytic cells. T-cell lymphoma may arise in skin, called mycosis fungoides.

Classification : The classification of non-Hodgkin's lymphoma is given in Table 26.1. Only the important types are enumerated in the next column.

SUBTYPES OF LYMPHOMA : See Fig. 26.30

Note : Only the most common types of NHL are briefly described below.

NON-HODGKIN'S LYMPHOMA

B-cell (90%)	T-cell (10%)
1. Small lymphocytic lymphoma (equivalent to B-cell)	1. T-cell prolymphocytic leukaemia
2. Lymphoplasmacytic lymphoma	2. Peripheral T-cell lymphoma
3. Mantle cell lymphoma	3. Adult T-cell leukaemia
4. Follicular lymphoma	4. Angioimmunoblastic T-cell lymphoma
5. Burkitt's lymphoma	5. Anaplastic large cell lymphoma (some do not express T-cell markers)
6. Diffuse large B-cell lymphoma	6. Enteropathy–type T-cell lymphoma
7. Extranodal marginal zone B-cell lymphoma	7. Mycosis fungoides (skin)
8. Myeloma/Plasma-cytoma	

Following general principles are applied to classification of NHL.

Cell morphology

Small cell : Size is that of a mature lymphocyte.

Large cell : 5-6 times larger than small cell.

Growth pattern

Follicular : Cells form aggregates that resemble lymphoid follicle but without germinal centres (Fig. 26.32).

Diffuse : Diffuse distribution of cells with no evidence of follicular aggregation (Fig. 26.33).

Lymphocyte maturation

Small mature B-lymphocytes undergo transformation to plasma cells.

In non-Hodgkin's lymphoma, there are several relatively common groups which have distinct clinical and pathological features as follows. Table 26.3 shows cell of origin, genotype and salient clinical features of lymphoma.

1. Small cell lymphomas (Fig. 26.31)

These behave as indolent low-grade lymphoma. Bone marrow involvement with associated leukaemia is common. They occur predominantly in

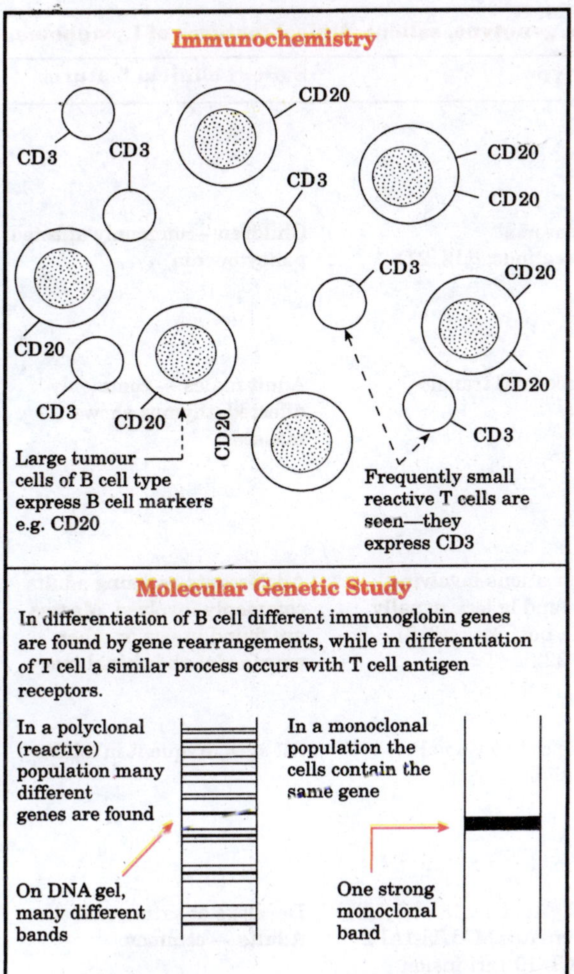

Fig. 26.30. Subtypes of lymphoma

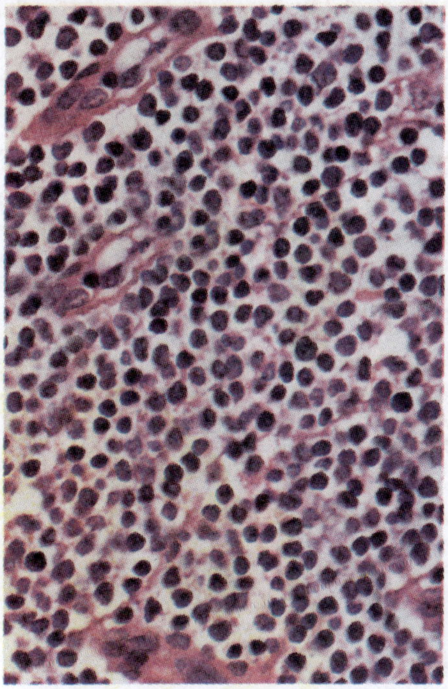

Fig. 26.31. Non-Hodgkin's lymphoma (small cell type), HE × 200

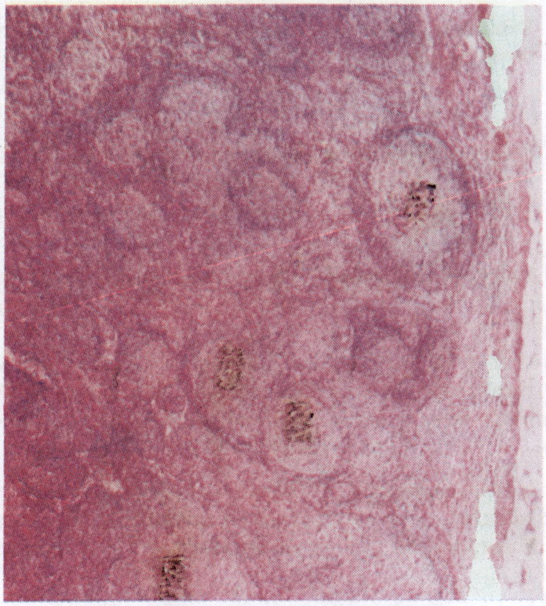

Fig. 26.32. NHL : Follicular lymphoma with small cell predominance, HE × 50

elderly patients with widespread disease. In this type, also called *Peripheral B-cell Neoplasm*, architecture of lymph node is diffusely effaced predominantly by small lymphocytes (6–12 µm) containing round to irregular nuclei.

These cases are diagnosed as small lymphocytic lymphoma/chronic lymphocytic leukaemia. The cells of origin are either naive B-cell or post-germinal centre memory B-cell which expresses CD 5. *Genotypically,* there is *Trisomy* 12, deletions of 11q, 13q and 17p.

2. Follicular lymphoma with small cell predominance (Fig. 26.32)

The disease runs a long indolent course and complete remission is difficult. This tumour occurs in older individuals associated with generalised lymphadenopathy.

Table 26.3 : Table showing summary of cell of origin, genotype, salient clinical features of Lymphoma

Diagnosis	Cell of Origin	Genotype	Salient clinical features
NON-HODGKIN'S LYMPHOMA : *Tumour of Immature B and T cells*			
Precursor B-cell : Acute lymphatic leukemia/lymphoma	Bone marrow precursor B-cell expressing TdT	Chromosomal translocations; t(12, 21)	Children—commonly affected, pancytopenia
Precursor T-cell : Acute lymphatic leukaemia/ lymphoma	Precursor T-cell (thymic origin) with TdT	Chromosomal translocations	Adult males — commonly affected, thymus shows masses
Tumour of mature B-cells			
Burkitt lymphoma	Germinal centre B-cell; with CD 10 expression	Translocations involving c-myc and lg loci; usually t(8; 14), but also t(2; 8) or t(8; 22).	Adolescents or young adults – commonly involved. Masses are found in jaw or other extranodal abdominal mass
Diffuse large B-cell lymphoma	Germinal centre or postgerminal centre B-cell	Diverse chromosomal aberrations	All ages, frequent in adults
Extranodal marginal zone lymphoma	Postgerminal centre memory B-cell	Trisomy 18, t(11;18), t(1;14); latter creates MALTI-IAP2 and BCL 10-IgH fusion genes, respectively	Develops at extranodal sites. Adults — common
Follicular lymphoma	Germinal centre B-cell expresses CD10, BCL2, and BCL6	t(14; 18) involving the *BCL2* gene.	Adults with lymphadenopathy
Hairy cell leukaemia	Postgerminal centre memory B-cell	Nothing particular	Older males with pancytopenia and splenomegaly; indolent
Mantle cell lymphoma	Naive B-cell; expressing cyclin D1 and (usually CD5)	t(11; 14) involving *BCL 1* (cyclin D1) and IgH	Elderly males suffering from disseminated disease
Multiple myeloma/ solitary plasmacytoma	Plasma cell derived from a postgerminal centre B-cell	Involves *IgH* rearrangements	Myeloma

Table 26.3 contd. to next page

Table 26.3 continued from previous page

Diagnosis	Cell of Origin	Genotype	Salient clinical features
Small lymphocytic lymphoma/chronic lymphocytic leukaemia	Naive B-cell or postgerminal centre memory B-cell; expresses CD5	There is trisomy 12, deletions of 11q, 13q, and 17p	Adults — commonly affected lymph nodes and bone marrow are involved
Tumour of mature T-cells or NK-cells			
Adult T-cell leukaemia/ lymphoma	Involving helper T-cell with CD25 (IL-2 receptor)	Tumour cells contain HTLV-1 provirus present	Adults — skin lesions + marrow lesion
Anaplastic large cell lymphoma	T-cell (cytotoxic)	*ALK* shows rearrangements	Young adults + children — affected often lymph nodes enlarged
Extranodal NK/T-cell lymphoma	Commonly from natural killer cell or cytotoxic T-cell (rare)	Nothing particular	Adults — commonly affected most common sinusoidal masses
Mycosis fungoides/ Sezary syndrome	Arises from helper T-cell	Nothing particular	Adults — commonly affected — shows cutaneous patches/ modules
T-cell granular lymphocytic leukaemia	Two types : (1) CD8+.T-cell, (2) NK-cell	Nothing particular	Adult — commonly involved. Splenomegaly
Hodgkin's lymphoma			
Hodgkin's lymphoma, lymphocyte-depletion subtype	Germinal centre or postgerminal centre B-cell	Nothing particular, about 70% EBV associated	Elderly people — common, also in HIV + patients
Hodgkin's lymphoma, lymphocyte-predominance subtype	Germinal centre B-cell	Nothing particular. It is not associated with EBV	15 to 40 years old — common lymphadenopathy +indolent
Hodgkin's lymphoma, lymphocyte-rich subtype	Germinal centre or postgerminal centre B-cell	Nothing particular, about 40% EBV associated	Males, lymphadenopathy + moderately aggressive
Hodgkin's lymphoma, mixed cellularity subtype	Postgerminal centre memory B-cell	Nothing particular, about 70% EBV associated	Males with lymphadenopathy + moderately aggressive
Hodgkin's lymphoma, nodular sclerosing subtype	Germinal centre or postgerminal centre B-cell	Nothing particular, but rarely EBV associated	Young females — common, mediastinal mass may be present

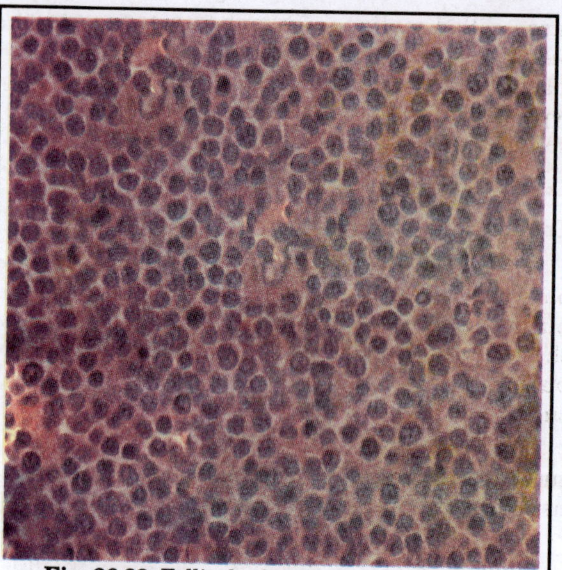

Fig. 26.33. Follicular lymphoma of lymph node *(diffuse)* (small cleaved cell pattern), HE × 200

Morphology : Lymph node under low power shows either nodular or nodular and diffuse growth pattern (Fig. 26.32). Two principal types of cells are found : (i) small cells with irregular or cleaved nuclear contours (known as small cleaved cells) and (ii) larger cells with open nuclear chromatin, several nucleoli and modest amount of cytoplasm, known as centroblasts. In most cases, small cleaved cells make up the majority of the cells (Fig. 26.33).

Cell of origin : Germinal centre B-cell, expresses CD 10, BCL 2 and BCL 6.

Genotype : t(14,18) involving the BCL 2 gene.

3. Large cell lymphomas (Fig. 26.34)

There is high cell proliferation rate in this type of NHL and it requires aggressive chemotherapy for regression. They occur particularly in adults.

4. Lymphoblastic lymphomas

They have high cell proliferation rate associated with large masses of tumour cells. This type requires aggressive chemotherapy to achieve remission. They present in childhood.

5. Burkitt's lymphoma (Fig. 26.35)

It is composed of cells intermediate in size between small lymphoid cells and immunoblasts. Burkitt's lymphoma predominantly affects children, and is often associated with extranodal tumour especially in the jaw and abdomen.

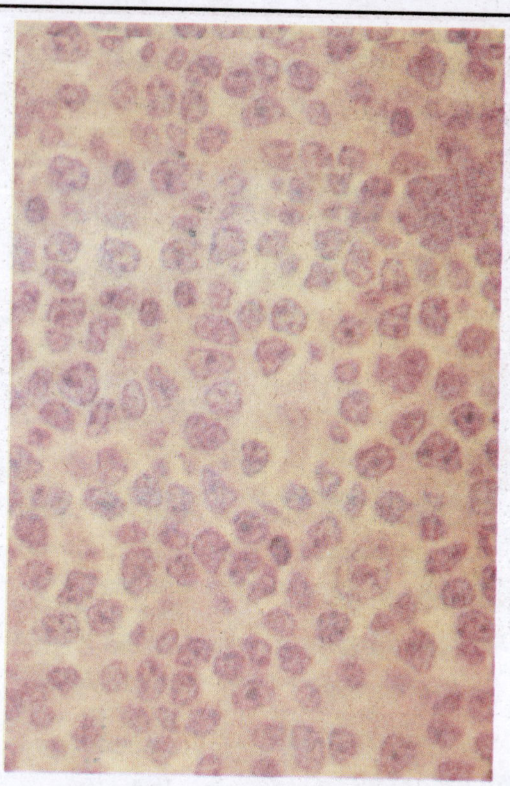

Fig. 26.34. NHL : Large cell lymphoma, HE × 200

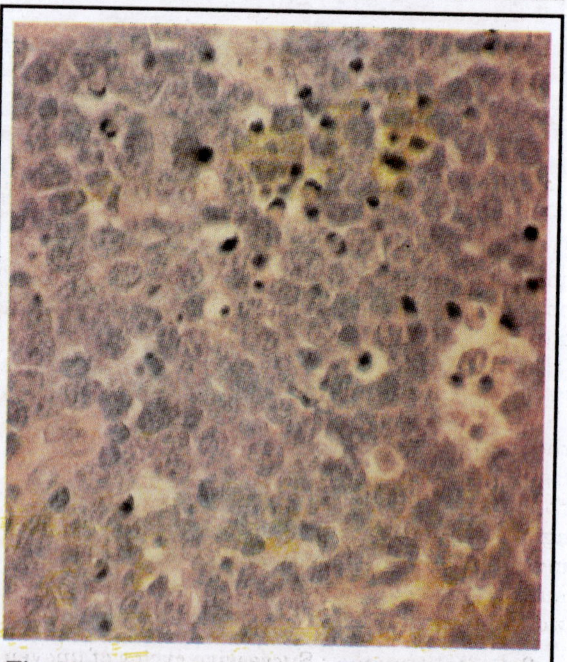

Fig. 26.35. Burkitt's lymphoma (lymphoblastic), Jaw (× 600)

Fig. 26.36. NHL : Diffuse pattern, HE × 65

Immunoblastic sarcoma

The term immunoblastic sarcoma is applied to a large celled malignant lymphoma composed of cells having the morphologic features of immunoblast (transformed lymphocytes). These are of two types, B-cell immunoblastic sarcoma and T-cell immunoblastic sarcoma.

Clinical diagnosis of NHL

This is made by :

(i) Identification of cytological features of neoplastic cells (size, shape, content and position of nuclei; amount and distribution of cytoplasm). On the basis of cytological findings, the type of lymphoma is determined. Then the pattern as follicular or diffuse (Fig. 26.36) is defined.

(ii) Then the cell of origin (B- or T-Cell) of the tumour is determined by immunological methods using antibodies, that stain specific cell markers.

The follicular and diffused patterns of lymphoma are further subdivided into small (Fig. 26.31) and large cell (Fig. 26.34) variants.

In the *small cell variant* the neoplastic cells are small lymphocyte type cells with round basophilic nuclei with a thin rim of cytoplasm. In *large cell variant,* the neoplastic cells exhibit less uniformity of nuclear shapes, size and staining intensity and the nuclei of majority of cells are large with an open chromatin pattern and large nucleoli.

SYSTEMIC DISEASES

THYROID

Nontoxic goitre

This is a simple enlargement of the thyroid gland not associated with increased secretion of thyroid hormone (T_3, T_4). The cause is lack of iodine in diet.

Classification

1. **Diffuse (simple) goitre** : In simple goitre, the thyroid gland is usually diffusely and more or less symmetrically enlarged due to an absolute or relative deficiency of iodine or to goitrogenic agents. In most instances, normal thyroid hormone is achieved. The condition may occur endemically *(endemic goitre)* and also sporadically in women *(sporadic goitre)*.

2. **Colloid goitre** : Successive cycles of uneven hyperplasia and involution occur in late stage of most diffuse hyperplasia, which gives rise to nodularity. Thyroid is enlarged and translucent due to large amount of stored colloid, which results from continuing iodine deficiency.

Colloid goitre may be *diffuse* or *nodular* (due to disproportionate hyperplasia, involution or fibrosis).

Histology (Fig. 26.37)

(i) Section shows the picture of thyroid tissue.

(ii) Gland acini are dilated and filled with deeply staining colloid material.

(iii) Lining epithelium of acini is flattened cubical.

Diagnosis : Colloid goitre.

HYPERPLASIA OF THYROID

Thyroid function is under the control of TSH that stimulates thyroid acinar cells to produce thyroxine. Circulating thyroxine then regulates TSH

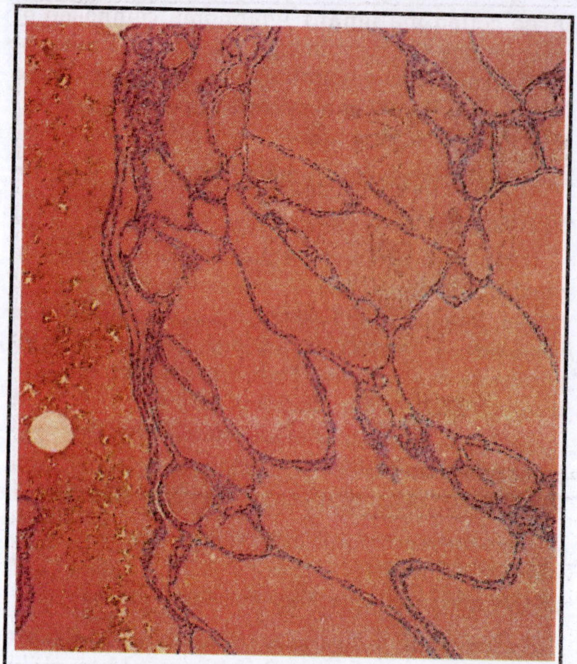

Fig. 26.37. Colloid goitre, HE × 100

production by a negative feedback mechanism. Under certain circumstances, when this balance is disrupted, there is excess production of TSH leading to hyperplasia and hypertrophy of acinar cells producing histological picture of thyroid hyperplasia.

Graves' disease

It is a common cause of pathological thyroid hyperplasia. It is an auto immune disease in which a circulating long acting thyroid stimulator (LATS) is produced that binds with thyroid acinar cells, mimicking the effects of TSH which results in excess secretion of thyroxine.

Histology (Fig. 26.38)

(i) Acinar cells are tall with large nuclei (evidence of greater metabolic activity).

(ii) Most of the acini are smaller than normal (because of increased amount of thyroxine, there is less colloid in acini).

(iii) There is a lymphocytic aggregate (lymphoid follicle) — right side.

KIDNEY

GLOMERULONEPHRITIS (Fig. 26.39)

Primary lesions of the glomerulus are most often referred to by the loose term glomerulonephritis. The old classification still persists : acute glomerulonephritis showing primary active proliferative and destructive lesions of the glomerulus and the term chronic glomerulonephritis which is best called end-stage kidney.

Basic changes in glomerulonephritis

The glomerulus shows following type of reaction in response to damaging stimuli.

(i) Swelling or proliferation of the normally flat endothelial cells lining the glomerular capillaries.

(ii) Proliferation of the epithelial cells investing the outer surface of the glomerular capillary tuft. Normally these epithelial cells remain attached to the basement membrane by foot processes separated by gaps of 30-60 nm diameter.

(iii) Thickening of basement membrane of glomerulus.

(iv) Proliferation of cells of mesangium and production of excessive mesangial material.

Nomenclature of patterns of primary glomerular lesions : Glomerular involvement is

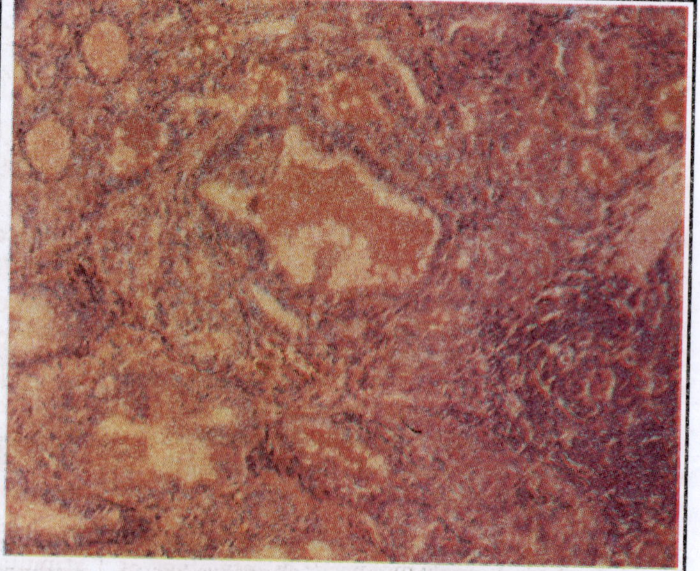

Fig. 26.38. Graves' disease, HE × 200

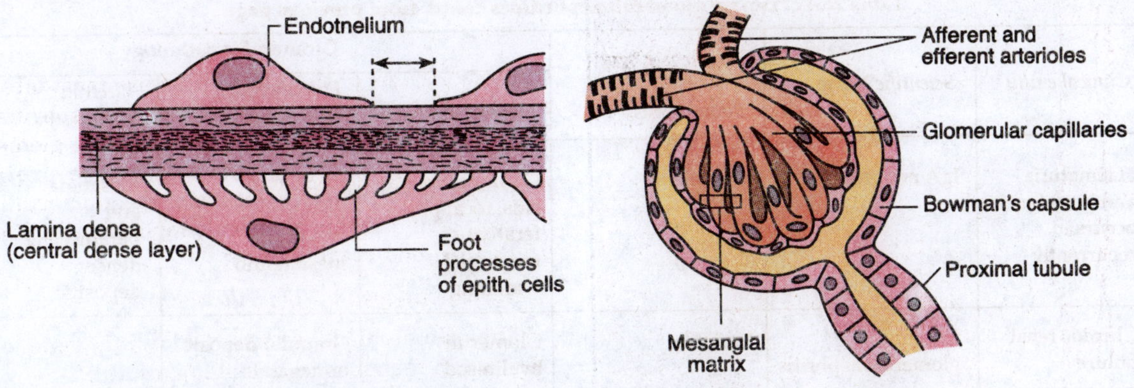

Fig. 26.39. Structure of glomerulus

Table 26.4 : Primary glomerulonephritides

Clinical entity	*Scientific Name*	*Pathogenesis*	Glomerular pathology		
			Light Microscopy	*Fluorescence Microscopy*	*Electron Microscopy*
Acute nephritis	Poststreptococcal glomerulonephritis	Antibody mediated; circulating/planted antigen	Glomeruli show diffuse proliferation; leukocytic infiltration	Immunoglobulin granular IgG and C3 in GBM and mesangium	Subepithelial humps
Rapidly progressive glomerulonephritis	Goodpasture syndrome	Ig anti-GBM, COL4-A3 antigen	Proliferation of glomerulus cells, crescents	Linear IgG and C3	No deposits; GBM disruption; fibrin
Rapidly progressive glomerulonephritis	Idiopathic RPGN	Formation of anti-GBM antibody immune complex ANCA-associated	Glomerular epithelium shows proliferation; focal necrosis; crescents	Granular IgG and C3	There is no deposit
Nephrotic syndrome	Membranous glomerulopathy	Antigen not known	Capillary wall shows thickening	Granular IgG and C3; diffuse	Usually subepithelial deposits
Nephrotic syndrome	Minimal change disease	Podocyte injury	Normal; lipid in tubules	Negative	Loss of foot processes; no deposits
Nephrotic syndrome	Focal segmental glomerulosclerosis	Unknown	Sclerosis and hyalinosis with focal and segmental	Focal; IgM C3	Foot processes are lost
Nephrotic syndrome	Membrano-proliferative glomerulonephritis (MPGN) Type I	(i) Immune complex	(i) Proliferation of mesangium	(i) IgG + C3; Clq + C4	(i) Subendothelial deposits
Hematuria Chronic renal failure	Dense deposit disease (MPGN) Type II	(ii) Autoantibody; alternative complement pathway	(ii) Basement membrane thickened	(ii) C3 ± IgG	(ii) Dense deposits

Table continued to next page

Table 26.4 : Primary glomerulonephritides contd. from previous page					
			Glomerular pathology		
Clinical entity	*Scientific Name*	*Pathogenesis*	*Light Microscopy*	*Fluorescence Microscopy*	*Electron Microscopy*
Haematuria and proteinuria occurs recurrently	IgA nephropathy	Unknown	Glomerulonephritis, focal proliferative — mesangial widening	Deposit of IgA +/- IgM, IgM, and C3 in mesangium	Mesangial and paramesangial dense deposits
Chronic renal failure	Chronic glomerulonephritis	Variable	Glomeruli hyalinised	Granular deposit or negative	

ANCA = antineutrophil cytoplasmic antibody, GBM = glomerular basement membrane, RPGN = rapidly progressive-glomerulonephrilis.

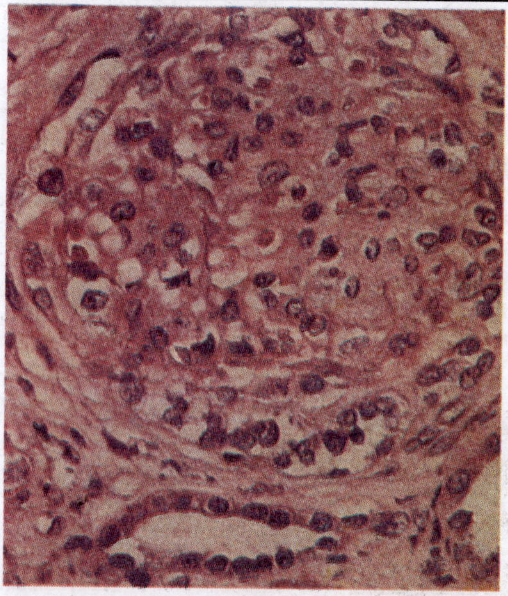

Fig. 26.40. Acute proliferative post-streptococcal glomerulonephritis

called *diffuse* when all the glomeruli of kidney are affected, whereas when only some glomeruli are involved, it is known as *focal* lesion. Based on the degree of involvement of each glomerulus, the lesion is called global when entire glomerulus are affected and segmental only when some segments of glomerular tuft is involved (Table 26.4).

Acute proliferative glomerulonephritis

Most common in children and often follows a streptococcal sore throat by *Streptococcus pyogenes*.

Histology (Fig. 26.40)

(i) Cellularity of glomerulus (endothelial cells) is increased and infiltrated with polymorphonuclear leucocytes.

(ii) Proliferated endothelial cells blocked the lumen of many capillaries.

(iii) Urinary passage is clear as there is no proliferation of podocytes.

END STAGE OF KIDNEY

Chronic glomerulonephritis is the end stage pool of various forms of glomerulonephritis. The patient is uraemic, hypertensive and in chronic renal failure.

Microscopical features (Fig. 26.41)

(i) Section shows the structure of kidney tissue.

(ii) Some glomeruli are atrophied with hyaline change.

(iii) There is marked atrophy of cortical tubules with hyaline change.

(iv) Marked periglomerular and interstitial fibrosis with scanty focal lymphocytic infiltration.

(v) Arterioles show evidence of elastosis.

(vi) A small percentage of glomerulus looks normal and may be hypertrophied.

Benign hypertensive nephrosclerosis

(arteriolosclerotic kidney) (Fig. 26.42)

Histological features of benign nephrosclerosis closely simulate those of chronic nephritis.

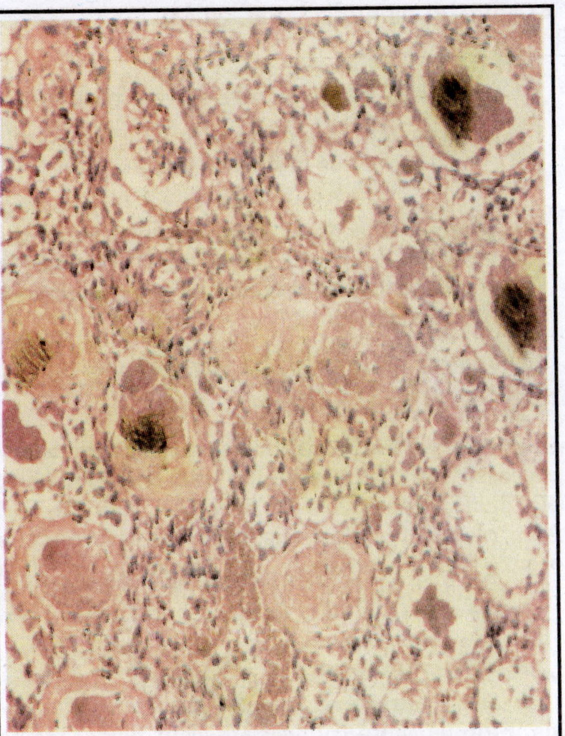

Fig. 26.41. End-stage kidney (chronic nephritis), HE × 65

Microscopically, many glomeruli become converted into hyaline masses as a result of chronic ischaemia, caused by thickening and hyalinisation of the walls of the afferent arterioles. Hyaline material is composed of plasma proteins lipids and basement membrane material. When sufficient nephrons have been affected, and eventually lead to chronic failure the morphologic state is known as end stage kidney.

LIVER

FATTY CHANGE : LIVER (Fig. 26.43)

The causes of fatty change (steatosis) include toxins (particularly alcohol and halogenated hydrocarbons such as chloroform), chronic hypoxia diabetes mellitus and obesity. The condition may progress to cirrhosis.

Microscopic features (Fig. 26.43)

This specimen was a wedge biopsy of liver from a chronic alcoholic.

(i) There are large vacuoles in the hepatocytes (ballooning degeneration) in the centrilobular region around a branch of hepatic vein. The nucleus in the fatty cells is displaced to the periphery of the cell.

(ii) Panlobular fatty change in the middle of the lobule is evident.

(iii) Hepatocytes near periphery of lobule are much less affected.

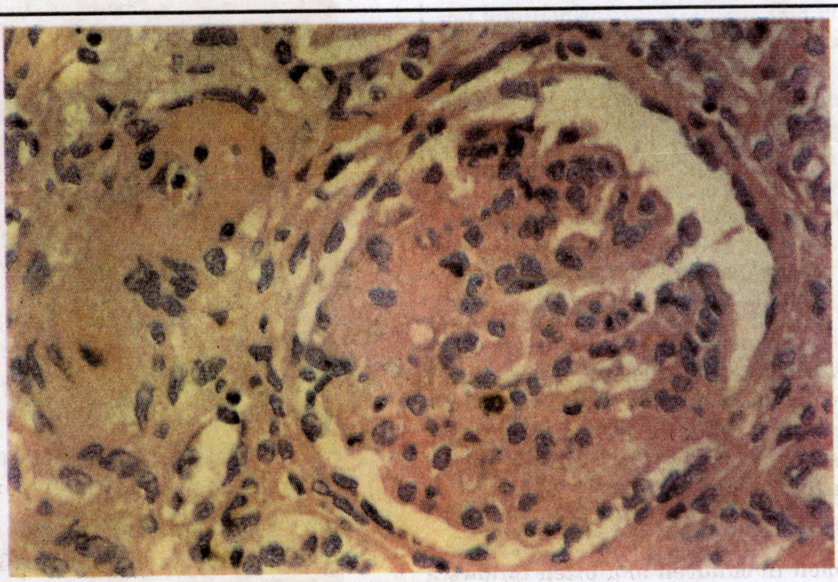

Fig. 26.42. Arteriosclerotic kidney (benign hypertension), HE × 250

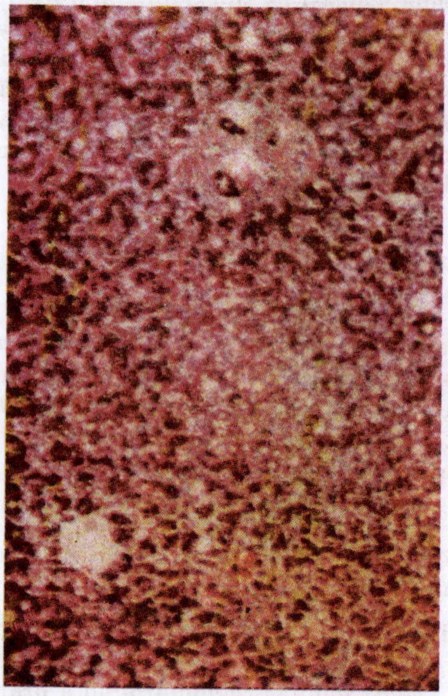

Fig. 26.43. Fatty change in liver (alcoholic hepatitis), HE × 350

Note : Fatty changes are most marked in the central and middle zones of the lobules.

CIRRHOSIS

Cirrhosis is the end result of long continued damage of liver cells, from a great many causes. Loss of liver cells is accompanied by compensatory liver cell hyperplasia and nodule formation. There is also chronic inflammatory reaction and progressive replacement fibrosis. It is characterised by fibrous septa which cut across the liver lobules. These septa form links between the portal tracts, between portal tracts and hepatic veins or between adjacent hepatic veins and enclosed regenerative liver nodules. Some nodules may be partially divided by irregular septa. Lymphocytes, and less commonly plasma cells are often present in fibrous septa and in portal tracts. The most important causes of cirrhosis are *alcoholic cirrhosis, post-viral cirrhosis* and *biliary cirrhosis* (primary and secondary to obstruction). In a large percentage of patients, the aetiology of cirrhosis cannot be established either clinically or morphologically, this is called *cryptogenic cirrhosis.* It is presumed that majority of cases of cryptogenic cirrhosis follow an episode of sub-clinical hepatitis.

ALCOHOLIC CIRRHOSIS (Fig. 26.44)

Histology

(i) Section shows picture of liver tissue.

(ii) Normal architecture of liver is completely lost by bands of fibrous tissue.

(iii) Increased fibrosis starting from portal triad to central vein, has subdivided the individual lobules in small islands of unaffected liver cells and some regenerating nodules.

Diagnosis : Micronodular cirrhosis of liver.

PRIMARY BILIARY CIRRHOSIS

In primary biliary cirrhosis, an inflammatory process, there is destruction of the intrahepatic bile ducts, hepatocytes are, however, also affected. As a result of cholestasis, necrosis of liver cells occurs which eventually leads to cirrhosis. With the destruction of the liver cells, portal tracts expand.

Microscopic features (Fig. 26.45)

1. Most characteristic is the regularity of fibrosis. Fibrous septa connect adjacent portal tracts but leaving the centrilobular region unaffected producing a pattern of monolobular fibrosis.

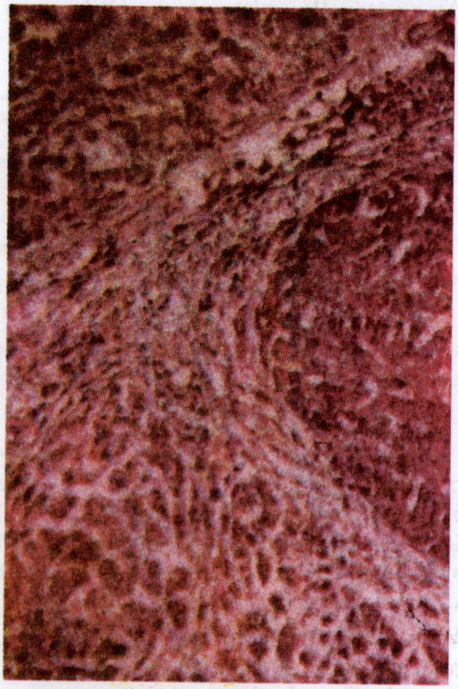

Fig. 26.44. Alcoholic cirrhosis, HE × 150

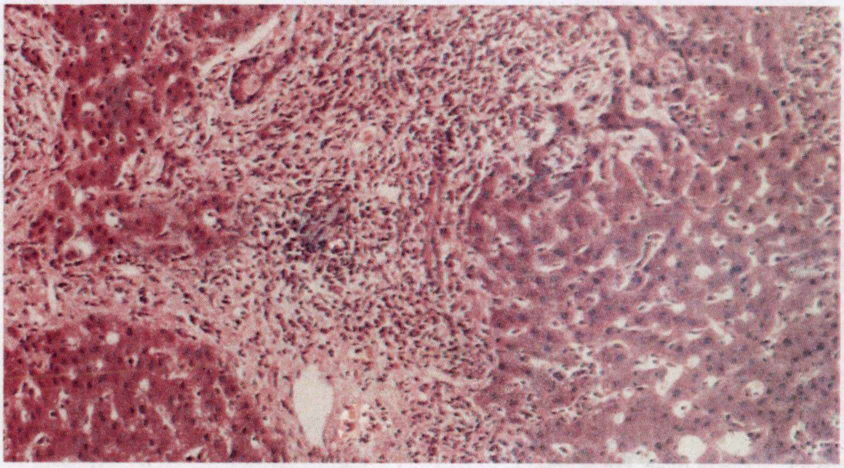

Fig. 26.45. Primary biliary cirrhosis, HE × 250

2. The most conspicuous change is the patchy lymphocytic infiltration of the portal tracts. Large bile ducts are not visible.

NUTMEG LIVER

In chronic heart failure (right sided), the inferior vena cava and hepatic veins become congested. The pressure is transmitted to the central veins resulting in congestion of sinusoids with blood. As a result, hepatocytes in the centrilobular zones frequently undergo atrophy.

Microscopic features (Fig. 26.46)

(i) Section shows structure of liver.

(ii) Central vein is distended with blood.

(iii) Hepatocytes surrounding the central vein show severe fatty changes and many hepatocytes are atrophied and necrosed.

(iv) Hepatocytes in mid-zone show fatty changes.

(v) Peripheral cells of the lobule surrounding central vein are normal (because of better oxygenation provided by hepatic artery).

Note :

1. In a very chronic case of passive venous congestion, lobular architecture is distorted by fibrous thickening of the walls of central veins. This fibrous tissue when extends to the surrounding lobules, the condition is called *cardiac cirrhosis*.

2. When the hepatic cells with fatty change undergo necrosis the surviving hepatocytes undergo regeneration producing nodular regenerated hyperplasia.

MALARIA LIVER

Microscopic features (Fig. 26.47)

(i) HE section shows the structure of liver.

(ii) Central veins and surrounding sinusoidal capillaries are dilated.

(iii) Kupffer cells lining the sinusoids are enlarged and contain slaty-coloured malarial pigment.

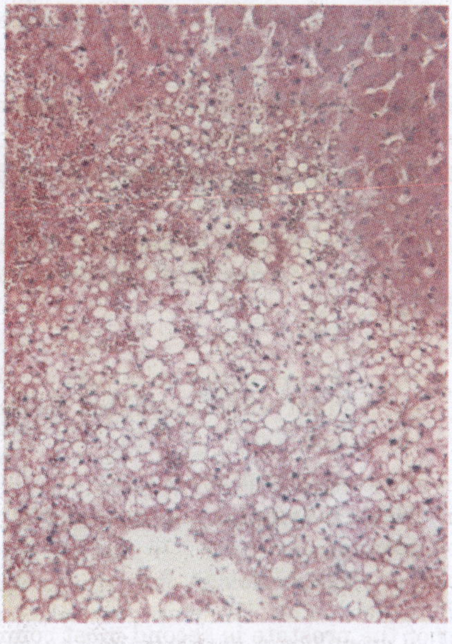

Fig. 26.46. Chronic passive venous congestion and fatty change (nutmeg) liver, HE × 60

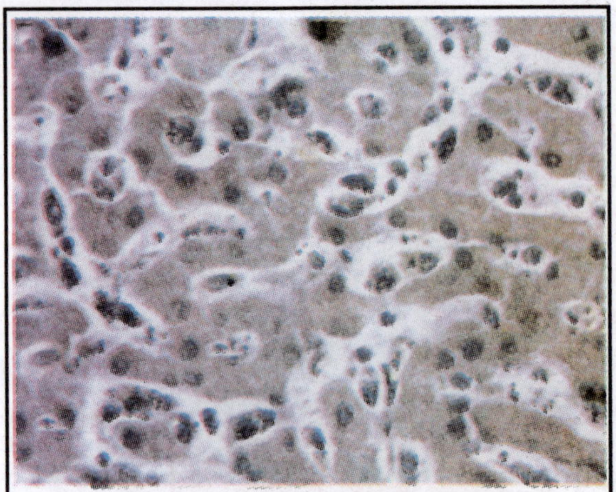

Fig. 26.47. Malaria liver, HE × 250

(iv) Parasitised red cells are found (sometimes) in the sinusoids.

(v) Parenchymal cells surrounding central vein may show some fatty change.

PROSTATE

Benign hyperplasia of prostate

Prostate enlarges from its normal weight of 15-20 g to 100 g or more. It is nodular and firm to woody hard. Cut surface shows a yellow white appearance with minute cysts containing milky fluid and tiny concretions (corpora amylacea).

Histology (Fig. 26.48)

(i) Section shows fibromuscular-glandular structure of prostate.

(ii) All the elements show evidence of hyperplasia.

(iii) There is marked epithelial proliferation and some glands show papillary buds and infoldings.

(iv) Glandular acini are lined by a single regular layer of tall columnar or cuboidal epithelium with vacuolated eosinophilic cytoplasm.

(v) Some acini contain corpora amylacea.

(vi) There is lymphocytic infiltration within stroma.

Adenocarcinoma of prostate (Fig. 26.49)

Cancer of the prostate is second most common in men, preceeded in frequency by lung cancer. It is rare below 40 and prevalence is high over the age of 80.

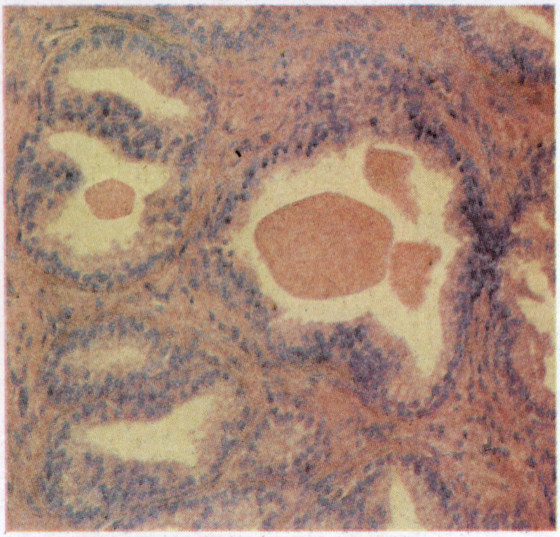

Fig. 26.48. Benign hyperplasia of prostate, HE × 150

Gross : Prostate is firm, fibrous and often enlarged. Cut section shows homogeneous appearance and contains irregular yellowish areas.

Histology : The neoplasm originates from the peripheral zone or in the transitional zone of the prostate. H.E. section shows : (i) Closely set small irregular acini lined by a single layer of epithelium. There is loss of intracinar papillary infoldings. (ii) There is little or no stroma between the malignant acini. (iii) Often intraprostatic perineural spaces show early invasion by cancer cells.

Latent carcinoma : Small capsular foci with so-called latent carcinoma of prostate with features of well differentiated carcinoma are discovered incidentally in a prostate showing benign hyperplasia. Incidence rises with age reaching 80% at the age of 80. *Prostatic intraepithelial neoplasia* **(PIN)** : This is analogous to CIN.

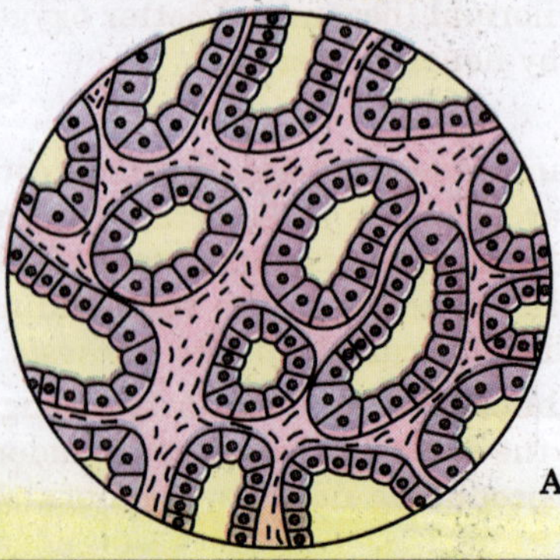

Fig. 26.49. Adenocarcinoma prostate

Section III

PATHOLOGICAL SPECIMENS (Systemic Pathology)

Section III contains

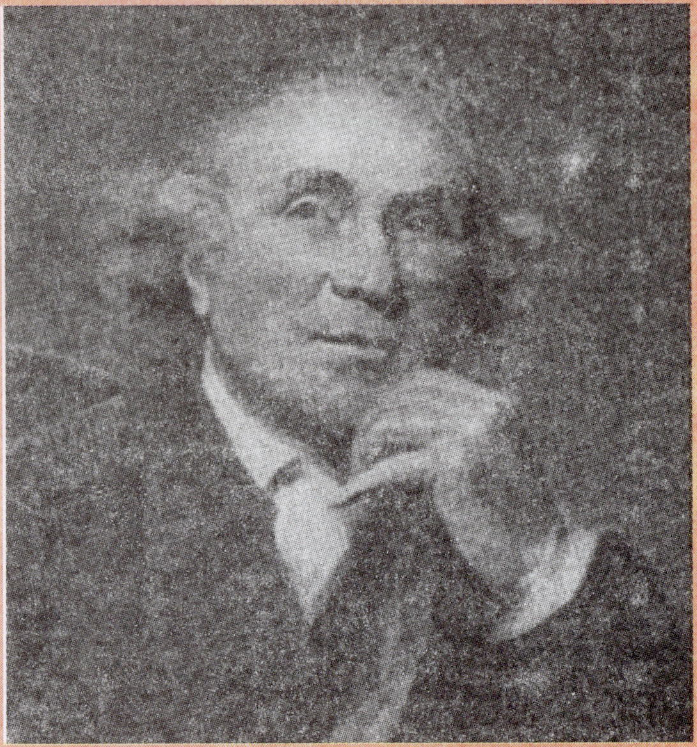

John Hunter (1728–1793)

Founder of Medical Museum Techniques — *He was a Scottish surgeon considered as the greatest surgeon-anatomist of all times. He made unique collection of various pathological specimens which resulted in Hunterian Museum of the Royal College of Surgeons, London. His description of syphilitic chancre (Hunterian chancre) and adductor canal (Hunterian canal) are known by his name. William Hunter, famous anatomist of his time was his brother.*

Chapter 27

Cardiovascular System

Normal

(i) Heart of an elderly person normally weighs 250-350 g (range 200-400 g). An increase in weight of heart is called *cardiomegaly.*

(ii) Normally, thickness of right ventricle is 3 mm and that of left ventricle ranges from 9-12 mm.

(iii) *Hypertrophy* (enlargement of myocardial cells) of heart occurs when cells are called upon to perform more work.

(iv) All valve cusps are smooth and translucent. Mitral and tricuspid valves are attached to papillary muscles by chordae tendinae.

(v) Shape of ventricles is normally of that of a pyramid with wider base at atrioventricular valves and pointed at the apex of heart. When the lumen is increased, the heart becomes round which is called *dilatation.*

(vi) Pericardium is normally smooth, glistening and transparent through which epicardial fat and myocardium is visible.

Cardiovascular diseases

(i) The most common underlying cause of heart diseases is atherosclerosis of the coronary arteries.

(ii) Most infections of pericardium *(pericarditis)* and myocardium *(myocarditis)* are viral and most infections of endocardium *(endocarditis)* and valves (valvulitis) are bacterial and fungal. However, in rheumatic fever they may develop pancarditis involving all the three layers.

RHEUMATIC FEVER

Rheumatic fever is a systemic disease following infection by group A β-haemolytic streptococci in throat. Systemic manifestations are attributed to disordered immunological response. It is believed that antibodies produced against the M proteins of certain strains of group A beta haemolytic streptococci cross react with glycoprotein antigens in the heart, joints and other tissues.

Aschoff body (rheumatic nodule) (Fig. 27.1)

It is the basic lesion in acute rheumatic fever. It is an oval or elongated microscopic nodule.

M.E. : There is central ill-defined area of fibrinoid necrosis surrounded by a mixture of lymphocytes, plasma cells and histiocytes. The histiocytes may be large and multinucleated. *Anitschkow myocyte* (A) is characterised by scanty eosinophilic cytoplasm and a ribbon-like elongated nucleus. These cells are thought to represent large modified fibro-histiocyte cells. Fibroblasts are very scanty (predominant in older scarred lesions).

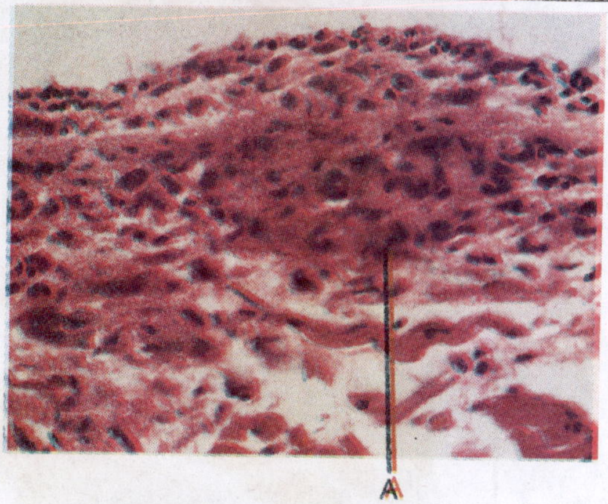

Fig. 27.1. ME Aschoff body (A), HE × 180

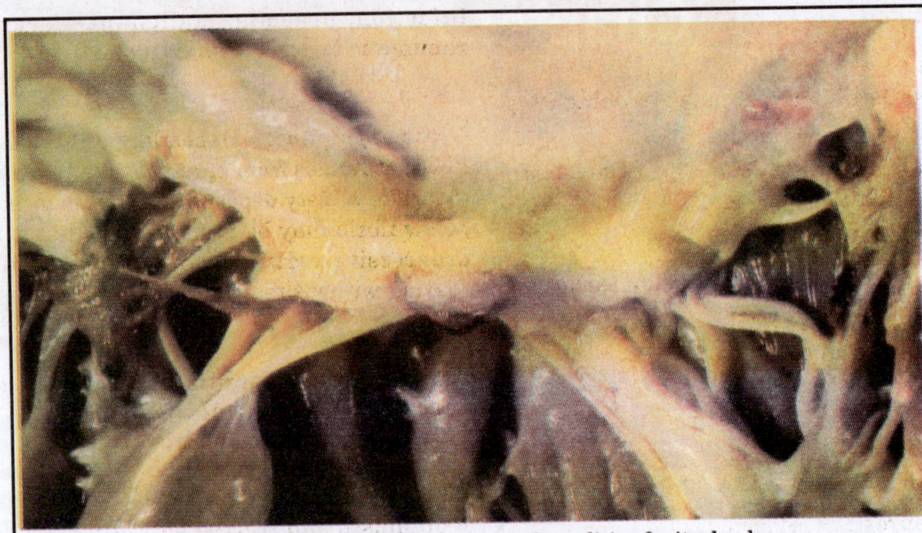

Fig. 27.2. Verrucous rheumatic endocarditis of mitral valve

Distribution : Aschoff bodies are seen in interstitial connective tissue of myocardium, particularly near blood vessels; in subpericardial fibrous tissue and in subendocardial connective tissue.

Verrucous rheumatic endocarditis of mitral valve (Fig. 27.2)

Rheumatic fever provides the prototype of verrucous endocarditis. Left side of the heart is affected, especially the mitral valve.

Macroscopically, the valves initially become oedematous and swollen in acute disease. Then small thrombi (fibrin and platelets) form on them which are called verrucae. They are greyish or reddish-brown, multiple warty masses arranged specially along the line of closure of the valve cusps and also on the rest of the valvular surface. These are firm and not easily wiped off and hence do not give rise to emboli.

Fate of rheumatic endocarditis

Healing of this acute inflammation leads to :

1. Mitral stenosis
2. Mitral regurgitation

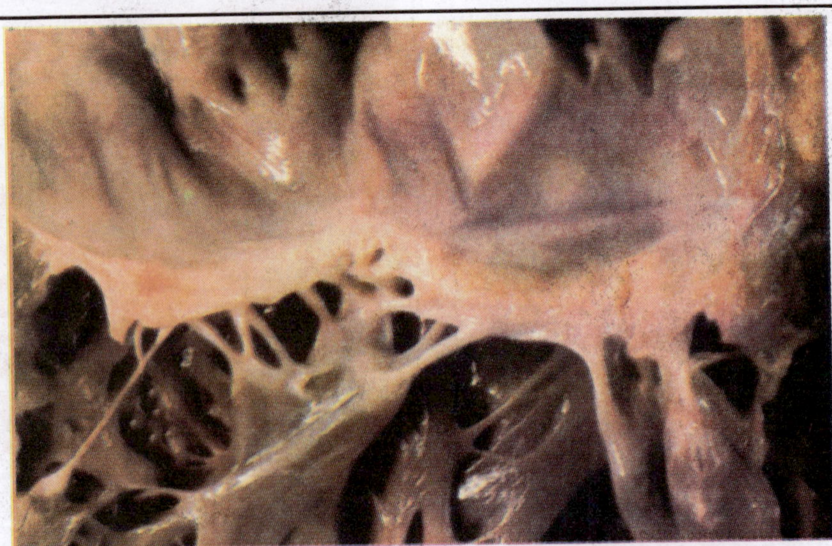

Fig. 27.3. Rheumatic endocarditis : Sclerosis of mitral valve

Mitral stenosis

Macroscopic features

1. Valve leaflets show fibrous thickening (Fig. 27.3).
2. Commissures are fused and fish-mouth looking mitral valve (Fig. 27.4).
3. Left atrium dilated.
4. Left ventricle — normal or, small (disused).
5. Jet lesion of endocardial sclerosis in the papillary muscle — *Zahn's pocket.*

Mitral regurgitation (incompetence)

Macroscopic features

1. Gradual retraction of free edges of leaflets.
2. Commissures are retracted.
3. Shortening and fusion of chordae tendinae.
4. Rupture of chordae and papillary muscles.
5. Formation of *MacCallum's patch.*

PERICARDITIS

Pericarditis may be acute or chronic.

Acute pericarditis

Common causes include acute myocardial infarction and viral infection (*Coxsackie B*), less frequent causes are secondary to bacterial infection, uraemia, malignant disease, SLE, rheumatic fever and tuberculosis.

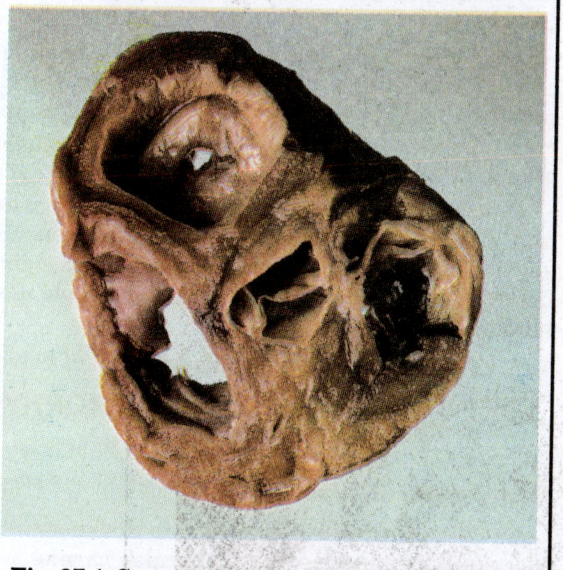

Fig. 27.4. Cross section of heart showing fish-mouth appearance of mitral valve in rheumatic endocarditis

Fibrinous pericarditis (Fig. 27.5)

Gross appearance : Depending on the amount of fibrin, it ranges from barely visible fibrin ridges to massive, velvety deposit. Sometimes mesothelium below fibrin may be destroyed, so that it becomes progressively difficult to pull off the fibrinous coating without tearing epicardial tissues.

Chronic pericarditis

True chronic pericarditis is more commonly seen as scars or adhesions of a previous acute pericarditis. The scars are whitish irregular areas of fibrosis on the anterior surfaces of the ventricles which are known as "milk spots". These are areas of organised and scarred pericardial exudate.

BACTERIAL ENDOCARDITIS (Fig. 27.6)

These are mainly caused by localisation of bacteria on a heart valve and sometimes the lining of a cardiac chamber. Left side of heart is more frequently affected. The disease may occur on

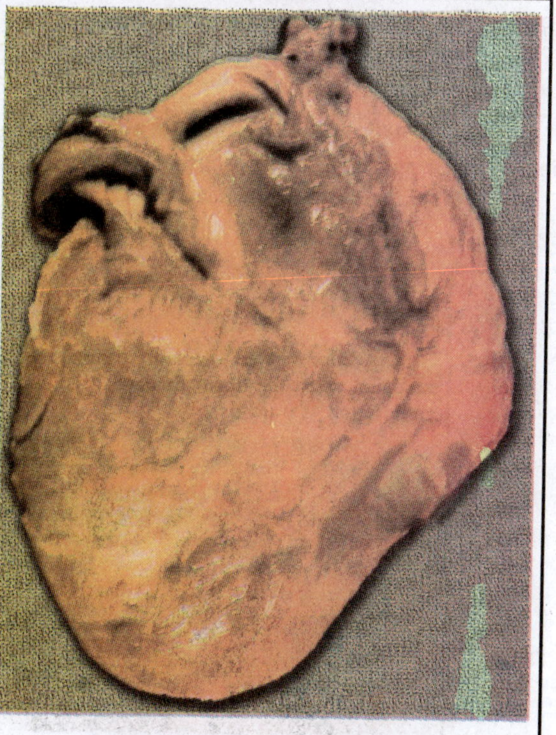

Fig. 27.5. Fibrinous pericarditis

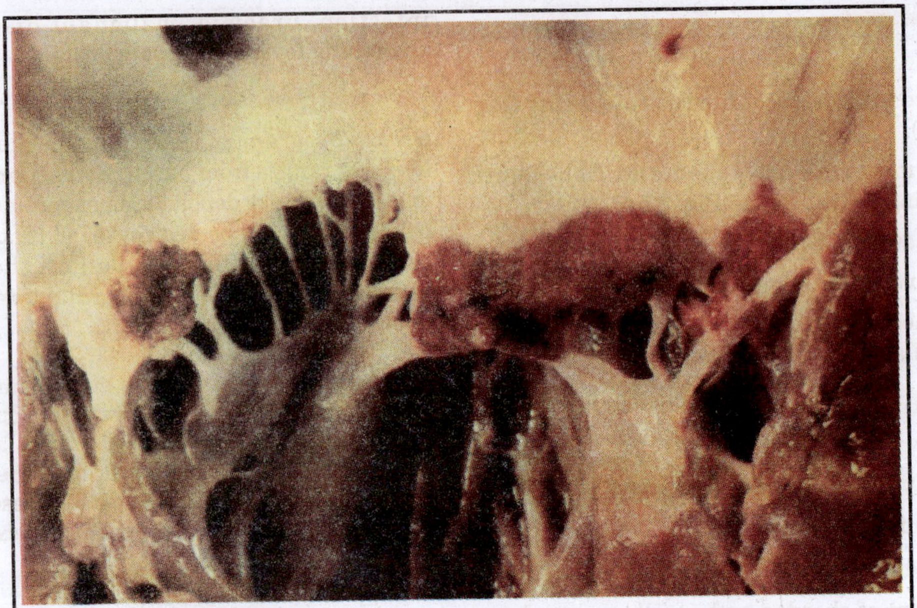

Fig. 27.6. Valvular endocarditis (bacterial). Vegetations accompanied by ulceration

normal valves, but commonly it involves previously damaged valves, either congenital or acquired (rheumatic fever, prosthetic valves). Infective endocarditis may also be caused by fungi. Clinically and pathologically endocarditis can be divided into *subacute, acute* and *post-operative.*

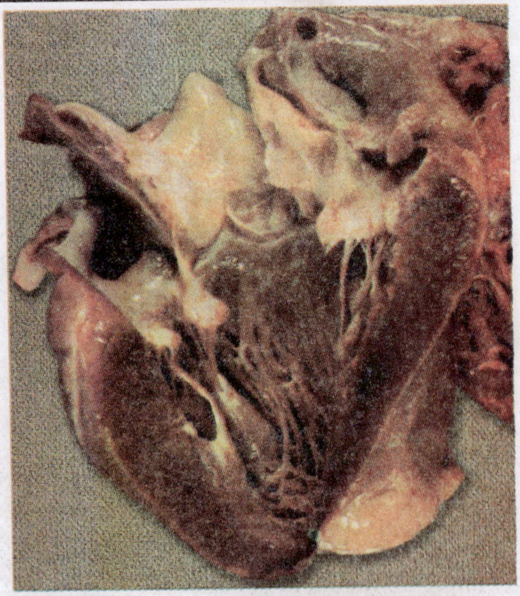

Fig. 27.7. Hypertrophy of left ventricle (left ventricle is opened)

Subacute endocarditis : The common organisms causing subacute endocarditis are less virulent organism like *Streptococcus sanguis* (viridans streptococci), others include *Str. milleri, Str. bovis, Coxiella burnetii.*

Acute endocarditis is caused by highly virulent and infective organism, usually *Staph.aureus,* less often *Str. pneumoniae, E. coli, Klebsiella, H. influenzae.*

Post-operative endocarditis : This is endocarditis following cardiac surgery in which prosthetic heart valves or other prosthetic materials are used. *Staph. albus* is the commonest offending agent.

Gross appearance : Vegetations vary in size and shape but they are larger than rheumatic vegetations (Fig. 27.6). Sometimes they are significantly large and polypoid. They are friable and tend to give rise to emboli.

M.E : There is non-specific inflammation of valve.

LEFT VENTRICULAR HYPERTROPHY

(Figs. 27.7 and 27.8)

Macroscopical examination

Left ventricular wall is increased in thickness and the papillary muscles and trabeculae carnae are prominent. Heart is sometimes massively enlarged *(corbovium).*

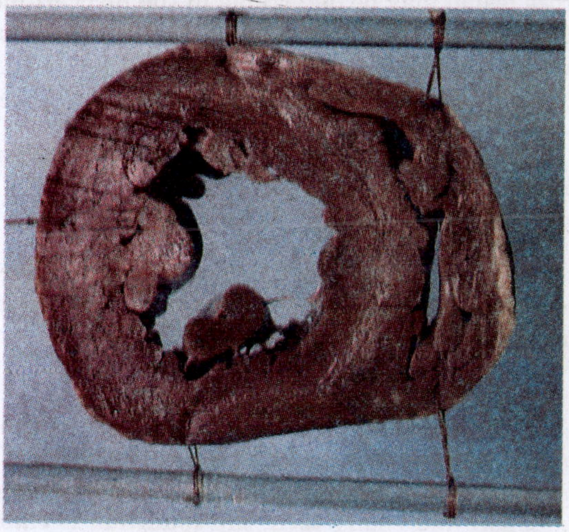

Fig. 27.8. Cross section of left ventricle showing hypertrophied ventricular wall

Causes : Most common in hypertension and also in disease of mitral or aortic valves with resulting incompetence or stenosis.

ISCHAEMIC HEART DISEASE

Most common cause of ischaemic heart disease and infarction is arteriosclerosis due to coronary artery atheroma. Depending on the rate of development of the ischaemia and its ultimate severity, one of the following four syndromes may develop : (i) angina pectoris, (ii) myocardial infarction, (iii) chronic ischaemic heart disease (IHD), and (iv) sudden cardiac death (SCD).

ARTERIOSCLEROSIS (Fig. 27.9)

Arteriosclerosis is a generalized progressive arterial disease associated with localised arterial occlusions and aneurysms. The pathology of arteriosclerosis has gained greater surgical importance with the development of direct operative therapy for lesions of major arteries.

Pathology

The pathology of arteriosclerosis primarily consists of the following :

(a) Formation of intimal *plaques,* made of lipid deposits and proliferated spindle cells; the latter appear to be of heterogenous nature, fibroblasts and smooth muscle cells predominating.

(b) There is reduplication and fragmentation of the interal elastic lamina.

(c) There is degeneration of the media, as evident from fragmentation of elastic tissue network by hyaline, mucinoid, and collagenous degeneration of the smooth muscle, and by medial calcification.

(d) There is adventitial fibrosis and chronic inflammatory cellular infiltration.

Arteriosclerosis may present as an occlusive disease when the disease attacks the intima more rapidly than the media and adventitia, but may present as an aneurysm when the reverse is true. Sometimes occlusive disease and aneurysm may co-exist in the same arterial system in same patient.

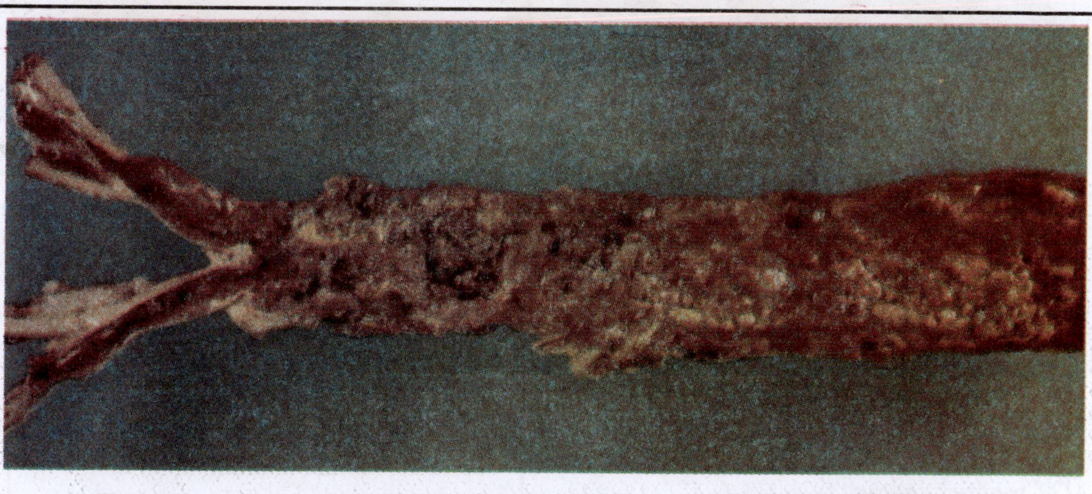

Fig. 27.9. Arteriosclerosis of aorta, ulceration plaques exposes atheroma to blood stream

Pathogenesis of arteriosclerosis

It is believed to be multifactorial. Important factors in its pathogenesis include :

(i) Changes in lipid metabolism.

(ii) Increased endothelial permeability to serum lipoprotein complexes.

(iii) Susceptibility of the intima to mechanical injury from flow turbulence at major bifurcations and in the presence of hypertension.

(iv) Elastic tissue fragmentation, and thrombosis or disruption of vasa vasorum.

Pathogenesis

More than 75% of IHD cases is due to severe coronary atherosclerosis with stenosing plaques leading to reduction in cross sectional area of arterial lumen (hence known as coronary heart disease).

Acute myocardial infarction

It should be remembered that when the patient dies quickly after infarction of myocardium no gross lesion may be detectable in the myocardium at necropsy. It is only after 8 to 10 hours that myocardial changes become apparent.

Evolution of ischaemic lesion

If the patient survives, the following changes in myocardium are observed.

(a) *After 8-10 hours*

Ischaemic muscle becomes swollen and lustreless in appearance in contrast to neighbouring unaffected area.

(b) *Older infarct*

As the age of the infarct increases, the morphological alterations become more recognisable. Within a few days, the infarcted muscle becomes pale, soft and easily torn, the condition is called *myomalacia cordis* by Zielger. The infarcted area is demarcated from the rest of the heart by a zone of confluent haemorrhages (Fig. 27.10).

Pathogenesis

More than 90% of patients IHD suffer from advanced coronary atherosclerosis. Although a

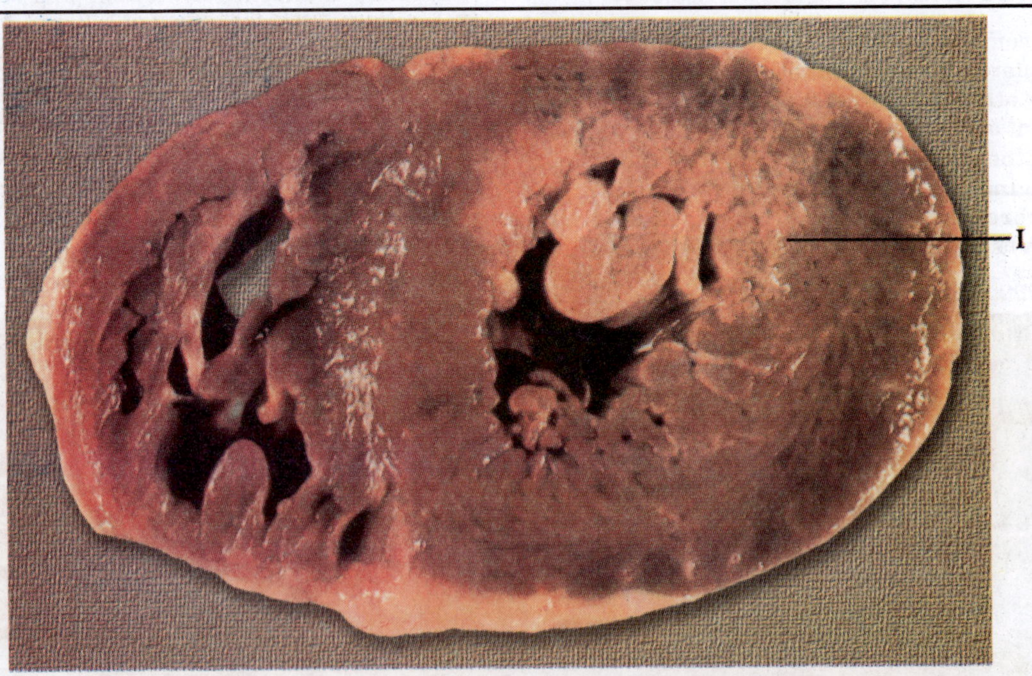

Fig. 27.10. Myocardial infarction. Infarcted area (I) is showing pale discolouration

Cross section of the heart shows : Visibly gross areas of pale discolouration of inner myocardium and papillary muscles.

single coronary trunk may be affected, but more often two or all three — left anterior descending (LAD), left circumflex (LC), right coronary (RC) or a first order branch of right coronary are affected. However, the left anterior descending branch (LAD) is most severally affected.

Types of myocardial infarction

1. *Transmural infarct* : This type is more common and severe type in which the ischaemic necrosis affects the full thickness, or nearly that, of the ventricular wall. Most lesions begin as subendocardial lesions. The subendocardial myocardium of the wall of left ventricle is commonly involved because it is least well perfused and subjected to compressive forces of the outer layers of ventricular wall during the systole.

2. *Subendocardial infarct* : It is less common and less severe than the intramural infarct. Subendocardium is most vulnerable to any reduction in coronary flow.

Sites of involvement in IHD

1. *Left anterior descending coronary artery* (40-50%)	Anterior wall of left ventricle near apex; anterior two thirds of interventricular septum.
2. *Right coronary artery* (30-50%)	Posterior wall of left ventricle; posterior one third of interventricular system.
3. Left circumflex coronary artery (15-20%)	Lateral wall of left ventricle.

Gross appearance (Fig. 27.10)

(i) Visibly gross areas of pale discolouration of inner myocardium.

(ii) Pale appearance of papillary muscles.

(iii) Dense white scar immediately under the endocardium at the site of the infarct (Fig. 27.10).

(iv) The blotchy appearance of myocardium to the scar is partly attributable to fresh infarction.

Histochemical studies

Enzyme succinic dehydrogenase is lost from infarcted muscle cells about 6-8 hours after infarction which can be dissected in gross as well as microscopical specimens. The finding is helpful in timing the onset of infarction.

Histological features

(i) *Within a few hours* of onset of local ischaemia, the muscle fibres die, histologically recognisable by swelling, blurring, cross-striation and deep eosinophilia.

(ii) *In second week,* a zone of proliferating granulation tissue surrounds the necrotic area.

(iii) *In third week*, formation of collagen fibres can be seen, first near the edges and later in deeper areas. From third week reparative reaction known as 'organization' occurs without interruption, unless a further ischaemic attack occurs.

(iv) *By the end of 2nd month*, in all but the largest infarcts replacement by collagen fibres provide a sufficient mechanical strength to prevent cardiac rupture. However, when bed-rest is succeeded at suitable intervals by ambulation and mild bodily exercise, patient resumes with safety and a more normal mode of life.

Chapter 28

Respiratory System

Normal

Right lung has 3 lobes and left lung has two lobes and lingula (equivalent to middle lobe of right), however, left lung is smaller than the right.

Microscopically, progressive branching of the bronchi form bronchioles and finally to terminal bronchioles (less than 2 mm in diameter) Fig. 28.2. Part of the lung distal to terminal bronchiole is called acinus. Cartilage is seen in section of bronchi and their branches but bronchioles lack of cartilage and submucosal glands within their walls.

NOSE

Nasal polyp

It is a product of chronic inflammation of nasal mucosa, commonly infective in nature and sometimes allergic.

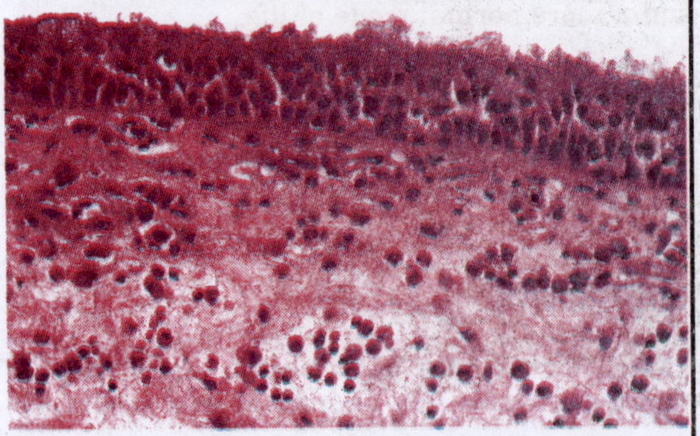

Fig. 28.1. Rhinosporidiosis showing spherules in nasal polyp (× 140)

Histology (Figs. 25.13, 28.1)

(i) Stroma grossly oedematous.

(ii) Plenty of inflammatory cells including plasma cells and eosinophils.

(iii) Large spherules with endosporulation are seen.

Diagnosis : Rhinosporidiosis caused by *R. Seeberi.*

LUNGS

Emphysema

It is defined as permanent enlargement of the air spaces distal to terminal bronchiole.

Pathogenesis

Middle and old aged smokers are mostly affected as a result of destruction of elastic recoil of alveolar walls caused by the loss of enzyme elastase and inflammation (α1–AT deficiency).

Types

A. Generalised	*B. Segmental*
Diffuse	Regular
Focal	Irregular

Each of generalised and segmental types are further subdivided as (Fig. 28.2) :

1. *Centrilobular or centriacinar*
2. *Panacinar*
3. *Paraseptal*
4. *Irregular*

Diagnosis of emphysema is established on clinical and radiological evidences.

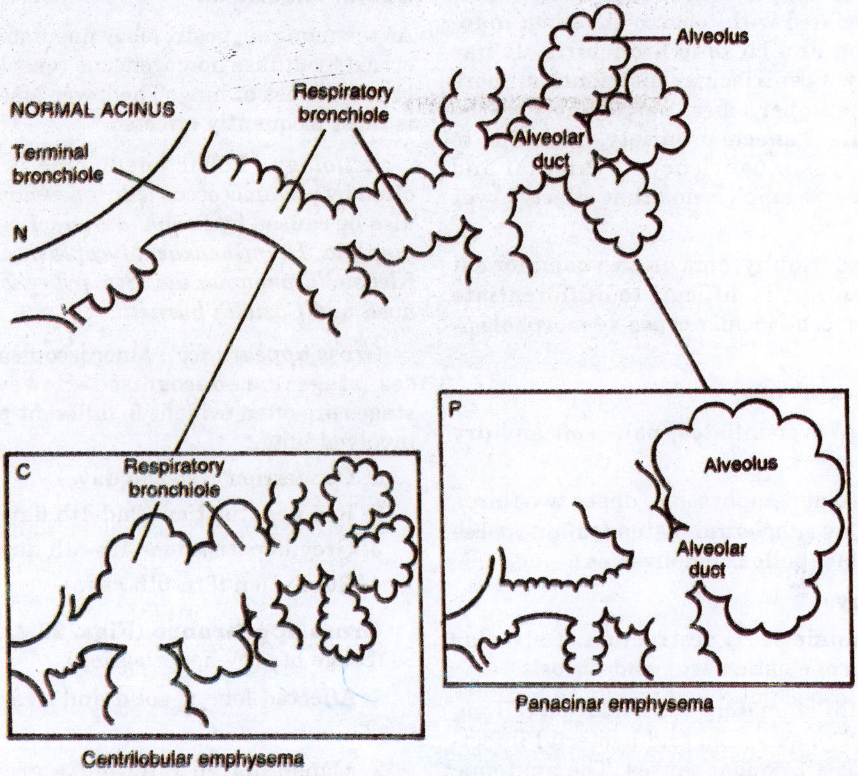

Fig. 28.2. N = Diagram of normal structures within the acinus, the fundamental unit of the lung. A terminal bronchiole is immediately proximal to the respiratory bronchiole. C = Centrilobular emphysema with dilation that initially affects the respiratory bronchioles. P = Panacinar emphysema with initial distention of the peripheral structures (i.e., alveolus and alveolar duct); the disease later extends to affect the respiratory bronchioles.

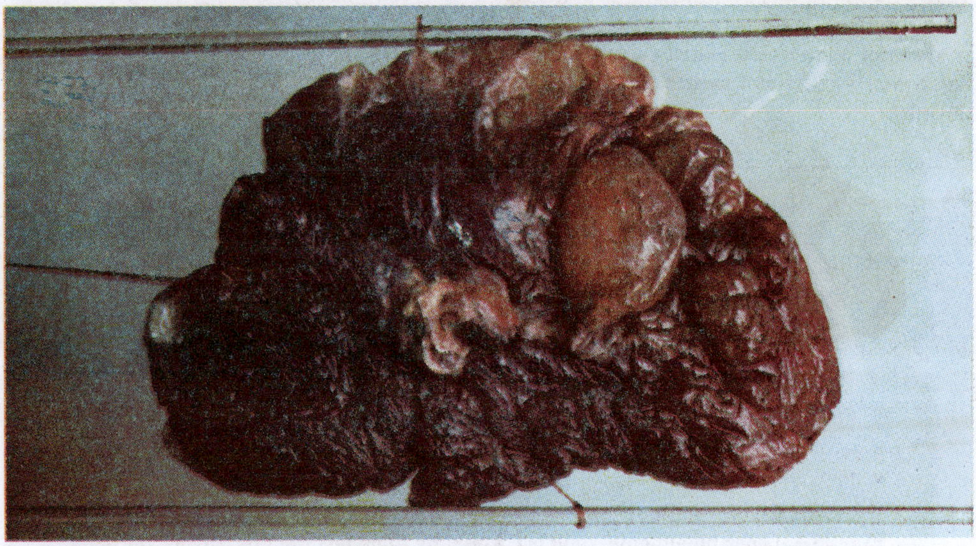

Fig. 28.3. Bullous emphysema

Generalised emphysema (Fig. 28.3) : Emphysema associated with tobacco smoking, industrial smoking and chronic bronchitis. It has predominantly a centriacinar distribution, more common in the upper lobes, particularly in the apical segments. Panacinar variety, often due to alpha-1-antitrypsin deficiency, is familial and gives rise to severe emphysema that affects lower lobes.

Generalised emphysema is the commonest type. In practice, it is difficult to dfifferentiate panacinar from centriacinar types by morphological pattern.

Gross apperarance

1. Lungs are over-inflated, pale, soft and dry with rounded edges.

2. In centriacinar emphysema, upper two thirds of the lung show subpleural distended air spaces producing bullae (bullous emphysema).

Microscopy

There is thinning and destruction of alveolar walls with loss of elastic tissue and fibrosis.

PNEUMONIA : Inflammatory consolidation of lung tissue is called pneumonia, and bacterial infections are the most frequent causes. The anatomic types are known as *lobar pneumonia, lobular or bronchopneumonia* and *interstitial* pneumonia.

LOBAR PNEUMONIA

As the name suggests, lobar pneumonia is characterised by diffuse homogeneous consolidation of one or more lobes of lung. The lower lobe of right lung is most frequently affected.

Aetiology : Lobar pneumonia is caused most often by pneumococcus *(Str. pneumoniae),* but may also be caused by *Staph. aureus, Legionella pneumophila, H. influenzae, Mycoplasma pneumoniae, Klebsiella pneumoniae, Str. pyogenes, Ps. aeruginosa* and *Coxiella burnetii.*

Gross appearance : Macroscopically four phases (stages) are recognised. However, different stages are often evident in different portions of the involved lung.

1. Congestion (1st-2nd days),
2. Red hepatisation (2nd-4th days),
3. Grey hepatisation (4th-8th days),
4. Resolution (8th-9th days).

Gross appearance (Figs. 28.4, 28.5)

(Stage of grey hepatisation)

1. Affected lobe is solid and liver-like consistency.

2. Consolidated lung looks grey because of disappearance of congestion and red cells in the alveoli and predominance of neutrophilic exudate.

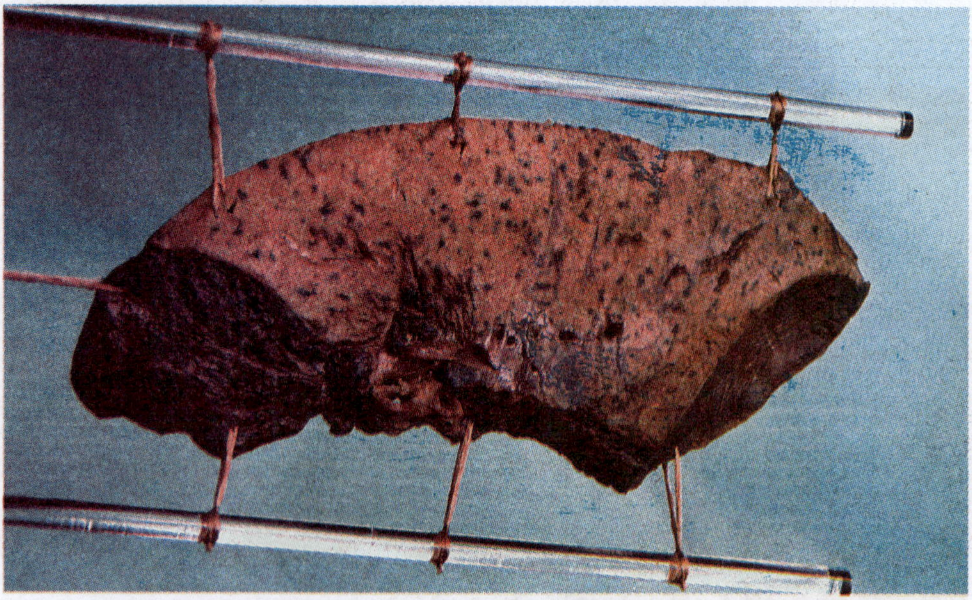

Fig. 28.4. Lobar pneumonia, lung is covered by thick layer of pus. Involved area is dark and consolidated

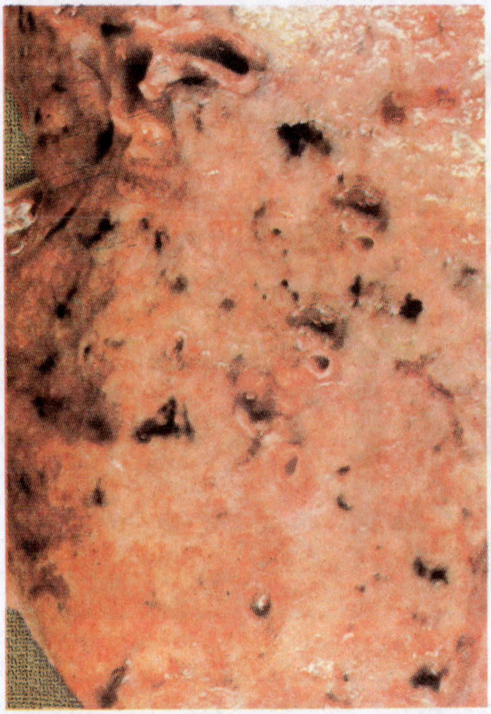

Fig. 28.5. Stage of grey hepatisation, cut section of lung

3. Pleural surface of affected lobe remains covered with a layer of fibrinous exudate.

M.E. : Vide Fig. 25.6.

BRONCHOPNEUMONIA (LOBULAR PNEUMONIA)

Bronchopneumonia is characterised grossly by nodules of consolidation, i.e., consolidation is patchy and irregular in distribution. The distribution is quite variable and lower lobes are more frequently involved.

Pathogenesis : Some abnormality of the respiratory tract is a predisposing factor of bronchopneumonia. The infection reaches the lung from upper respiratory tract or mouth by aspiration or inhalation.

Causative agents : *Streptococcus pyognes, Str. pneumoniae, H. influenzae,* certain anaerobic bacteria.

Gross appearance (Figs. 28.6, 28.7) :

1. Multiple, patchy consolidated areas are distributed throughout both lungs, but unequally.

2. The consolidated areas are firm, nodular and palpable.

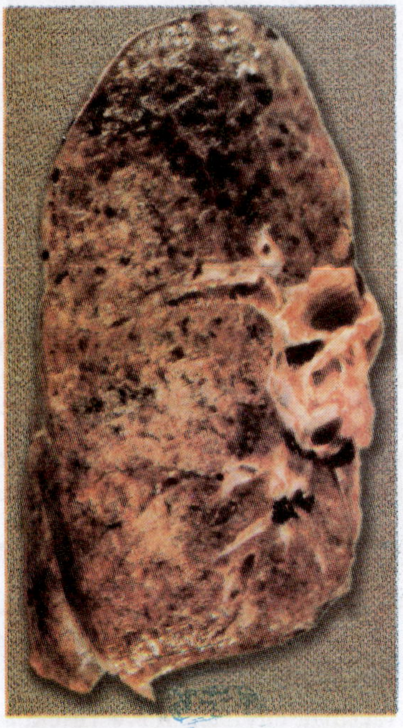

Fig. 28.6. Bronchopneumonia : cut surface shows nodular consolidation

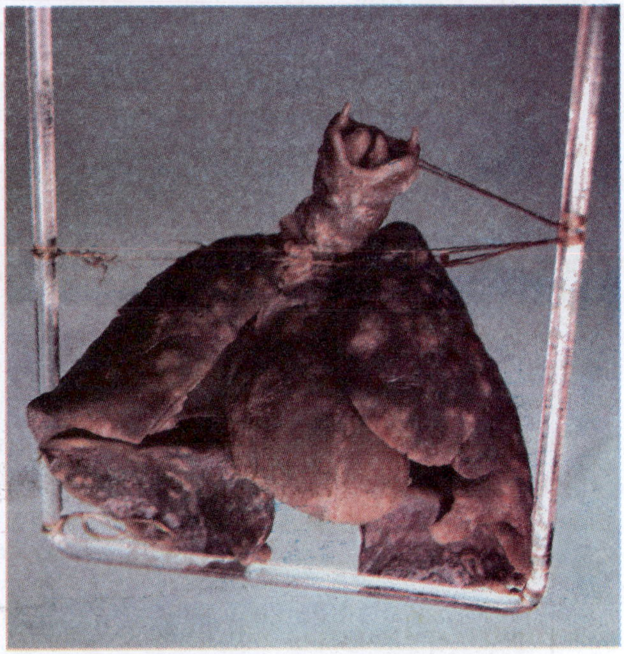

Fig. 28.7. Bronchopneumonia (infant) showing patchy consolidations in both lungs

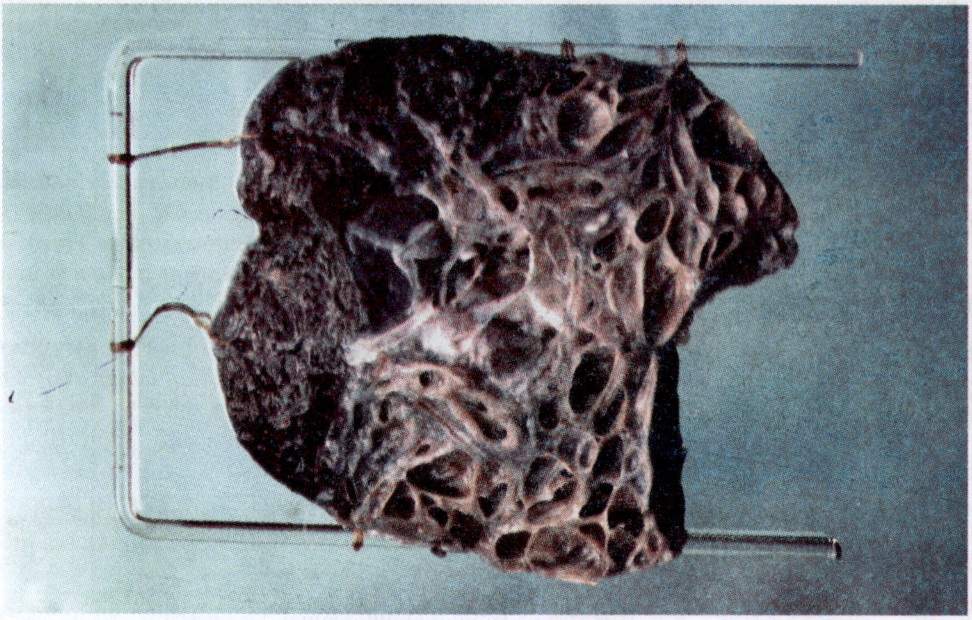

Fig. 28.8. Bronchiectasis, saccular type

3. The lesions are more extensive in the lower lobes in their posterior and basal parts.

4. Cut surface shows patchy consolidated areas surrounding the bronchioles, which are filled with pus.

5. Some bluish areas of collapse and lighter areas of emphysema often accompany the lesion.

Note : There is little or no exudate on the pleural surface of lung.

M.E. : Vide Figure 25.8.

BRONCHIECTASIS

Bronchiectasis is an abnormal dilatation of the bronchi. Depending upon gross or, bronchographic appearance, bronchiectasis is sub-classified into :

(a) *Cylindrical*

(b) *Fusiform* (or, *pyriform*)

(c) *Saccular*

(d) *Morbilliform* (or, varicose)

Two main anatomical varieties are described below :

(a) **Cylindrical dilatation** with extensive involvement throughout the length of the bronchus. Bronchi are greatly dilated throughout their length.

(b) **Saccular** dilatations which are more localised and exaggerated.

Causes

Bronchiectasis may be congenital or acquired. There is a *congenital abnormality* in bronchial development, particularly in the muscle and elastic component which include ciliary dysfunction syndrome and cystic fibrosis. *Acquired bronchiectasis* may be secondary to repeated pulmonary infection, bronchial obstruction and pulmonary fibrosis.

Gross appearance (Fig. 28.8)

1. Lung shows widespread involvement characterised by numerous dilated bronchioles; lower lobe is more extensively involved.

2. Bronchial dilatations are predominantly cylindrical with a few saccular dilatations in upper lobe.

3. The dilated bronchi are filled up with pus, and appear to be crowded together with reduction of intervening lung substance, and appear as cavities.

4. Bronchiectatic cavities have thick, white fibrous walls with tortuous lumens.

Histology : Damage or destruction of muscle

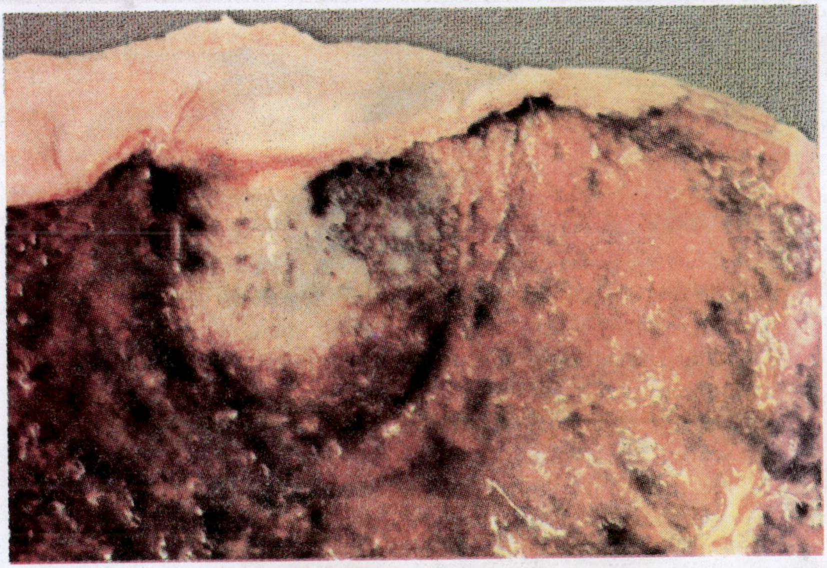

Fig. 28.9. Sub-pleural primary complex

and elastic fibres occur accompanied by inflammation.

Tuberculosis

Lungs are more frequently affected by tuberculosis followed by lymph node than any other organ. Causative agents include *M. tuberculosis, M. bovis* and atypical mycobacteria.

I. Primary infection (Fig. 28.9)

Primary infection may occur in any organ such as lung, tonsil, intestine or skin but in children the usual site is lung and is called primary tuberculosis, characterised by formation of *"primary complex"* (Fig. 28.9). It consists of a (i) small subpleural midzonal focus (tuberculous nodule measuring 1–2 cm) and (ii) a lymphatic component with involvement of draining lymph nodes and (iii) connecting channel (lymphangitis). In most cases, the tubercle undergoes healing with fibrosis and calcification. Occasionally, the primary lesion may progress by direct extension (caseous pneumonia) or disseminate by bronchus, lymphatics or blood stream producing miliary tuberculosis and distant organ tuberculosis.

II. Secondary or adult type infection

It is mainly caused by reinfection or reactivation of an old infection. Most often lungs in the apical region are affected.

Types of adult type pulmonary tuberculosis : (i) Fibrocaseous, (ii) Cavity (ulcerative) type, (iii) tuberculous bronchopneumonia, (iv) haematogenous miliary tuberculosis in lungs.

Fibrocaseous type

Gross appearance (Figs. 28.10 and 28.11)

(1) Section of lung shows cavitating lesions, foci of caseous necrosis accompanied by fibrosis in the apical region.

(2) Acute cavities have ragged, irregular, yellow-grey walls. Chronic cavities have a smooth, regular and fibrous lining.

(3) Cavity is surrounded by atelectatic lung.

M.E. : Wall of cavity is composed by fibrin layer, a layer of necrotic tissue, and more peripherally epitheloid cells, Langhans' giant cells, lymphocytes and fibroblasts are found (Fig. 25.10).

Miliary tuberculosis in lung (Fig. 28.12)

Cut section of lung grossly shows small (1-3 mm dia.) yellowish lesions visible both in subpleural location and in section. M.E. shows scattered tubercles in lung. These are foci of yellow white consolidation. The term miliary is derived from the resemblance of these foci to "millet" seeds. Central caseation is often absent.

BRONCHIAL CARCINOMA

Bronchial carcinomas arise from the bronchial epithelium or mucous glands. They can be divided into two groups : *carcinoma of bronchus* and *bron-*

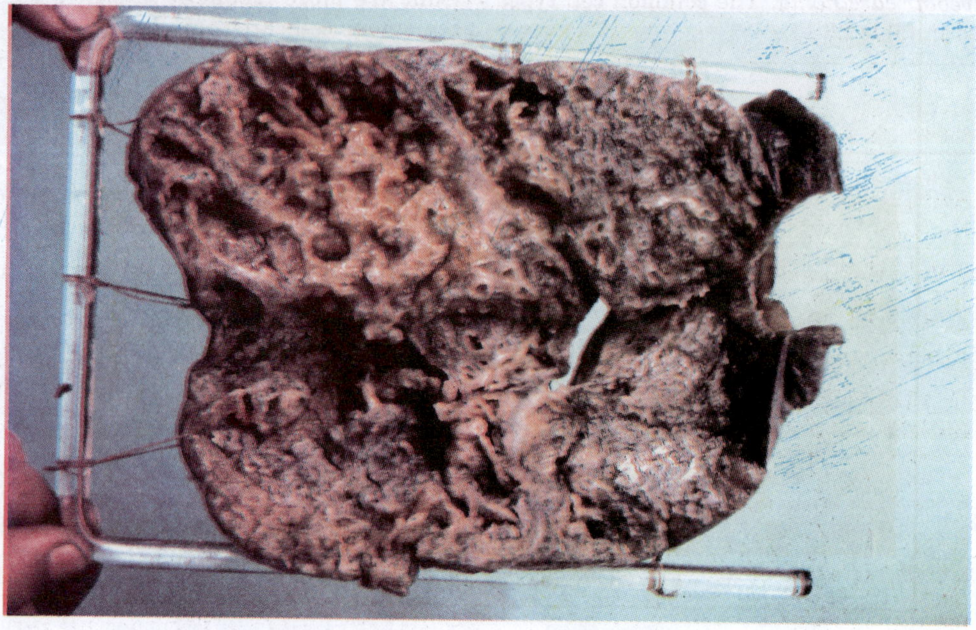

Fig. 28.10. Chronic fibrocaseous tuberculosis of lung : cut surface

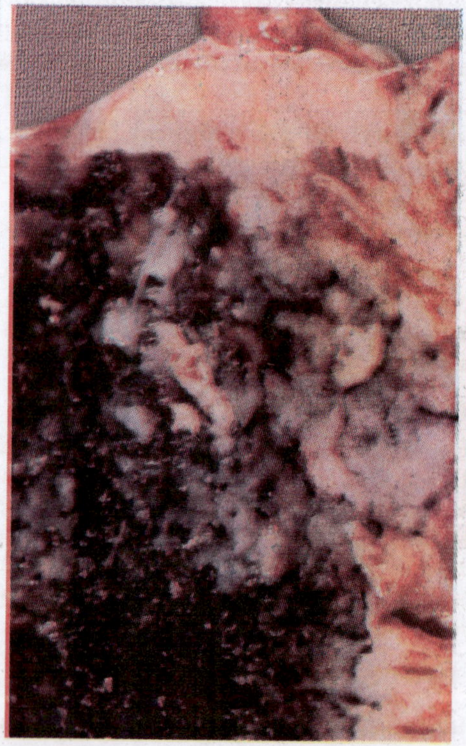

Fig. 28.11. Detail of fibrocaseous tuberculosis in cut surface of right apex

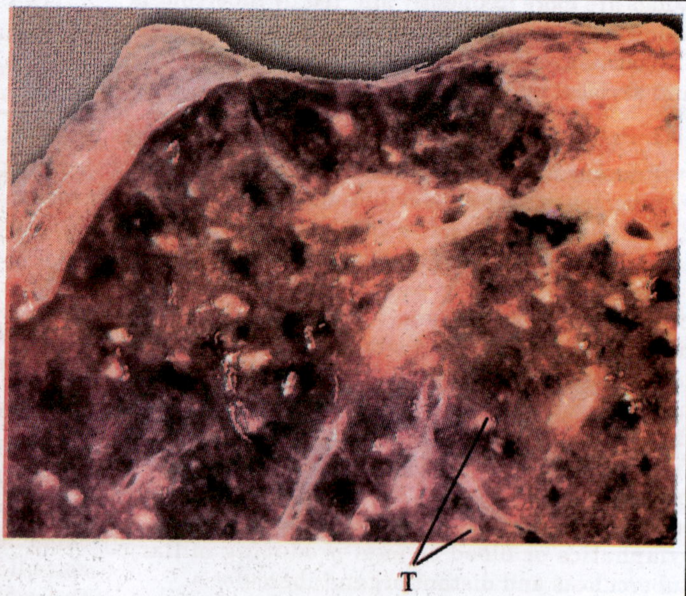

Fig. 28.12. Miliary tuberculosis lung : Small yellowish lesions of milary tubercles (T) are visible in section

chioloalveolar carcinoma. The common cell types are listed in table 28.1.

Table 28.1
Common cell types of bronchial carcinoma

Cell type	%
Differentiated carcinoma	
Squamous cell	50
Adenocarcinoma	15
Undifferentiated carcinoma	
Small cell (oat cell)	25
Large cell	10

SQUAMOUS CELL CARCINOMA (Figs. 28.13, 28.14)

Gross appearance

(i) Most often it is located near hilum, arising in large bronchi (Fig. 28.13).

(ii) The tumour is firm and whitish with an irregular infiltrating outline.

(iii) It often shows areas of haemorrhage and necrosis.

Squamous metaplasia, hyperplasia and atypical proliferative changes of bronchial epithelium are more frequent in cigarette smokers. Squamous cell carcinoma is associated with cigarette smoking and arises most frequently from major bronchi near hilum.

Histology

It shows characteristic squamous cell carcinoma (Fig. 28.14) but tend to vary widely in degree of differentiation.

SMALL CELL (OAT CELL) CARCINOMA

Gross appearance

The tumour is small, located almost always centrally having necrosis and haemorrhage.

Histology

Section (Fig. 28.15) shows small, tightly packed, darkly stained, ovoid tumour cells that are somewhat larger than lymphocytes and have darkly staining nuclei and very scant cytoplasm.

Ultrastructural features and hormonal secretion (ACTH, HCG, ADH) suggest that the tumour arises from argyrophilic cells belonging to the APUD system. These are rapidly metastasing tumours.

Oat cell is believed to originate from pulmonary neuroendocrine cells normally scattered within the bronchial mucosa.

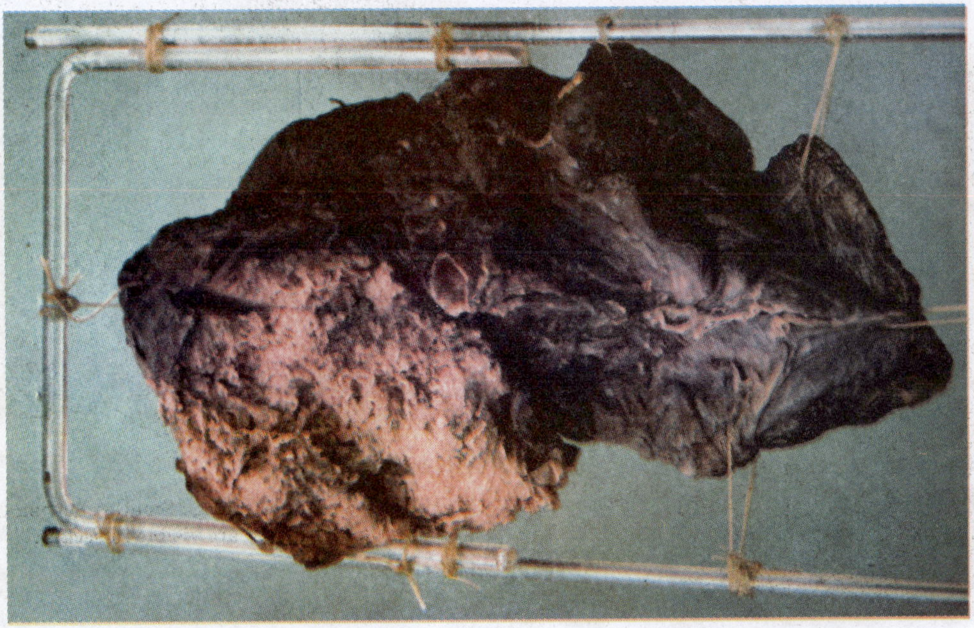

Fig. 28.13. Primary squamous cell carcinoma of bronchus arising near hilum

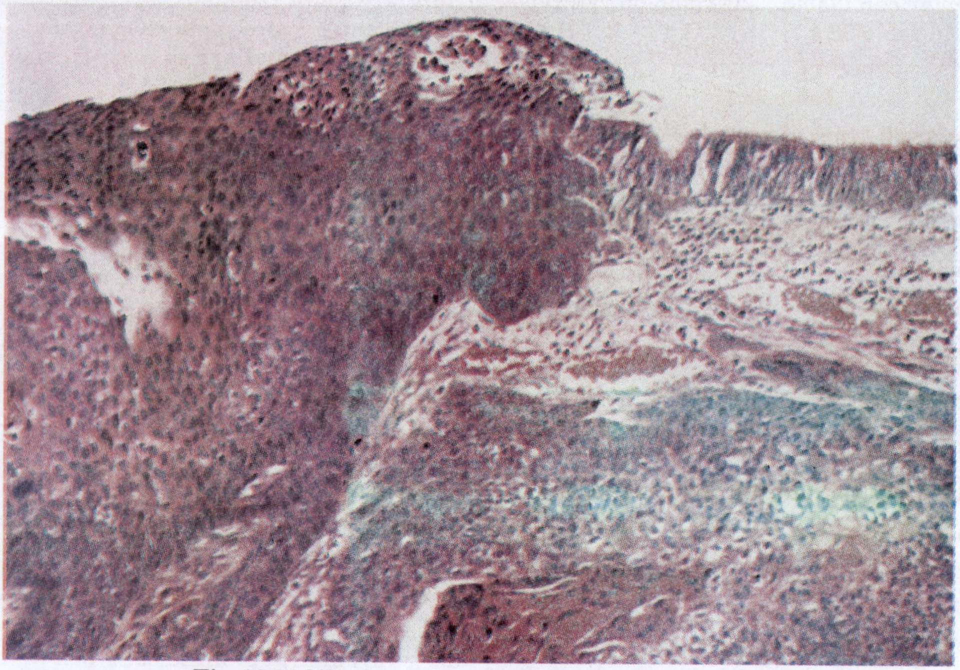

Fig. 28.14. ME : Squamous cell carcinoma of lung (× 200)

METASTATIC CARCINOMA LUNG

Metastatic deposits in the lung may be derived from breast, GIT, genito-urinary tract (uterus, prostate, kidney), malignant melanoma and sarcoma of bone.

Gross appearance

Secondary deposits are often multiple (Fig. 28.16) and bilateral. Patients often do not have respiratory symptoms, and diagnosis is made by radiological examination.

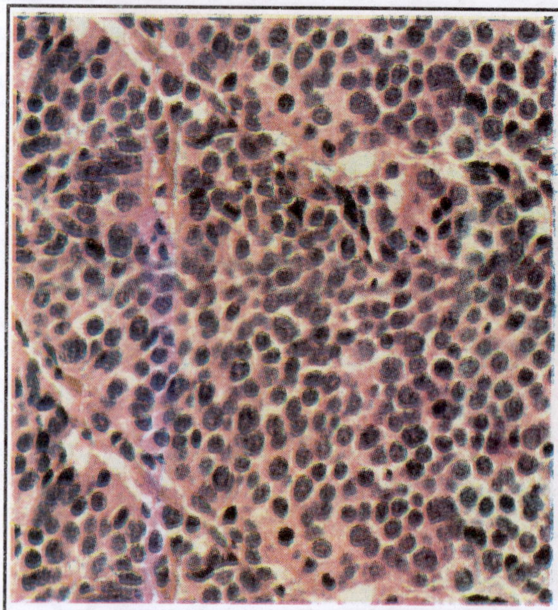

Fig. 28.15. ME : Oat cell carcinoma (× 200)

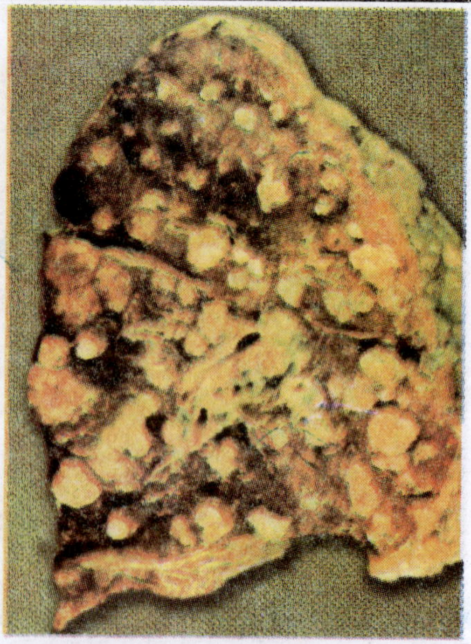

Fig. 28.16. Metastatic carcinoma in lung

Chapter 29

Alimentary System

ORAL TISSUES

Many benign and malignant tumours may arise in the oral tissues, the most common lesions include squamous cell carcinoma of lips, oral mucosa and tongue. Salivary gland tumours, both benign — pleomorphic salivary adenoma (Fig. 29.1), adenolymphoma, and malignant tumour (adenocystic carcinoma) are relatively common.

BENIGN PLEOMORPHIC ADENOMA (MIXED TUMOUR) OF SALIVARY GLAND

The tumour occurs most commonly in the parotid gland, more common in women. It has an epithelial and mesenchymal element. It is round, often irregular in shape and poorly circumscribed. It is surrounded by a thin capsule that may form a cleavage plane between the tumour and surrounding gland.

Histology (Fig. 29.1)

(i) Section shows well stained neoplastic glandular epithelia and

(ii) Pale blue loose connective myxomatous tissuc stroma somewhat resembling cartilage.

(iii) There is a thin capsule outside indicating the circumscribed nature of the tumour.

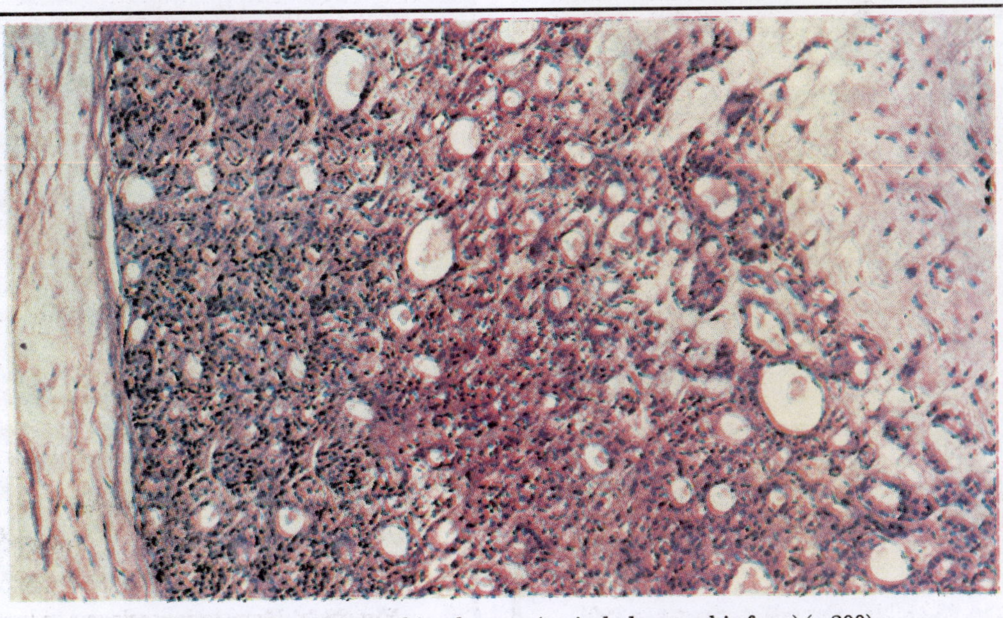

Fig. 29.1. Benign pleomorphic adenoma (typical pleomorphic form) (× 200)

Occasionally the tumour is entirely made of glandular component without any myxomatous stromal component, this variety is referred to as *monomorphic salivary adenoma*.

OESOPHAGUS

Lower oesophagus often becomes inflamed as a result of gastric acid reflux that may produce either oesophagitis or chronic peptic ulcer.

Most common neoplasm of oesophagus is squamous cell carcinoma (Fig. 29.2). Adenocarcinoma may occasionally arise in metaplastic glandular epithelium at lower end of oesophagus.

Macroscopy appearance

(i) A diffuse infiltrative type of growth in lower third of oesophagus.

(ii) Oesophageal stenosis is produced due to abundant connective tissue reaction.

STOMACH

Histology : Stomach is made of four layers with gastric type of mucosa. Gastric pits in mucosa are lined by columnar mucous secreting cells. Crypts show chief cells with pale cytoplasm and parietal cells (oxyphil cells with pink granular cytoplasm).

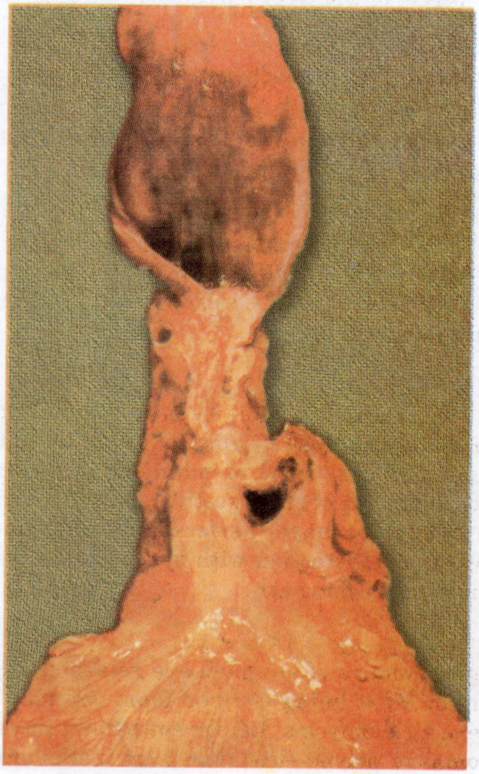

Fig. 29.2. Stenosing squamous cell carcinoma of oesophagus (of lower third)

GASTRITIS

Inflammation of the stomach is called gastritis and is of two types :

(i) *Acute gastritis* : It is associated with aspirin or anti-inflammatory drugs, excessive alcohol and severe stress.

(ii) *Chronic gastritis* : It is associated with both autoimmune causation and several well established environmental factors. *Helicobacter pylori* is an important cause of gastritis as well as of gastric ulcer.

CHRONIC PEPTIC ULCER

Sites : Peptic ulcers develop in areas exposed to acid-pepsin secretion : duodenum, stomach, lower part of oesophagus, jejunum at the site of gastrojejunostomy, or rarely in the ileum adjacent to Meckel's diverticulum.

Pathogenesis : Action of acid pepsin gastric content causes necrosis of surface epithelium, possibly resulting from loss of normal protective surface barrier.

In addition to the action of acid and pepsin, *Helicobacter pylori* infection of antral and duodenal (1st part) mucosa serves as an important predisposing factor. In most instances of gastric and duodenal ulcers, there is an associated antral gastritis caused by *H. pylori.* Thus, irritant gastric secretion reaches submucosal tissue which leads to formation of *acute ulcer* (punched out ulcer involving mucosa and submucosa). Most often the destructive process is arrested by an acute inflammatory response which dilutes and buffers the toxic effects of acid-gastric secretions and limits tissue damage. However, gastric acid may cause continuing tissue destruction, and concurrent organisation and repair may go on. A dynamic balance between tissue damage and repair is reflected in *chronic peptic* ulcer. When the reparative responses weaken, the ulcer progresses with risk of perforation of stomach wall.

CHRONIC GASTRIC ULCER

Chronic gastric ulcer is usually single, 90% are situated in lesser curvature within the antrum or at the junction between body and antral mucosa,

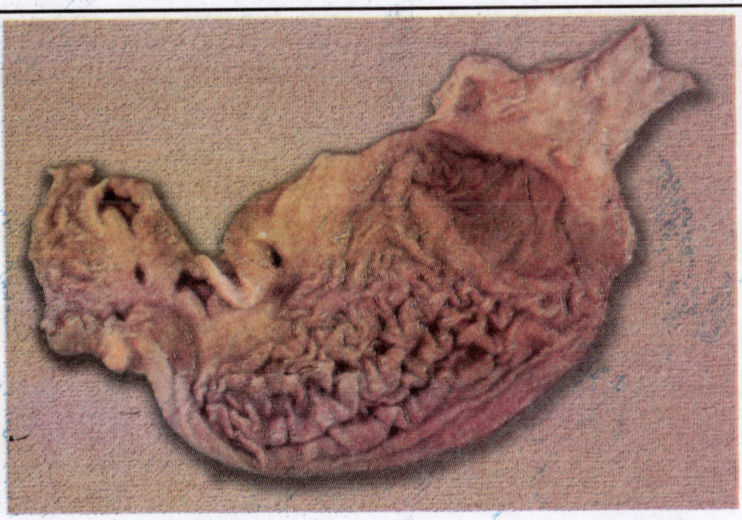

Fig. 29.3. Multiple peptic ulcer of lesser curvature areas of cardia and duodenum of stomach

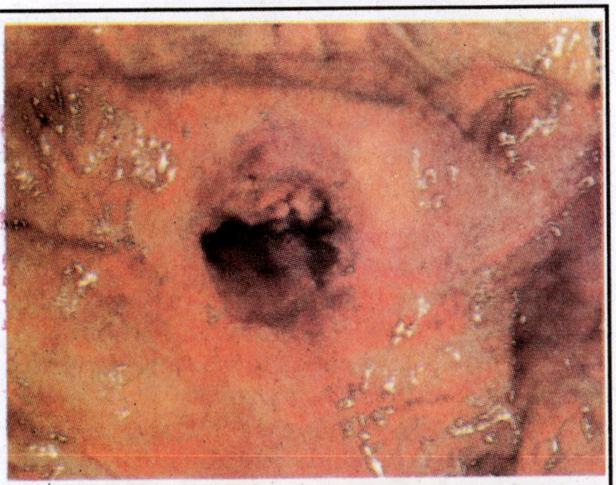

Fig. 29.4. Peptic gastric ulcer at lesser curvature of stomach penetrating pancreas

and only a few occur near the cardiac end close to junction with the oesophagus.

Macroscopic appearance (Figs. 29.3 & 29.4)

1. It is indurated, deep, punched out (or funnel shaped).
2. Base of ulcer is covered by roughened necrotic material.
3. Ulcer bed is usually brownish due to the presence of digested blood.
4. Surrounding mucosa is reddened due to hyperemia.
5. Variable degrees of fibrosis and distortion develop.
6. Margin of the ulcer is regular.

Histology (Figs. 29.5 & 29.6)

(1) Mucosal and muscle layers end abruptly at the edge of ulcer.

(2) Base is composed of fibrous scar tissue, muscle layers are usually completely gone.

(3) Over the fibrous base there are successive layers of granulation tissue, necrotic and hyalinised materials and inflammatory exudate.

(4) Blood vessels in base show intimal thickening and narrowing.

Complications

Spontaneous healing has been described and confirmed by autopsy findings (Figs 29.5, 29.6). The use of drugs seems to enhance the healing with cicatrization of many gastric ulcers. Sequelae include haemorrhage, perforation, malignant change, scar contraction with pyloric stenosis or deformity of the stomach.

TUMOURS OF STOMACH

Benign tumours of stomach are relatively uncommon. Most being derived from connective tissue, e.g., leiomyoma. Benign epithelial tumours adenomas or polyps—less than 2 cm in diameter, are occasionally seen. Malignant tumours of stomach are common and ranks as the fourth commonest tumour in females and third in males.

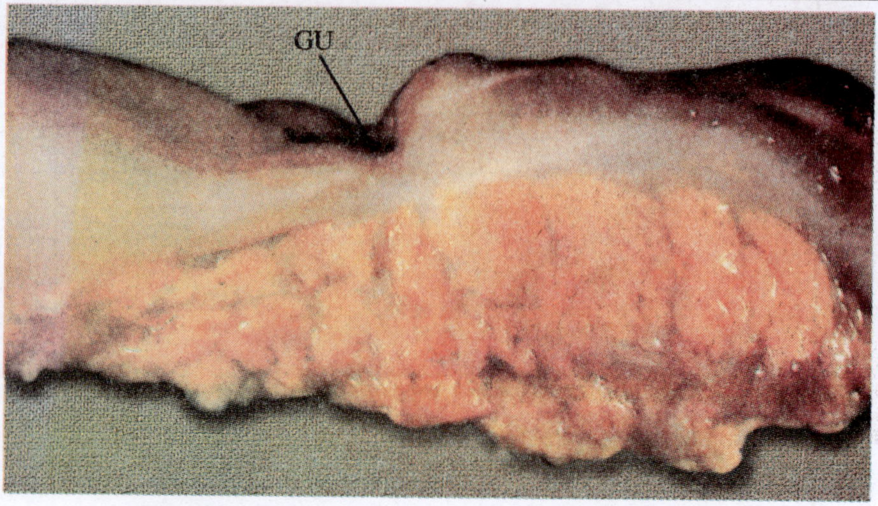

Fig. 29.5. Healed peptic gastric ulcer (GU) by cicatrization

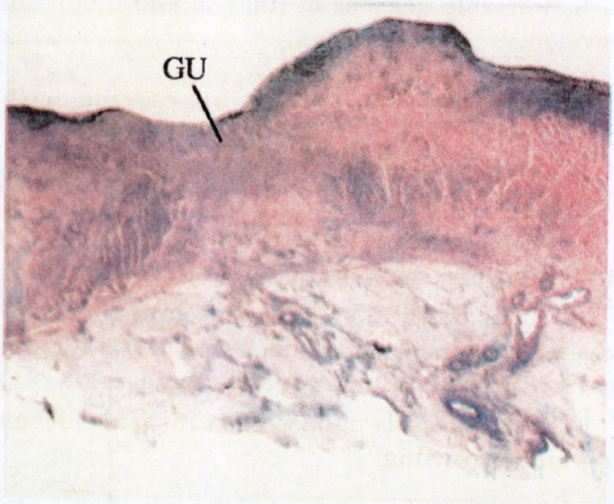

Fig. 29.6. Peptic gastric ulcer (GU) healed by cicatrization : Sclerotic bed of ulcer penetrating to serosa

CARCINOMA OF STOMACH

Site : Almost 60% gastric cancers occur at pylorus, 20% in body and 5–15% in cardiac region.

Gastric dysplasia : It is a precancerous lesion and recognised by cytological changes in the epithelial cells.

Early gastric cancer : It is defined as a cancer confined to the mucosa or mucosa and submucosa, regardless of the metastasis in lymph node. Such lesions represent only a depressed area and diagnosed by biopsy during gastroscopy.

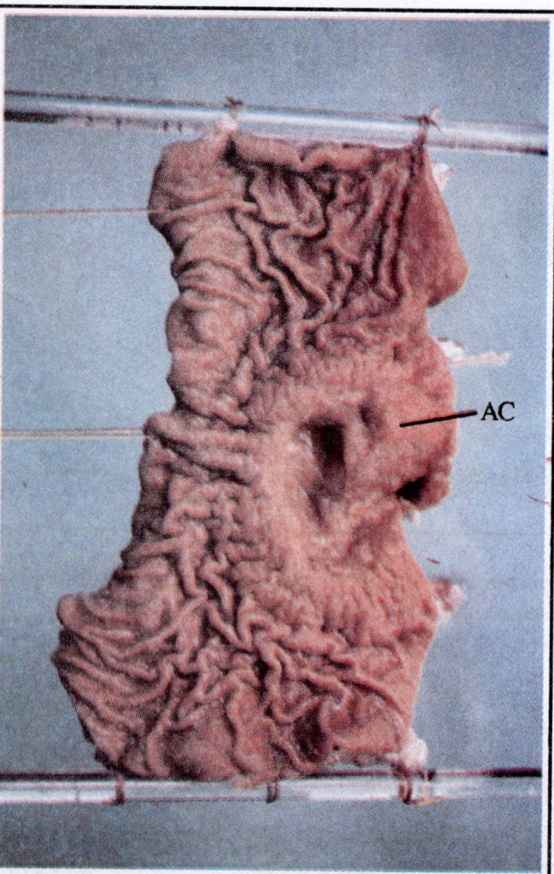

Fig. 29.7. Gastric adenocarcinoma (AC) with plaque-like penetrating growth (ulcerative carcinoma)

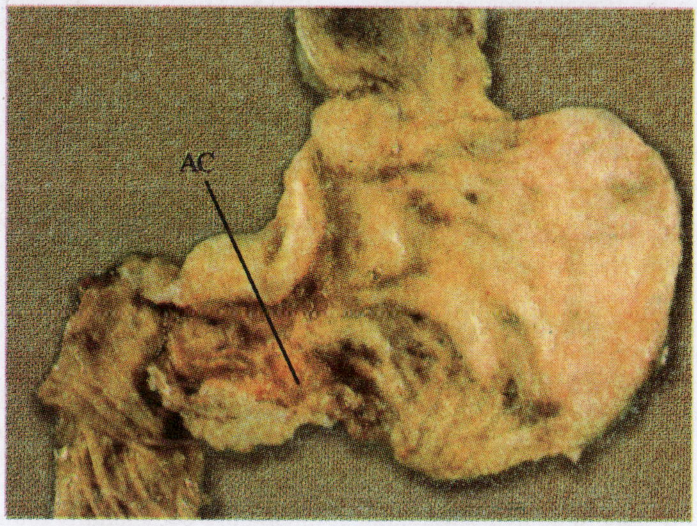

Fig. 29.8. Mucous adenocarcinoma (AC) of stomach with peritoneal invasion

Gastric carcinoma

Macroscopically several types are described :

1. Fungating polypoid tumour (Fig. 29.9).
2. Carcinoma with diffuse infiltration (scirrhous carcinoma) which may be localised (in pylorus) or diffuse. In diffuse type (Fig. 29.10), stomach is reduced in size with a thickened firm wall (leather bottle stomach or *linitis plastica*).
3. Mucoid carcinoma (Fig. 29.8).
4. Superficial spreading carcinoma.
5. Ulcerative or penetrating carcinoma (Fig. 29.7).

Microscopically, carcinoma of stomch are adenocarcinomas arising from mucous-secreting and glandular cells, with varying degrees of differentiation. Mucous production may occur in

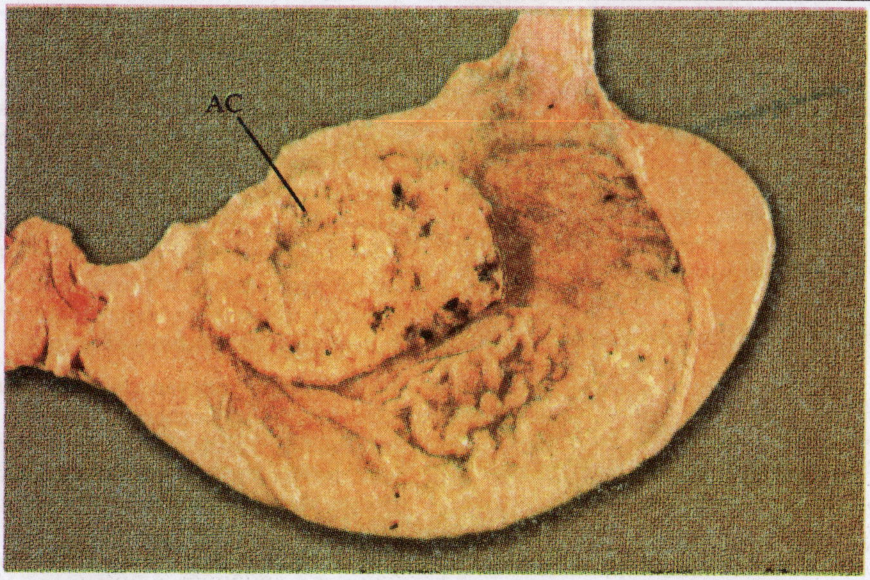

Fig. 29.9. Adenocarcinoma (AC) of the body of stomach (polypoid growth on posterior wall)

any variety but when the tumour predominantly contains translucent and gelatinous areas, it is called *mucoid carcinoma* (Fig. 29.8). Mucous accumulates in cytoplasm of tumour cells that displaces and flattens the nucleus of the cell, producing signet ring appearance.

Fungating polypoid carcinoma (Fig. 29.9)

It is a soft bulky tumour (Fig. 29.9) projecting into the cavity of the stomach. Necrosis is common and the surface is often ulcerated and infected, and it tends to bleed easily. It remains superficial for a considerable time but eventually penetrates the muscle wall and spreads to adjacent structures. It is usually a typical adenocarcinoma.

Ulcerative or penetrating carcinoma (Fig. 29.7)

It is the most frequent form of gastric carcinoma (30%). It appears as a large shallow ulcer and bowl shaped. The margins are irregular, raised and covered by neoplastic vegetations (nodules).

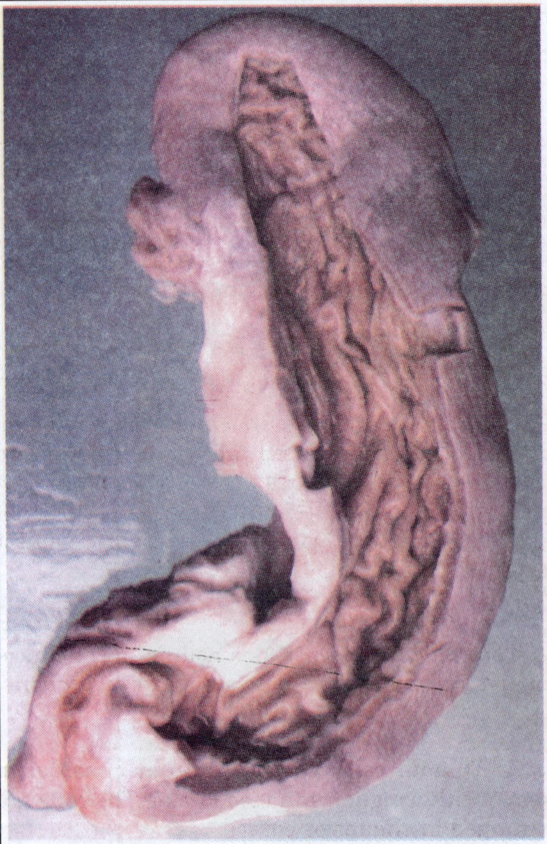

Fig. 29.10. Adenocarcinoma of stomach with diffuse infiltration of stomach (linitis plastica)

Diffuse spreading or infiltrating (Scirrhous) carcinoma (Fig. 29.10)

The tumour appears to arise from deeper glands and the surface is not involved. The tumour (Fig. 29.10) grows by infiltrating the gastric wall without endoluminal expansion, sometimes extending to the whole stomach (called *linitis plastica*). The stomach is reduced in size with a thickened firm wall. Rugae are prominent. *Histologically* malignant cells in groups are found in the midst of abundant connective tissue stroma.

SMALL INTESTINE AND APPENDIX

Primary tumours of small intestine and appendix are very rare with exception of carcinoid tumour. Appendicitis is an acute inflammation and is very common (Fig. 29.11). Leiomyosarcoma and lymphoma are occasionally found in ileum.

Structure of Intestine and colon

Macroscopic identification

(i) *Small intestine* has narrower lumen, mucosal folds are perpendicular to long axis and there is mesenteric attachment.

(ii) *Large intestine / colon* possesses wider lumen. There are three straps of taenia coli on serosal surface with flat band or strip of soft tissue along their borders (appendices epiploicae) and sacculation or bulges of the wall between taenia.

Histology : Both small and large intestine show four layers :

(a) *Small intestinal mucosa* shows villi on the surface which extend into the lumen as finger-like projections covered by epithelial cells. Between the bases of the villi, there are pit-like crypts of Liberkuhn which contain stem cells that replenish and regenerate the epithelium. Surface of epithelium of crypt contain three cell types : *columnar* epithelial cells of microvilli (absorptive cells), interspersed between absorptive cells are mucous secreting *Goblet cells* with eosinophilic cytoplasm and *Paneth* cells at the base of crypts.

(b) *Colonic mucosa* : Unlike mucosa of small intestine, colonic mucosa is devoid of villi and is flat. Surface epithelium is of columnar absorptive cells, have shorter and less abundant microvilli. Crypts have abundant Goblet cells. Paneth cells are occasionally present.

ACUTE APPENDICITIS

Aetiology — See Chapter 25 (p. 193).

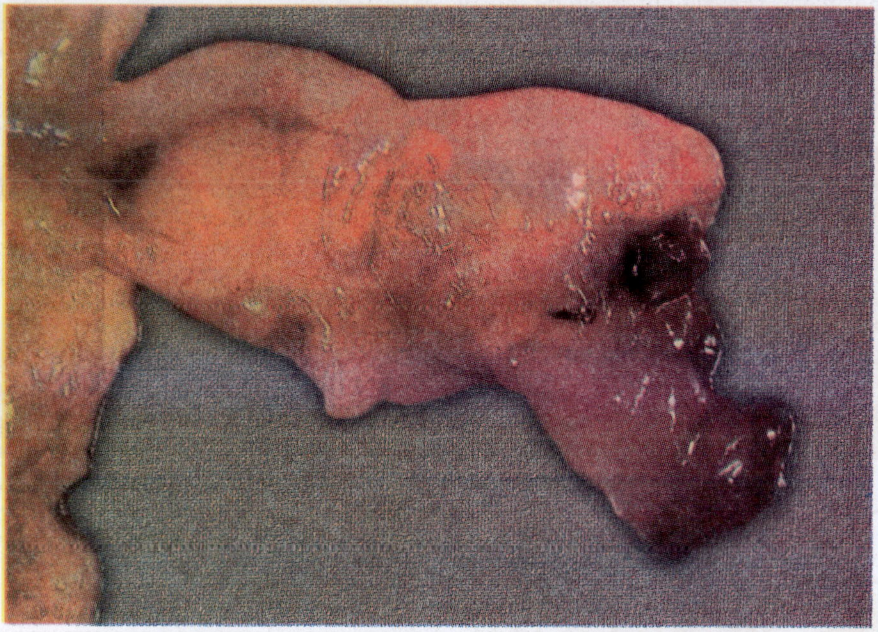

Fig. 29.11. Recurrent acute appendicitis with perforation

Gross appearance (Fig. 29.11)

1. Appendix is swollen.
2. Serosal blood vessels are congested.
3. Surface of serosa is dull-looking due to deposition of fibrin or purulent exudate.
4. Muscular walls are thick and oedematous.
5. Lumen : Mucosal surface is swollen, congested and may show areas of haemorrhage and ulceration.
6. Lumen may be obstructed by faecolith (firm dried faecal concretion), lymphoid tissue or calculus.

Figure 29.11 is that of recurrent acute appendicitis with perforation. The form of appendicitis gives rise to acute attacks of pain every few months, and majority of them end in severe acute attacks. Such type of appendicitis is also called subacute appendicitis, and appendix in most of these cases show obliterative appendicitis.

For microscopic features refer Figs. 25.2, 25.3.

Mucocele : Complete obstruction of the proximal portion of the appendix sometimes results in dilatation (mucocele) of the distal part. It may be :

(a) *Benign mucocele* : Mild infection may cause obstruction leading to retention of secreted mucus.

(b) *Malignant mucocele* : Progressive distension of appendix occurs by mucus secreted by mucus secreting tumour cells, e.g., mucinous cystadenocarcinoma of appendix. The rupture of the mucocele may give rise to *(pseudo) myxoma peritonei,* although it is more commonly due to ovarian mucinous cystadenocarcinoma of ovary.

CARCINOID TUMOUR OF APPENDIX

Carcinoid tumours arise from mucosal neuroendocrine APUD cells (amine precursor uptake and decarboxylation) and are normally found in thyroid, parathyroid, adrenal medulla and paraganglionic tissue. Carcinoid tumours are commonest in appendix and small bowel.

Macroscopic Examination (Fig. 29.12)

The tumour presents as a nodule in the mucosa and submucosa. Cut surface looks yellowish.

Histologically (Fig. 29.13)

(i) Tumour cells are polygonal or cuboidal in shape with irregular rounded nuclei. The cells are arranged in clumps or cords.

(ii) The cytoplasm of tumour cells is brightly pink and granular.

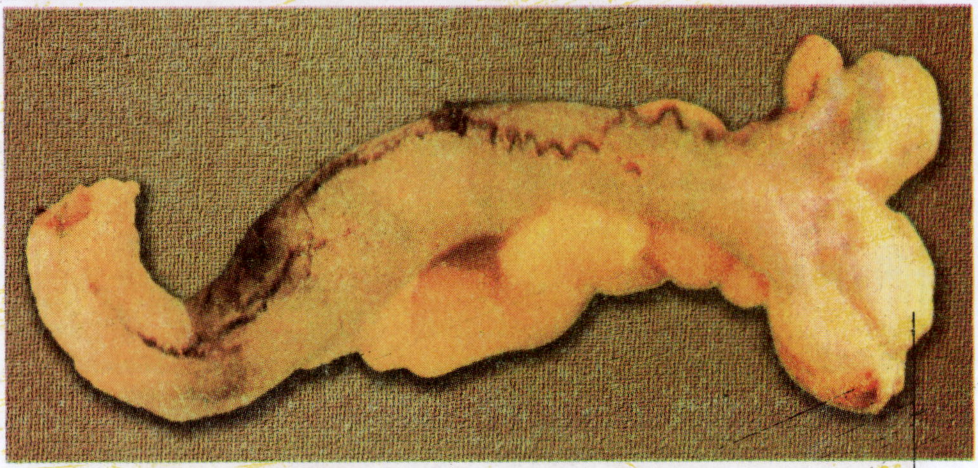

Fig. 29.12. Carcinoid tumour of appendix (C)

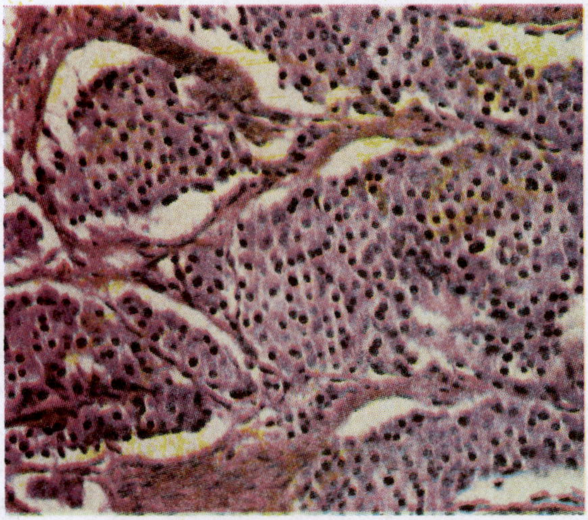

Fig. 29.13. Carcinoid tumour (× 300)

ENTERITIS

TYPHOID ULCER

The lower ileum and caecum, where lymphoid tissue is most abundant, are affected by *S. typhi* but lesions may be found in jejunum and colon.

Pathogenesis

Following ingestion of salmonellae with food or drink, there is invasion of intestinal lymphoid follicle and proliferation of bacteria. The phase lasts for 2 weeks and is virtually asymptomatic. Then bacteraemia follows. After a few days of bacteraemia, the bacteria localise in lymphoid tissue of small intestine, mesenteric nodes, gall bladder, liver and spleen. The typical lesion is in the *Peyer's patches* and follicles.

Gross appearance (Fig. 29.14)

(i) *Lesions* : The Peyer's patches swell at first, then tiny necrotic areas slough off, leaving small

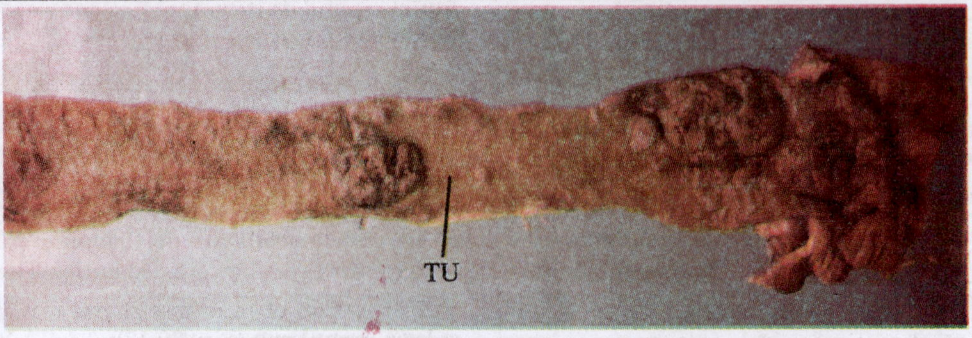

Fig. 29.14. Salmonella : Multiple typhoid ulcers (TU) in small intestine

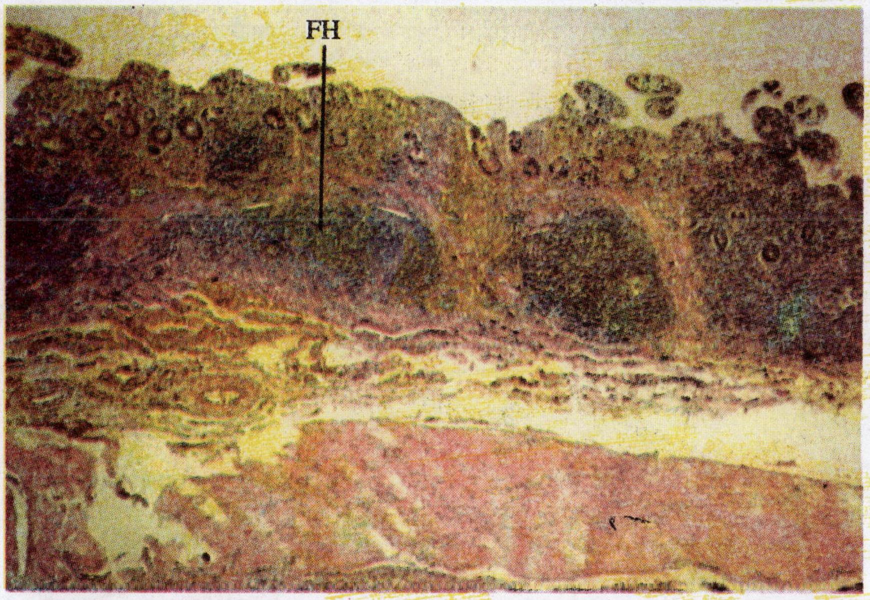

Fig. 29.15. Salmonella enteritis : lymphatic follicular hyperplasia (FH) (HE × 10)

ulcers that, by their coalescence, form rounded areas of ulceration having the size, shape and situation of Peyer's patches.

(ii) Long axis of ulcers is in the direction of long axis of bowel, which in contrast encircle the gut in tuberculous ulcer.

(iii) The ulcers are brownish-black with undermined edges.

(iv) The ulcers only involve the mucosa and submucosa, but deeper extension and perforation may occur.

Microscopy (Fig. 29.15) : There is lymphoid follicular hyperplasia in early stage and then the lymphoid tissue shows necrosis, which is infiltrated by large mononuclear cells and plasma cells.

Complications : Haemorrhage, perforation may occur at the end of 2nd week. Septicemic complications, e.g., cholecystitis, pneumonia, myocarditis, arthritis, osteomyelitis and meningitis may develop.

Other salmonellosis

The lesions produced by *S. paratyphi* A, *S. paratyphi* B, *S. enteritidis* and *S. typhimurium* resemble pathological changes of typhoid fever but are much less severe and are commonly limited to a small portion of the bowel. Frequently, there is an absence of ulceration.

Tuberculosis

Aetiology : (i) Intestinal tuberculosis may be primary, the organisms being ingested with milk or other food. (ii) More commonly, it is secondary which generally follows a pulmonary infection due to swallowing of infected sputum.

Morphological types

The lesion is most common in lower ileum and from there extends upward to upper ileum and downward to colon. **Macroscopically**, there are two forms :

1. Ulcerative

It is mainly seen in secondary tuberculosis, but primary infection due to ingestion of infected and unpasteurised cow's milk may occur. The lesions start in the Peyer's patches and solitary lymphoid follicles, and yellow areas of caseous necrosis develop in mucosa and submucosa.

***Macroscopically* (Fig. 29.16)**

(i) Ragged ulcer develops following sloughing of the necrotic material.

(ii) Since the lesions extend by lymphatic vessels, which encircle the gut, the lesions are transverse in location.

Microscopic features

HE section of intestine shows typical tuberculosis granuloma (Fig. 29.17).

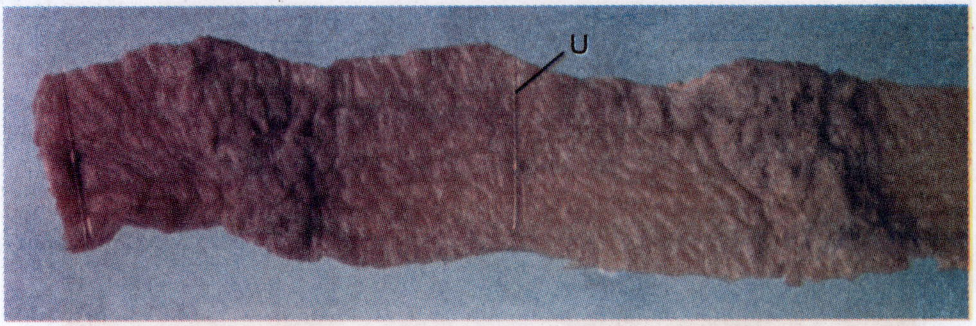

Fig. 29.16. Intestinal tuberculosis : transverse ulcers (U) of ileum

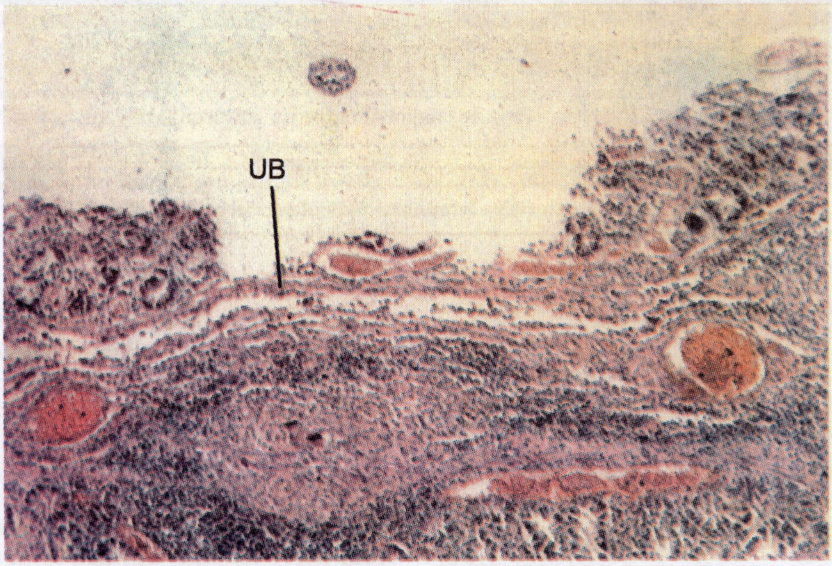

Fig. 29.17. Tuberculosis granuloma on ulcerated bed (UB) of ileum (HE × 12)

2. Hyperplastic

Occasionally, tuberculosis occurs in marked thickening of wall of caecum and ascending colon with fibrosis extending to the surrounding structures. There is irregular ulceration and caseation in the mucosa which extends into the wall. Pulmonary lesion is usually present in these cases. *Histologically* the two forms are similar.

Crohn's disease (Regional enteritis)

Crohn's disease (Crohn, 1932) is a chronic non-tuberculous, granulomatous disease affecting terminal 10-20 cm of colon but may be found in any part of the alimentary tract from mouth to anus.

Aetiology : Aetiology is unknown but several potential factors have been considered which include various bacterial and viral agents and hypersensitivity.

Gross appearance (Fig. 29.18) : The wall of GIT is greatly thickened, especially in the sub-mucosa with corresponding stenosis of the lumen, mucosal ulceration and enlargement of mesenteric lymph nodes.

Histology : It is a non-caseating granuloma and consists of focal aggregates of epitheloid cells and giant cells in the involved intestine and mesenteric lymph node.

LARGE INTESTINE

Bacillary dysentery (Shigella infections)

It is an acute inflammation of large intestine caused by shigella endotoxin which has a local

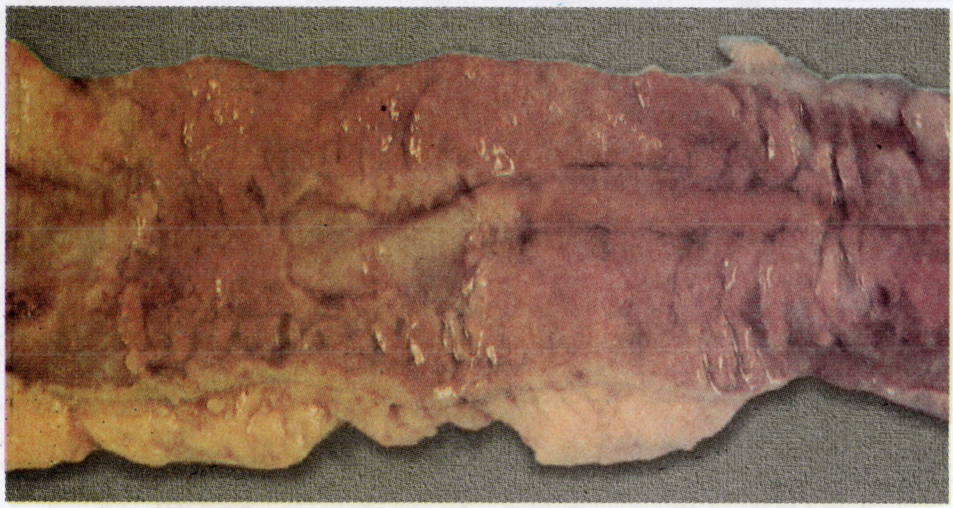

Fig. 29.18. Crohn's disease (regional enteritis) in terminal ileum

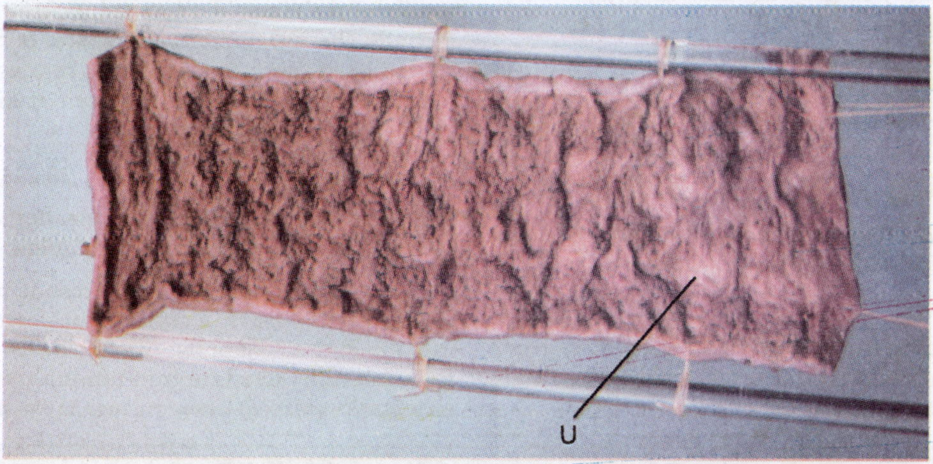

Fig. 29.19. Bacillary dysentery (U) in large intestine (colon)

effect on mucosa (loss of epithelium and abscess formation). The bacteria invade mucosal cells but do not go beyond lamina propria. Severity of illness depends on the type of infecting species of shigella. *S. shigae* (*S. dysenteriae* type 1) causes most severe and fulminating form of dysentery which produces exotoxin in addition to endotoxin. The exotoxin acts as enterotoxin and neurotoxin. *S. sonnei* causes mild form and *S. flexneri* and *S. boydii* cause moderate type of acute inflammation.

Histologically

(i) There is necrosis and desquamation of surface layers.

(ii) The ulcer surface is then covered by a pseudomembrane made of fibrin, leucocytes, cell debris, necrosed epithelia and bacteria.

Macroscopic appearance (Fig. 19.19)

(i) The ulcers are usually shallow, not undermined and vary in size and shape (Fig. 29.19).

(ii) The small ulcers coalesce forming large ulcers leaving only occasional islands of intact mucosa on gut wall.

Amoebic Dysentery

Amoebiasis usually involves colon, especially caecum, but may be found as far down as anal canal and above to terminal ileum. Cysts of *E. histolytica* ingested with food and drink reach

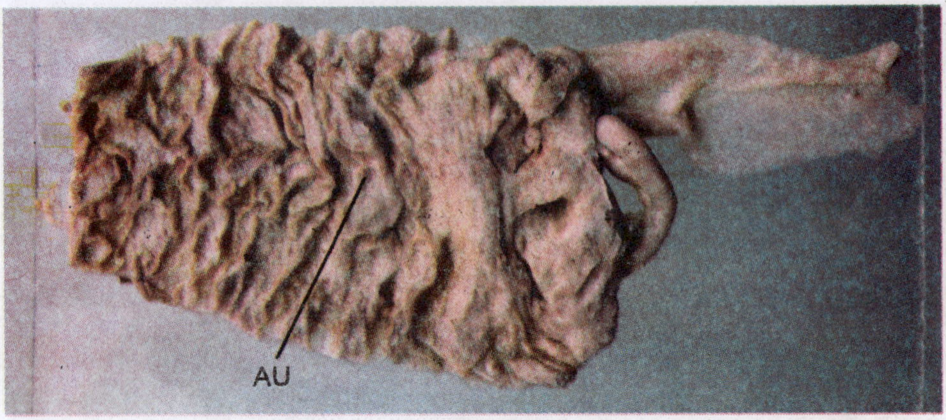

Fig. 29.20. Amoebic ulcer (AU) in wall of colon

colon, where vegetative trophozoite forms emerge from the cysts. Some amoeba invade mucous membrane of large bowel by the aid of digestive enzymes and spread and multiply in submucosa. By digesting the submucosa, the blood supply to the mucosa is cut off causing necrosis. Then ulcers are formed and finally large areas may be denuded of mucosa.

Gross appearance (Fig. 29.20)

The ulcers are flask-shaped, vary greatly in size and are surrounded by healthy mucosa.

Histology

It is a necrotic process with modest cellular reaction rich with granulocytes, with pathognomic finding of amoebae.

Ulcerative Colitis (UC)

It is an inflammatory condition of the mucosa, primarily of the sigmoid colon and rectum. Although initially the inflammation is acute. It becomes a typically chronic disease with remissions and relapses. The aetiology is unknown. It may be due to hyperimmune state.

Macroscopic features (Fig. 29.21)

These are large ulcerations beginning in rectum and extending to sigmoid colon.

(a) ***Acute stage*** : (i) The mucosa is congested. (ii) Abscess appears in crypts which contain polymorphs and eosinophils. (iii) With the spread of inflammatory exudate into lamina propria, the abscesses coalesce. Then mucosa is destroyed and

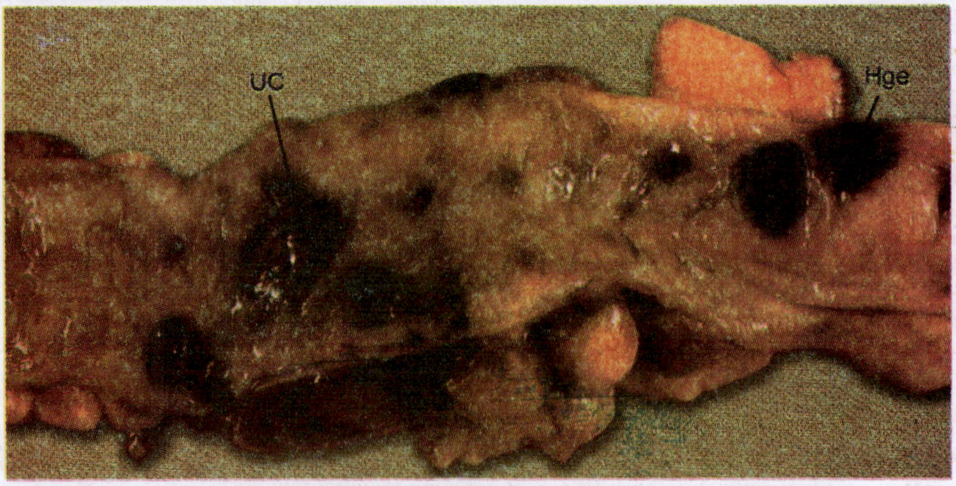

Fig. 29.21. Ulcerative colitis (colon) (UC) with intraparietal haemorrhage

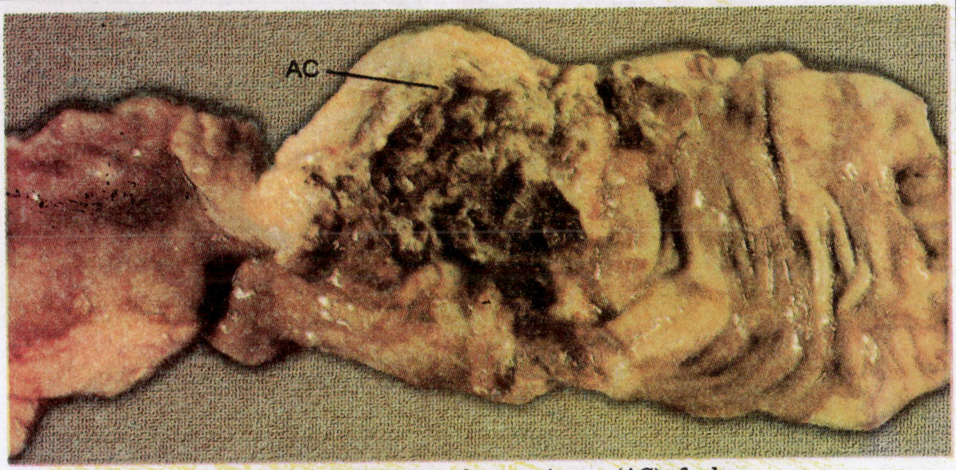

Fig. 29.22. Infiltrative adenocarcinoma (AC) of colon

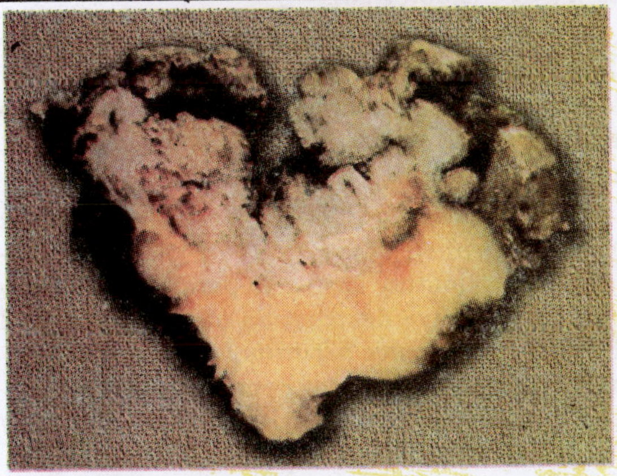

Fig. 29.23. Fungating polypoid carcinoma of colon

ulcer forms. (iv) The ulcer extends into submucosa but no further. (v) The base is formed by granulation tissue which contains large number of plasma cells. (vi) The surviving islands of oedematous and congested mucosa are called Wechselmann's pseudopolyps.

(b) *Periods of remission* occur when many of the ulcerated areas heal, but the crypts of Leiberkuhn do not reform completely. Ultimately the surface may be covered by a simple layer of mucus secreting epithelium without glands. In indolent *chronic disease*, progressive mucosal atrophy occurs.

COLORECTAL CARCINOMA

Malignant epithelial tumours are found frequently in large intestine and in particular in rectum and colon.

Macroscopic types

1. *Fungating polypoid carcinoma (Fig. 29.23)* :
   (i) It is found mainly in colon and appendix.
   (ii) Margin of attachment is irregular.
   (iii) Most often cauliflower type of growth.
2. *Infiltrative (or ulcerative) (Fig. 29.22)* : It is composed of a rigid ulcerated plaque with raised border, predominant in colon and ileum.

Microscopic types

1. Adenocarcinoma — most frequent;
2. Squamous carcinoma — rare tumour;
3. Undifferentiated carcinoma.

Histology (Fig. 29.24)

1. Section shows well defined glandular pattern.
2. The tumour has infiltrated into submucosa.
3. Moderately well differentiated adenocarcinoma.

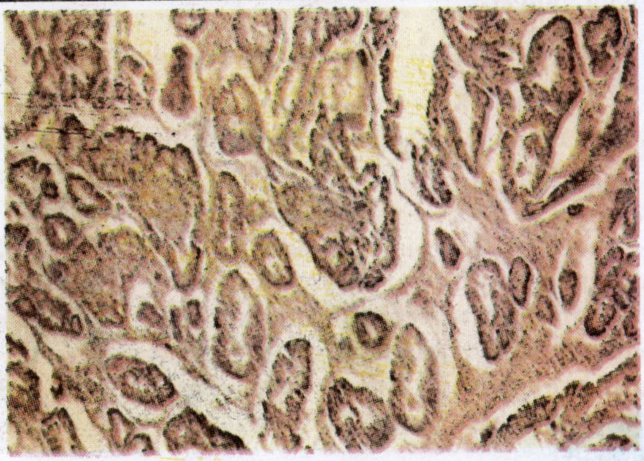

Fig. 29.24. Adenocarcinoma of colon (× 100)

Chapter 30

Liver, Gall Bladder and Pancreas

LIVER

Normal adult liver weighs 1400 to 1600 gm. It is capsulated, reddish brown in colour and firm in texture. Lobar and lobular venous radicles can be seen on cut surface of liver.

Structure of liver

Classically the liver has been divided into 1-2 mm diameter lobules, each arranged round a central vein (terminal tributaries of hepatic vein), with portal tracts at the periphery of the lobules. Accordingly, hepatocytes in the vicinity of the central vein are called *centrilobular* (or centrolobular) and those near the portal tract are *periportal.*

Recent evidence shows liver as a 3-dimensional structure and the view of lobular pattern is not quite true. Now, the smallest unit of liver is considered as acinus of varying shape. In the acinus, the liver parenchyma is divided into three zones :

(i) Zone–1 closest to vascular supply with good blood supply,

(ii) Zone–2 with a reasonable blood supply and

(iii) Zone–3 with the poorest blood supply which makes it most vulnerable to hypoxia.

Microscopically

Section of liver is diagnosed by : (i) the cords of hepatocytes that are polygonal with abundant pink granular cytoplasm and a central vesicular nucleus with a nucleolus, (ii) portal tracts containing radicles of hepatic artery, portal vein and bile duct are seen, (iii) thin-walled central venous radicle.

Diseases of liver

1. **Sublethal injury** to liver leads to *fatty change* (see chapter 23).

2. **Acute hepatitis** ; Four important causes are — (i) *viral hepatitis,* (ii) *toxins-induced* (e.g., alcohol), (iii) *drug-induced* such as anaesthetic gas halothane and (iv) *systemic infections (Leptospira, Toxoplasma).*

3. **Chronic inflammations of liver** include : (i) *chronic persistent hepatitis* (a prolonged relapsing but self-limiting form of hepatitis without any evidence of active destruction of liver cells, and (ii) *chronic aggressive hepatitis* which is an insidiously progressive form of hepatitis showing evidence of active destruction of liver cells that may lead to cirrhosis and liver failure.

4. **Cirrhosis** : It is the end stage of a variety of chronic liver diseases having the common features of diffuse persistent destruction of hepatocytes, regeneration of hepatocytes to form abnormal nodules and the development of fibrosis.

5. **Other important liver disorders** include : (i) *right-sided heart failure,* (ii) *amyloidosis,* (iii) *inborn errors of metabolism,* (iv) *secondary metastasis* in liver and (v) *primary malignancy (hepatoma).*

Fatty changes in liver

The terms *steatosis* and *fatty change* describe abnormal accumulations of fat *(triglycerides)* in non-fatty tissues, especially within parenchymal cells. Fatty change is often seen in liver because it plays a central role in fat metabolism. However, it also occurs in skeletal muscles, heart and kidney, which have a high metabolic rate.

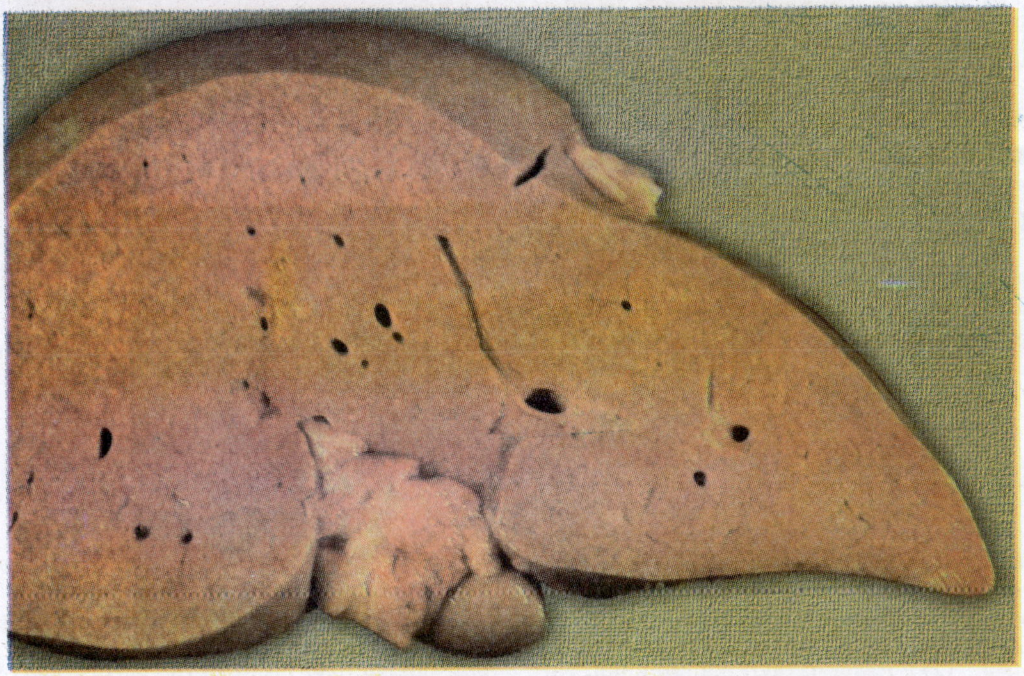

Fig. 30.1. Fatty liver (*cross section*), the liver shows yellow discolouration

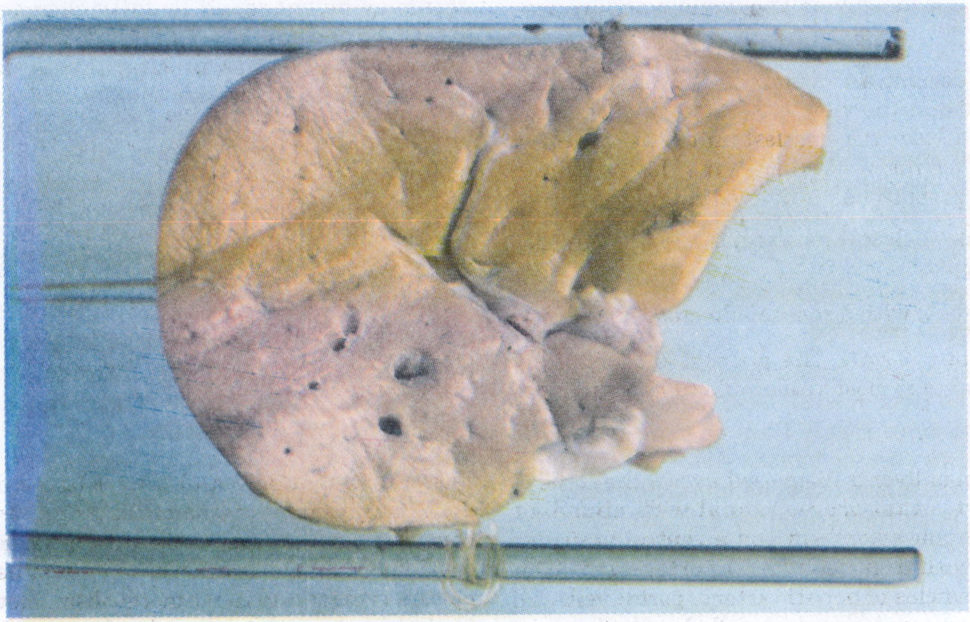

Fig. 30.2. Fatty liver

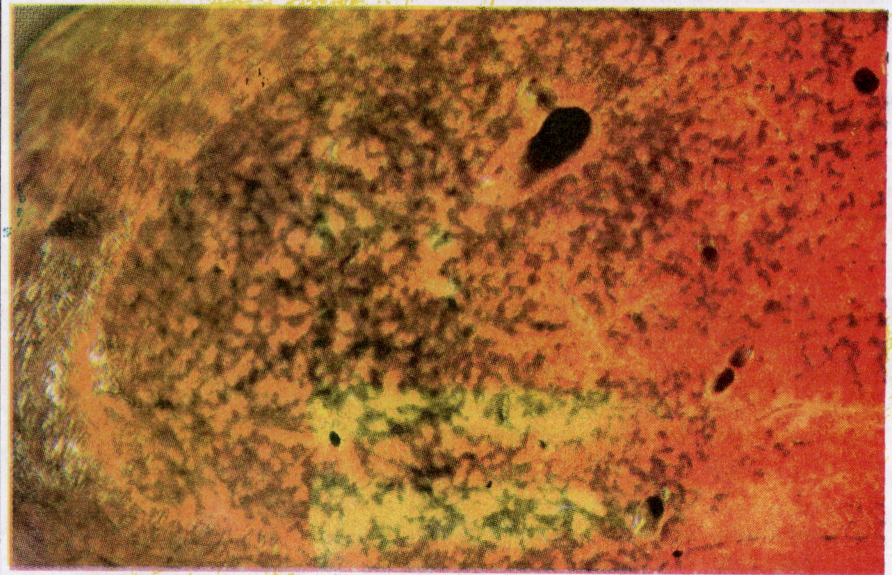

Fig. 30.3. Nutmeg liver (*cut section*) in chronic passive venous congestion

Causes : (1) Lack of oxygen e.g., anemia, cardiac failure. (2) *Poisons, toxins* etc. e.g., alcohol, infection, organic solvents.

Macroscopic appearance (Figs. 30.1, 30.2) : Cross section of the liver shows yellow discoloration (severe fatty change). Mild fatty change may not affect the gross appearance.

M.E. : In HE stained section the fat appears like clear vacuoles in cytoplasm of liver cells (Figs. 23.4A & B)

Special stain : Definite identification for fats is made by special stains such as *Oil Red O and Sudan IV* on frozen sections prepared from either fresh or aqueous formalinised tissues.

Passive Venous Congestion (or passive hyperemia)

Cause : Acute and chronic passive venous congestion of the liver results from *right sided heart failure* or, more rarely from *obstruction of the inferior vena cava* or hepatic vein. It is brought about by diminished venous blood flow from an area and is characterised by dilatations of the veins and capillaries. Passive hyperemia (congestion) may be acute, but is often prolonged, with resultant chronic passive congestion.

Morphology

(a) *Early stage* : Dilatation of central veins and sinusoids of liver occur in the early stage of chronic heart failure.

(b) *Later stage* : Atrophy and disappearance of liver cells occur later which lead to formation of large pools of blood and the architecture around the central vein changes (Fig. 30.3). This may be enhanced by fatty changes at the border of centrilobular atrophy giving a pale colour. This results in alternating dark red (caused by dilated hepatic venules and sinusoids) and yellow (liver cells with fatty change) areas giving the appearance of cut surface of nutmeg (**nutmeg liver**). Long-standing congestion results in so-called cardiac cirrhosis.

Histology : Vide chapter 26 (Fig. 26.46).

Amoebiasis in Liver

Amoebiasis involves mainly colon and is caused by trophozoites of *E. histolytica*. Infection of the liver is a secondary complication of intestinal amoebiasis via portal venous system.

Types

1. **Chronic amoebic hepatitis** : Liver is grossly enlarged with fibrosis and cholestasis. Microscopically, there is mononuclear cell infiltration in portal tracts and within lobules along with epitheloid and giant cells.

2. **Amoebic liver abscess** : It may be single or multiple and have a diameter of few millimetres

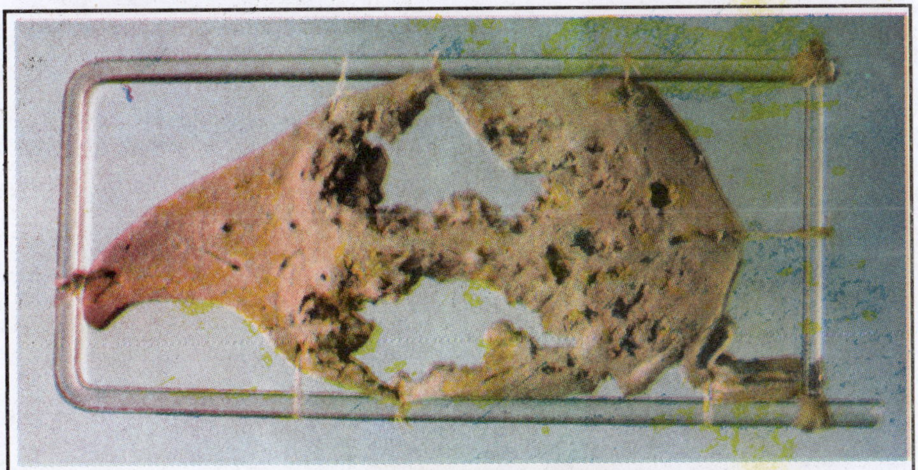

Fig. 30.4. Amoebic liver abscess

to few centimetres. Right lobe is most commonly affected. Central necrosis may be caused by ischaemia secondary to amoebic obstruction of small vessels.

Macroscopic examination (Fig. 30.4)

Wall : Rough and shaggy; in older abscess the wall consists of connective tissue.

Content : Anchovy sauce like (semi-fluid and chocolate coloured) but can be yellow or green. True pus is not present unles secondary bacterial infection occurs.

Microscopic examination

Low grade response of lymphocytes, macrophages and fibroblasts are seen in abscess wall. *E. histolytica* can be seen in the edge of living tissue and in the adjacent necrotic material.

Hydatid disease

It is caused by *Echinococcus granulosus.* Dog is the definitive host of adult worm. Eggs swallowed by intermediate hosts (sheep, cattle, accidentally — man) lead to development of hydatid cysts in various organs and tissues.

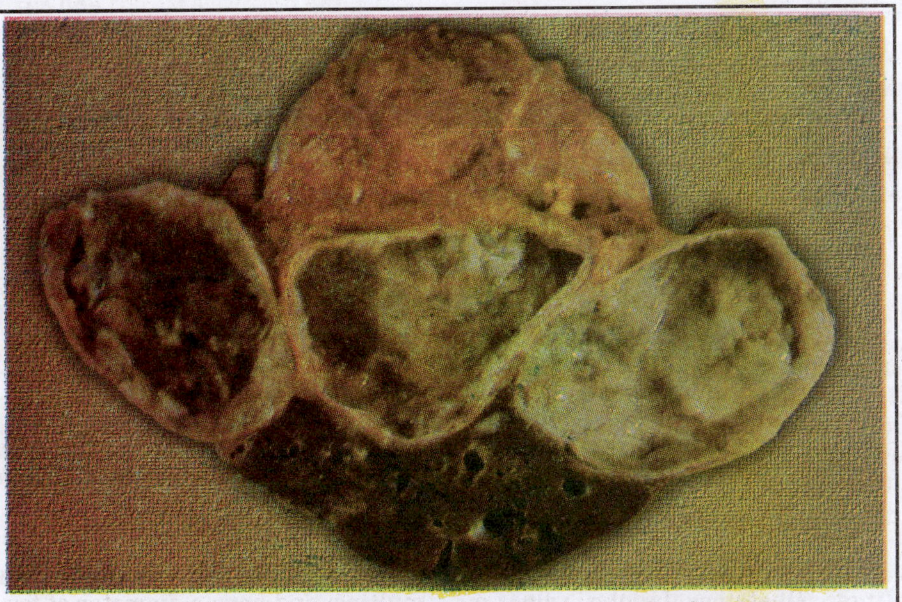

Fig. 30.5. Hydatid disease liver, cut surface showing daughter cysts

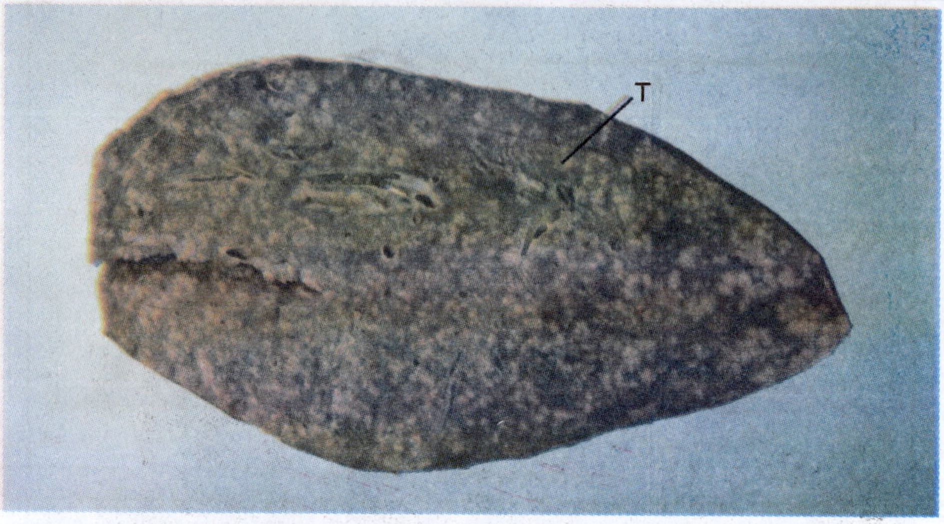

Fig. 30.6. Miliary tuberculosis of liver showing sago-grain-like tuberculosis throughout the liver. T = Tubercle

Sites : Mainly in liver but can be seen in lung, brain, kidney and heart.

Gross examination (Fig. 30.5) : Cyst measures up to 20 to 30 cm in diameter. The cyst is unilocular in case of infection by *E. granulosus*, but multilocular cyst is produced by *E. multilocularis.* The cyst consists of spongy mass of minute irregular cavities. It tends to grow peripherally into adjacent tissue.

Content : Transparent fluid rich in sodium chloride with scolex.

Diagnosis :

(1) *Casoni test* by intradermal injection of sterile hydatid fluid.

(2) Latex agglutination test (negative with calcified cyst).

MILIARY TUBERCULOSIS LIVER

It is a manifestation of systemic dissemination of tubercle bacilli, most prominent in liver, bone marrow, spleen, adrenals, meninges, kidneys, etc.

Macroscopic appearance (Fig. 30.6)

There are small, visible (2-4 mm) foci of yellow-white lesions distributed throughout the liver.

CHRONIC VIRAL HEPATITIS

When acute viral hepatitis does not resolve within six months, it can be assumed that the disease has become chronic (chronic hepatitis).

Classification

There are 4 main causes :

1. *Chronic persistent hepatitis due to persistent hepatitis B, D and C* : The inflammation is confined to portal tracts with predominance of lymphocytes with little or no piece meal necrosis. Lobular architecture is preserved. The condition may last for many years but the prognosis is good and cirrhosis develops in very few patients.
2. *Auto-immune hepatitis* : This occurs especially in young women. Anti-nuclear and anti-smooth muscle antibodies are found in serum of classic type I disease. Liver specific auto-antibodies, e.g., to a sialoglycoprotein receptor (ASGP-R) on periportal hepatocyte cell surface have also been detected. In type II (smaller sub-group), anti-Liver Kidney Microsomal Antibodies (anti-LKM-I) has been found and it is more aggressive.
3. *Drugs* : Methyl dopa, nitrofurantoin.
4. *In metabolic disorders* like α_1 anti-trypsin deficiency, Wilson's disease.

Pathologically all above four are similar conditions and severity varies. A grading system devised by Ishak is followed and the clinical entity is divided in two forms (Table 30.1).

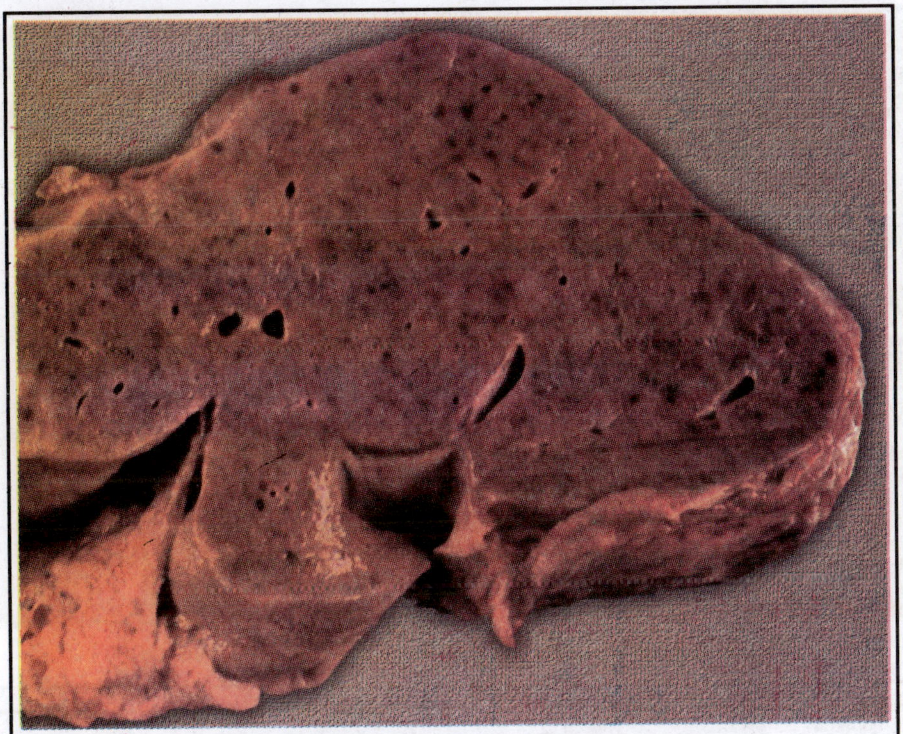

Fig. 30.7. Chronic active hepatitis

Table 30.1 : Ishak's device of subdivision of chronic hepatitis

	Mild	Severe
Former name	Chronic persistent hepatitis	Chronic active hepatitis
Prognosis	Good	Poor if untreated
Type of lesion	Inflammation largely confined to portal tract and limiting plate preserved	Inflammation spills into periportal area.
	Occasional liver cell necrosis	Liver cell necrosis interface hepatitis (piece-meal necrosis)
fibrosis	Usually no fibrosis	There is often

Macroscopically (Fig. 30.7)

(i) Irregularly sized nodules separated by variable but mostly broad scars.

(ii) Such cases progress to post-necrotic cirrhosis.

CIRRHOSIS OF LIVER

Cirrhosis refers to a fibrosis or scarring of the liver that is a progressive and diffuse process; and conversion of the normal architecture into structurally abnormal nodules. The two key elements in diagnosis are :

1. *Fibrosis* : Increase of the connective tissue component.

2. *Diffuse nodular hyperplasia* : Distortion of the lobular architecture by nodules of regenerative or hyperplastic liver parenchyma.

Aetiological classification

1. Alcoholic cirrhosis;
2. Viral cirrhosis, e.g., post-necrotic cirrhosis;
3. Toxins and drugs;
4. Biliary disorders — primary biliary cirrhosis, secondary biliary cirrhosis;
5. Metabolic disease, e.g., haemochromatosis, alpha-1-antitrypsin deficiency, Wilson's disease;
6. Venous outflow obstruction;
7. Indian childhood cirrhosis;
8. Cryptogenic.

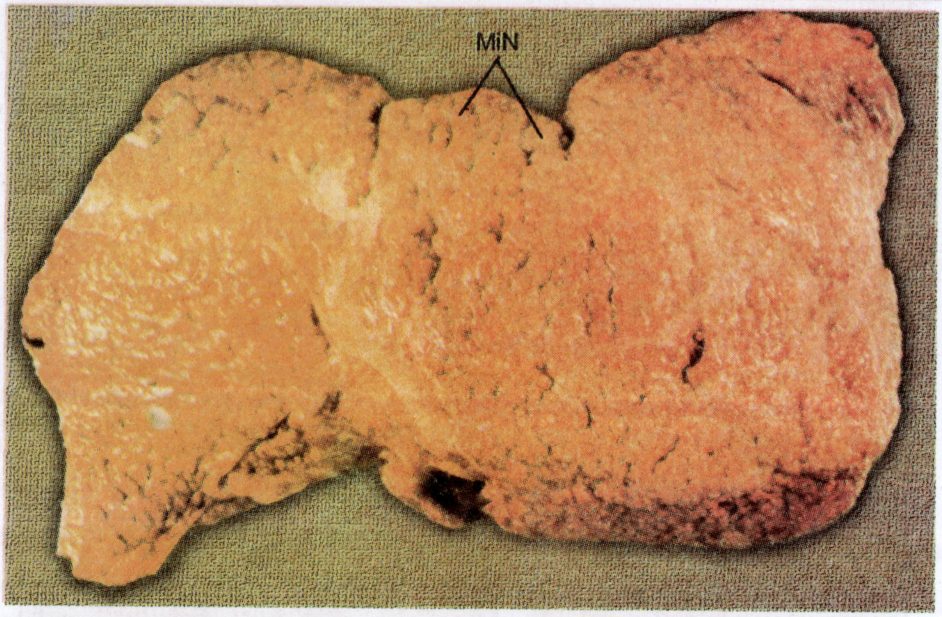

Fig. 30.8. Alcoholic cirrhosis, entire liver shows micronodules (MIN)

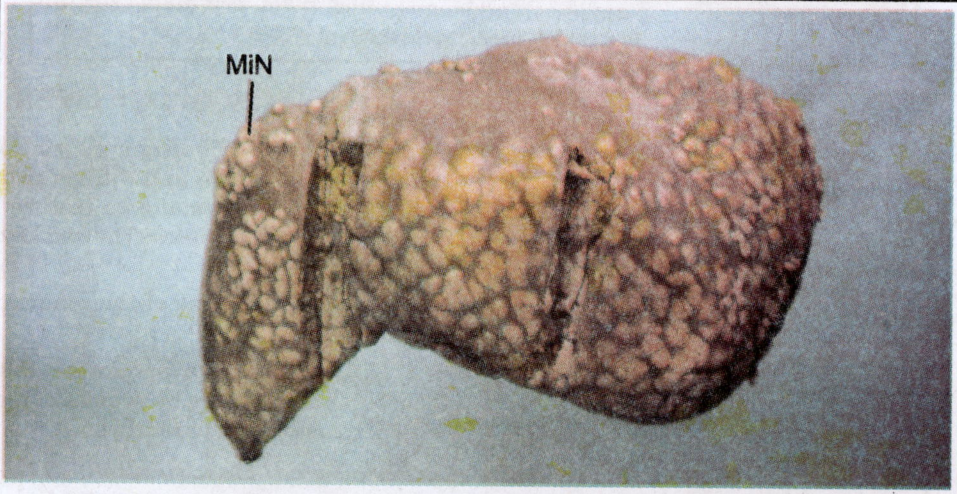

Fig. 30.9. Alcoholic cirrhosis(portal cirrhosis) showing micronodules (MIN) in liver

Alcoholic cirrhosis

It is also called Lannec's cirrhosis, and has in the past been called nutritional cirrhosis. Most common cause is alcohol and usually develops slowly and insiduously.

Excessive alcohol consumption is associated with several distinct pathological conditions in the liver : (i) *fatty liver,* (ii) *alcoholic hepatitis,* (iii) *hepatic fibrosis,* (iv) *cirrhosis.* When there are attacks of alcoholic hepatitis, sometimes fibrosis becomes progressive leading to cirrhosis.

Gross examination (Figs 30.8, 30.9)

1. Liver — atrophic, 600-700 gm (Normal 1,440-1,600 gm).

2. Surface is irregular and nodular (2-5 mm in diam.), which are projecting masses of liver cells.

3. Colour is reddish-brown or yellowish if there is associated fatty change.

4. Consistency is firm. Cut surface shows interlacing network of grey translucent connective tissue that separate prominent nodules of liver cells.

Microscopical features : See chapter 26 (Fig. 26.44).

POSTNECROTIC CIRRHOSIS

Postnecrotic cirrhosis (macronodular cirrhosis) is characterised by irregularly sized nodules separated by variable but mostly broad scars.

Aetiology : A history of long-standing chronic active hepatitis usually precedes postnecrotic (posthepatic) cirrhosis. Frequency of cirrhosis complicating viral hepatitis ranges from 2–4%. HBV is encountered in about 20–25%, HCV in 25-30% cases of postnecrotic cirrhosis.

Gross appearance (Fig. 30.10)

1. Liver is smaller than normal.

2. Capsule is thick.

3. Liver is characterised by large grey-brown nodules (1 cm or more in diam.) irregularly distributed in the liver, which are separated by broad bands or areas of depressed scarring (fibrous tissue).

4. On cutting, there is resistance to the knife and cut surface shows numerous macronodules.

Microscopic feature

1. Irregular macronodular pattern with regeneration of new nodules.

2. Fibrous septa surrounding the nodules are often broad, resulting in approximation of portal tracts.

3. Stenosis of biliary duct occurs due to scarring which leads to cholestasis.

4. Hepatocytes look normal in some nodules while they are irregular in others with dysplasia.

Hepatocellular carcinoma often arises in macronodular cirrhosis.

Morphological classification of cirrhosis

1. **Micronodular cirrhosis** : The nodules of liver tissue, 1-2 mm in diam. are of fairly uniform size outlined by grey fibrous tissue as seen *in alcoholic cirrhosis, Wilson's disease* and *pigmented cirrhosis, biliary cirrhosis.* Nodules are separated by a fine framework of connective tissues.

2. **Macronodular cirrhosis** : The nodules are larger, usually more than 5 mm diam. The liver has a coarsely nodular appearance and there is considerable variation in the size of nodules. It is a typical of postnecrotic cirrhosis. Incidence of hepatocellular carcinoma originating in large nodules is higher.

BILIARY CIRRHOSIS

Types :

Biliary cirrhosis may be primary and secondary.

1. ***Primary biliary cirrhosis*** **(PBC)** : It is a relatively uncommon disease that occurs mostly in middle aged women. The essential lesion is a chro-

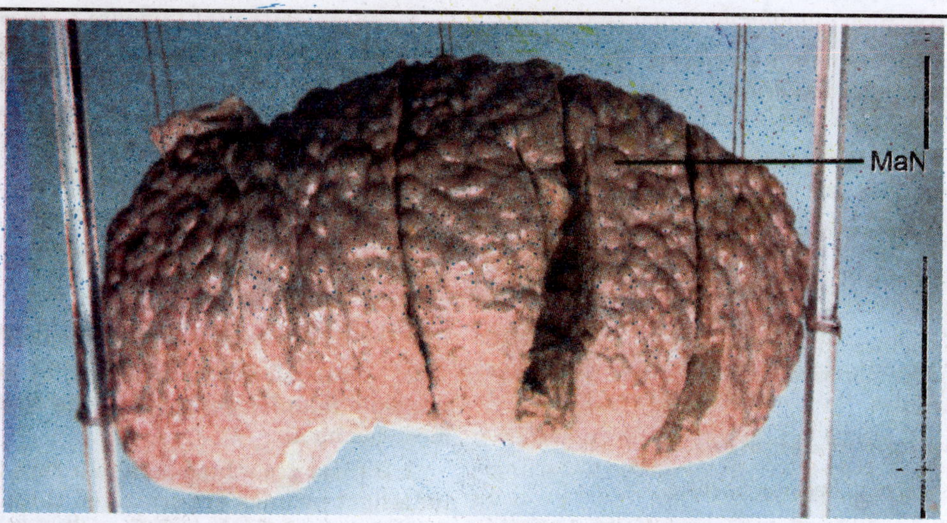

Fig. 30.10. Post-necrotic cirrhosis of liver showing large irregular macronodules (MaN)

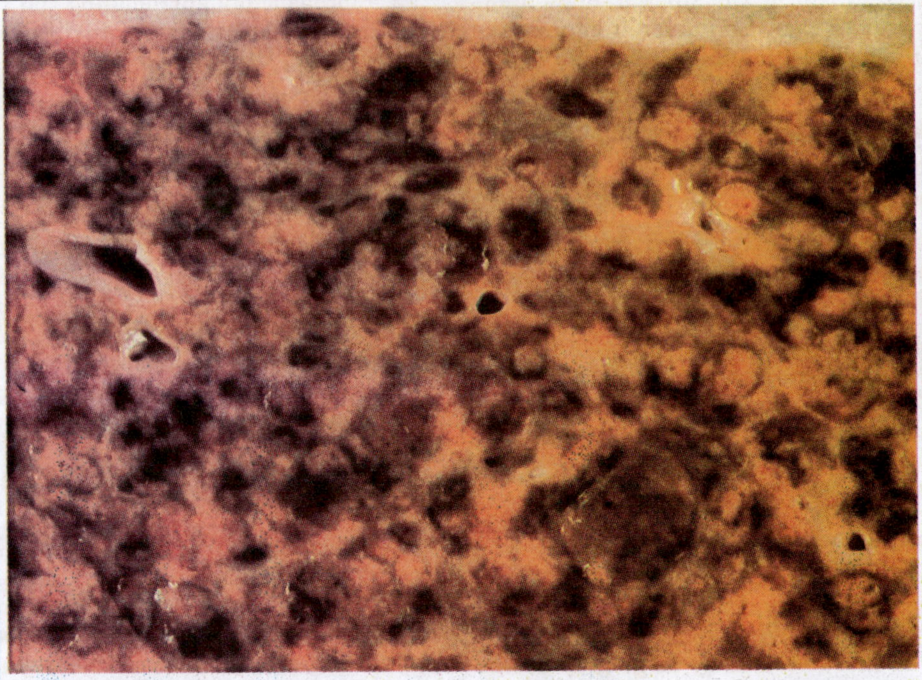

Fig. 30.11. Secondary biliary cirrhosis due to cholestasis. Liver shows greenish colour with micronodular cut surface

nic inflammation which destroys small intrahepatic bile ducts. Both inflammation and cholestasis leads to irregular loss of hepatocytes and nodular regeneration producing *micronodular cirrhosis*. The cause is unknown, however, immunological abnormalities such as elevated IgM and anti-mitochondrial antibody accompanying the disease suggest an immune-mediated mechanism.

2. ***Secondary biliary cirrhosis*** : It is a relatively uncommon complication of prolonged extra hepatic obstruction of bile duct system.

Causes : Lithiasis, cholangitis, parasitosis and tumours compressing extra-hepatic biliary ducts.

Gross appearance (Fig. 30.11)

1. Liver is deep green colour (bile stained) and is usually increased in size and weight.

2. Cut surface shows a characteristic appearance with fine fibrotic bands and green parenchymatous nodules.

Microscopic examination

1. Portal tracts become fibrotic.

2. Large and small ducts are distended and frequently contain inspissated bile.

3. Hyperplasia of bile duct occurs.

4. Fibrosis extends between portal tracts and lobules.

TUMOURS OF LIVER

Types

Primary :

1. *Benign epithelial tumours* : Liver cell adenoma, bile duct adenoma, bile duct cystadenoma, and papilloma.

2. *Malignant epithelial tumours* (primary carcinoma) : Cholangiocarcinoma (25%), Hepatocellular carcinoma (75%) (Fig. 30.12).

Secondary : Metastatic carcinoma

HEPATOCELLULAR CARCINOMA (HCC)

Macroscopic types

1. Solitary (massive) large tumour (Fig. 30.12).

2. Nodular form characterised by presence of multiple nodules throughout the liver. This is most common.

3. Diffuse growth pattern is a rare type. Tiny indistinct nodules are scattered throughout the liver and are difficult to differentiate from regenerative nodules of cirrhosis.

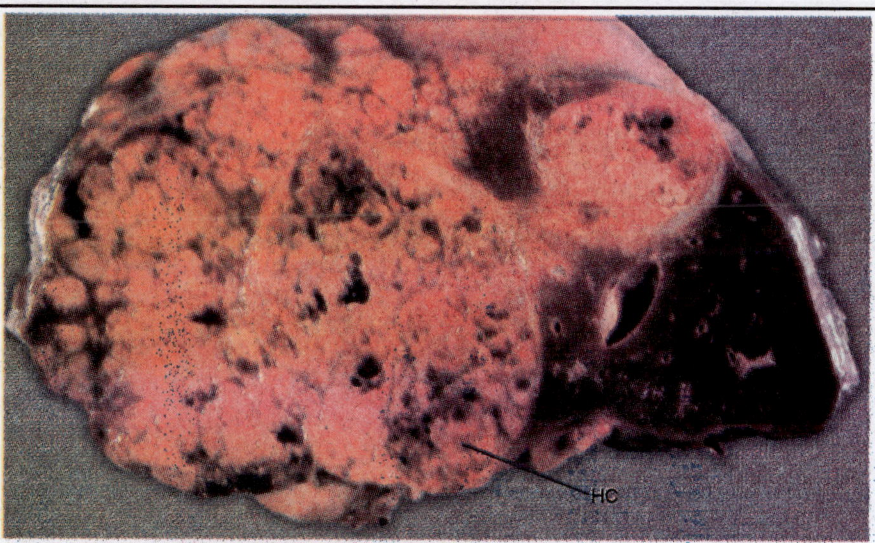

Fig. 30.12. Primary hepatocellular carcinoma (HC)

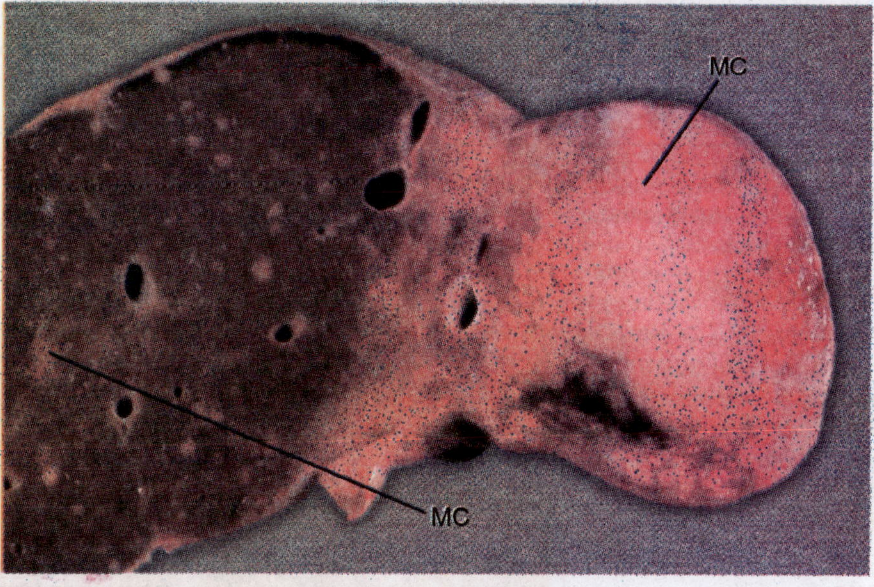

Fig. 30.13. Metastatic carcinoma in left lobe liver (MC) (primary : carcinoma oesophagus)

Microscopic feature

HCCs range from well differentiated to highly undifferentiated tumours. Picture in well-differentiated lesions includes :

1. Cells grow in columns resembling normal liver.
2. The tumour cells are often hyperchromatic and multinucleated or are of giant size.
3. Atypical lobule may be formed, and there is often some bile in or near the tumour cells.
4. Supporting connective tissue is minimal or absent.

Histological pattern may be of three types — *trabecular, macrotrabecular* and *papillary.*

METASTATIC TUMOURS

Malignancy within the liver is most frequently metastatic and the liver happens to be the most

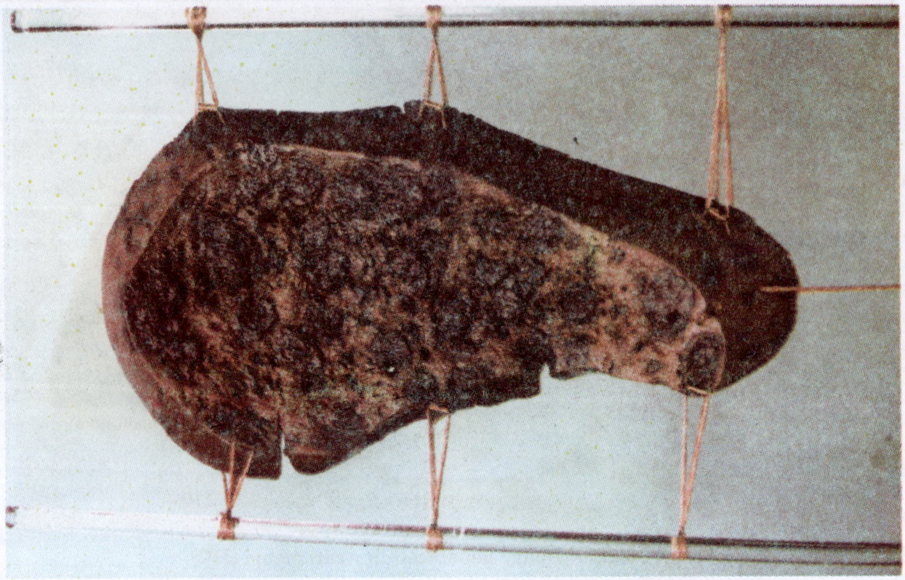

Fig. 30.14. Metastatic carcinoma liver (malignant melanoma)

frequent site for metastasis. Portal venous drainage is the main cause for this.

Gross examination (Figs. 30.13, 30.14)

(i) Metastases are often multiple but may be single. Metastatic nodules are grey-white except with melanoma. (ii) Metastatic nodules in malignant melanoma look black.

GALL BLADDER

Gall bladder disease is often associated with stone formation (Fig. 30.15) and chronic obstruction of the cystic duct leading to chronic cholecystitis (Fig. 30.16). Tumours of biliary system are rare and usually adenocarcinoma (e.g., cholangiocarcinoma of bile duct epithelium).

CHOLELITHIASIS

Principal function of gall bladder is to concentrate and store bile. About 10-20% western adults suffer from gall stone trouble. Basically three factors are involved in stone formation : *abnormalities in composition of bile, bile stasis and infection.*

Types of stone

These are of three main types :

1. *Mixed stone* (Fig. 30.15) — in 80% cases, multiple stones and faceted due to contact with one another.

2. *Cholesterol stone* — 2-3 cm × 1.5-2 cm, oval, associated with excessive cholesterol in bile.

3. *Bile pigment stone* — multiple and results from chronic haemolysis with excess bilirubin production.

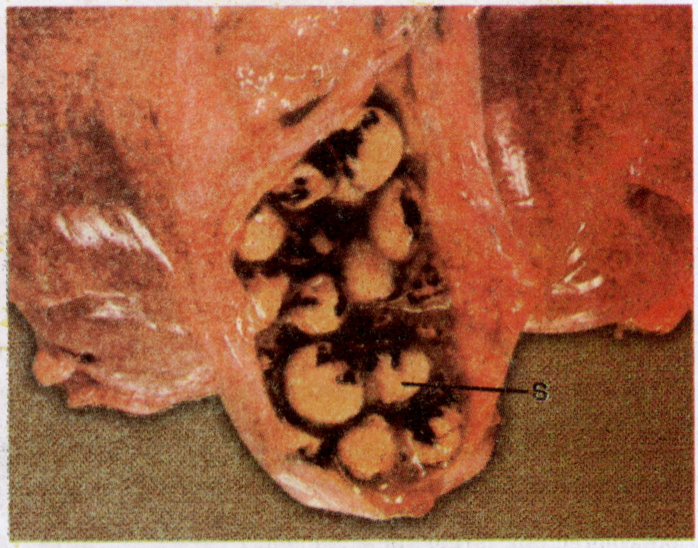

Fig. 30.15. Cholelithiasis : Gall bladder shows large number of stones (S) with their surfaces faceted (mixed stones)

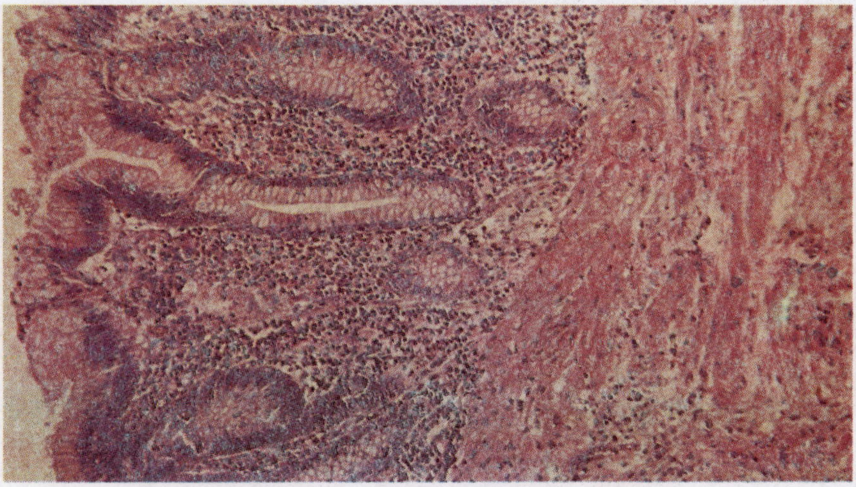

Fig. 30.16. Chronic cholecystitis of gall bladder (× 110)

CHRONIC CHOLECYSTITIS

Macroscopically

(1) Gall bladder may be small.

(2) Usually contains mixed stones.

(3) Mucosa is thickened and inflamed.

Histology (Fig. 30.16) :

(i) Epithelial cells are full of mucus.

(ii) Normal mucosal folds are lacking and there is infiltration by lymphocytes, plasma cells and eosinophils.

(iii) Muscle coat shows hypertrophy and infiltrated by few lymphocytes.

TUMOURS OF GALL BLADDER

Types

1. **Benign** : Benign tumours and tumour-like conditions of gall bladder, though infrequent, include :

(a) *Adenomas* which resemble the adenomas of GIT, they may be sessile or pedunculated. They may exhibit tubular, tubulovillous, or villous patterns of growth. There is always some degree of atypia present, and a few show evidences of carcinoma in situ. Like colorectum, larger the adenoma, more likelihood of presence of an area of malignant change.

(b) *Tumour-like polyps* include cholesterol polyp, inflammatory polyp etc.

(c) *Paragangliomas* may develop from small paraganglia in the gall bladder serosa.

2. **Malignant** : Most cancers of gall bladder are adenocarcinomas (90%) and abaout 5-10% are squamous cell carcinomas or adenoacanthomas. Grossly 70% cancer show *diffuse* growth pattern and 30% as polypoid mass.

***Gross examination* (Fig. 30.17)**

(i) Polypoid growth.

(ii) Exophyting lesion fungating into lumen.

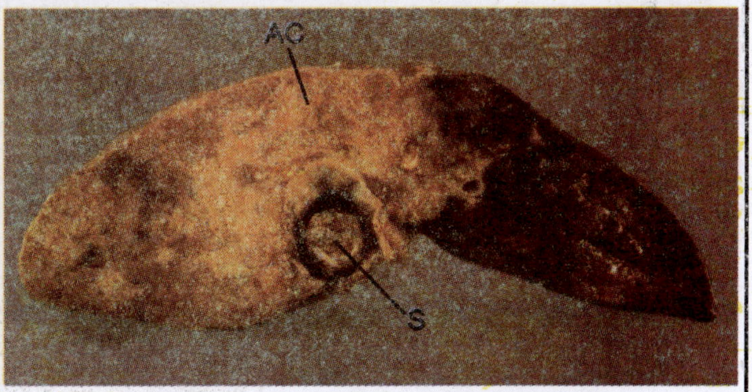

Fig. 30.17. Adenocarcinoma (AC) gall bladder with gall stones (S)

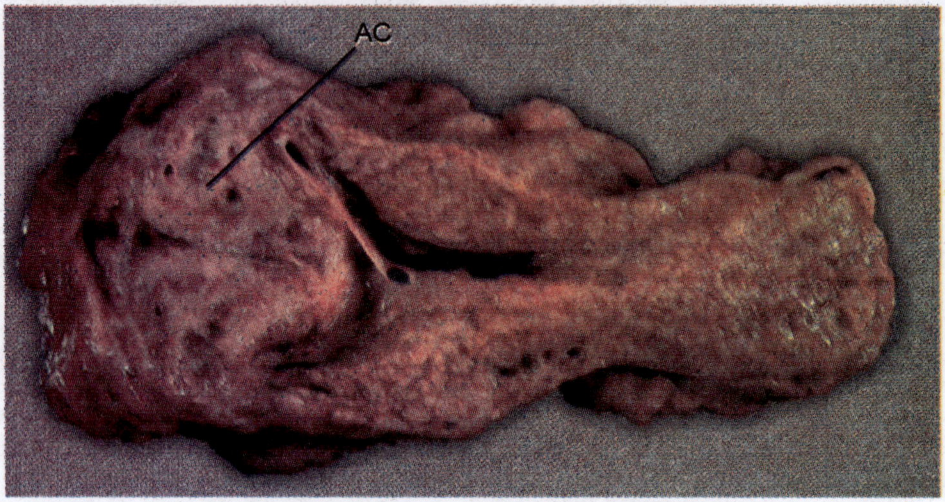

Fig. 30.18. Adenocarcinoma (AC) of head of pancreas

Microscopic appearance

Most cancers of GB are adenocarcinoma with varying degree of differentiation. Some display papillary surface which may be deeply invasive.

PANCREAS

Inflammation of pancreas (pancreatitis) may present in acute or chronic form resulting in high mortality as a result of release of pancreatic enzymes in surrounding tissues causing severe local tissue destruction. Chronic pancreatitis often causes intractable pain.

Malignant tumours are almost always adenocarcinoma that usually arises from the pancreatic ductal epithelium. Most tumours arise in head although they may arise in body and in tail. They grow insiduously and remain undetected until a very advanced stage.

ADENOCARCINOMA

Macroscopically (Fig. 30.18)

(i) Specimen of pancreas shows a hard lardaceous mass poorly delineated from the surrounding tissues.

(ii) Tumour is hard and white.

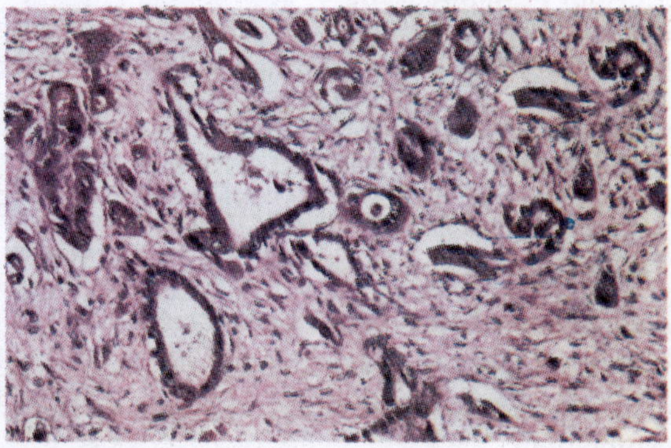

Fig. 30.19. Adenocarcinoma of pancreas (× 135)

Histology (Fig. 30.19)

It is usually scirrhous tumour, histologically an adenocarcinoma.

(i) Tumour shows a ductular pattern.

(ii) Tumour cells are pleomorphic and forms cords and acini.

(iii) Tumour cells are lying in abundant densely fibrous stroma.

Chapter 31

Urinary System

Urinary system comprises of kidneys, pelvicalycal systems, ureters, bladder and urethra. Kidney is responsible for the excretion of waste products of the body.

Kidney

Each human adult kidney weighs about 150 gm. It is bean-shaped and the ureter arises from the pelvis at the hilum. Normally, the external surface is covered by a thin translucent capsule. When the capsule is stripped off, the renal surface is smooth, occasionally foetal lobulation markings may persist.

On the cut surface, the kidney is made of pale *cortex* (1.2 to 1.5 cm thick) and a darker *medulla*. The medulla consists of renal *pyramids*, the apices of which are known as *papillae*, each related to a calyx. From the point of view of diseases, kidney can be divided into four components : blood vessels, glomerulae, tubules and interstitium.

Urinary bladder

The lower urinary tract comprising of renal pelvis, ureters, bladder and urethra (except for its terminal portion) is lined by a special transitional epithelium. Urinary bladder is a muscular organ looking like an inverted pyramid.

Microscopically

Kidney is made of glomeruli and the tubules that are lined by cuboidal epithelium. Normally, glomeruli and tubules are interspersed with blood vessel and stromal tissue but stroma is not normally visible. For histological structure of glomerulus, see chapter 26 and fig. 26.39. The present classification of primary glomerulonephritis are given in chapter 26 (Table 26.4).

Bladder is lined by transitional epithelium. It has also lamina propria and muscle coat.

GLOMERULAR DISEASE

Glomeruli may be injured by a number of factors and also in the course of systemic diseases. A tentative classification of glomerular diseases is given in Table 31.1.

Table 31.1
Classification of glomerular disease

A. Primary glomerulonephritis
1. Acute diffuse (endocapillary) proliferative glomerulonephritis (a) Post-streptococcal (b) Non-streptococcal
2. Rapidly progressive (crescentic) glomerulonephritis
3. Membranous glomerulonephritis
4. Minimal change disease
5. Mesangiocapillary (membranoproliferative) glomerulonephritis
6. Focal segmental glomerulopathy
7. IgA nephropathy
8. Chronic glomerulonephritis
B. Systemic diseases
1. SLE
2. Diabetes mellitus
3. Amyloidosis
4. Goodpasture's syndrome
5. Polyarteritis nodosa
6. Henoch-Schonlein purpura
7. Bacterial endocarditis
C. Hereditary disorders
1. Alport's syndrome
2. Fabry's disease

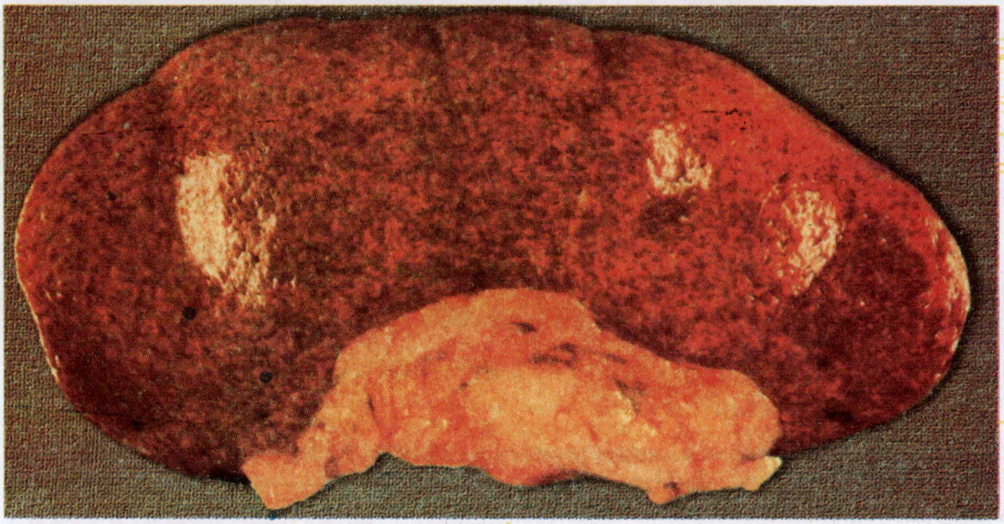

Fig. 31.1. Kidney in acute diffuse post-streptococcal glomerulonephritis

Glomerular damage leads to :

1. *Reduced urinary output* as a result of endothelial swelling.
2. *Proteinuria* following inflammation and alteration of permeability of layers of glomerulus.
3. *Haematuria* as a result of focal loss of epithelium and endothelium.

Hypercellularity : There is hypercellularity in the glomerular tufts in some inflammatory diseases which is characterised by one or more combinations of the following :

1. ***Cellular proliferation*** : Proliferation of mesangial or endothelial cells.
2. ***Leucocyte infiltration*** : Infiltration by neutrophils, monocytes and in some cases lymphocytes occur.
3. ***Formation of crescents*** : Crescents are accumulations of proliferating parietal epithelial cells and infiltrating leucocytes.

GLOMERULONEPHRITIS (GN)

Pathogenesis : Pathogenesis of glomerulonephritis is mediated by immune mechanisms which may act in two ways :

1. Injury by antibodies reacting in situ within the glomerulus, either with insoluble fixed (intrinsic) glomerular antigens or with molecules planted in the glomerulus, and
2. Injury resulting from deposition of soluble circulating antigen-antibody complexes in the glomerular basement membrane.

ACUTE STREPTOCOCCAL (Proliferative) GLOMERULONEPHRITIS

This type of nephritis classically appears 1 to 4 weeks after a streptococcal infection of pharynx or skin. It occurs most frequently in children of 4-6 years of age, but adults of any age may also be affected.

Gross appearance (Figs. 31.1, 31.2)

Lesions are found in both kidneys :

1. Kidneys — slightly increased in volume.
2. Subcapsular surface is smooth and grey, on which tiny haemorrrhagic petechiae are sometimes visible. Capsule strips off easily.
3. Cut surface shows pale cortex and a congested medulla with sharp demarcation between the two zones.

Microscopic examination (Figs. 31.3A& B)

1. Glomeruli are enlarged and oedematous, so that Bowman's capsular space is practically eliminated. Tubules show cloudy swelling.
2. Hypercellularity is caused by :
   (a) Proliferation of endothelial and mesangial cells and, in many cases, epithelial cells.
   (b) Infiltration by inflammatory cells mostly neutrophil granulocytes.

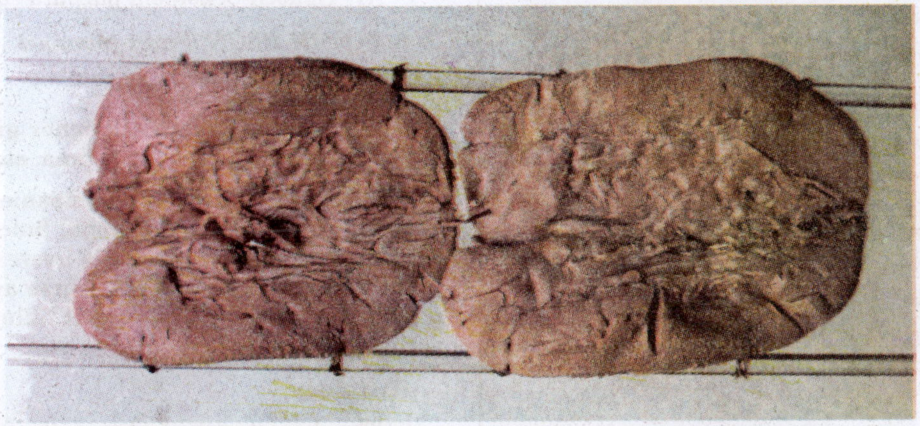

Fig. 31.2. Kidney (cut surface) in diffuse proliferative glomerulonephritis

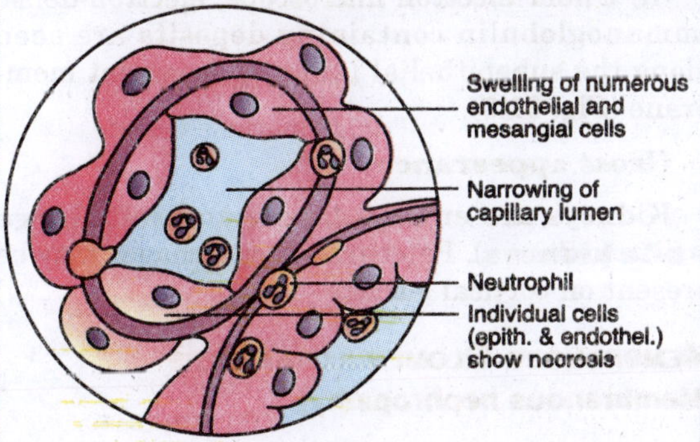

Fig. 31.3A. Acute diffuse post-streptococcal glomerulonephritis (electron microscopy)

3. By electron microscopy — electron-dense granular deposit is present in subepithelial postion.

Acute non-streptococcal glomerulonephritis

A similar form of GN occurs sporadically which apparently has no incidence of preceding streptococcal infection, although it is possible that, in some instances, such infection existed previously but was undetected. It has been reported in association with various non-streptococcal bacterial (staphylococcal, pneumococcal), viral (HBV, mumps, infectious mononucleosis) and parasitic infections (malaria, toxoplasmosis).

Rapidly progressive (crescentic) glomerulonephritis (RPGN)

The condition is also known as diffuse extra-capillary proliferative glomerulonephritis, crescentic glomerulonephritis. There is crescent formation in 50% of glomeruli.

As the name suggests, RPGN may be caused by a number of different diseases, some of which are restricted to kidney while others are systemic. RPGN may be classified into three groups.

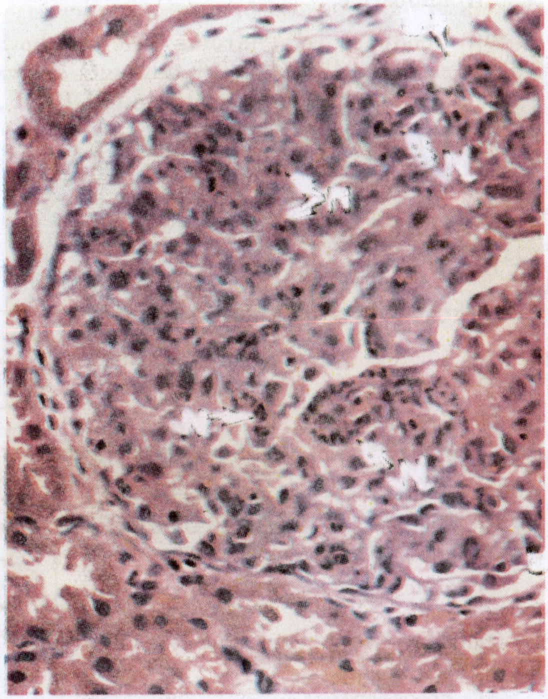

Fig. 31.3B. M. E. Acute diffuse proliferative glomerulonephritis with increase in glomerular tuft and red cells in tubules (haematuria) (× 400)

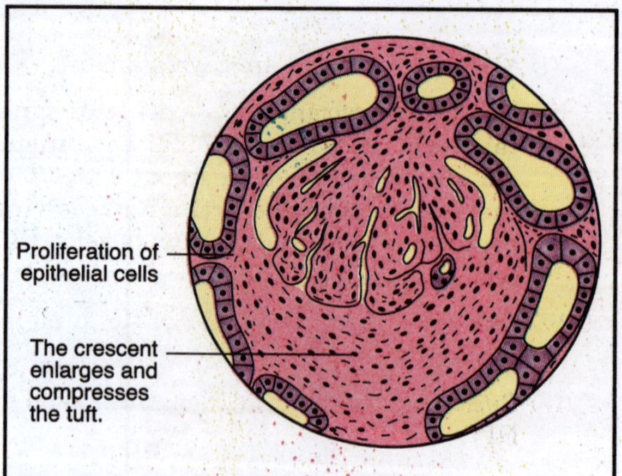

Fig. 31.4. RPGN showing proliferation of epithelial cells, enlargement of crescents and compression of glomerular tuft (*Schematic*)

In each group, RPGN may be associated with a known disorder or it may be idiopathic.

Types :

1. *Type I RPGN (Anti-GBM antibody)*
   (i) Idiopathic.
   (ii) Goodpasture syndrome. There is both renal and pulmonary damage; shows antibody to type IV collagen in GBM.
2. *Type II RPGN (Immune complex)*
   (i) Idiopathic
   (ii) Post-infectious
   (iii) SLE
   (iv) Henoch-Schonlein purpura (IgA)
3. *Type III RPGN (Pauci-immune)*
   (i) Idiopathic
   (ii) NCA associated, Wegner granulomatosis, polyarteritis nodosa, etc.

Glomerular damage is accompanied by rapid and progressive decline in renal function, often with anuria, usually resulting in irreversible acute renal failure. It has a rapid course and usually terminates in death from renal failure usually within 3-12 months.

Histology

(i) The characteristic feature is the formation of epithelial 'crescents' by proliferation of Bowman's capsule epithelial cells (Fig. 31.4).

(ii) Under electron microscope, electron-dense immunoglobulin containing deposits are seen along the subepithelial lining of basement membrane (Fig. 31.5).

Gross appearance

Kidneys are enlarged, pale and soft (**large white kidneys**). Petechial haemorrhages may be present on cortical surface.

Membranous Glomerulonephritis (Membranous nephropathy)

It is characterised by diffuse thickening of glomerular capillary wall (basement membrane) and accumulation of electron-dense subepithelial deposits in the basement membrane. The deposit contains immunoglobulin (Fig. 31.5).

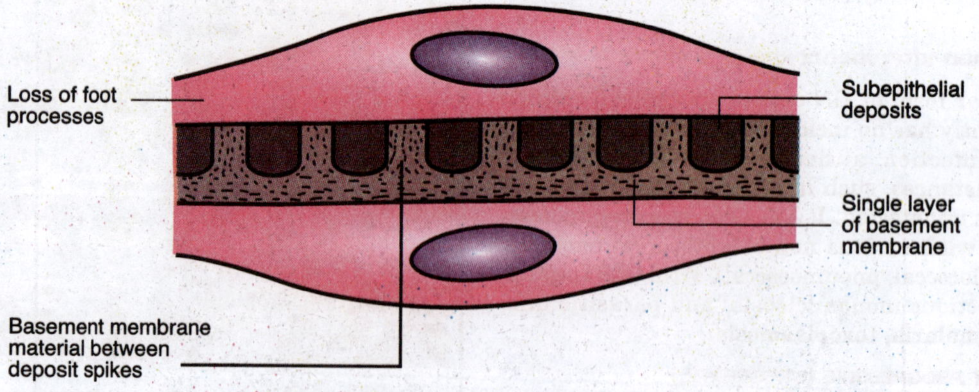

Fig. 31.5. Membranous glomerulonephritis. Electron-dense immunoglobulin containing deposits along subepithelial lining of basement membrane (*Schematic*)

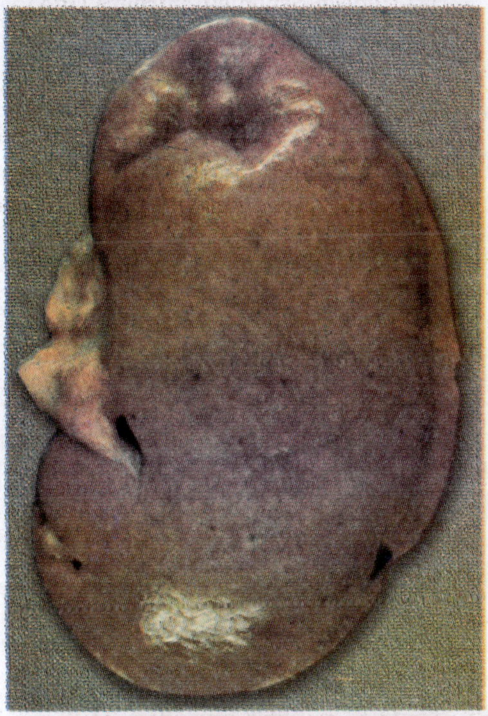

Fig. 31.6. Membranous glomerulonephritis *(large white kidney)*

This accounts for approximately 30% of cases of nephrotic syndrome in adults, some patients, however, present with asymptomatic proteinuria.

Aetiology

(i) About 85% of cases are asymptomatic.

(ii) *Drugs* involved include — penicillamine, captopril, gold, non-steroidal antiinflammatory drugs (NSAIDs). About 1 to 7% of cases of rheumatoid arthritis receiving penicillamine or gold therapy develop this type of nephritis.

(iii) *Tumours,* e.g., carcinoma of lung, melanoma.

(iv) *Infections,* e.g., malaria, hepatitis B and C, HIV.

Macroscopy (Fig. 31.6)

The appearance of kidney varies from a large white as much as 400 gm to normal or shrunken size.

(i) Here the kidney is mostly large white.

(ii) Cortex is yellowish and medulla is almost normal.

Histopathololgy (Fig. 31.7)

(i) Generalised thickening of capillary basement membrane.

(ii) Loss of foot processes.

(iii) There is no proliferation of endothelial or mesangial cells.

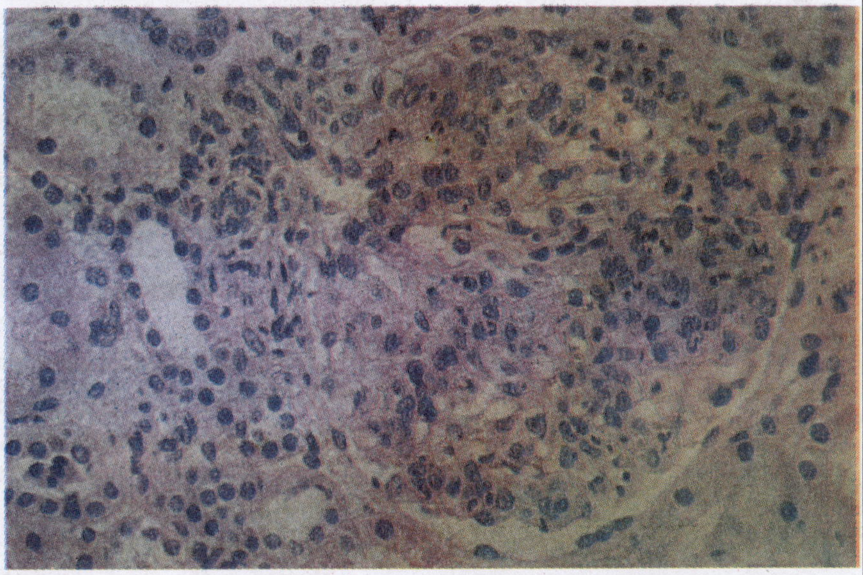

Fig. 31.7. Membranous glomerulonephritis : Diffuse hyaline thickening of glomeruli. Glomeruli do not show hypercellularity (× 350)

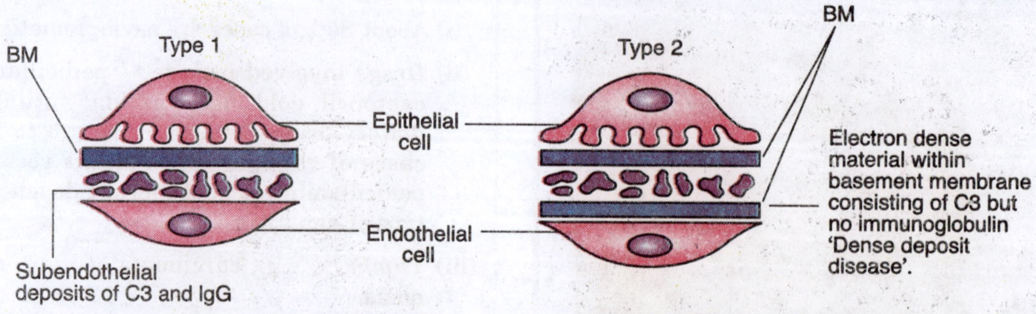

Fig. 31.8. Mesangiocapillary glomerulonephritis : Electron microscopy showing deposit in basement membrane of glomerulus. Basement membrane = BM.

Prognosis

(i) 35% cases — shows spontaneous remission.

(ii) 65% cases — continue having proteinuria and in 40% cases eventually chronic renal failure supervenes.

Mesangiocapillary Glomerulonephritis (Membranous proliferative glomerulonephritis)

Mesangiocapillary glomerulonephritis is characterised by alteration in the basement membrane, proliferation of glomerular cells and leucocyte infiltration.

Aetiology

The disease is of two major types — type I and type II. They differ in ultrastructural patterns, in type I — there is subendothelial deposit of C3 and IgG, while in type II — there is duplication of basement membrane and accumulation of C3 (but no Ig) between two layers of basement membrane. Type II is, therefore, called *Dense deposit disease.* Type II disease is relatively rare.

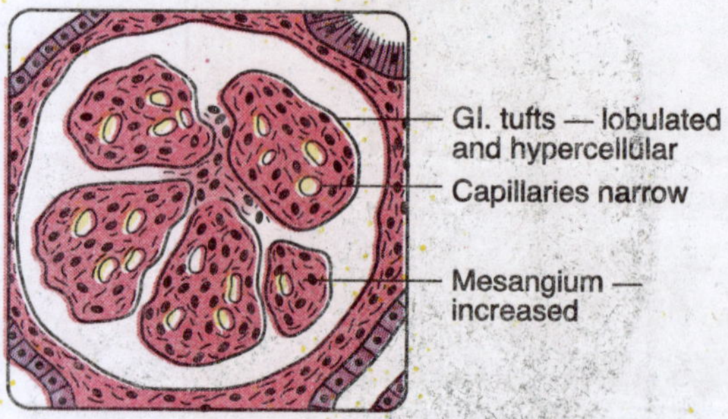

Fig. 31.9A. Mesangiocapillary glomerulonephritis (× 350), Type I

(i) Complement activation — a common feature of both forms.

(ii) Type I disease — results from immune complexes by the classical pathway.

(iii) In type II disease — there is activation of complement by the alternative pathway by an autoantibody which stabilises C3 converting enzyme.

By electron microscopy (Fig. 31.8)

(i) Glomeruli are large and hypercellular.

(ii) Hypercellularity results from proliferation of mesangial cells and capillary endothelium and infiltrating leucocytes. Parietal epithelial cells are swollen and occasionally crescents are formed.

(iii) In type I disease, there is subepithelial electron-dense deposits of C3 and IgG and C1 and C4.

(iv) In type II disease, the lamina dens of basement membrane is transformed into an irregular ribbon-like structure. C3 is present (but no IgG) in the deposit but there are Clq and C4.

Clinical features

(i) Children and young adults are usually affected.

(ii) All patients present nephrotic syndrome cr proteinuria.

(iii) About 50% cases progress to renal failure (often with hypertension) within a decade.

Histopathology (Figs. 31.9A, 31.9B)

(i) H.E. section shows diffuse proliferative change in the glomerus, with increase in the number as well as the size of the endothelial and the mesangial cells.

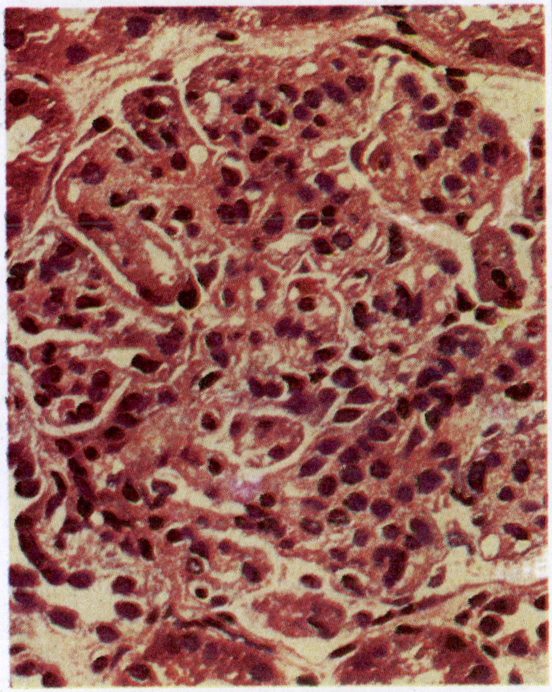

Fig. 31.9B. Mesangiocapillary glomerulonephritis (× 350), Type I

(ii) Glomerulus shows diffuse eosinophilic sclerosis by marked proliferation of mesangial cells.

Causes of large white kidney

1. Rapidly progressive glomerulonephritis.
2. Membranous glomerulonephritis.
3. Nephrotic syndrome.

Note : Flea-bite haemorrhages on the surface of decapsulated kidney is common in malignant nephrosclerosis.

Acute nephritic syndrome

It is characterised by acute onset of haematuria, proteinuria, hypertension, oedema and oliguria. It may be produced by systemic disorder, e.g., SLE or by primary glomerular disease, e.g., proliferative GN.

Chronic glomerulonephritis (CGN)

Chronic GN is an **end-stage pool of glomerular disease** fed by a number of streams of specific types of glomerulonephritis.

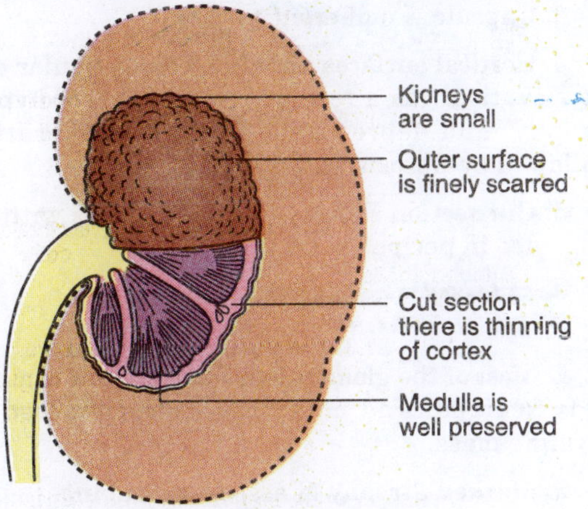

Fig. 31.10. Granular contracted kidney (chronic glomerulonephritis) or renal arteriosclerosis

1. *Post-streptococcal GN* : It is a rare antecedent of chronic GN in children, except in adults.

2. *Rapidly progressive GN* : When patients with RPGN survive the acute episode, they usually pass on to chronic GN.

3. *Focal segmental glomerulosclerosis* also progresses to RPGN.

Gross appearance (Figs. 31.10 and 31.11)

1. Kidneys are symmetrically contracted.

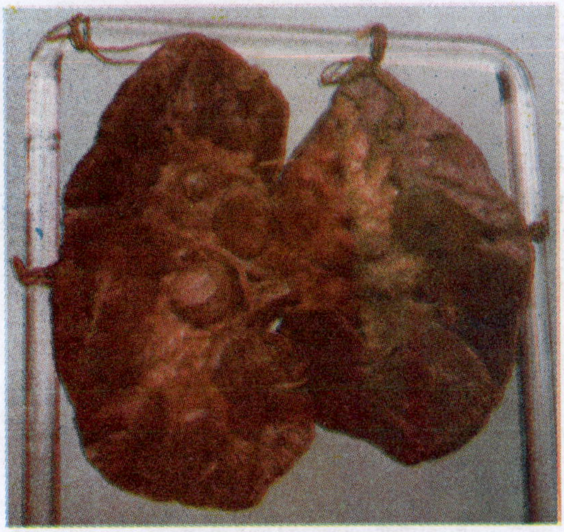

Fig. 31.11. Cut section of granular contracted kidney

2. Small contracted kidneys are firm.

3. Capsule — adherent to cortex.

4. Cortical surfaces are diffusedly granular due to elevations (as a result of compensatory hypertrophy) and depressions (due to degeneration followed by fibrosis and scarring).

5. Cut section shows — thinned cortex with an increase in peripelvic fat.

Microscopical examination (Figs. 31.12A& B)

1. Most of the glomeruli are partially or completely scarred, and many become converted to hyaline mass.

2. Marked atrophy of associated tubules.

3. Irregular interstitial fibrosis.

4. Lymphocytic infiltration.

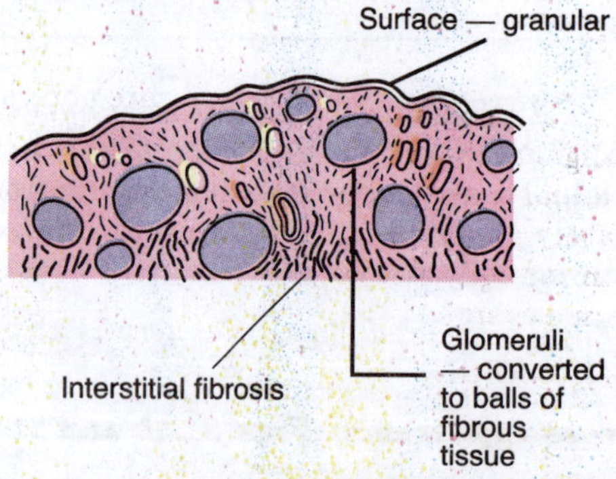

Fig. 31.12A. Microscopy of chronic glomerulonephritis *(schematic)*

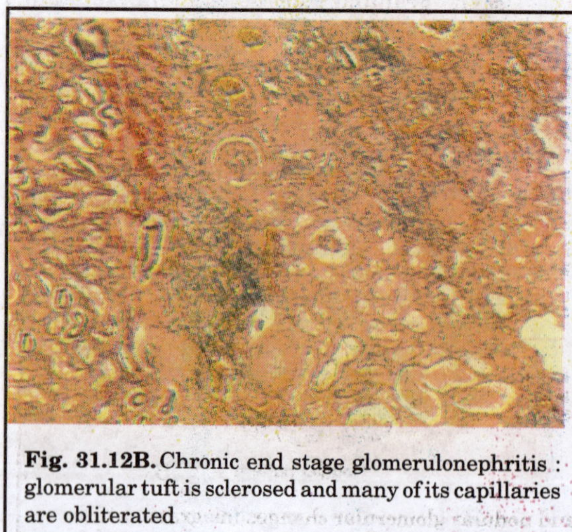

Fig. 31.12B. Chronic end stage glomerulonephritis : glomerular tuft is sclerosed and many of its capillaries are obliterated

Causes of granular contracted kidney

1. Chronic GN
2. Benign nephrosclerosis
3. Chronic pyelonephritis — nodules are broad, coarse, patchy, unilateral.

Nephrotic Syndrome (NS)

Nephrotic syndrome is characterised by massive proteinuria, hypoproteinaemia (hypoalbuminaemia); generalised oedema and hyperlipidaemia (hypercholesterolaemia). Underlying the clinical complex may be one of a number of distinct diseases, and they all have in common an increased glomerular membrane permeability.

Causes

A. *Primary glomerulonephritis*

1. Membranous glomerulonephritis
2. Lipoid nephrosis
3. Focal glomerulosclerosis

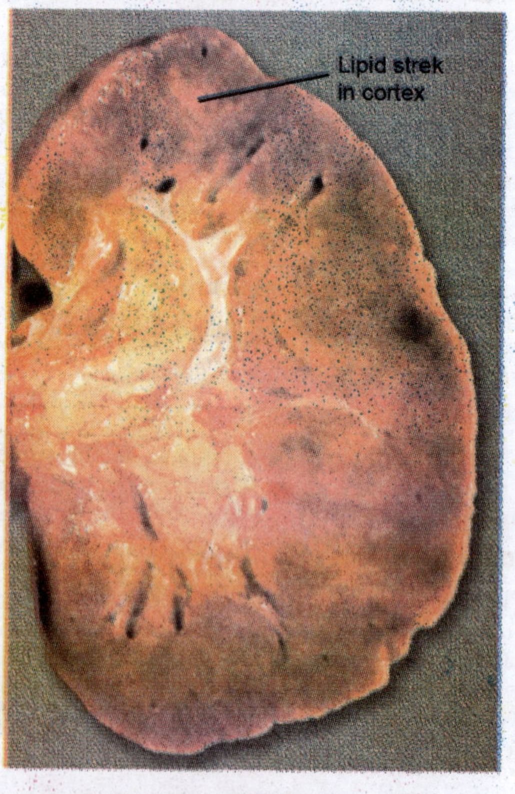

Fig. 31.13. Kidney in nephrotic syndrome (membranous glomerulonephritis)

B. *Associated with systemic disease*

1. SLE
2. Polyarteritis
3. Diabetes mellitus
4. Amyloidosis

Gross appearance (Fig. 31.13). There is enlargement and general pallor of kidney. Cut section shows yellow streaks of lipid in cortex.

SYSTEMIC CAUSES OF RENAL DISEASE

Kidney is commonly involved in systemic diseases particularly of the blood vessels, e.g., diabetes mellitus, arterial hypertension, amyloidosis, systemic lupus erythematosus, polyarteritis nodosa, sclerodema, etc.

DIABETIC GLOMERULOSCLEROSIS

Up to 30% of diabetics develop proteinuria. In addition to predisposition to urinary tract infections, papillary necrosis and the effects of arteriosclerotic vascular disease in kidney, diabetes cause glomerulosclerosis.

In diabetic glomerulosclerosis, pathological changes take place in the glomeruli (glomerulosclerosis) and also in the walls of afferent and efferent arterioles. Diabetic glomerulosclerosis takes one of two forms — nodular or diffuse (Fig. 31.14). Nodular form is also called Kimmelstiel-Wilson lesion.

Histopathology

Base membrane of glomerulus is thickened. In addition, a hyaline material is deposited in the mesangium.

(i) When the eosinophilic hyaline material is deposited diffusely and more or less evenly throughout the glomerulus, the condition is called *diffuse form* of diabetic glomerulosclerosis (Figs. 31.14A, 31.15). In time, many glomeruli may get hyalinized.

(ii) When the eosinophilic hyaline material is deposited unevenly in segment form in the mesangium as one or more nodules, it is referred to as *nodular form* (Fig. 31.14B).

Clinical effects

(i) Screening test for microalbuminuria is useful in detecting early disease.

(ii) Proteinuria may result in nephrotic syndrome.

(iii) Hypertension leads to further damage of kidney. Hence control of diabetes and blood pressure is important to delay the onset of renal failure.

HYPERTENSIVE NEPHROSCLEROSIS

Pathological changes in the kidney differ in benign and malignant hypertension. Benign hypertension is of gradual onset and progressive, reaching only moderately elevated diastolic pressure. In contrast, in malignant hypertension, rise in BP is rapid and severe.

BENIGN HYPERTENSIVE NEPHROSCLEROSIS

Macroscopy (Fig. 31.16)

(i) Usually smaller kidneys.

(ii) Surface granular with depressed dark red scars (granular contracted kidney, similar to that of chronic glomerulonephritis).

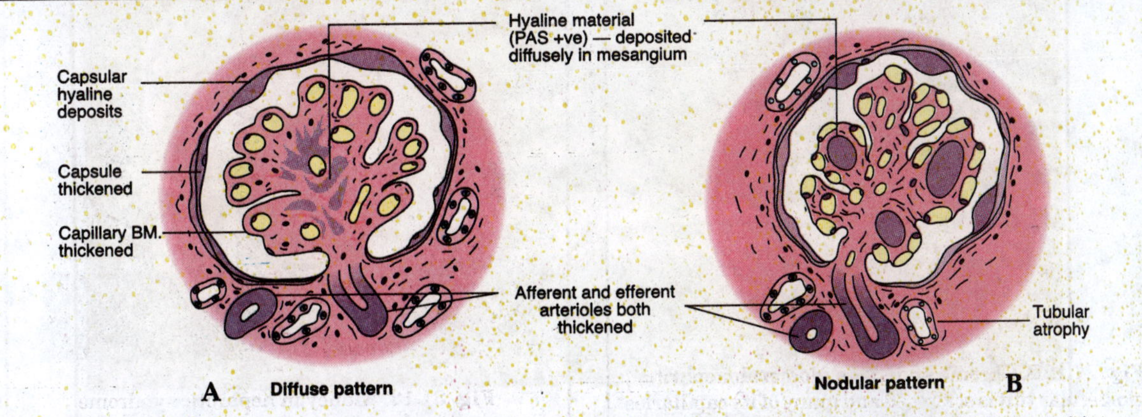

Fig. 31.14A& B. Diabetic glomerulosclerosis : diffuse and nodular glomerular changes (diagrammatic)

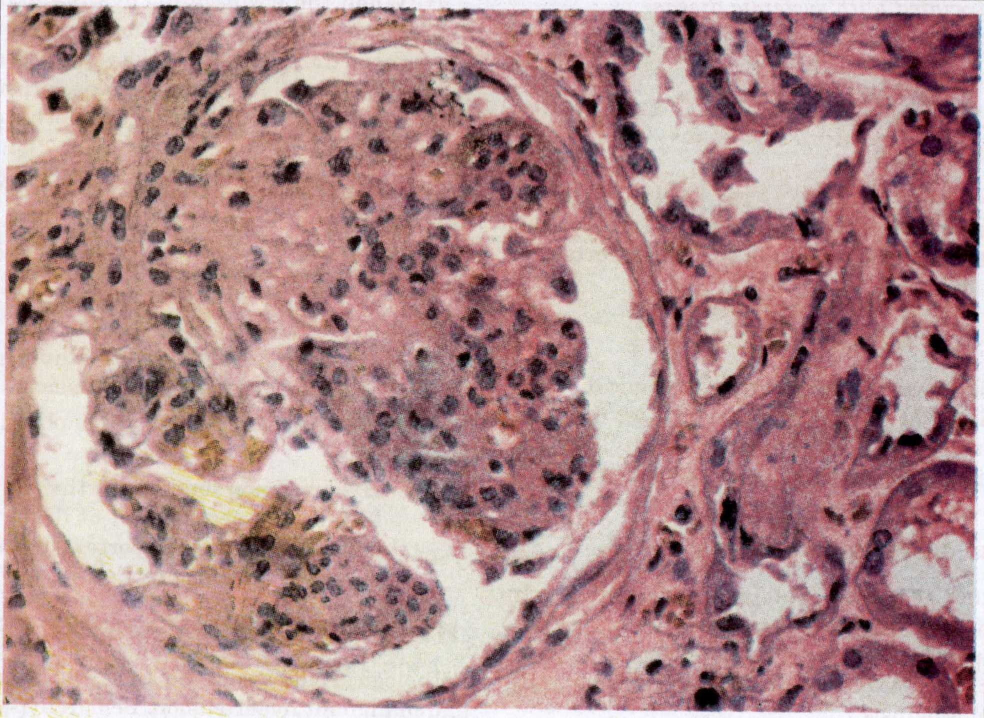

Fig. 31.15. Diabetic diffuse glomerulosclerosis, HE × 250

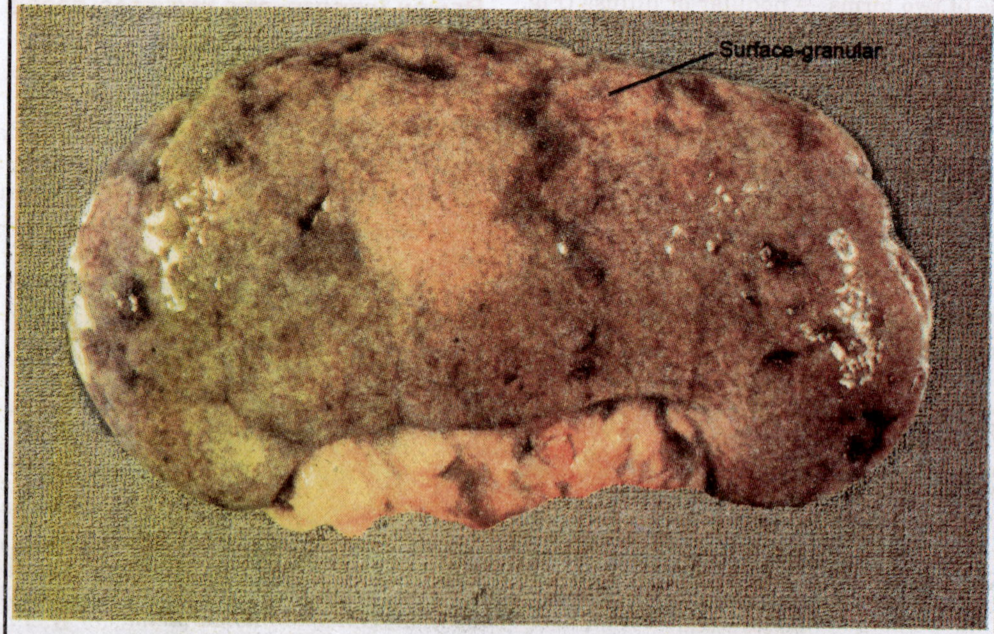

Fig. 31.16. Kidney in benign nephrosclerosis

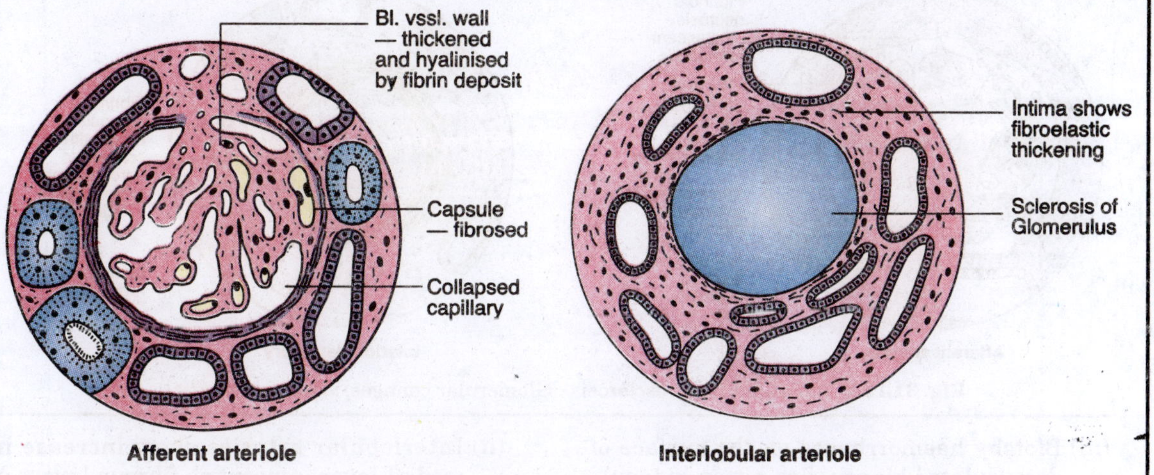

Fig. 31.17. Microscopy : Benign nephrosclerosis

Histology (Figs. 31.17, 26.42)

(i) The wall of afferent arterioles become thickened and hyalinized due to deposition of fibrin and basement membrane matrix.

(ii) Glomerulus is diffusely sclerosed with greatly reduced cellularity.

(iii) Fibrosis of media and fibroelastic thickening of intima occur in intertobular arteries.

(iv) Glomerulus is adherent to Bowman's capsule at several points.

MALIGNANT HYPERTENSIVE NEPHROSCLEROSIS

Macroscopy (31.18)

(i) Kidney size is almost normal.

(ii) Surface is smooth.

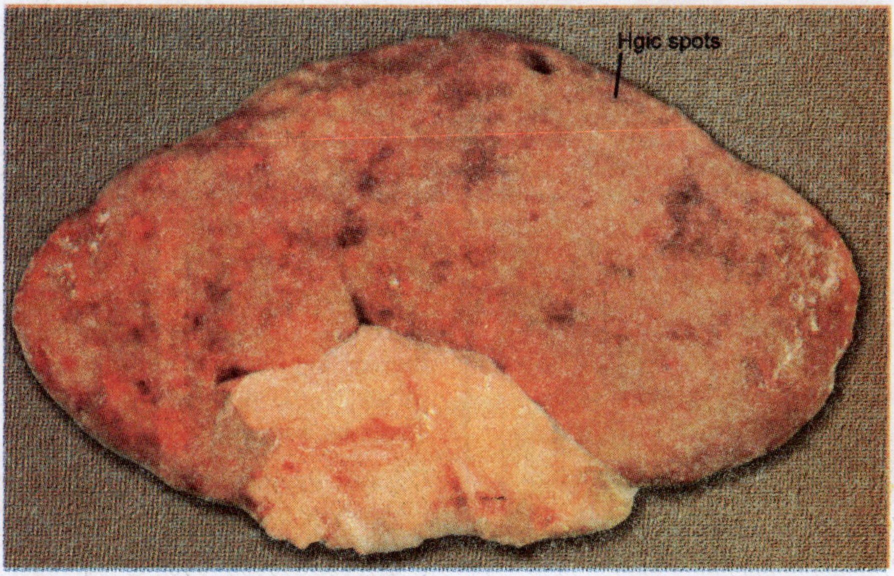

Fig. 31.18. Kidney in Malignant nephrosclerosis *(Flea-bitten kidney)*

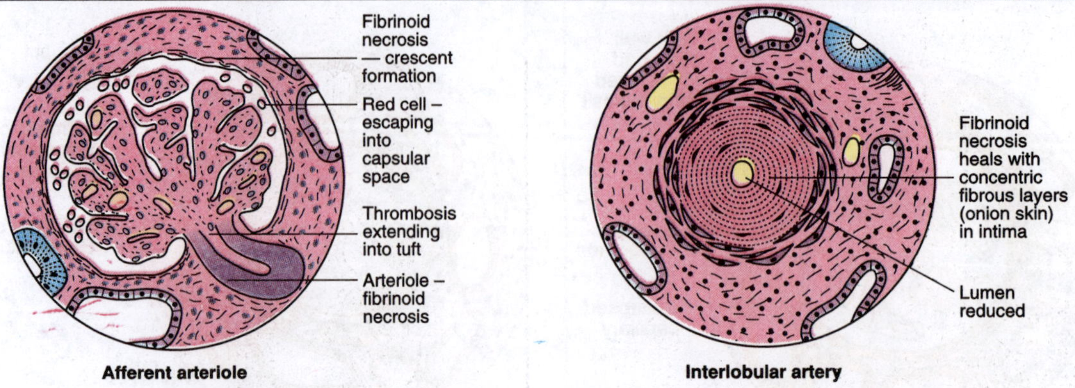

Fig. 31.19A. Malignant nephrosclerosis : Glomerular changes, × 200 *(schematic)*

(iii) Blotchy haemorrhages on the surface of decapsulated kidney (flea-bitten kidney).

(iv) Cut surface shows cortical haemorrhages and occasional infarct in cortex.

Histology (Figs. 31.19A & B)

(i) Afferent arterioles : The hall mark is firbinoid necrosis, afferent arterioles and adjacent part of glomerular tuft also show necrosis. Rest of the tuft is shrunken, lobulated and slightly fibrosed.

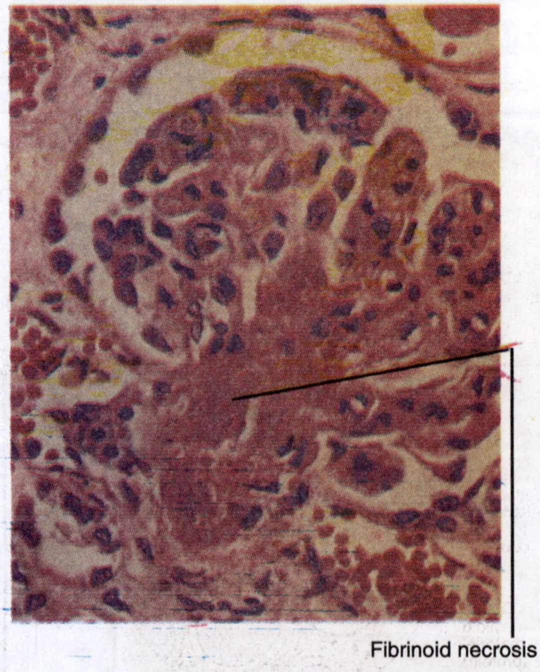

Fig. 31.19B. Kidney : Malignant hypertensive nephrosclerosis (× 350)

(ii) Interlobular arteries show increase in medial layer, concentric fibrous layers in intima (onion-skin like) and narrowed lumen.

INFECTIONS OF KIDNEY

Pyogenic infections of kidney produce predominantly tubulointerstitial nephritis which may be acute or chronic.

ACUTE PYELONEPHRITIS

Acute pyogenic nephritis is an acute suppurative inflammation of kidney caused by pyogenic bacteria and sometimes virus (e.g., polyoma virus). Most of the involved bacteria are normal commensals in the lower intestinal tract, they gain access to kidney either by ascending infection from lower urinary tract or by blood stream spread.

The hallmarks of acute pyelonephritis is patchy interstitial suppurative inflammation which is externally seen as small superficial abscesses that are yellow and raised. There is also intratubular aggregates of neutrophils and tubular necrosis.

Generally glomerular and vascular compartments are spared. The lesion may regress with therapy but leave interstitial retracting scars in the parenchyma.

CHRONIC PYELONEPHRITIS

Chronic pyelonephritis is a tubulointerstitial disease in which both parenchyma and renal pelvis are involved. Chronic pyelonephritis is a diffuse lesion with a surreptious course, sometimes develops after recurrent attacks of acute pyelonephritis and sometimes without any

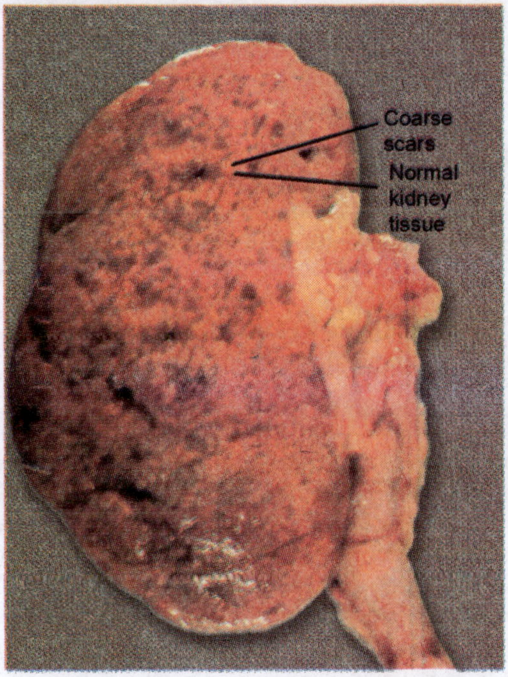

Fig. 31.20A. Kidney in chronic pyelonephritis

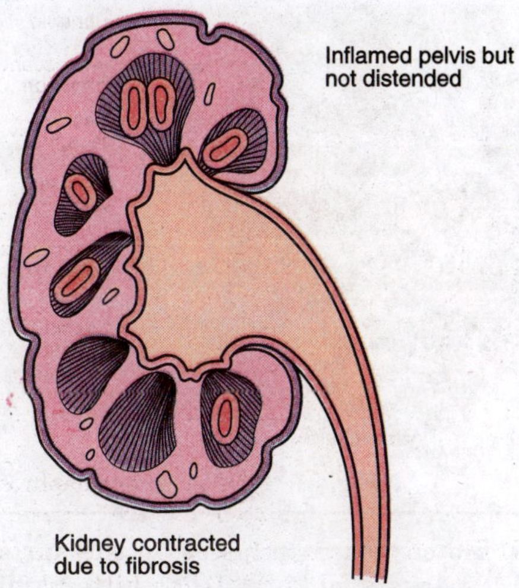

Fig. 31.20B. Cut section of kidney in chronic pyelonephritis

evidence of past infection. Congenital anomalies of the urinary tract is now regarded as important. The lesion may be unilateral and females are affected more than males.

Macroscopically (Figs. 31.20A & B)

(i) Kidney is small and contracted (weighs less than 100 gm each).

(ii) Outer surface shows **coarse wedge-shaped** scars that alternate with areas of normal kidney tissue to the shrunken fibrous tissue. Kidney is irregularly scarred and the scar areas show irregular depression on the surface.

(iii) Cut section shows dilated pelvis and blunted calyces. Pelvis is inflamed but not distended (Fig. 31.20B).

Microscopically (Figs. 31.21A, 31.21B)

(i) Interstitium shows heavy chronic inflammatory infiltrate consisting of lymphocytes, plasma cells and macrophages. There is extensive interstitial fibrosis.

(ii) Tubules : Many tubules are atrophied (advanced case). Some tubules show either atrophy or dilatation. Dilated tubules often contain densely eosinophilic (colloid) casts producing thyroidisation of the tubules.

(iii) The wall of pelvicalyceal system shows evidence of chronic inflammation and scarring.

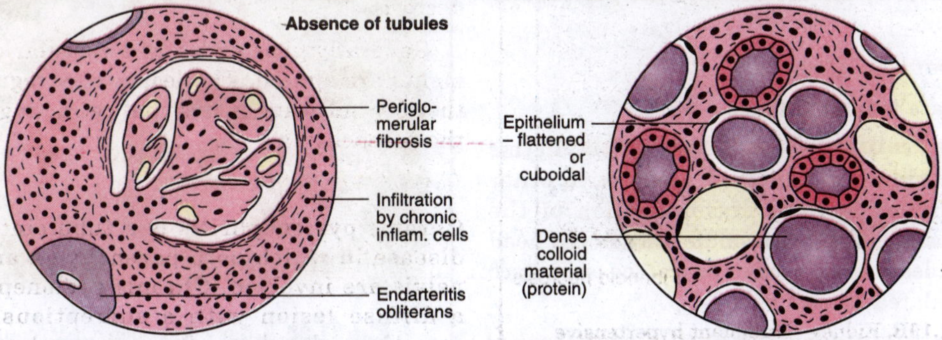

Fig. 31.21A. Histopathological appearance of kidney in chronic pyelonephritis *(schematic)*

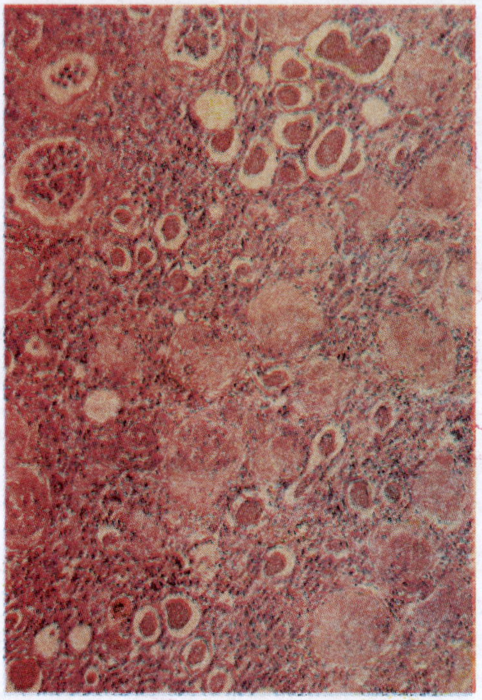

Fig. 31.21B. Chronic pyelonephritis microscopic picture (× 70)

(iv) There is usually periglomerular fibrosis and hyalinisation of some glomeruli. In Fig. 31.21B, the glomeruli are nearly all fibrosed and avascular.

RENAL TUBERCULOSIS

Pathogenesis

Renal tuberculosis is almost always blood-borne and secondary to an active tuberculous lesion elsewhere. Infection starts at cortex and then spreads within the glomeruli. At a later stage the bacilli may progress to the tubules and the peritubular tissues.

Macroscopic types

There are two main types :

1. **Acute miliary renal tuberculosis**: In this type, the kidney is involved along with other organs during miliary dissemination of the tubercle bacilli. There are small whitish pin head sized nodules both on section as well as on surface of decapsulated kidney.

2. **Chronic ulcerative and caseous renal tuberculosis** : This is the more frequent form of renal tuberculosis. Lesions spread to mucosa of pelvis, ureter and bladder.

Gross examination (Fig. 31.22)

Cut section of kidney shows cavitations of varying size containing caseous material within renal parenchyma. The wall of the hydronephrotic cavities are ragged, hard and whitish in colour. They rarley communicate with pelvis.

Diagnosis

Special culture in L.J. medium (3 consecutive morning samples) for tubercle bacilli.

OBSTRUCTIVE DISEASE

This group of disorder is usually caused by stenosis or defects in organogenesis. Obstruction in flow of urine, especially when its onset is rapid, usually results in urinary stasis and dilatation of the outflow tract upstream of the obstruction. The phenomenon is known as *hydronephrosis* when the pelvis is involved, and *hydroureter* if the stenosis is at a lower level.

Common causes of obstruction

1. *Congenital anomalies* : Posterior urethral valves and urethral strictures, meatal stenosis, bladder neck obstruction, ureteropelvic junction narrowing or obstruction, severe vesicoureteral reflux.

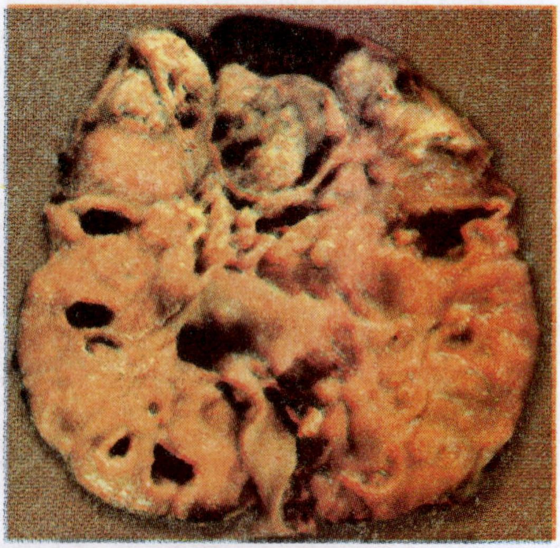

Fig. 31.22. Kidney (cut open) in caseous and ulcerative tuberculosis

2. *Benign prostatic hyperplasia*

3. *Urinary calculi*

4. *Tumours* : Carcinoma of prostate, tumour of bladder, contiguous malignant disease (e.g., retroperitoneal lymphoma), carcinoma of cervix or uterus.

5. *Inflammation* : Prostatitis, ureteritis, urethritis, retroperitoneal fibrosis.

6. *Sloughed papillae* or *blood clots*

7. *Pregnancy*

8. *Uterine prolapse* and *cystocele*

9. *Functional disorders* : Neurogenic (spinal cord damage) and other functional abnormalities of ureter or bladder (called *dysfunctional obstruction).*

Hydronephrosis

Hydronephrosis is a dilatation of the renal pelvis and calyces associated with progressive atrophy of renal tissue resulting from an obstruction to the outflow of urine.

The degree of hydronephrosis depends on the degree and duration of obstruction. When the obstruction is partial and intermittent, glomerular filtration is not suppressed, and progressive dilatation ensues resulting in greater degree of hydronephrosis than do sudden complete obstructions. The latter tends to produce atrophy with mild dilatation of the pelvis and calyces. With obstruction of one ureter only, hydronephrosis occurs in corresponding kidney, whereas obstructions at or below outlet of bladder lead to bilateral hydronephrosis.

Gross examination (Fig. 31.23)

1. Kidney may be slightly or massively enlarged.

2. Renal pelvis distended, calyces flattened. Renal tissue becomes atrophic and then the dilated pelvis assumes a saccular and rounded form.

3. In severe cases, outer surface of kidney is lobulated and kidney may be transformed into a thin wall sac.

Note : The atrophy and fibrosis of renal parenchyma affect tubules more rapidly than the glomeruli.

Microscopic examination

1. Cortical tubular atrophy with interstitial fibrosis.

2. Progressive blunting of apices of pyramids.

Polycystic Disease of Kidney

This appears in two main forms — *adult type* and *infantile type,* both inherited autosomally; but in the former it is a dominant trait and recessive in the latter. Infantile type is rare.

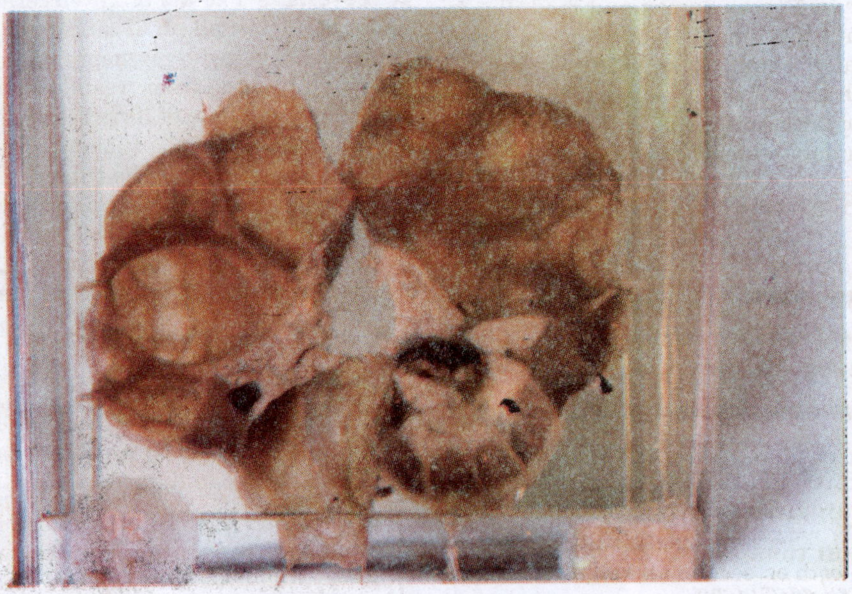

Fig. 31.23. Hydronephrosis of kidney

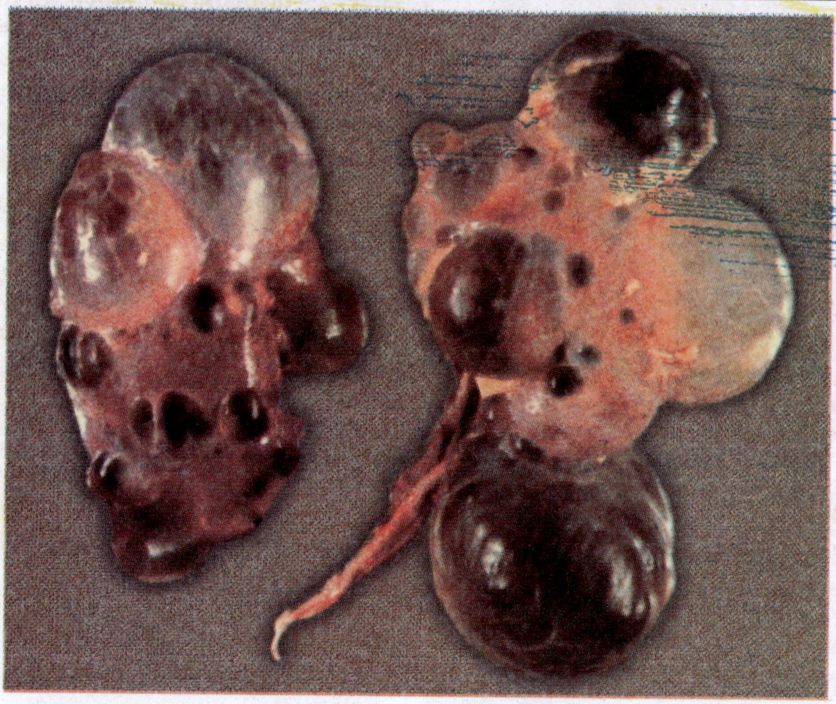

Fig. 31.24. Polycystic kidney in adult

Gross appearance (Fig. 31.24)

Kidney of an adult shows marked multicystic nodulations with transparent walls, visible on the surface. In cut section (the figure), almost entire renal parenchyma (both cortex and medulla) is replaced by multiple smooth-walled cysts. Cysts may occasionally communicate with one another but never with the pelvis of kidney. The content may be thin or thick and viscid fluid, clear amber or dark brown due to presence of blood.

RENAL TUMOURS

Classification

I. Benign tumours

1. *Adenoma* is quite common, greyish yellow (0.5 to 2 cm) in the cortex.
2. Renal *fibroma* or hamartoma is commonly found in medulla; there may also develop interstitial cell tumour.
3. *Angiomyolipoma*. 4. *Oncocytoma*.

II. Malignant tumours

1. *Renal cell carcinoma*
2. Wilms' tumour (nephroblastoma)

RENAL CELL CARCINOMA

(Hypernephroma or Adenocarcinoma of kidney, Grawitz's tumour)

It represents 1 to 3% of all visceral cancers and about 85-90% of all renal cancers in adults. It was erroneously called hypernephroma as it had been supposed to arise from "rests" of adrenal cells in the kidney because of its gross yellow colour and the resemblance of the tumour cells to clear cells of the adrenal cortex. The tumour is composed of large clear cells with abundant pale foamy cytoplasm, which is now believed to have originated from convoluted tubular epithelium, as evidenced by electron-microscopic studies of the tumour cells.

Gross appearance (Fig. 31.25)

1. It may arise in any part of kidney, but more commonly it affects the poles, usually upper pole.

2. *Size* : It is usually a solitary large, rounded tumour, 3-15 cm in diameter.

3. *Capsule* : At first, the tumour is well encapsulated and separated from the renal tissue. However, the tumour being microscopically invasive, it is not easily separated from surrounding tissue.

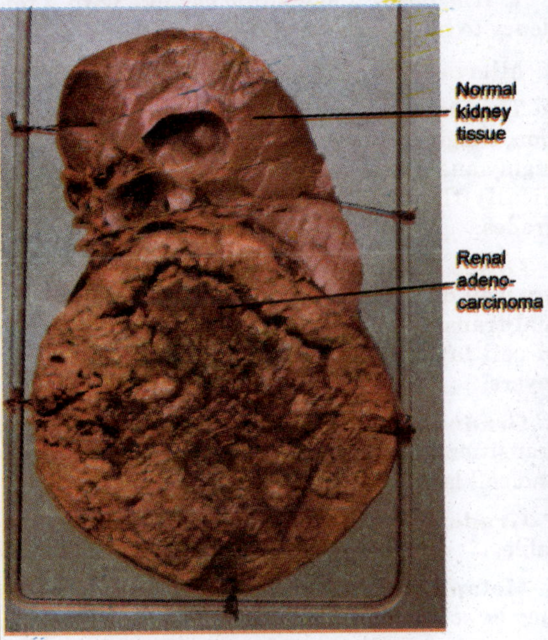

Fig. 31.25. Renal adenocarcinoma

4. *Cut surface* is yellow grey and connective tissue trabeculae traverse irregularly through the tumour.

5. *Haemorrhage* and *necrosis* are common.

Microscopic examination :

See chapter 26 Fig. 26.18.

Metastasis

Local spread is by penetration of renal capsule and invasion of renal veins.

The tumour is vascular and metastasises to regional lymph nodes, bone, lung and liver. Spread to opposite kidney occurs by veins. The tumour metastasises widely giving rise to any local symptoms or signs.

NEPHROBLASTOMA (Wilms' tumour)

It is a common primary renal tumour of childhood (approximately 1 per lakh children under age 15 years). This embryonic type of tumour is derived from kidney rudiments (nephrogenic nests) and produces a large solitary well-circumscribed mass (10% are bilateral). Microscopically, the classic triphasic combination of blastemal, stromal and epithelial cell types is commonly seen (Fig. 31.26). There may be skeletal differentiation. The tumour rapidly invades blood vessels leading to pulmonary metastasis. Long-time survival rate is 90% with nephrectomy and chemotherapy. It appears that mutation a gene (WT-1) is responsible for development of the tumour.

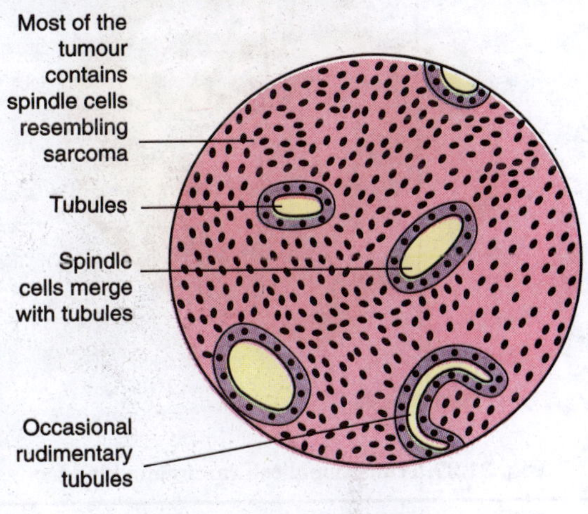

Fig. 31.26. Nephroblastoma

TUMOURS OF RENAL PELVIS

Pelvis of kidney gives rise to same type of tumours as found in bladder, the commonest types being transitional cell papilloma and transitional papillary carcinoma.

TUMOURS OF URINARY BLADDER

I. Benign tumours

1. *Transitional cell papilloma*
2. *Inverted transitional cell papilloma*

II. Malignant tumours

Transitional cell carcinoma.

Differentiation of benign and malignant tumours

The benign transitional cell papilloma of bladder is extremely difficult to differentiate from grade I papillary carcinoma (Fig. 31.27) and hence some experts consider transitional cell papillomas to be transitional cell carcinoma (TCC) grade I. Inverted transitional cell papilloma differs from transitional cell papilloma by its endophytous growth.

TRANSITIONAL CELL CARCINOMA

About 90% of bladder tumours are TCC grades I to IV and the rest show phenomena of metaplasia that can be squamous, glandular or mixed.

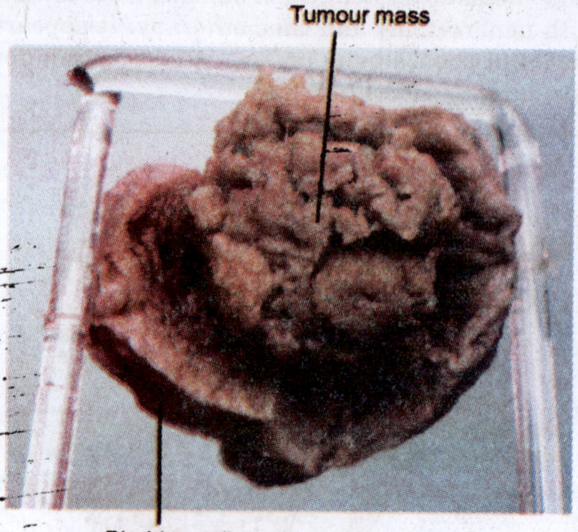

Fig. 31.27. Transitional cell carcinoma bladder

Gross appearance (Fig. 31.27)

1. The tumour may be papillary or flat and invasive or non-invasive.

2. It is bulky and cauliflower-like with a tendency to haemorrhage and necrosis.

Microscopic examination (Fig. 31.28)

The tumours vary in the degree of differentiation, ranging from normal transitional cell type to highly anaplastic and pleomorphic type. Microscopically they can be distinguished into three grades.

Grade I : Tumour cells display some atypia but are well differentiated and closely resemble normal transitional cells. Mitosis are rare. Number of cell layer is increased to more than seven layers.

Grade II : Tumour cell still recognisable as of transitional origin. Both the numbers of mitosis and cell layers increase (often more than ten).

Grade III : Tumour cells are barely recognisable.

Metaplastic growth : Metaplastic phenomena may be so striking that some forms are defined as squamous carcinoma or adenocarcinoma. The origin of adenocarcinoma of bladder may also be connected with embryonal residues.

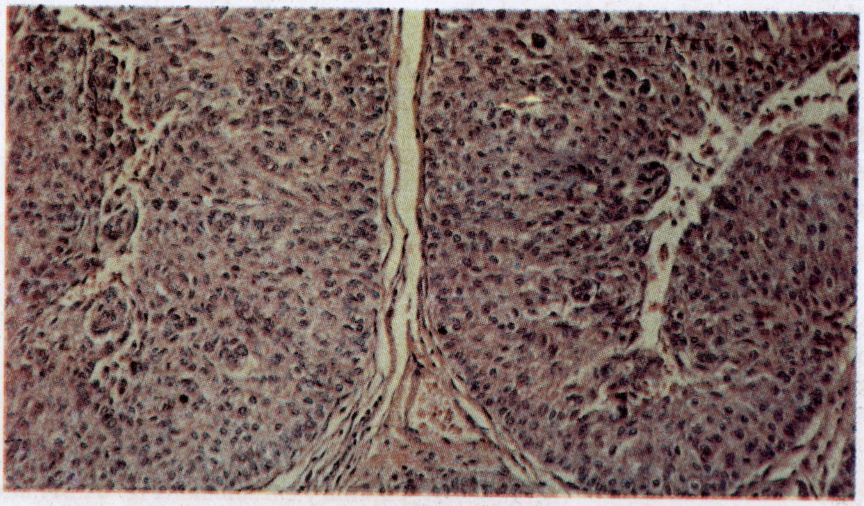

Fig. 31.28. Transitional cell carcinoma of bladder — grade II, HE × 250

Chapter 32

Male Reproductive System

DISORDERS OF PROSTATE

1. *Prostatis* : Acute and chronic bacterial type. Sometimes abacterial in nature.
2. *Benign hyperplasia* — see chapter 26.
3. *Prostatic carcinoma* : Adenocarcinoma.

ADENOCARCINOMA PROSTATE

A. Diagnostic tests in carcinoma of prostate

1. *Measurement of prostate specific antigen* (PSA) using immunohistochemical technique or ELISA is a useful marker.
2. Blood *alkaline phosphatase* is raised when metastases are present.

B. Differentiation (grading)

Geleason system (Grades 2 through 10) — well differentiated to aggressive anaplastic tumours, grading correlates with prognosis of disease (vide chapter 26).

DISEASES OF PENIS

TUMOURS OF PENIS

Tumours of penis are not very common and most tumours include carcinoma and a benign epithelial tumour — condyloma acuminatum.

I. Benign tumours

Condyloma acuminatum

It is caused by human papilloma virus (HPV) type 6 and 11. It is a sexually transmitted disease and can occur on moist cutaneous surface of external genitalia in either sex. *Giant condyloma* is much larger than condyloma acuminatum.

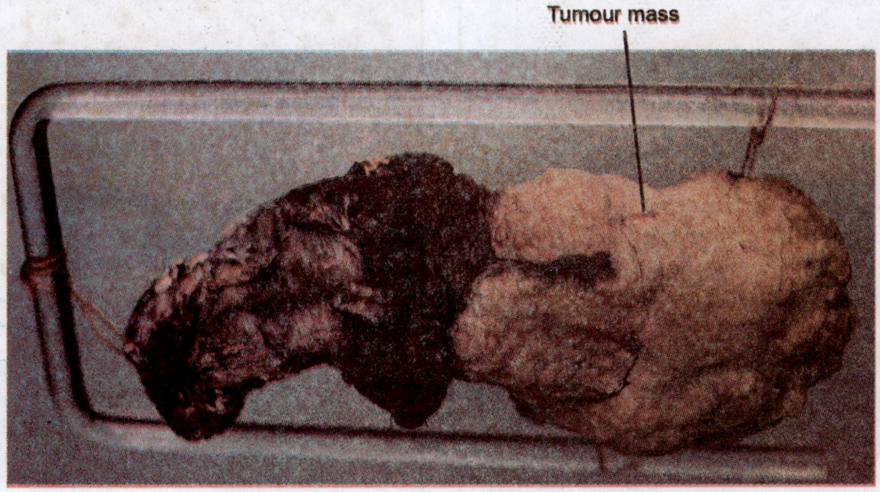

Fig. 32.1. Squamous cell carcinoma of penis

Macroscopic appearance

The tumour occurs on coronal sulcus and inner surface of prepuce. They are single or multiple sessile or pedunculated, red papillary excrescence of one to several mm in diameter.

Microscopic examination

Branching villous papillary connective tissue is covered by a thickened hyperplastic epithelium.

II. Carcinoma of penis

Squamous cell carcinoma of penis represents about 1% of cancers in males. HPV type 16 is implicated in its causation. The lesion begins usually on the glans or inner surface of the prepuce near coronal sulcus. Incidence is extremely rare among Jews and Moslems and common in uncircumcised people. Smegma is believed to be a source of yet unidentified carcinogen. Metastasis occurs to inguinal, and, later, retroperitoneal lymph nodes.

(a) ***Carcinoma in situ***
(Bowen's disease, Queyrat's erythroplasia)

The epithelial cells show cytologic changes of malignancy confined to the epithelium.

(b) ***Invasive squamous cell carcinoma***

Macroscopic appearance (Fig. 32.1)

It begins as a small warty growth. In advanced cases, the tumour appears as an ulcerative fungating mass which has virtually destroyed the entire tip of the penis or large part of the shaft. Sometimes papillary growth also occurs.

Histology : Squamous cell carcinoma.

DISEASES OF TESTIS

A. Epididymitis and Orchitis

1. Acute inflammation
2. Chronic granulomatous orchitis :
   (a) Tuberculosis (b) Gamma

B. Tumours

Germ cell Tumours include :

1. Seminoma. 2. Malignant teratoma

SEMINOMA

It corresponds to dysgerminoma in the female. It accounts for 50% of all testicular tumours. Growth is extremely radiosensitive. It occurs in early middle age (around 40).

Gross appearance (Fig. 32.2) : Tumour is uniform and pale creamy colour. It has a faint lobular appearance and often looks like a potato.

Microscopy (Fig. 32.3)

1. Tumour cells — uniformly large and polyhedral and closely packed.

2. Cells have a clear foamy cytoplasm (containing glycogen). Nucleoli are prominent in round to ovoid nucleus.

3. Delicate fibrous stroma passing through groups of tumour cells are heavily infiltrated by lymphocytes.

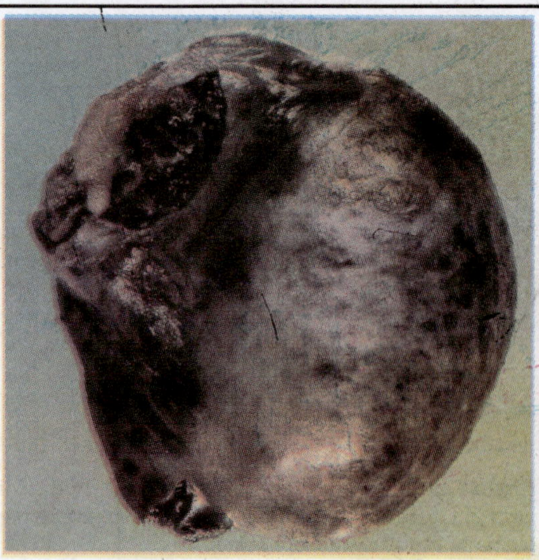

Fig. 32.2. Seminoma testis

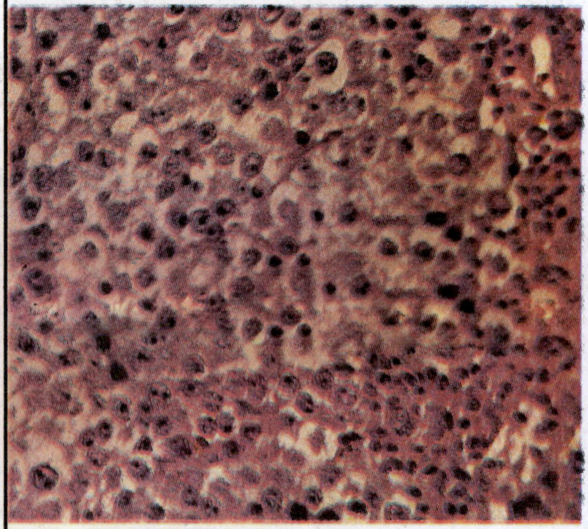

Fig. 32.3. Seminoma testis, HE × 250

Chapter 33

Female Reproductive System

HYDATIDIFORM MOLE

It is a benign condition of placental tissue but it has the potentiality for developing choriocarcinoma.

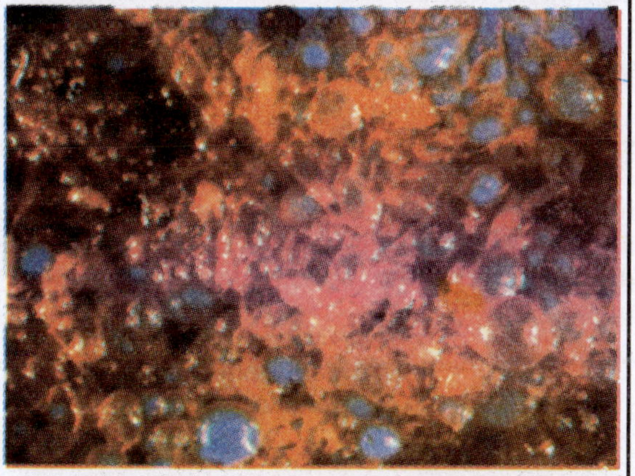

Fig. 33.1. Hydatidiform mole suspended in saline showing numerous swollen villi

Macroscopy (Fig. 33.1)

Molar tissue looking grape-like vesicles up to 3 cm in diameter. There is clear watery fluid within the vesicles.

Microscopically (Fig. 33.2)

Chorionic villi markedly swollen and expanded due to hydropic swelling of villous stromal core. Surface of each villous is covered with a thin layer of trophoblast.

UTERUS

TUMOURS OF CERVIX

I. Epithelial tumours

A. *Benign*
   1. *Endocervical polyps*
   2. *Viral warts*

B. *Malignant*
   1. *Squamous cell carcinoma,* intraepithelial and invasive.
   2. *Adenocarcinoma*
   3. *Adenoacanthoma*

II. Non-epithelial tumours

A. *Benign*
   1. *Leiomyoma*

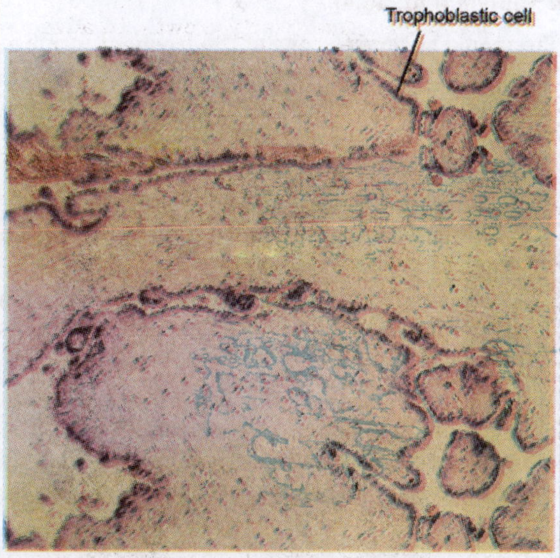

Fig. 33.2. Photomicrograph of partial hydatidiform mole revealing swollen villi and slight hyperplasia of the surface trophoblast

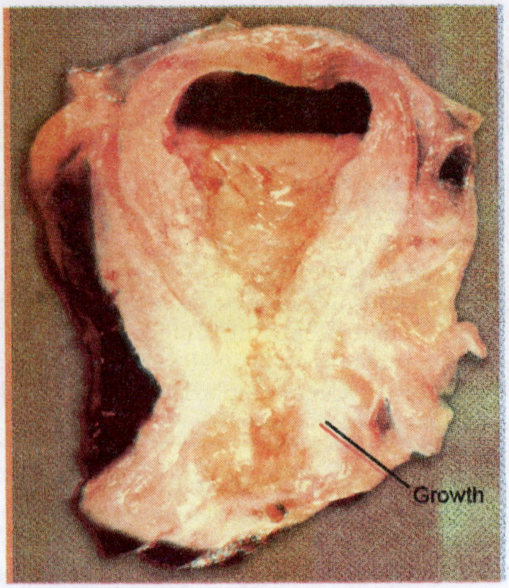

Fig. 33.3. Squamous cell carcinoma of cervix invading uterine body and bladder

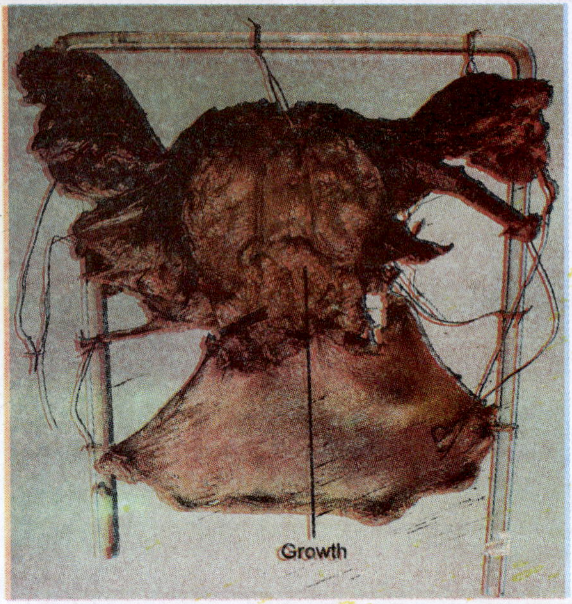

Fig. 33.4. Squamous cell carcinoma of cervix

B. *Malignant*

1. *Leiomyosarcoma*
2. Embyronal rhabdomyosarcoma

Squamous cell carcinoma of cervix (Fig. 33.4)

Carcinoma of cervix is one of the frequent forms of cancer in women. The incidence has fallen in developed countries due to detection of early cancers. About 95% of cervical cancers are *squamous cell carcinoma* and the remainder being *adenocarcinoma.*

Squamous cell carcinoma mainly arises from ectocervical mucosa; its incidence is related to :

(1) early age at first intercourse, (2) multiple sexual partners, and (3) a male partner with multiple previous sexual partners.

The tumours seems to develop from pre-invasive neoplastic lesions (*see below*). Human papilloma virus (HPV) is currently considered as an important factor in cervical carcinogenesis. *Herpes* simplex *virus*–2 (HSV-2) may also play an aetiologic role.

Gross appearance (Figs. 33.3 and 33.4)

Invasive carcinomas manifest in 3 distinctive forms : (a) *fungating* (or exophytic), (b) *ulcerating* and (c) *infiltrative.*

The most common type is fungating (exophytic vegetating) tumour that projects above the surrounding mucosa (Figs. 33.3 and 33.4). The ulcerating type, in its early stage, can be confused with an inflammatory process, and infiltrating type is difficult to recognise. However, the typing has got no relationship to the histological pattern.

Microscopic examination

It can differentiate into 3 types :

1. Keratinising squamous cell carcinoma, which is a well-differentiated carcinoma (Grade I).

2. Poorly differentiated squamous carcinoma, the most common type (Grade II).

3. The small-celled undifferentiated carcinoma, with less favourable prognosis (Grade III).

Cervical Intraepithelial Neoplasia (CIN)

Papanicoloau's smear screening is very effective in preventing cervical cancer because majority of cancers are preceded by a precancerous lesion.

Cervical intraepithelial neoplasia (CIN) was formerly known as dysplasia, CIN is now the accepted term of cervical precancers. The degree of cellular abnormality is variable and is graded I (mild dysplasia), grade II (moderate dysplasia) and grade III (severe full thickness atypia). CIN III includes grade III dysplasia and squamous cell carcinoma in situ. CIN begins almost always at the squamo-columnar junction, in the transformation zone (vide chapter 37, p. 331).

Adenocarcinoma of cervix

It is less common and accounts for 5% of all cervical cancers. By biopsy examination it is difficult to be certain, whether the tumour represents a primary cervical malignancy or an extension of endometrial cancer.

Adenoacanthoma

Mixed form of adenocarcinoma and squamous cell carcinoma has been described.

TUMOURS OF UTERUS

I. ***Tumours of endometrium***

- A. *Benign* : Endometrial polyps.
- B. *Malignant* : Adenocarcinoma, adenosquamous carcinoma.

II. ***Non-epithelial tumours***

- A. *Benign* : Leiomyoma (Fibroid)
- B. *Malignant* : Leiomyosarcoma, endometrial stromal sarcoma.

Leiomyoma (also called fibroid, fibroma, fibromyoma, myoma)

These are the most common tumours found in women (about 25%) in their active reproductive life. Leiomyoma is benign tumour composed of interlacing bundles of smooth muscle and fibrous tissue.

Gross examination (Figs. 33.5 and 33.6)

The tumours are often multiple grey-white, discrete, spherical, and of variable size (barely visible to 10-15 cm massive size). They are encapsulated and mostly found within myometrium (intramural), but can also be submucous or subserous. Consistency of tumour is rubbery. Large leiomyomas show central necrosis and haemorrhage due to scant vascularisation. There can be cystic degeneration.

Microscopic examination

The tumour is composed of whorled bundles of well differentiated smooth muscle cells. The individual muscle cells are usually uniform in size and shape with oval nucleus and long, slender, bipolar cytoplasmic process. Mitosis is scarce.

Adenocarcinoma (Fig. 33.7)

Endometrial adenocarcinoma, most common malignancy of body of uterus, usually arises at about the time of menopause.

Gross appearance (Fig. 26.10)

1. *Vegetative type* : Exophytic growth that fills the endometrial cavity (Fig. 33.7). Uterus may be

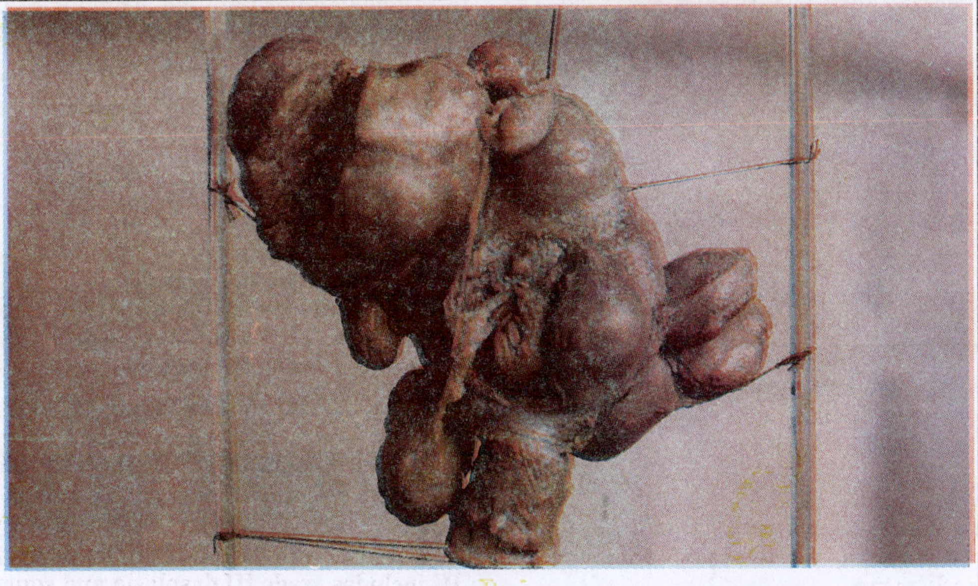

Fig. 33.5. Uterine leiomyoma — multiple fibroids (*Note : A foetus*)

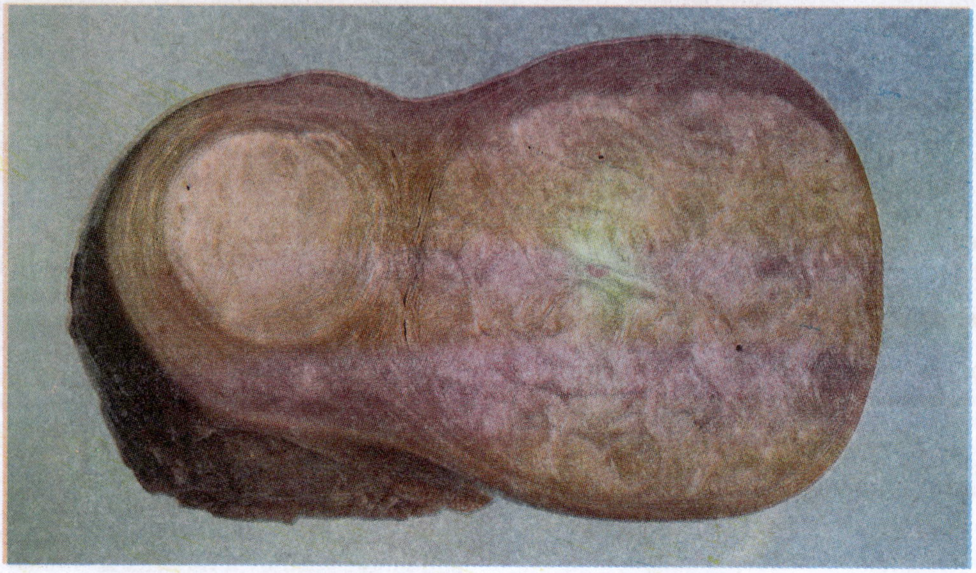

Fig. 33.6. Leiomyoma uterus (cross section)

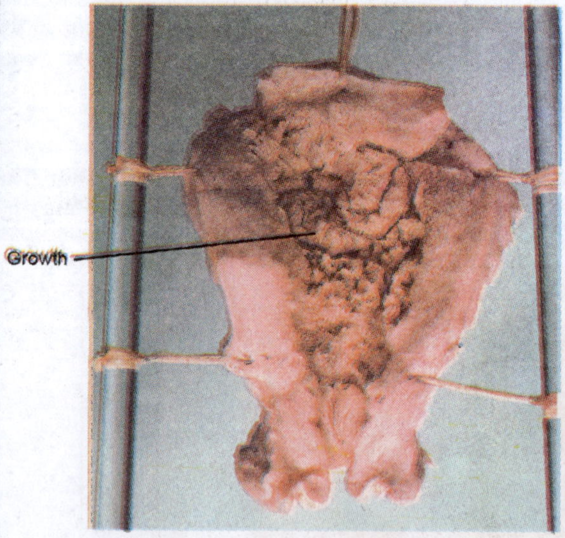

Fig. 33.7. Adenocarcinoma of endometrium

of normal size or enlarged. There is abundant necrotic material in uterine cavity.

2. *Infiltrative type* : The tumour infiltrates the myometrium in such a manner that the primary site may not be recognised.

Microscopical features

The tumour is composed of atypical glands, arranged back to back that have a tendency to form folds and/or papillae. Tumour cells invade the underlying myometrium.

The tumour can be well differentiated, poorly differentiated or undifferentiated. Well differentiated forms bear many similarities to the atypical adenomatous hyperplasia.

Adenoacanthoma

There are benign squamous metaplasia in some cases of well differentiated adenocarcinoma which are called adenoacanthoma or adenosquamous carcinoma.

Chapter 34

Breast

TUMOURS OF BREAST

Tumours of breast are mostly confined to women.

Classification

I. *Benign*

1. Fibroadenoma
2. Cystosarcoma phyllodes
3. Intraduct papilloma

II. *Malignant*

A. *Non-infiltrating* (non-invasive)

1. Intraduct carcinoma (papillary, cribriform and solid carcinoma in situ).
2. Lobular carcinoma in situ.

B. *Infiltrating* (invasive)

1. Infiltrating ductal carcinoma *not otherwise specified* (carcinoma NOS) (scirrhous carcinoma).
2. Medullary carcinoma.
3. Colloid or mucinous carcinoma.
4. Paget's disease (infiltrating ductal carcinoma with Paget's disease).
5. Infiltrating lobular carcinoma.

FIBROADENOMA OF BREAST

Fibroadenomas are very common benign tumours of breast of young women (20-35 years old). It mostly arises in the breast as a solitary lesion but

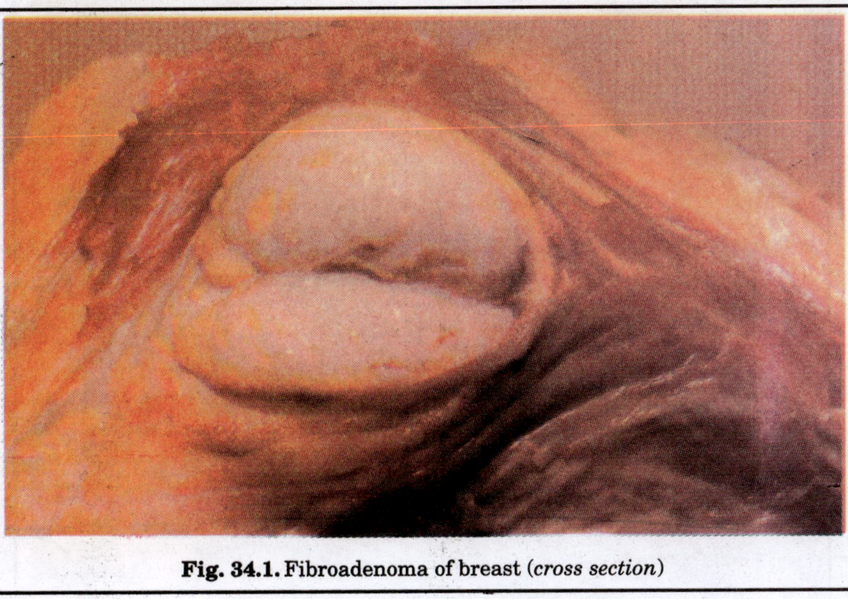

Fig. 34.1. Fibroadenoma of breast (*cross section*)

may occur as a component of fibroadenosis particularly in older women about the time of menopause.

Macroscopic appearance (Fig. 34.1)

A fibroadenoma forms a well circumscribed mass, up to about 3 cm diameter, formed by condensation of connective tissue. It is greyish white in appearance and firm in consistency.

Microscopical examination (Figs. 26.6, 26.7)

See chapter 26. Fibroadenoma is a mixed tumour comprising of epithelial (mammary duct type epithelium) and fibrous stromal components.

CARCINOMA OF BREAST

Breast cancer causes about 20% of cancer deaths in females. Breast carcinomas may originate in the epithelium of mammary ducts or the breast lobular glands *(ductal* and *lobular carcinoma,* respectively), vast majority (90%) are of ductal origin. Both ductal and lobular carcinoma may be in situ stage (malignant cells confined to the gandular component of the organ by the epithelial basement membrane of duct or lobule).

Non Infiltrating Carcinoma

In intraduct carcinoma, the malignant cells fill and distend the duct. *Histologically* these are divided into 5 subtypes : *comedocarcinoma, solid, cribriform, papillary* and *micropapillary carcinoma.*

Comedocarcinoma is characterised by rapidly proliferating high grade malignant cells that have filled the duct and tumour cells at the centre are necrotic.

Microscopical examination

The ducts are filled with malignant cells (large and pale staining with large nuclei). The cells have abundant cytoplasm with round or oval nuclei. Many of the nuclei are hyperchromatic with evidence of increased mitosis. Sometimes, distension of the duct is marked and the neoplastic cells at the centre undergo necrosis (*comedo carcinoma*). The tumour cells have not infiltrated the surrounding stroma and the epithelial basement membrane of the duct is intact. However, infiltration eventually supervenes with development of infiltrating ductal carcinoma.

Infiltrating Duct Carcinoma (Scirrhous Carcinoma)

This is the most common type of breast carcinoma (65-80%). They mostly exhibit a marked increase in dense, fibrous tissue stroma, giving the tumour hard consistency, hence called *scirrhous carcinoma* (Fig. 34.2). Glandular/tubular differentiation may be well developed, barely detectable or altogether absent (for this reason the term adenocarcinoma is not advisable as a synonym for invasive ductal carcinoma).

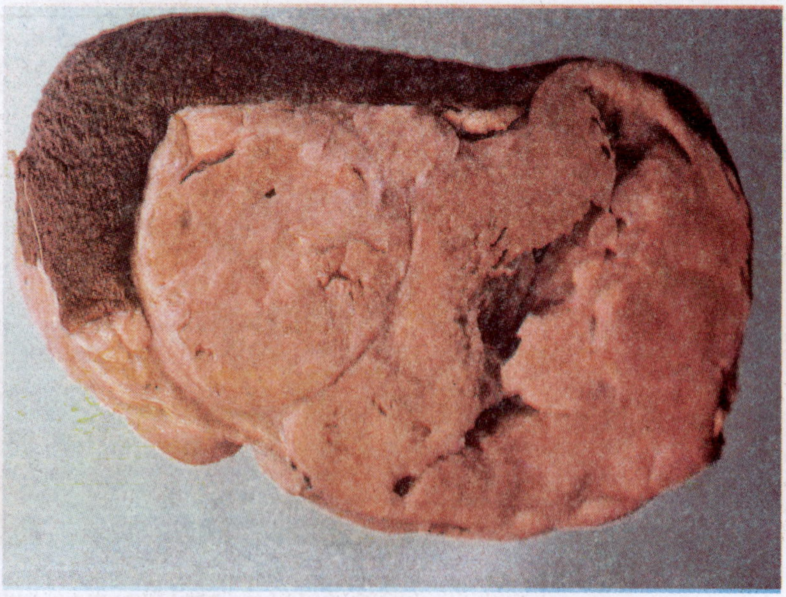

Fig. 34.2. Scirrhous carcinoma of breast

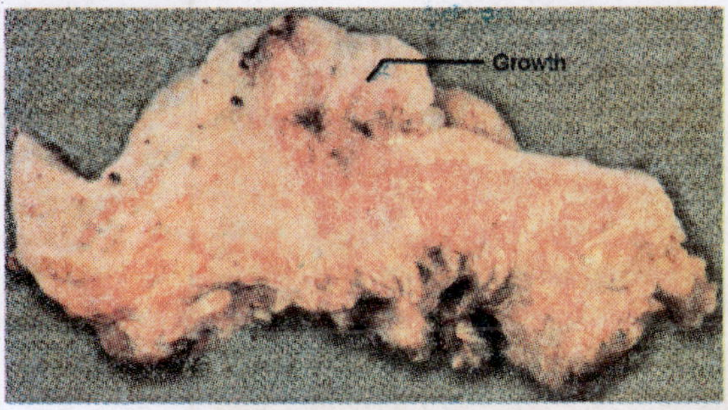

Fig. 34.3. Ductal carcinoma of breast (*cross section*)

Gross appearance (Figs. 34.2 and 34.3)

In typical case, the tumour is 1-2 cm in diameter and rarely exceeds 5 cm, firm, poorly circumscribed, cuts with a resistant gritty sensation, shows yellowish grey cut surface. Trabeculae of tumour radiate through surrounding parenchyma into fat (crab-like configuration).

Histological examination (Fig. 26.17)

The tumour is composed principally of a dense fibrous stroma in which there are nests or cords of tumour cells. Glandular or tubular differentiation may develop or may not develop. The cells are round to polygonal and vary in size and shape but they are larger and more pleomorphic than those of invasive lobular carcinoma. The neoplastic cells infiltrate surrounding fibrofatty tissue.

Medullary Carcinoma

Medullary carcinoma of breast accounts for 1 to 5% of breast carcinomas.

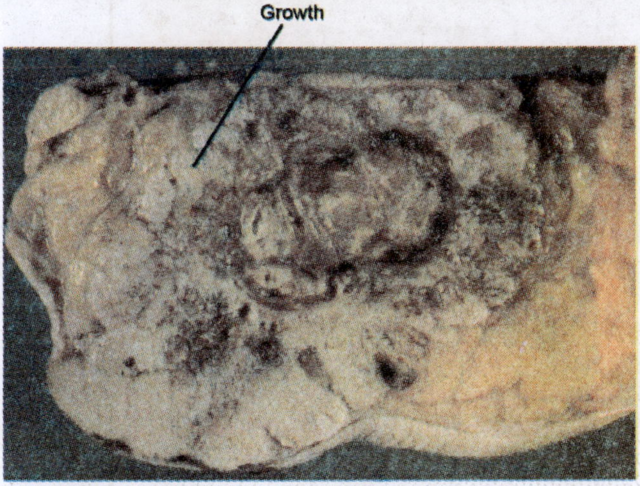

Fig. 34.4. Medullary carcinoma of breast (ulcerated)

Gross appearance (Fig. 34.4, 34.5)

1. Size 2-3 cm, solitary nodule of soft consistency and fairly well demarcated.
2. Cut surface—solid, homogeneous grey.

Histology

1. Solid, syncytium like sheets of large cells with vesicular, often pleomorphic nuclei, containing prominent nucleoli and frequent mitosis. There is minimal or no glandular differentiation or intraductal growth, and absence of mucin secretion.
2. Moderate to marked lymphocytic infiltrate between these sheets and at the periphery. Most lymphocytes are T cells.
3. Scanty fibrous component.

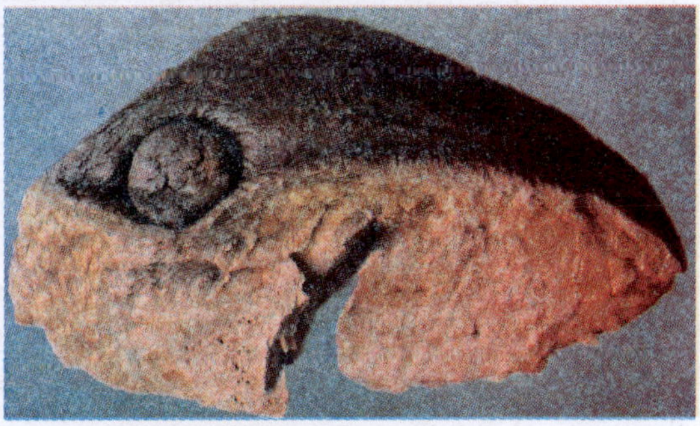

Fig. 34.5. Breast carcinoma (*cross section*) : infiltrating ductal medullary carcinoma

Paget's Disease

Paget's (*James Paget, 1874*) disease of the nipple is the name given to a crusted eczema-like lesion of the nipple and areola associated with an underlying carcinoma of excretory duct (Fig. 34.6).

Histology : The epidermis of nipple and areola becomes infiltrated by large, pale, vacuolated cells (Paget cells) with hyperchromatic nuclei and pale cytoplasm (Fig. 34.7).

Origin of Paget's cells

The Paget's cells are breast carcinoma cells that extend intraepithelially along the epithelium of the mammary and nipple ducts to surface from an intraduct or infiltrating ductular carci-

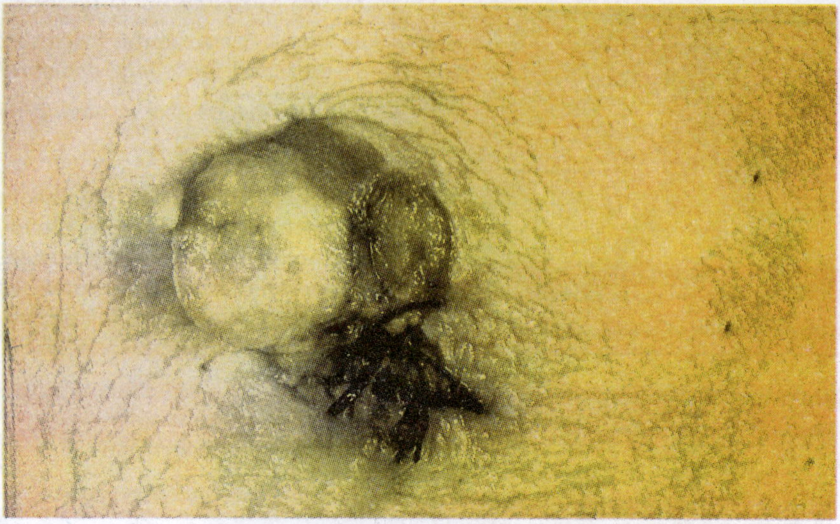

Fig. 34.6. Paget's disease of the nipple

noma, which is invariably present in the underlying breast tissue.

LOBULAR CARCINOMA

Invasive lobular carcinoma arises from the lobules and their terminal ductules. Its prognosis is as bad as invasive duct cell carcinoma.

Gross examination : The tumour is rubbery and poorly circumscribed.

Histology : The tumour cells are small, sometimes innocuous appearing neoplastic cells found singly or at most in small clusters in the form of an 'Indian file' in stroma.

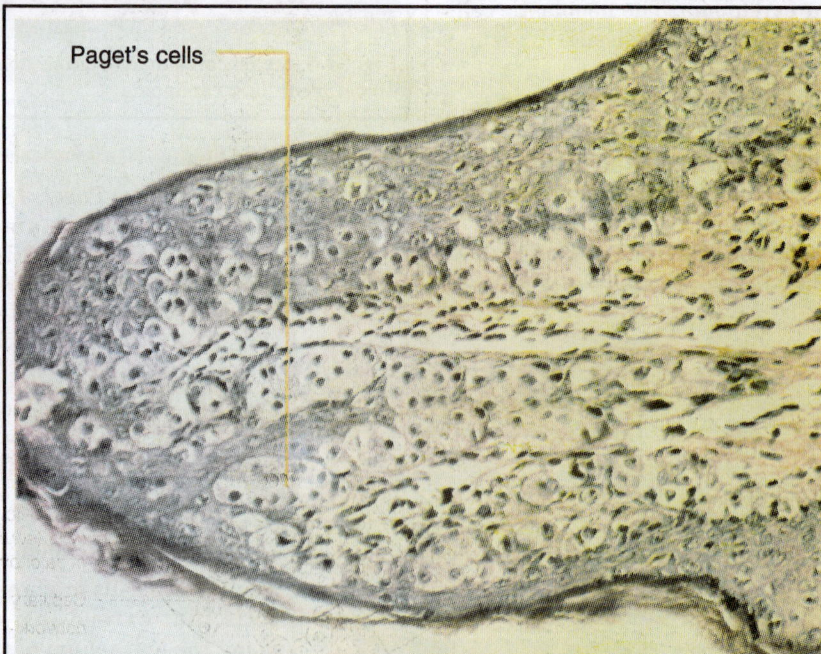

Fig. 34.7. ME : Paget's disease of nipple, HE × 250

Chapter 35

Thyroid

Normal structure

Thyroid is a bilobed organ and the two lobes are connected by isthmus. It has a smooth external surface covered by a thin transparent capsule. Variations in the structure of thyroid gland include the presence of a pyramidal lobe, a remnant of the thyroglossal duct above the isthmus (Fig. 35.1).

NON TOXIC GOITRE

This is a simple enlargement of the thyroid gland not associated with increased secretion of thyroid hormone (T_3, T_4). The cause is lack of iodine in diet.

Classification

1. **Diffuse (simple) goitre** : In simple goitre, the thyroid gland is usually diffusely and more or less symmetrically enlarged due to an absolute or relative deficiency of iodine or to goitrogenic agents. In most instances, normal thyroid hormone is achieved. The condition may occur endemically *(endemic goitre)* and also sporadically in women *(sporadic goitre)*.

2. **Collolid goitre (Fig. 35.2)** : Successive cycles of uneven hyperplasia and involution occur in late stage of most diffuse hyperplasia, which gives rise to nodularity. Thyroid is enlarged and translucent due to large amount of stored colloid, which results from continuing iodine deficiency.

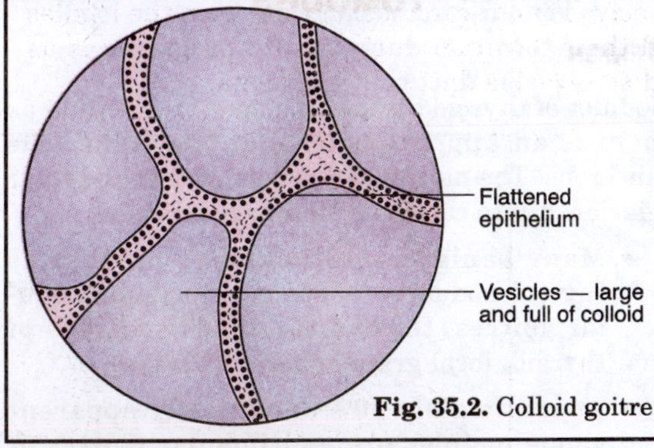

Fig. 35.2. Colloid goitre

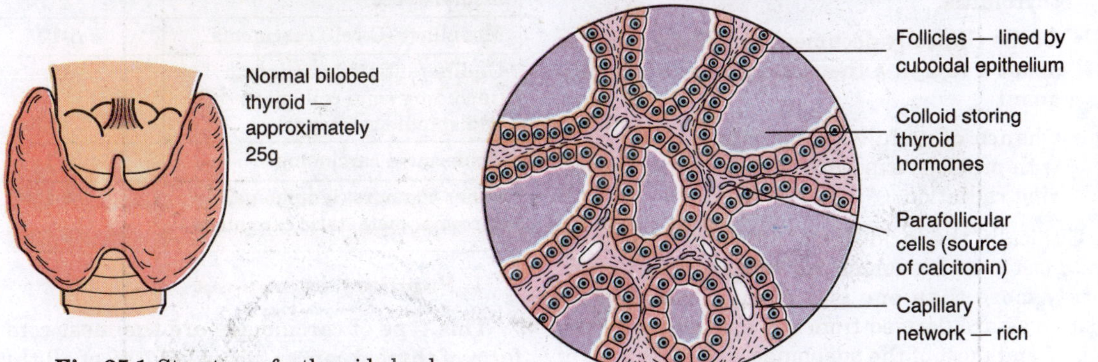

Fig. 35.1. Structure of a thyroid gland

Colloid goitre may be *diffuse* or *nodular* (due to disproportionate hyperplasia, involution or fibrosis).

Histology (Figs. 26.37, 35.2)

(i) Section shows the picture of thyroid tissue.

(ii) Gland acini are dilated and filled with deeply staining colloid material.

(iii) Lining epithelium of acini is flattened cubical.

Diagnosis : Collolid goitre.

Hyperplasia of thyroid

Thyroid function is under the control of TSH that stimulates thyroid acinar cells to produce thyroxine. Circulating thyroxine, then, regulates TSH production by a negative feedback mechanism. Under certain circumstances, when this balance is disrupted, there is excess production of TSH leading to hyperplasia and hypertrophy of acinar cells producing histological picture of thyroid hyperplasia.

Graves' disease : See chapter 26 (Fig. 26.38).

TUMOURS

Benign

Nodules of thyroid command a special attention as there is an apprehension that they might be cancerous. The nature of thyroid nodules and their relationship to cancer is summarised below.

- Many benign conditions may present as thyroid nodule — adenomas, multiple nodular goitres, thyroiditis, malformations of thyroid, focal granulomatous disease.
- Approximately 50% of clinically apparent single nodules are multilobular goitres or thyroiditis.
- Of the clinically documented solitary nodules about 1 to 2 in a thousand prove to be malignant.
- Chance of nodule harbouring cancer rises with previous exposure of neck region to ionizing radiation.

Clinically the incidence of adenoma is 1 to 3% and most true adenomas are solitary lesions, but rarely more than one is present. True thyroid adenomas are derived from the epithelium of the follicle and most of the adenomas show presence of follicles on microscopy, so almost all could be designated follicular adenomas.

Follicular adenoma

This fairly common benign tumour is usually single and is encapsulated with compression of the surrounding gland. Very occasionally there may be found hypersecretion with thyrotoxicosis. Degenerative changes including haemorrhage into the tumour are common.

Microscopic examination

(i) The tumour exhibits complete fibrous encapsulation.

(ii) The tumour cells are benign follicular epithelial cells which form follicles of varying size.

(iii) There may be variety of pattern of growth seen most commonly being microfollicular pattern characterised by small follicles containing little or no colloid.

Malignant

Carcinoma of thyroid is an uncommon tumour and accounts for about 1% of all forms of cancer. There are several histological variants (Table 35.1). The two most prevalent variants are papillary and follicular patterns which are collectively referred to as well-differentiated cancers accounting for 80 to 85% of cancers of thyroid. Anaplastic and medullary carcinomas are responsible for about 10% and 5% of cancers respectively.

Table 35.1 : Classification of cancers of thyroid

Type	Frequency (%)
Papillary carcinoma (including mixed papillary and follicular types)	60-70
Follicular carcinoma (including clear cell, Hürthle cell and insular types)	20-25
Medullary (C-cell) carcinoma	5-10
Undifferentiated carcinoma (including smal cell, giant cell, and spindle cell types)	10
Epidermoid carcinoma	< 1
Other tumours (lymphoma, sarcoma, metastatic carcinoma)	< 1

1. Papillary carcinoma

This type of carcinomas are the most common form of thyroid cancer, about 60-70% of all thyroid cancers. Particularly young women are most frequently affected. The tumours are usually small

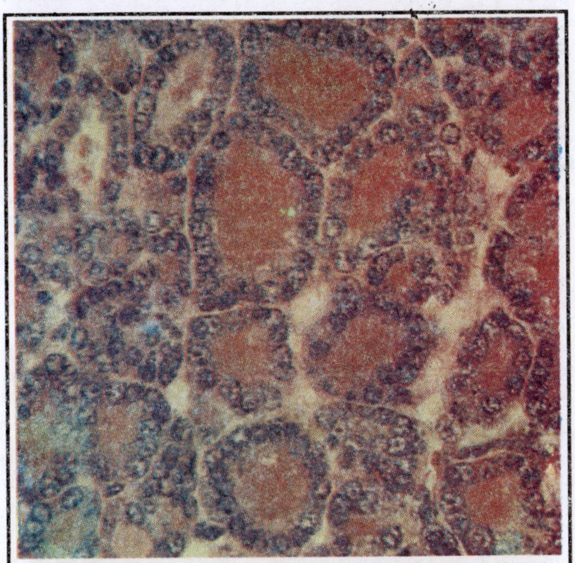

Fig. 35.3. Papillary adenocarcinoma thyroid

and may be multiple within the thyroid. They metastasise readily to local lymph nodes and the first clinical sign of metastasis be an enlarged cervical lymph node containing metastatic papillary tumour.

The tumour is so named because it has pure papillary or mixed papillary or follicular architecture or to all cancers made of cells having ground-glass optically clear nuclei.

Histological variants

These may be of several histological features which include :

Microscopic examination (Fig. 35.3)

(i) *Papillary pattern* : Papillae are composed of fibrovascular stalk and covered by single layer of tumour cells.

(ii) *Tumour cells* : The neoplastic cells have overlapping pale nuclei and clear or oxyphil cytoplasm.

(iii) *Invasion* : The tumour cells invade the capsule, and intrathyroid lymphatics.

(iv) *Psammoma bodies* : Near about half of papillary carcinomas exhibit typical, small concentric calcified spherules in the stroma.

2. Follicular carcinoma

The term follicular carcinoma is applied to cancers composed of cells that form follicles or are disposed in cords or islands with microfollicles in which there is no papillae, no ground-glass nuclei, nor psammoma bodies. When any of these three features is present, the lesion is considered a papillary carcinoma, both anatomically and biologically.

Macroscopical examination

They may take the fom of — (i) either an encapsulated grey-white nodule of several centimeters in diameter, (ii) or a massive, invasive growth that shows extension into perithyroid structures (Fig. 35.4).

Microscopical features

The encapsulated pattern mimics an adenoma. Histologic variation among these cancers is marked . The cells range from well-differentiated to markedly anaplastic. Neoplasms composed largely or entirely of Hürthle cells are rarely seen. The better levels of differentiation tend to occur in lesions which produce follicles. Vascular and capsular invasion may be seen in both types — encapsulated and infiltrative viariants, but it is more characteristic of the infiltrative lesion.

3. Anaplastic carcinoma

In contrast to the two types of well-differentiated carcinoma of thyroid described above, this is a poorly differentiated, highly malignant tumour that causes death usually within 2 years. Older persons between the ages of 60 and 80 years are frequently affected. About 10% of thyroid carcinomas belong to this category. By the time the patient is brought to medical attention, anaplastic carcinoma is usually a bulky mass that has obviously extended beyond the thyroid capsule.

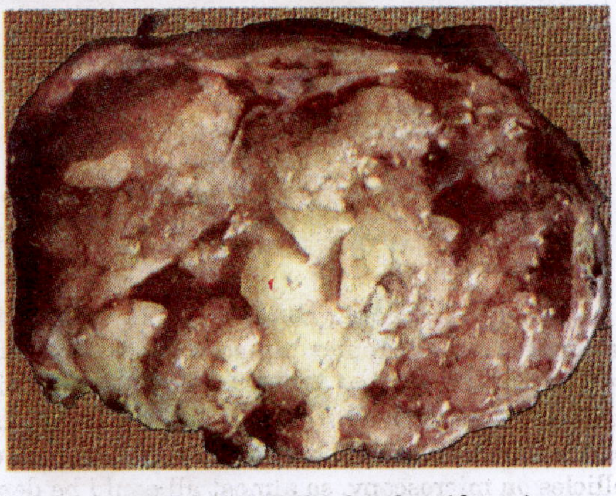

Fig. 35.4. Thyroid : Follicular thyroid carcinoma (infiltrative pattern)

Microscopic features

(i) The histologic pattern is extremely variable, but three variants can be recognised — giant cell, spindle cell and squamoid.

(ii) So-called small cell undifferentiated tumours are likely to be lymphomas or medullary carcinomas. (iii) In about 30% of the tumours, areas reminiscent of better-differentiated carcinomas are found, suggesting origin of the anaplastic cancer in a papillary or follicular carcinoma. (iv) Cytokeratin or CEA is often be identified within the tumour cells which confirms the epithelial origin of even the most anaplastic lesions.

4. Medullary carcinoma

It is a rare tumour derived from the calcitonin producing cells of the thyroid. Blood calcitonin level is high. In addition, there may be production of other hormones which result in a carcinoid or Cushing's syndrome. There is a familial form of the tumour in which there are multiple tumours of a number of endocrine organs.

Gross appearance (Fig. 35.5)

(1) Tumour is a single sharply circumscribed mass.

(2) Light greyish-white colour.

Microscopical features (Fig. 35.6)

(1) The tumour is composed of solid masses of cells, most of which are rounded, eosinophilic with central hyperchromatic nucles. (2) The tumour cells are found in a rich connective tissue stroma. (3) Sometimes amyloid deposits are found within the tumour mass. (4) Medullary carcinomas are composed of polygonal to spindle-shaped cells, which may form nests, trabeculae, and even follicles. (5) Small, more anaplastic cells are present in some tumours and may be the predominant cell type.

5. Lymphoma

B cell lymphoma occasionally arises in long-standing autoimmune thyroiditis (particularly in Hashimoto's disease).

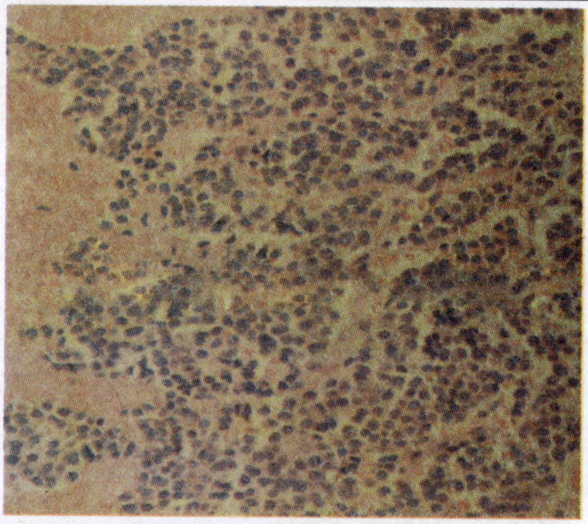

Fig. 35.6. Medullary carcinoma thyroid, ME × 200

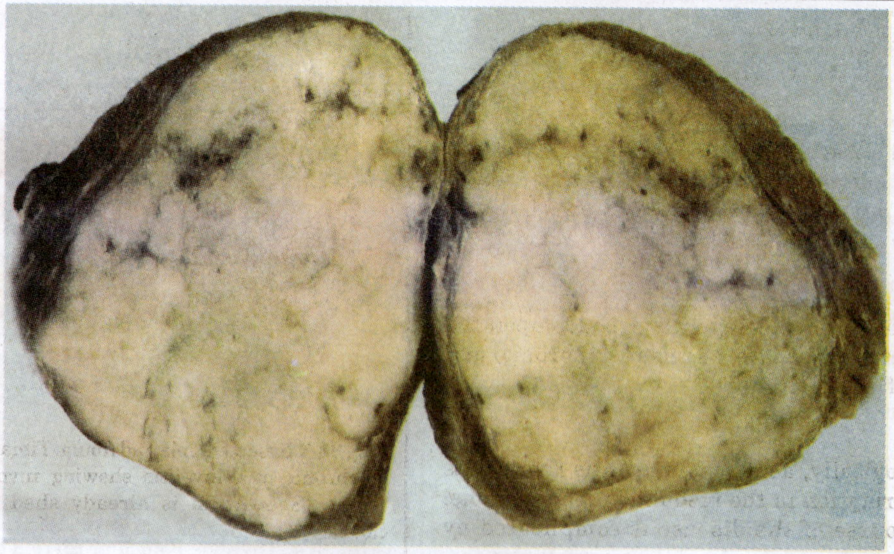

Fig. 35.5. Medullary carcinoma of thyroid

Chapter 36

Bones

INFECTIONS

Osteomyelitis means inflammation of bone and marrow and is essentially of two types : *acute purulent* and *chronic granulomatous.* All infective agents (virus, parasite, fungi, bacteria) can produce osteomyelitis, but infections caused by pyogenic bacteria and mycobacteria are the most common.

Pyogenic osteomyelitis

Causative organisms

1. *Staphylococcus aureus* — 80–90%
2. *Escherichia coli*
3. *Pseudomonas aeruginosa*
4. *Klebsiella* spp.
5. *Haemophilus influenza*
6. *Group D streptococci*

(2–6: 10–20%)

7. *Salmonella* spp.

Pathogenesis

In most cases the bacterium gains access to the marrow cavity by blood stream; it may also follow penetrating trauma. Long bones or vertebral bodies are mostly affected.

Morphology

Morphology of osteomyelitis depends upon the stage of infection (acute, subacute or chronic) and location of infection.

Acute osteomyelitis

Pathologically, acute osteomyelitis represents abscess formation in the medullary space of bone, but the course of the disease is complicated by several factors.

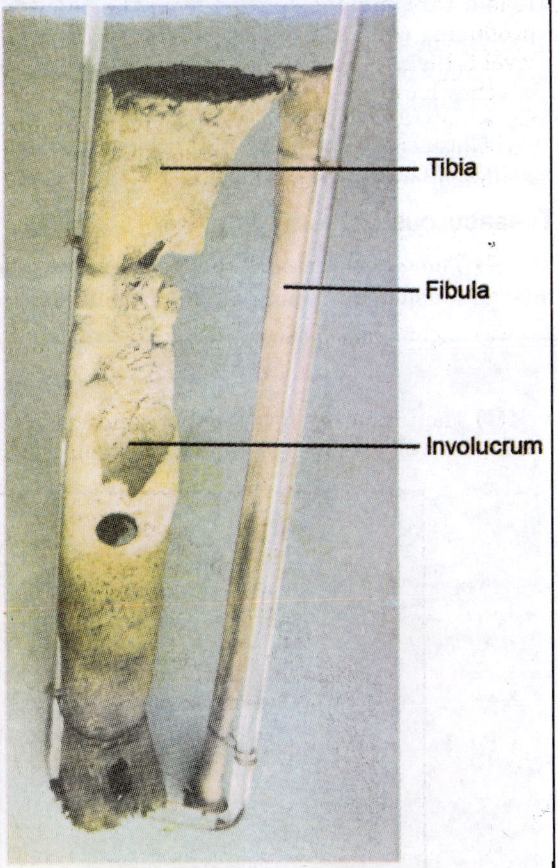

Fig. 36.1. Resected tibia and fibula. Tibia with features of chronic osteomyelitis showing involucrum with cloaca. Squestrum is already shed through the cloaca

The released toxins and destructive enzyme of the bacteria reduce local pH and oxygen tension, increase the intraosseous pressure which leads to segmental bony necrosis, known as *sequestrum*.

The spread of purulent exudate occurs through the Haversian system beneath the lifted periosteum causing its rupture and formation of a soft tissue abscess and eventually a draining sinus.

Involucrum is a sleeve of living reactive bodies or lamellar bone deposited around a sequestrum (Fig. 36.1).

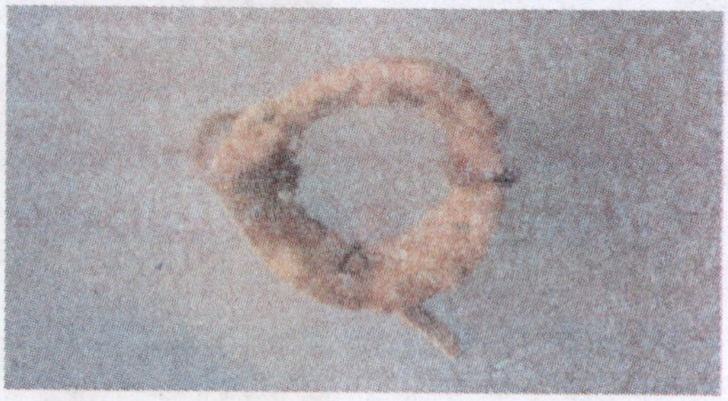

Fig. 36.3. Specimen showing ring-like sequestrum found in amputation stump

Sequelae

(a) Sequestrum (Figs 36.2, 36.3) crumbles and form free foreign body which usually passes out through the sinus tract.

(b) *Brodie's abscess* is a small intraosseous abscess mainly of cortex, walled off by reactive bone (involucrum).

(c) Chronic osteomyelitis, e.g., sclerosing osteomyelitis of Garre that develops typically in jaw.

TUBERCULOUS OSTEOMYELITIS

Tuberculous osteomyelitis is a haematogenous infection, usually of young adults or children. In developing countries, 1-3% individuals with pulmonary or extra pulmonary tuberculosis develop the lesion.

Pathogenesis

The spine (especially the thoracic and lumbar vertebrae) is the most common site of infection followed by bones of the hip, knee, ankle, elbow and wrist. In HIV infected individual, the infection is frequently multifocal.

In long bones, either the epiphysis or diaphysis is involved and spread often occurs to the adjacent joint *(tuberculous arthritis)*.

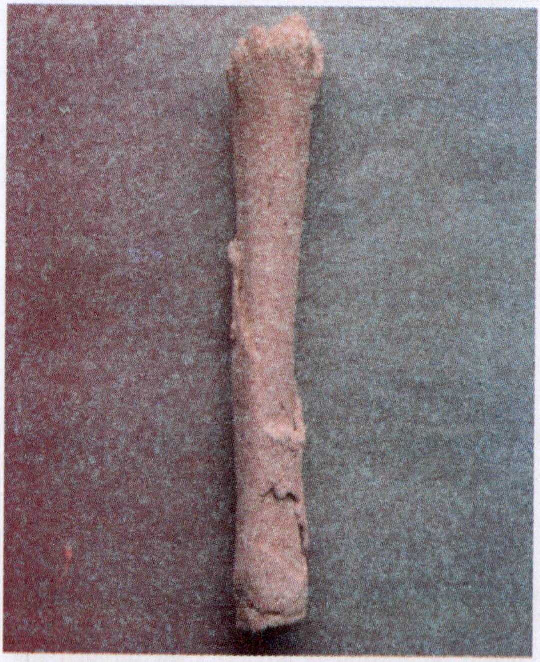

Fig. 36.2. Specimen showing tubular sequestrum involving whole diaphysis partially covered by involucrum

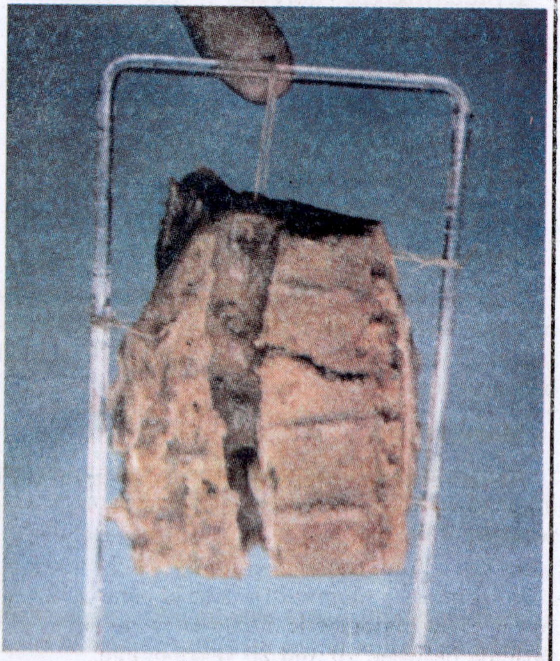

Fig. 36.4. Dorsal lumbar kyphosis to vertebral tuberculosis (*Pott's disease*)

Pott's disease (Fig. 36.4) : Tuberculosis of the vertebra usually occurs in childhood. The lesion starts in the bodies and spread through medullary cavity and breaks through intervertebral discs involving multiple vertebrae *(Pott's disease of spine)* and extends into soft tissues forming *cold abscesses*. The affected vertebrae become weak and tends to collapse, producing an acute antiflexion or angular kyphosis and neurological deficits secondary to spinal cord and nerve compression.

TUMOURS OF BONE

Bone tumours are classified into two large categories : *primary* and *secondary* (metastatic).

Classification of primary tumours

The primary bone tumours are classified according to their presumed tissue of origin and histology (Table 36.1).

Table 36.1
Primary bone tumours

Origin	*Benign*	*Malignant*
Cartilaginous (Chondrocyte)	Chondroblastoma Chondromyxoid fibroma Enchondroma	Chondrosarcoma
Osteoblastic (Osteoblast)	Osteoid osteoma Osteoblastoma	Osteosarcoma
Fibrous tissue (Fibrocyte)	Non-ossifying fibroma Fibrous dysplasia Xanthofibroma	Fibrosarcoma
Bone marrow (Plasma cells)	—	Plasmacytoma (myeloma)
Uncertain origin (Osteoclast)	Giant cell tumour (mostly benign, rarely malignant)	
Uncertain	—	Ewing's sarcoma

OSTEOSARCOMA

Osteosarcoma is a malignant mesenchymal tumour composed of osteoblastic (bone forming) cells that may be derived from the inner layer of periosteum or from the endosteum. It is the most frequent primary malignant tumour of bone (20%), exclusive of haematopoietic malignancy and occurs in patients between 10 and 25 years of age.

Location

Most tumour arising *de novo* are located in metaphyseal area (growing end) of long bones, particularly the lower end of femur, upper end of tibia, and upper end of humerus.

General consideration

The tumour grows centrally. By the time it is first discovered, the cortex has been eroded, medullary cavity infiltrated and replaced by tumour tissue proliferating and extending to periosteum. The proliferative neoplastic tissue elevates the periosteum, perforates and spreads to neighbouring soft structures. New bone formation is seen under the periosteum where periosteum is being stripped, a radiographic sign known as *Codman's triangle* develops. It metastasises by blood stream to distant organs.

Gross appearance (Fig. 36.5)

1. The gross appearance of osteosarcoma varies greatly. It may be white, soft and fleshy or gritty, or dark red and haemorrhagic.

2. The tumour often destroys overlaying cortex and produces a soft tissue mass.

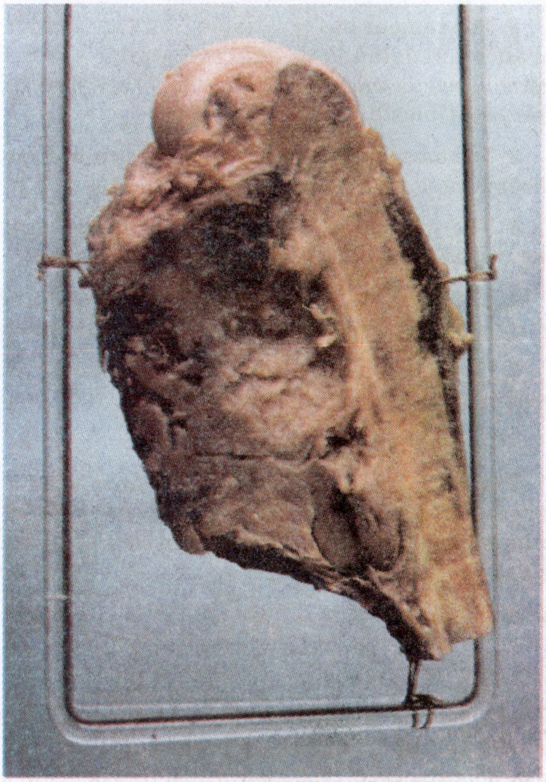

Fig. 36.5. Osteosarcoma of humerus

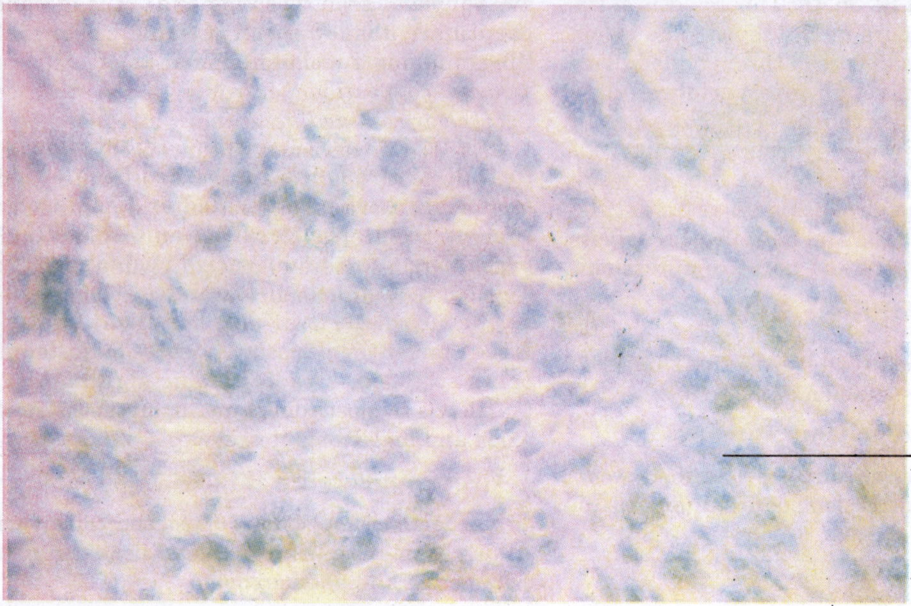

Fig. 36.6. ME : Osteosarcoma of humerus, HE × 250

Microscopic appearance (Fig. 36.6)

1. The tumour has a variable histological appearance but islands of delicately pink stained osteoid are usually present, which are derived from osteoblasts.

2. The osteoblasts are poorly differentiated and pleomorphic with much mitotic activity.

3. The tumour cells may grow in diffuse, nesting or pseudopapillary arrangements.

4. Blood vessels are usually numerous and early blood stream metastasis to lung is common.

5. Osteoclast-like multinucleated giant cells are seen in one fourth of the cases.

Microscopic variants

The important histological variants include *osteoblastic, chondroblastic, fibroblastic, telangiectatic* (blood filled cyst formation), *small cell* and *giant cell* subtypes.

GIANT CELL TUMOUR (*Syn* : Osteoclastoma; Myelogenic giant cell tumour)

Osteoclastoma is a synonym for giant cell tumour of bone because it contains a profusion of multinucleated, osteoclast type giant cells. Osteoclastoma is a relatively uncommon benign lesion (5% of bone tumours), but locally aggressive. It is usually seen in adults of more than 20 years of age (3rd and 5th decades) with a slight female preponderance.

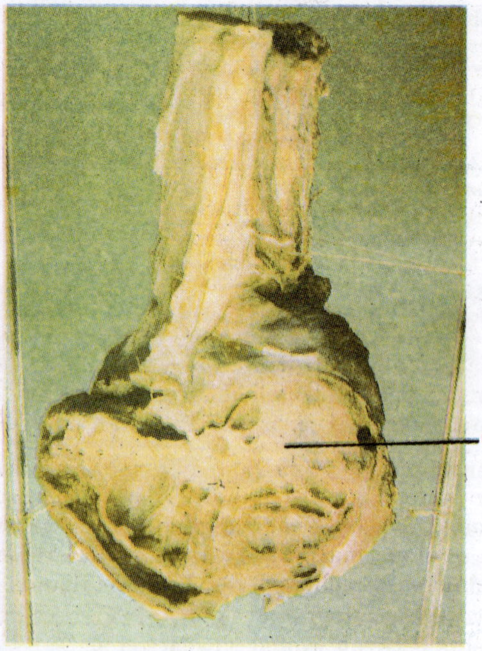

Fig. 36.7. Giant cell tumour of bone

Location

The tumour, usually a solitary lesion, almost always arises from epiphysis of long bones especially from the distal epiphysis of femur and proxymal epiphysis of tibia, particularly around the knee joint, where it forms an expansile locally destructive mass that may invade the joint. It also occurs in humerus, fibula and skull particularly the sphenoid bone.

Origin

Giant cell tumour is believed to have a monocyte macrophage lineage and giant cells are presumed to form by fusion of mononuclear cells.

Gross appearance (Fig. 36.7)

1. It appears as a red-brown, friable mass with areas of cystic degeneration secondary to necrosis.

2. Cortex is thinned and may be eroded, and there may be extension of the tumour to the neighbouring soft tissues.

Histology (Fig. 26.19)

The tumour is made of ovoid or spindle shaped cells interspersed with giant cells in a vascularised stroma.

Radiography

The tumour is entirely a lytic expansile solitary lesion. The overlying cortex is usually lost producing a bulging soft tissue mass delineated by a thin shell of reactive bone (soap bubble appearance).

Behaviour

1. Most of the giant cell (GC) like tumours of bone are benign (96%) and some of them tend to recur after removal. The recurrence rate varies between 35-40%.

2. About 4% GC tumours metastatise to the lungs usually after prior surgery, suggesting dislodgement of tumour emboli. The morphology of the metastic growth is the same as primary tumour.

The actively growing spindle cell stromal tissue determines the degree of malignancy of the lesion. In an obvious malignant tumour, the stroma shows increased cellularity and mitotic figures.

CHONDROSARCOMA

It is the second in frequency among the primary malignant bone tumours (12%) and occurs usually in the 4th decade of life.

Chondrosarcomas comprise a group of tumours that have a broad spectrum of pathological findings and are subclassifed morphologically into 5 types : *conventional intramedullary, juxta-cortical, clear cell, dedifferentiated* and *mesenchymal* variants. Conventional variants occurs in 2nd and 3rd decade. It is more frequent in males than in females. There is production of neoplastic cartilage. Chondrosarcoma may be primary or may result from a malignant change in a preexisting benign tumour (chondromyxoid fibroma, chondroma, or cartilaginous exostosis).

Location

Pelvis is most commonly involved, followed by ribs and long bones (femur, tibia and humerus).

Gross appearance (Fig. 36.8)

Large bulky tumour composed of grey-white, somewhat translucent glistening tissue. It is predominantly an intraosseous growth. The adjacent cortex is thickened or eroded, and the tumour grows with broad "pushing front" into surrounding soft tissue.

Histological features

Morphologically it resembles a benign chondroma, composed of an abundant basophilic and metachromatic cartilaginous matrix of adult hyaline type in which fully differentiated chondrocytes lie encased within lacunae. Several areas of lesion need examination for detecting locally malignant tumours. In malignancy, there is

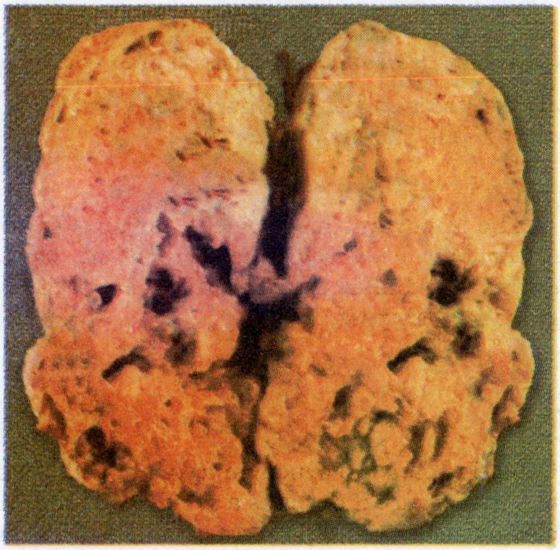

Fig. 36.8. Chondrosarcoma of femur (*resected specimen*)

increased cellular density, general increase in size of cell nuclei, presence of binucleated cells and cells with multiple nuclei, irregularity to nuclear size and nuclear hyperchromatism.

Behaviour

Chondrosarcomas are less malignant than osteosarcomas and prognosis is better than the other malignant tumours of skeleton. Tumours greater than 10 cm diameter behave more aggressively and metastasise preferentially to the lungs and skeleton.

Ewing's sarcoma and PNET

Ewing's sarcoma, also called Ewing's tumour, develops mostly in children and young adults (5 to 20 years old). It arises in diaphyses of long tubular bones, especially the femur and the flat bones of pelvis, ribs and scapulae. It is aggressive and metastasises to lungs and other bones.

Histogenesis : Current evidence suggests that both Ewing's sarcoma and primitive neuroectodermal tumour (PNET) are neuroectodermal in origin and associated with translocation and fusion of genes, typically *EWS* and *Fli-1* genes, on chromosomes 11 and 22.

Macroscopic appearance : Arising in medullary cavity, Ewing's sarcoma and PNET usually invade the cortex and periosteum, producing a soft tissue mass of varying consistency, depending on the amount fibrocalcific stroma which usually shows extensive haemorrhagic necrosis.

Microscopic appearance : It is composed of sheets of uniform small, round, lymphocyte-like cells. The sheets or cords of tumour cells are separated by thin and sometimes highly vascularised fibrous septa. The cells possess scant cytoplasm and the cytoplasm may appear clear as they contain glycogen. Necrosis may be prominent and there are few mitosis.

Microscopically, if the tumour cells are arranged in a circle about a central fibrillary space (Homer-Wright rosettes), it is indicative of neural differentiation. There is very little stroma.

Tumours with neural differentiation are labelled PNETS and those that are undifferentiated are called Ewing's sarcoma.

Metastatic bone tumours

More than 80% of all metastasis originate in kidney, breast, lung, prostate or thyroid; nearly 50% of these tumours ultimately develop metastasis in bone. The important sites of metastasis include pelvis, femur, skull, ribs and humerus. Spread occurs mainly by blood stream.

Section IV

CYTOPATHOLOGY

Section IV contains

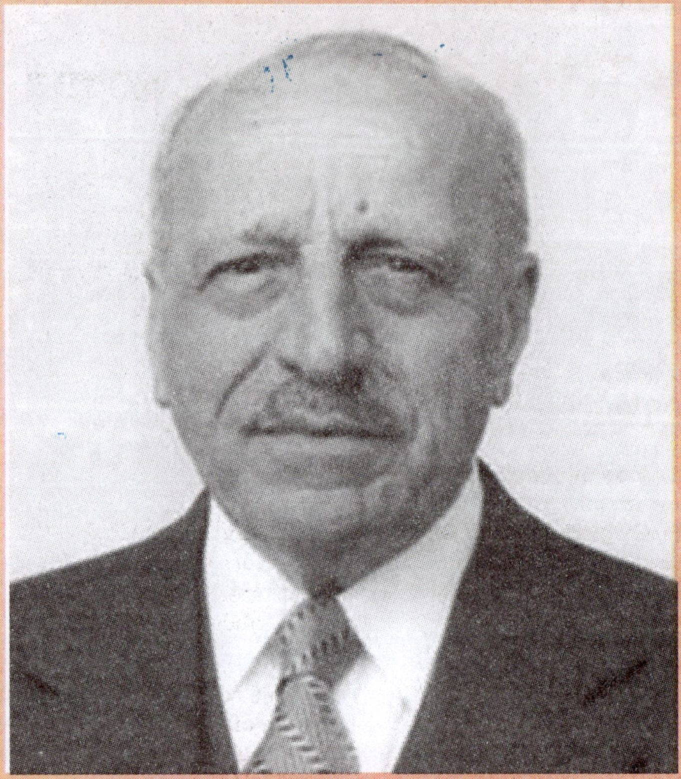

George N. Papanicolaou (1883–1962)

***Father of Exfoliative Cytopathology** — Papanicolaou, an American pathologist, first developed Pap test for detection and early diagnosis of cervical cancer.*

Chapter 37

Vaginal Exfoliative Cytopathology

CYTOPATHOLOGY

Cytopathology is the study of body cells which are exfoliated spontaneously from various body sites (mostly from epithelial surfaces), or obtained from various body cavities or various organs/masses by fine needle aspiration (FNAC). Cytology involves :

(a) Exfoliative cytology
(b) Aspiration/Interventional cytology
(c) Imprint cytology

Exfoliative cytopathology is dealt here in two chapters : Vaginal exfoliative cytopathology (chapter 37), Cytology of body cavity fluids (chapter 38). Fine needle aspiration cytology is dealt in chapter 39.

IMPRINT CYTOLOGY

In such study, touch preparations of fresh unfixed surgically excised tissues are prepared on glass slides. Preparations are then fixed, stained and studied immediately. Imprint cytology is regarded as complementary to frozen section.

EXFOLIATIVE CYTOPATHOLOGY

Exfoliative cytopathology is the study of normal and disease-altered desquamated cells from the various sites. Majority of the desquamated cells are epithelial, but some are mesodermal (connective tissue) in origin. These labile cells are shed (exfoliated) spontaneously and replaced by new cells. The rate of desquamation varies with each tissue. Some of the exfoliated cells accumulate in natural cavities (peritoneal and pleural) and in recesses. Most of the desquamated cells are lost from the surface or through the gastrointestinal tract.

Types of exfoliation

(a) *Natural spontaneous exfoliation* — The examples are :

(i) vagino-cervical cells in posterior vaginal fornix.
(ii) mesothelial cells in effusion of pleural and abdominal cavities.

(b) *Artificial exfoliation* : Artificial exfoliation of viable cells from the lesion takes place when the surface of mucosa is scraped by spatula or aspirated using a fine needle. This is exemplified by the scraping taken from cervical carcinoma where the deep basal cells are needed, whereas superficial cells are required for hormonal study.

Role of cytology

1. Early detection of cancer is done in screening. Unsuspected diseases can be detected with high degree of precision.

2. Nature of suspected diseases can be confirmed without any injury to tissue.

3. Cause of the disease and therapeutic response can be monitored simply.

Use of cytopathology

Exfoliative cytology is of little value for lesions that are readily accessible to incisional biopsy, e.g., skin or oral cavity.

It is a valuable tool for cervicovaginal cytology for screening of cervical carcinoma.

Screening for other cancers in high risk groups such as bronchial cytology in heavy smokers, nipple aspiration cytology in women and gastric cytology in pernicious anaemia are less than encouraging.

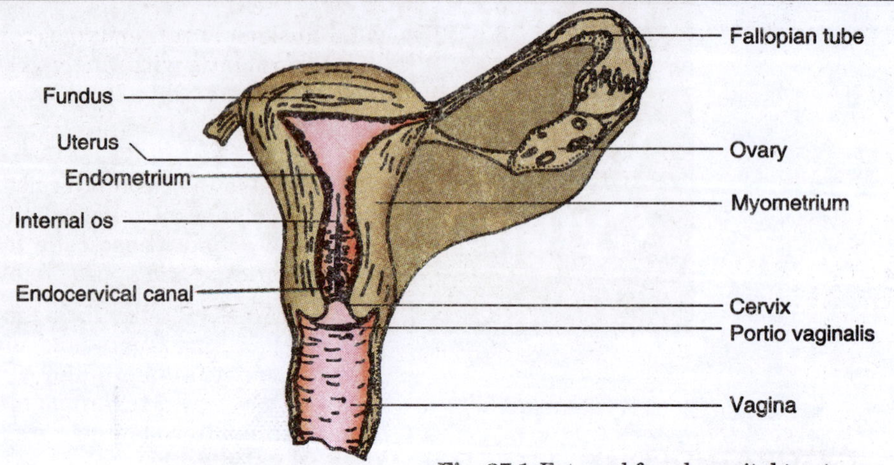

Fig. 37.1. External female genital tract

VAGINAL EXFOLIATIVE CYTOPATHOLOGY

Cytology of Normal Female Genital Tract

The different parts of female genital tract are illustrated in Fig. 37.1. The vagina and ectocervix (portio vaginalis) are normally covered by non-keratinised stratified squamous epithelium. This mucosa terminates at the external os of cervix where it is replaced by simple columnar epithelium (Fig. 37.2). The location of *squamocolumnar junction* varies with age. It is located on ectocervix in reproductive age group, but slowly recedes after menopause into cervical canal. This zone of transformation is of clinical significance, because majority of the cervical carcinomas and their precursors arise in this location.

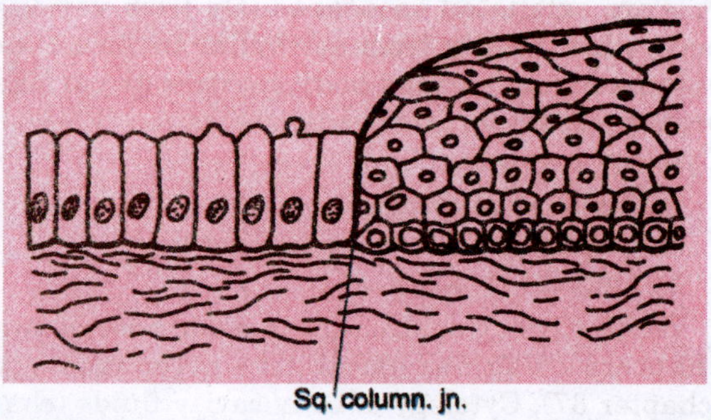

Fig. 37.2. Squamo-columnar junction of uterine cervix

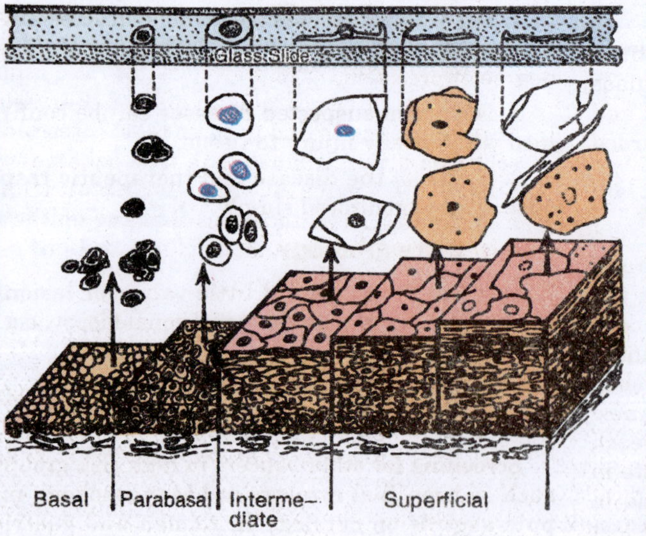

Fig. 37.3. Different histologic layers of a cervico-vaginal stratified squamous epithelium

The junction between the endocervical and endometrial mucosa occurs in internal os. As in the ectocervix, the location varies with age.

Squamous cells of ectocervix

In sexually active women, the non-keratinised stratified squamous epithelium covers the ectocervix. The vagino-cervical squamous epithelium is composed of *basal cell* layer, *parabasal cell* layer, intermediate cell layer and *superficial cell* layer (Fig. 37.3).

Germinal or basal cells : This is the

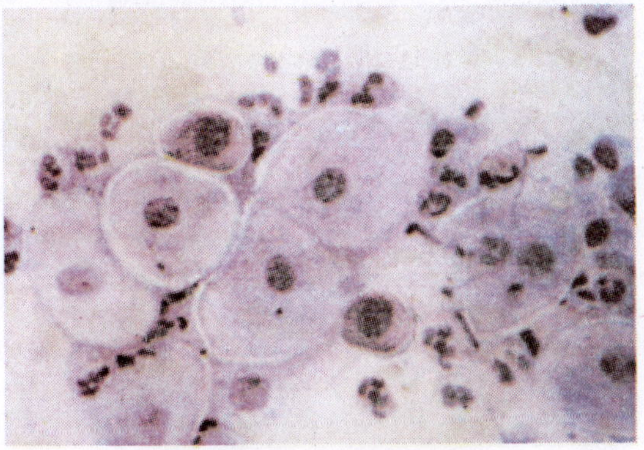

Fig. 37.4. Parabasal cells

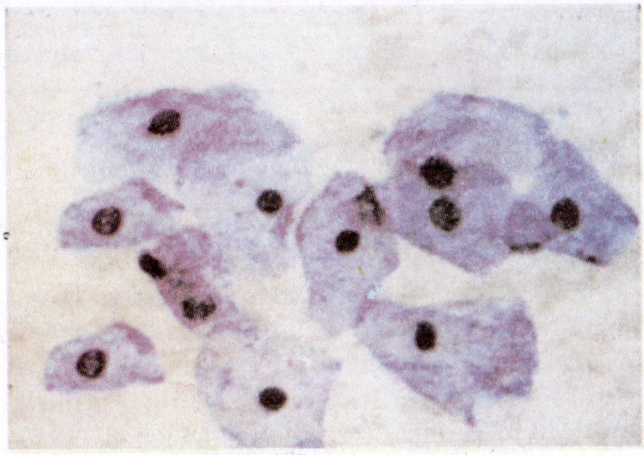

Fig. 37.5. Intermediate cells

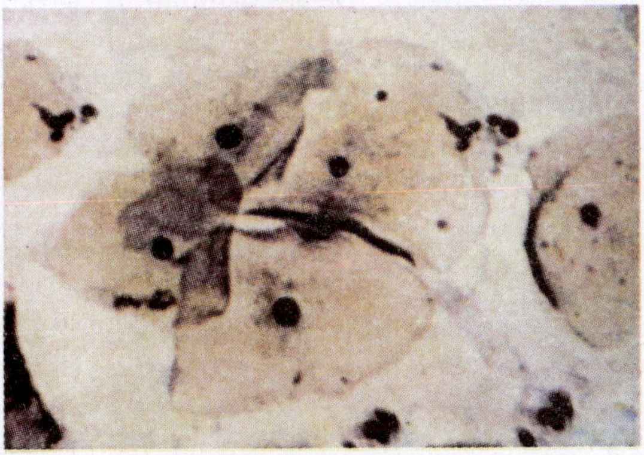

Fig. 37.6. Superficial cells

single cell layer lying upon basement membrane. Basal cells are not normally exfoliated and rarely seen in smear. They are almost always traumatically exfoliated. Basal cells are the smallest cells (10-12 μm diameter) of squamous epithelium and are round or oval. Cytoplasm is scanty, stain dark to deep blue with Papanicolaou stain (Fig. 37.3). The nucleus is rather large, round or oval, and hyperchromatic with finely granular chromatic pattern (Fig. 37.3).

Parabasal cells

Superficial to the basal layer lies a zone of several rows of polyhedral cells, called parabasal cells. When detached, these cells loose their intercellular bridges and appear round or oval.

The parabasal cells, 15-25 μm in diameter, are larger than basal cells and uniform in shape. Cytoplasm stains blue and contains vesicular nucleus. Nuclear-cytoplasmic ratio is about 1 : 3. Chromatin pattern is finely granular (Fig. 37.4).

Parabasal cells are either traumatically exfoliated in sheets (ulceration or post-irradiation) or singly from atrophic epithelium (prepuberty, lactation, post-menopausal mucosa or in oestrogen deficiency).

Intermediate cells

Originating from the parabasal cells, intermediate cells form the most common intermediate cell layer usually composed of several rows of slightly larger cells (Fig. 37.5).

The size of intermediate cells varies from 30-60 μm in diameter depending on the degree of maturation; those from the lower rows are smaller in size and stain bluish green, whereas those nearer the surface are larger and may take up the eosinophilic stain. The abundance of the cytoplasm and the smaller size of nuclei differentiate them from parabasal cells. Nuclear cytoplasmic ratio is about 1:100. Female sex chromatin masses (Barrbodies) are often easier to find in these cells. Intermediate cells has a thin wafer-like (a true squame) cytoplasm and vesicular nucleus. Exfoliation of intermediate cells indicates that the epithelium has reached only that stage of maturation.

Superficial cells

Originating from the uppermost layer of intermediate cell layer, the superficial cells are usually physiologically exfoliated (Fig. 37.6). They are the largest epithelial cells (40-46 mm in diameter) with pyknotic nuclei and found in the vaginal smear at the preovulatory time often after oestrogen therapy, or in case of functioning ovarian tumour.

The superficial cells in the smear occur usually singly, polyhedral in shape, translucent cytoplasm usually acidophilic (yellow to orange to pale pink to blue). The nucleus is pyknotic, stains uniformly dark without a recognisable structure. In anucleate squames (Fig. 37.7), the area formerly occupied by the nucleus appears as a pale zone (nuclear ghost).

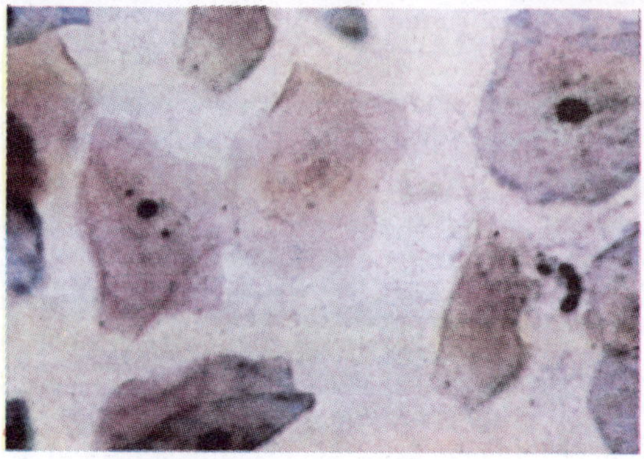

Fig. 37.7. Anucleate squames

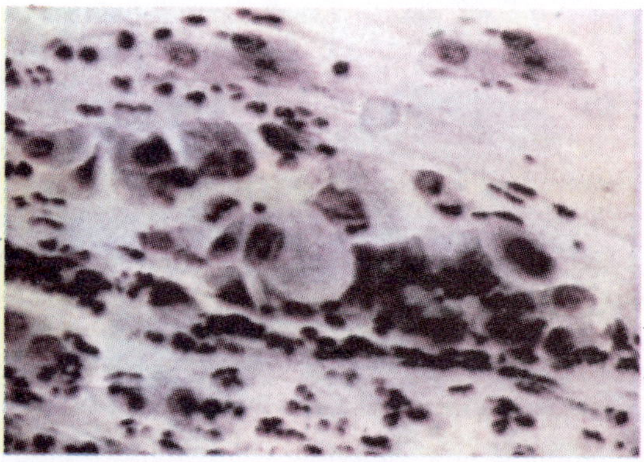

Fig. 37.8. Endocervical cells (lateral aspect). Tall prismatic cells, with distinct cell borders and round or oval nuclei of uniform size, are in palisading arrangement

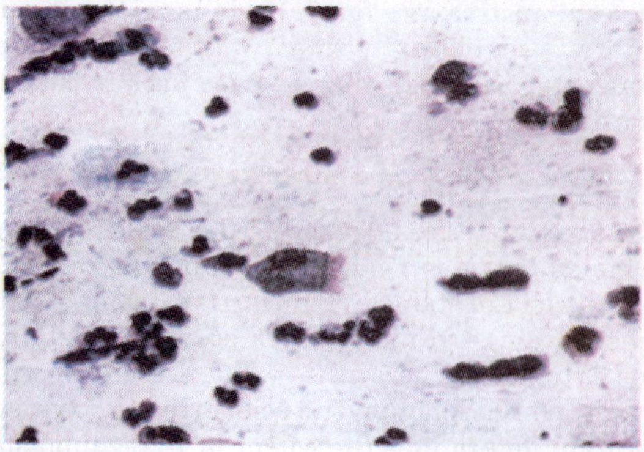

Fig. 37.9. Ciliated endocervical cells showing oval nuclei and blind chromatin pattern

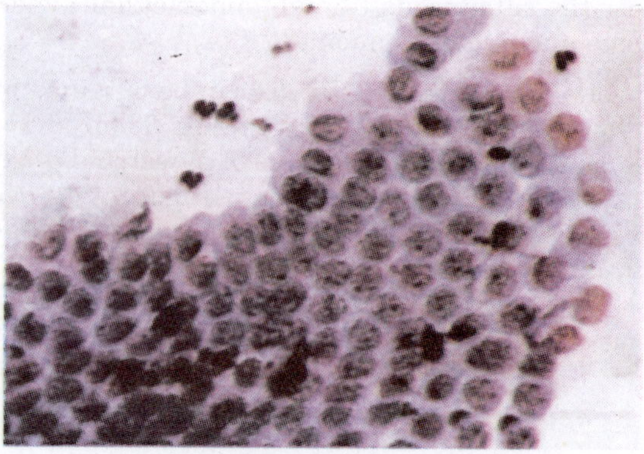

Fig. 37.10. Endocervical columnar cells; showing irregular bizarre, pseudohyperchromatic nuclei and clear cyanophilic vacuolated cytoplasm with partially blurred cell margins. Endocervical cells are larger than endometrial cells

Columnar cell of endocervix (Figs 37.8 to 37.10)

Three types of endocervical cells can be identified: *secretory, ciliated and non-ciliated cells.* Endocervical cells are not usually found in vaginal smear and are seen only in endocervical aspirations and endocervical scrapings. Their presence in vaginal pool is indicative of inflammatory condition of endocervix.

Secretory cells (15–60 μm) are tall columnar epithelia with basally located oval nucleus. They stain irregularly and cytoplasm often contains secretory vacuoles (Fig. 37.8). The *ciliated columnar cells* (Fig. 37.9) are somewhat smaller (10–25 μm) and look cylindrical or pyramidal in shape in smear. Cilia are present on luminal surface. Ciliated cells stain darker than the mucous secreting cells. *Non-secretory* endocervical cells (20-30 μm) probably represent secretory cells that have been compressed by surrounding cells.

It is difficult to differentiate endocervical from endometrial cells, the former is 4-5 times the size of a lymphocyte while the latter is 2-3 times as large as lymphocyte. Endocervical cells may occur singly, in groups or in sheets (Fig. 37.10).

Columnar endometrial cells (Fig. 37.11)

In posterior fornix aspirations, endometrial cells may be found normally only during menstrual flow and the following few days, early in pregnancy, and during abortion and postpartum period. Their presence at other times or after menopause indicates an abnormal endometrium e.g., polyp, endometritis, submucous fibroid, endometrial hyperplasia and adenocarcinoma.

However, endometrial cells can be obtained by endometrial aspiration or scraping. Their shape and size depends on the phase of menstrual cycle. In smear, cells are often round with scanty green to pink cytoplasm. Nucleus is round, dark blue and hyperchromatic (Fig. 37.11).

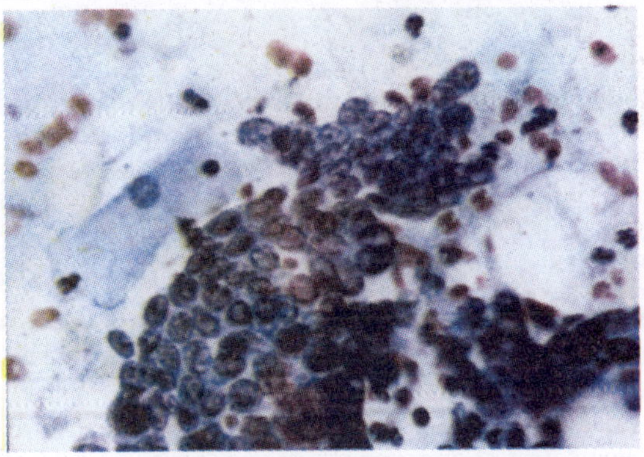

Fig. 37.11. Endometrial cells in clusters with tightly packed oval or round nuclei with a scant rim of cytoplasm. Nucleus shows finely granular chromatin. Nuclear membrane is intact.

Endometrial stromal cells

The superficial stromal cells are round cells with round or spindle-shaped nucleus while deep stromal cells are spindle-shaped.

PREPARATION OF SMEAR AND STAINING

Specimen (Figs 37.12A & 37.12B)

1. *Aspiration from posterior fornix* pool contains cells from the whole genital tract. Specimen obtained from the lateral wall of vagina is preferable to posterior fornix pool smears.

2. *Scraping from cervix* with Ayre's spatula (Fig. 37.12A) provides an aggregate of cells derived from cervical surface only. By using an Ayre's spatula of wooden or plastic make, specimen is collected from cervical os. The spatula, after introduction into vagina, is rotated through 360° to get the material from exocervix and squamo-

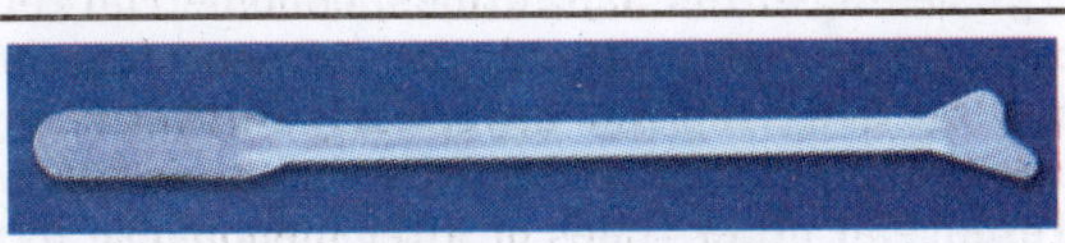

Fig. 37.12A. Ayre's spatula

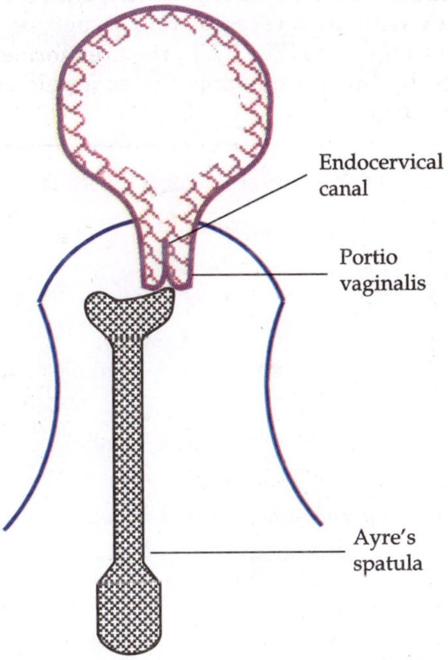

Fig. 37.12B. Method of collection of cervical smear

columnar junction. Smears on glass slides are made from spatula.

3. *Scraping from lateral vaginal wall* (Fig. 37.12B) is useful for hormonal study and for studying inflammatory conditions.

4. *Aspiration from endocervical canal* helps to detect lesions of endocervix and endometrium.

Fixation of slide

Smear made on albuminised slides are immersed in fixing fluid (equal parts of alcohol and ether) in a Couplin's jar and left for 15 minutes. Slides may be kept in fixative for 7-10 days without any deterioration. Usually smear is made on 2 slides from one patient and may be fixed back to back in fixative.

Staining of slide

The staining technique now used is essentially the same as that described by Papanicolau in 1942. The nuclei are stained with Harris's haematoxylin (basic stain), cytoplasm with eosin (acid stain), and cytoplasmic keratin — when present — with orange G. Phosphotungstic acid added to the eosin solution determines the colour of the cytoplasm. All stains ready for use are available commercially.

Preparation of stains

1. *Harris's haematoxylin* : For preparation of stain, see histopathology technique.
2. *Orange G* :

Orange G stock solution (0.5% solution in ethyl alcohol)	100 ml
Phosphotungstic acid	0.015 g

3. *Polychrome stain EA (Eosin-azure)* 36 or 65 :

Light green SF (yellowish) (0.1% solution in 95% alcohol)	45 ml
Bismarck brown (0.5% solution in 95% alcohol)	10 ml
Eosin (yellowish) (0.5% solution in 95% alcohol)	45 ml
Phosphotungstic acid	0.2 g
Lithium carbonate (saturated aqueous solution)	1 drop

Since these stains dissolve more easily in water than in alcohol, it is convenient to prepare 10% aqueous stock solution and then to dilute them with appropriate volume of alcohol.

Staining technique

1. Slides are removed from fixative and then dehydrated by successively passing through descending grades of alcohol (80%, 70% and 50% with 10 dips in each) to water.
2. Stain with Harris's haematoxylin 2 to 5 minutes.
3. Rinse in tap water.
4. Differentiate in 0.25% aqueous hydrochloric acid until the cytoplasm is decolourised and only the nuclei retain the stain.
5. Rinse in tap water and "blue" in ammoniated water (for preparation, see histopathology technique) until the desired staining density is attained.
6. Wash in running tap water for 5 minutes.
7. Dehydrate the slide passing through ascending grades of alcohol — 50%, 70% and 95% (6 dips in each).
8. Stain in orange G for 2 minutes.
9. Rinse in 95% alcohol in 2 separate containers — (5 dips each).
10. Stain in EA 36 or EA 65 for 2 minutes.
11. Rinse in 2 changes of 95% alcohol (5 seconds or dips each).
12. Dehydrate by passing through absolute alcohol.
13. Clear by rinsing in xylene (2 changes), and dry.
14. Mount in mounting media (DPX or Canada balsam).

CYTOLOGY OF UTERUS IN HEALTHY WOMAN

Aspiration smear from posterior fornix contains epithelial cells, which are almost exclusively squamous type, derived from upper one-third of vagina and ectocervix. Endocervical cells are usually absent and endometrial cells are only seen during menstruation or immediately before and after period.

The degree of maturation and glycogen storage of squamous cells of vagina and ectocervix is hormone-dependent. In the first half of menstrual cycle (proliferative phase), ripening follicle secretes oestrogen alone; while in second half (secretory phase), the corpus luteum produces progesterone as well as oestrogen but the effect of oestrogen is no longer detectable cytologically.

Indices and values

Maturation Index (MI)

The maturation index represents a differential count of the squamous cell population. It is expressed as a percentage of parabasal, intermediate and superficial cells; for example, MI = 10/20/70 indicates 10% parabasal cells, 20% intermediate cells and 70% superficial cells.

Karyopyknotic index (KI)

It is the percentage of superficial squamous epithelial cells (with sharp, squared-off cytoplasmic edges and with pyknotic nuclei) expressed as a percentage of total mature squamous epithelial cells. The parabasal cells are excluded. The percentage of acidophilic squamous cells are termed *cornification index* (CI) or *eosinophilic index* (EI). Table 37.1 shows the cytohormonal averages in different age groups.

Table 37.1
Cytohormonal average in different age groups

Age group	Maturation index	Variation (±)
Newborn	0/90/10	10
Infancy	80/20/0	20
Preovulatory	0/40/60	10
Post-ovulatlory	0/70/30	15
Menopause	0/80/20	20
Post-menopause	50/50/0	45
Oestrogen therapy	0/10/90	10
Progesterone therapy	0/90/10	10
Androgen therapy	20/80/0	10

Sex chromosome determination

The sex chromosome or Barr body (found in 1949 by Barr and his co-workers), is the small basophilic body present in the nuclei of epithelial cells of female. It is located next to the inner surface of nuclear membrane (Fig. 37.13) and it is believed that one of the two X chromosomes becomes inactive early in embryonic life. Ideally, sex chromatin should be found in the interphase in all female cells, but because of generally poor preservation of many cells, artefacts etc., it can be identified in only 30-60% well-preserved and immediately wet-fixed cells.

Specimen : After brushing teeth, mouth is rinsed several times. The inner surface of cheek is energetically scraped by the edge of a tongue depressor or Ayre's spatula. Material is smeared on two clean glass slides and immediately transferred to fixative solution. A control smear is prepared from normal female attendant and fixed as above.

Staining of Barr body (Fig. 37.13)

Orcein stain (freshly prepared)

Orcein	....	0.1 g
Warm 50% solution of glacial acetic acid	....	10 ml

Solution is cooled and mixed by shaking the bottle under running tap water and filtered several times to eliminate debris and precipitate.

Procedure

1. Smears are fixed in at least 2 hours in acetic acid alcohol mixture (1 ml acetic acid + 9 ml alcohol/ methanol).

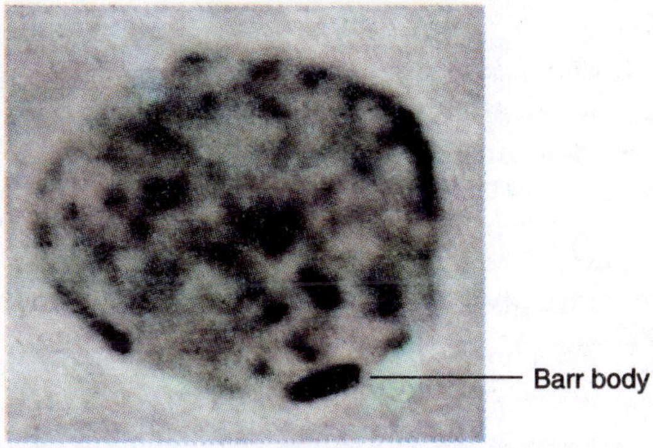

Fig. 37.13. Barr body. Chromosomal mass is lying in relation to the inner surface of nuclear membrane

2. Fixed smears are covered with orcein stain for at least 10 minutes and coverslips are placed very lightly to allow by oil immersion studies.

Examination : Only the chromatin components of nucleus are stained, leaving the remainder of the cells transparent. Control smear and patient's smear are examined, 200-300 epithelial cells are studied and cells with well-stained chromosome masses are also counted.

Indication : Various sex-related congenital abnormalities may be indicated when there is no Barr body, or more than one Barr body is present in cells. The number of sex chromatin equals the number of X chromosomes minus one.

HORMONAL CYTOLOGY

It is estimated by performing cytological examination of vaginal pool material or lateral vaginal wall material. Response of cervical epithelium to hormonal effect is slower than that of vaginal epithelium. Hormonal study should not be undertaken in the presence of vaginal or cervical inflammation because hyperaemia accompanying inflammation leads to excessive maturation of epithelium, unrelated to hormonal state.

Differential cell count

Three types of squamous cells of ectocervix are counted :

1. *Superficial cells* : eosinophilic cells and cyanophilic cells.
2. *Intermediate cells* : large intermediate cells and small intermediate cells.
3. *Parabasal cells.*

Identification of cell types

If the cytoplasm is thick, it is parabasal cell; if it is "wafer-thin", the cell is a squame of either intermediate or superficial type which is distinguished by nuclear status. Intermediate cell possesses a plump vesicular nucleus with an intact chromatin pattern, whereas superficial cell has a shrunken, pyknotic, hyperchromatic nucleus that lacks a chromatin pattern. A total of 200-300 squamous cells have to be counted. Thus a MI 0/70/30 represents that the patient is exfoliating no parabasal cells, 70% intermediate cells and 30% superficial cells; it reflects their ratio on the surface of intact vaginal epithelium at the time of their exfoliation. A shift of MI to the left (35/65/0) indicates the release of less mature cells, whereas a shift to the right (0/35/65) denotes a greater degree of cellular maturation before exfoliation.

At least 200 superficial and intermediate squamous cells are counted and those with pyknotic nuclei (superficial cells) are expressed as a percentage of the total (*Karyopyknotic index*). KI value of 70% indicates that 70% mature cells are superficial type. The value varies from day to day during normal menstrual cycle. It provides a useful and reliable information of oestrogen effects.

Indications for cytology evaluation

1. *Assessment of ovarian function* : After hysterectomy, during menstrual disorders and in premature menses (childhood).
2. *Assessment of abnormal hormonal production* : Before, during, and after pregnancy (e.g., threatened abortion); fertility study; hormone producing tumours and various endocrine disorders.
3. Assessment and guidance for hormone therapy.

Normal cytohormonal patterns

Oestrogens (MI = 0/10/90 ± 10)

It produces an increase of cellular maturation and proliferation of all layers of squamous epithelium, most markedly in the intermediate and superficial cells. With administration of increasing doses oestrogen (systemically or vaginally) to a patient with MI = 100/0/0, MI shifts to the right (MI = 0/50/50) (Table 37.1).

In patients with oestrogen deficiency, parabasal cells predominate. This is true when no inflammatory condition is present because bacterial infection may cause erosion of superficial cells leading to exposure of parabasal cells. In infective condition, the parabasal epithelial cells will be found in an inflammatory background of neutrophils, lymphocytes, histiocytes, etc. On the other hand, the mucosa becomes thin, and superficial layer is absent in deficient oestrogen stimulation.

Progesterone (MI = 0/90/10 ± 10)

Progesterone produces a proliferation of the intermediate layer of the squamous epithelium, at which time exfoliation takes place. Thus, predominant cell on surfaces and in vaginal smear is the intermediate cell and MI shifts toward the midzone (0/100/10).

Androgenic hormones (MI = 20/80/0 ± 10)

Androgens are male sex hormones (testosterone), mainly produced by adrenal cortex. Although they are present physiologically in small amounts throughout the menstrual cycle, this small amount does not influence smear pattern materially.

With administration of a high dose of androgen or in cases of masculinising tumours (arrhenoblastoma, adrenal rest tumour), the parabasal cells proliferate and mature with almost pyknotic nuclei and a dense glycogen containing cytoplasm, with MI shift to the left 90/10/0. In a post-menopausal patient, with atrophic mucosa, androgen causes proliferation of parabasal and intermediate cells (MI = 50/50/0) (Table 37.1).

CELLULAR CHANGE DUE TO INFLAMMATION, DEGENERATION, RADIATION OR ALKYLATING AGENTS

Degeneration

Decrease or cessation of the cellular function usually results in death of cell which usually occurs gradually. The degree of degenerative change depends on the nature and extent of injury. Degeneration occurs both in benign and malignant cells.

Causes — There are many causes, e.g.,

(i) in tissues prior to exfoliation — due to infection, inflammation, presence of blood cell, aging and cell death;

(ii) after exfoliation — due to drying before fixation and inadequate fixation after collection.

***Morphologic changes* (Fig. 34.14)**

(i) *Cytoplasm* : Clear, cyanophilic, foamy or

vacuolated cytoplasm with partially blurred cell margins. Cells are arranged in groups.

(ii) *Nuclei* are irregular, bizarre and pseudo-hyperchromatic. In benign cells, degeneration may mimic atypical or malignant features.

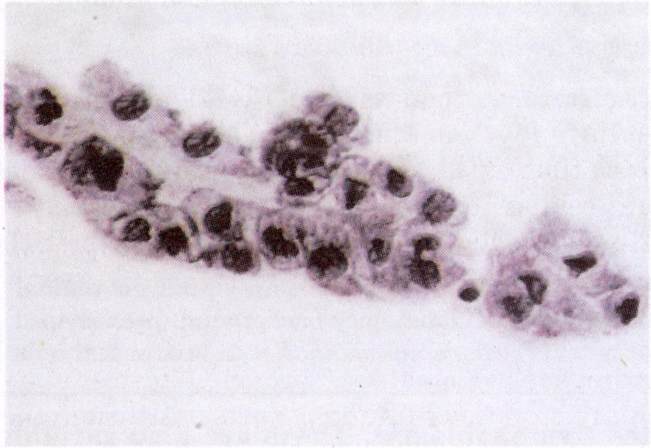

Fig. 37.14. Degenerated endocervical columnar cells with irregular and vacuolated foamy, cyanophilic cytoplasm

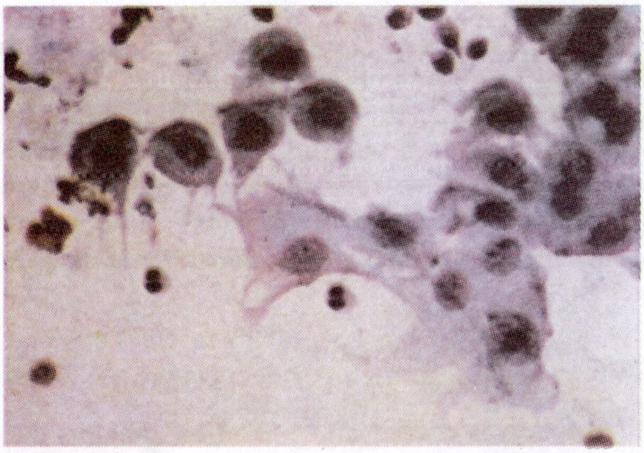

Fig. 37.15. Tissue repair. Sheets of large hyperactive basal cells with cyanophilic cytoplasm, slightly enlarged nuclei and well defined cell borders. Few elongated cells are also seen

Regeneration (Fig. 37.15)

Regenerating tissues are found in the healing process of inflammations, ulceration, biopsy etc. The repair or spider cells are abundant. They exfoliate singly or in clusters and appear as large hyperactive basal cells with cyanophilic cytoplasm and enlarged nuclei with uniformly finely granular chromatin pattern. Many cells are elongated. Nuclear cytoplasmic ratio is slightly altered.

Non-specific inflammation

Senile vaginitis (epithelial atrophy)

In senile vagina, lack of oestrogenic stimulation leads to parabasal cell maturation with consequent thinning of mucosa. The epithelial change invites secondary bacterial infection.

Microscopic examination

(i) Parabasal cells predominate and constitute more than two-thirds of epithelial cells.

(ii) Variation in size of parabasal cells, some are large with hyperchromatic nuclei and pale cytoplasm, while others are small resembling endometrial cells.

(iii) Some inflammatory cells consisting of neutrophils and histiocytes are present.

Post-radiation changes **(Fig. 37.16)**

Following large doses of radiation to the vaginal epithelium, such as therapy for carcinoma of cervix, nucleus and cytoplasm of epithelium are equally affected. Maturation index shifts to the left 100/0/0. In general, marked enlargement of the entire cell is the rule with occurrence of bizarre forms, e.g., tadpole cells or other unusual forms. Cytoplasm shows marked vacuolation, nuclei are enlarged and show signs of degeneration. Multinucleation is caused by impairment of mitotic activity.

Cancer cells exhibit similar alterations after radiation as their normal counterparts : enlargement and vacuolisation of nucleus and cytoplasm and karyorrhexis.

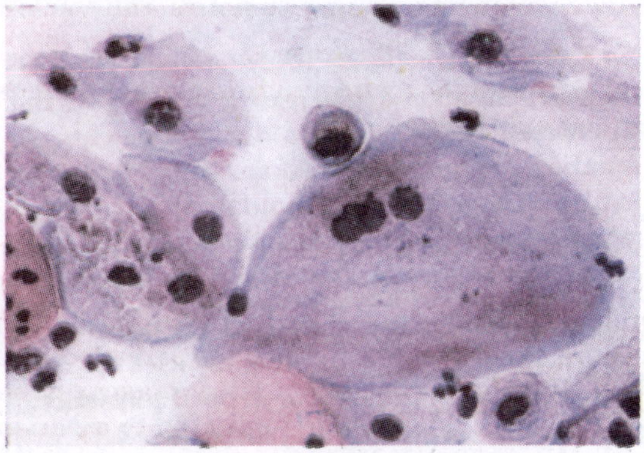

Fig. 37.16. Enlarged benign squamous cells with radiation changes having amphophilic or eosinophilic cytoplasm. Almost normal nuclear size, finely vacuolated cytoplasm. There are also polymorphs

Metabolic disorders

Patients with hypothyroidism (MI = 100/0/0) and *diabetes mellitus* frequently develop fungal and bacterial infection which takes more severe form than in a non-diabetic individual.

Infections

Most infections are polymicrobial, and both aerobic and anaerobic organisms are involved.

Causes

(a) *Bacterial infections : Esch. coli,* staphylococci, micrococci, actinomyces, gonococci and anaerobes *(bacteroides)*.

(b) *Protozoal infection* : *Trichomonas vaginalis.*

(c) *Miscellaneous infection* : *Candida albicans.*

(d) *Virus* : *Herpes simplex virus* Type 1 and 2.

Pathology

An acute infection of vagina and ectocervix may lead to loss or disruption of vaginal and cervical epithelium, resulting in ulceration. With destruction of surface layers, deeper layers are exposed and may be exfoliated. Following cell destruction and tissue damage, numerous leucocytes (polymorphs) emigrate producing an exudate. Dyskeratotic cells (cells with normal mature cytoplasm but with abnormal nuclei) derived from any of the squamous cell layers may be found. The acute phase is followed by regeneration and tissue repair. Variable number of histiocytes and foreign body giant cells containing inflammatory debris are found. When acute infection passes on to chronic stage, various amounts of plasma cells and lymphocytes are found along with polymorphs.

In infections of endocervical canal and endocervical glands, endocervical cells are also found in significant number.

The specific infective agent, e.g., trichomonas, bacteria and fungi are usually found in smears. Special stains can be used when required.

Chronic inflammation may affect columnar epithelium, squamous epithelium and metaplastic epithelium, and the underlying stroma. In some chronic inflammations, there is a localised or diffuse collection of lymphocytes, occasionally forming lymphoid follicles in the stroma next to the basement membrane of the cervical epithelium. The rupture of these follicles by an ulceration or energetic scraping leads to exfoliation of large number of mature and immature lymphocytes (lymphoblasts). There are also variable number of reticulum cells with large nuclei, granular chromatin and prominent nucleoli. Fair number of naked nuclei and endocervical cells are also found.

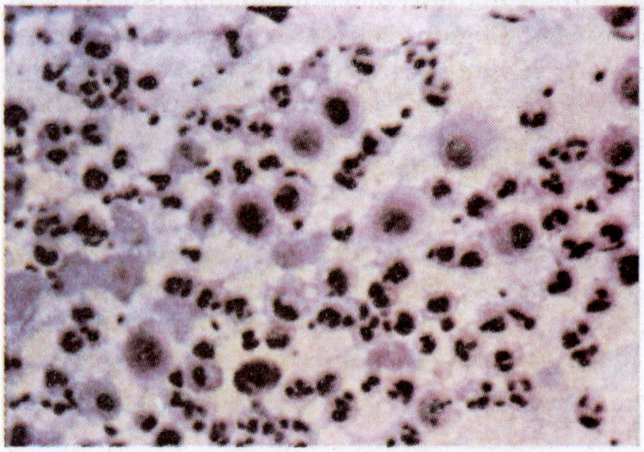

Fig. 37.17. Atrophic vaginitis. Pap. staining of vaginal smear shows inflammatory background, pear-shaped parasites *(Trichomonas vaginalis)* and parabasal cells

Microscopical features

Trichomonas vaginitis (Fig. 37.17): Pap. smear shows inflammatory background with exudate, numerous polymorphonuclear leucocytes, several degenerating parasites and naked nuclei. Intermediate cells show inflammatory cell changes (polychromasia) and the parabasal cells show eosinophilic cytoplasm with enlarged and hazy nuclei.

Herpes simplex genitalis (Fig. 37.18): Pap. smear shows inflammatory background of exudate

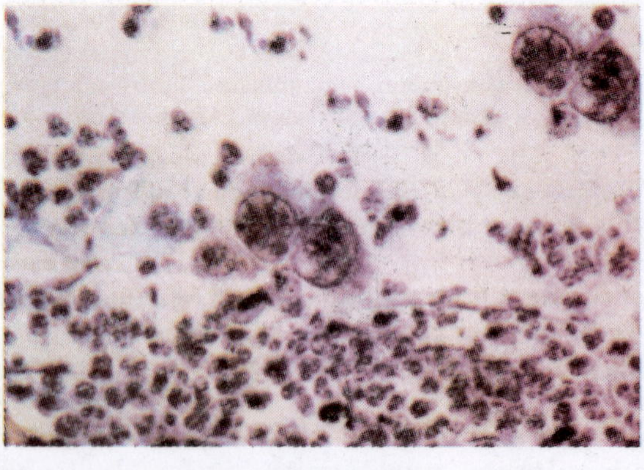

Fig. 37.18. Herpes simplex genitalis. Inflammatory background, multinucleated giant cells and cyanophilic inclusion bodies of type *B*

with numerous polymorphonuclear leucocytes, multinucleated giant cells with cyanophilic, transparent cytoplasm and ill-defined cell borders. Several inclusion bodies of type *B* with cyanophilic appearance are present.

Follicular cervicitis (Fig. 37.19) : Pap. smear shows large number of polymorphonuclear leucocytes, lymphocytes and lymphoblasts. There are groups of endocervical cells with inflammatory reaction (anisocytosis, polychromasia) and degenerative cell changes (cytoplasmic vacuolisation) and several reticulum cells with macronuclei.

Endocervicitis (Fig. 37.20) : Pap. smear shows inflammatory background and cluster of secretory endocervical cells with features of degeneration (polychromasia and vacuolated cytoplasm). Some nuclei are markedly enlarged with prominent anisokaryosis, hyperchromasia and nucleoli.

BENIGN PROLIFERATIVE REACTIONS

Squamous metaplasia : The glandular epithelium, mainly of the endocervix but also of endometrium, are sometimes transformed and replaced by stratified squamous epithelium. This is a protective mechanism of exposed cervical mucosa against irritation from chronic inflammation and vaginal acidity. Malignant potentiality of the metaplastic cells is very low and is only slightly higher than that of the normal epithelium. The cells gradually mature from immature to mature squamous epithelium.

M.E. : In immature squamous metaplasia, Pap. smear (Fig. 37.21) shows loose aggregate of immature metaplastic cells with prominent cell borders with dense cyanophilic cytoplasm. Nucleus shows uniform granular chromatin. Cells have rounded outlines.

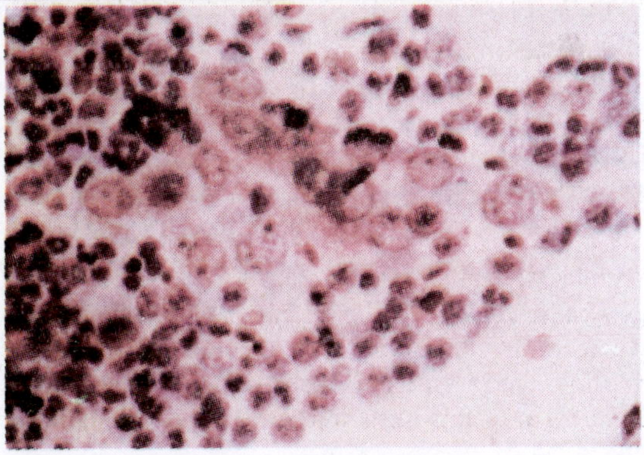

Fig. 37.19. Follicular cervicitis : Inflammatory background with lymphocytes and groups of endocervical cells with inflammatory and degenerative changes

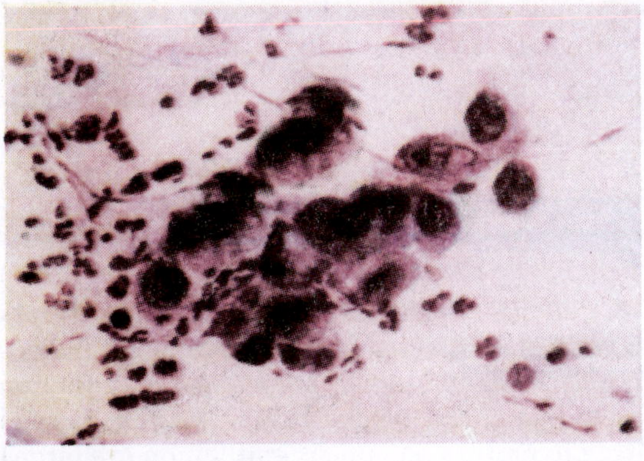

Fig. 37.20. Endocervicitis. Inflammatory background with cluster of endocervical cells with features of degeneration

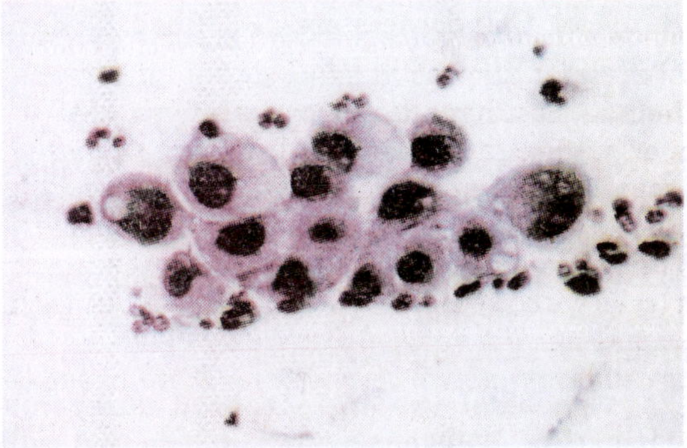

Fig. 37.21. Immature squamous metaplasia. Loose aggregates of immature metaplastic cells. Cell borders are prominent. Cytoplasm is cyanophilic and nucleus contains fine granular chromatin

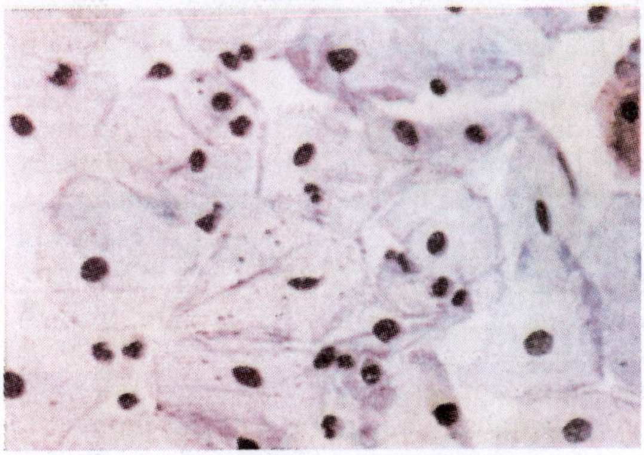

Fig. 37.22. Mature squamous metaplasia. Large, polygonal, cyanophilic cells closely resembling normal intermediate cells

In mature squamous metaplasia (Fig. 37.22) there are several large polygonal cyanophilic cells resembling normal intermediate cells. The clues for metaplastic origin are : rounded cell borders and small distinct rim of cytoplasm.

Reserve cell hyperplasia

One or several layers of immature small cells called *reserve cells* are located between the basement membrane and mature endocervical columnar epithelium. These basal cells have the potential to develoop into either squamous or glandular epithelium. They are most common during pregnancy and during use of contraceptive hormones (pills). Abundant diagnostic cells are found in direct cervical and endocervical scrapings than in vaginal pool smears.

M.E. : Vaginal Pap. smear shows clean background with squamous cells and a group of very small reserve cells with cyanophilic cytoplasm and dark nuclei. Cell borders are ill-defined. Nucleus shows chromatin clumping.

Leukoplakia (hyperkeratosis, white patch)

The hyperkeratinisation and increase in thickness of the superficial layer occurs mainly due to chronic irritation (e.g., uterine prolapse) or hormonal disturbance. A zone of granulated cell present between intermediate and superficial cell layers contains keratohyaline granules.

Pap. smear shows an increased number of hypermature, polygonal, often anucleated cells shed singly (80%) in sheets or in pearl formation.

Parakeratosis

Parakeratosis is closely related to leukoplakia.

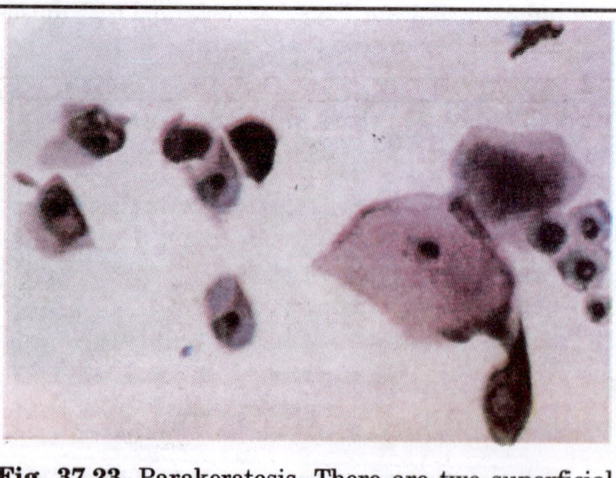

Fig. 37.23. Parakeratosis. There are two superficial cells and 8 so-called miniature superficial cells with eosinophilic cytoplasm and pyknotic nuclei

The surface of normal or atypical epithelium is covered by one or more layers of small keratinised cells with small pyknotic nuclei.

Microscopic picture : *Pap smear* (Fig. 37.23) shows clean background with two superficial cells, several miniature superficial cells with polygonal shape having eosinophilic, hyperkeratinised cytoplasm and pyknotic nuclei.

DYSPLASIA
(Precursors of squamous cell carcinoma)

The term *dysplasia* designates the presence of atypical features in the cervical squamous epithelium short of carcinoma in situ. Dysplasia — considered as precursor of carcinoma — is usually classified as *mild*, *moderate* and *severe* or marked dysplasia. All the lesions are considered to represent different stages of the same precursor of an invasive carcinoma. All dysplastic states are considered to be neoplastic and are called *cervical intraepithelial neoplasia* (CIN), grades I to III, depending on the degree of cellular abnormality present. CIN I is the equivalent of mild dysplasia, CIN II of moderate dysplasia and CIN III of marked dysplasia and/or in situ carcinoma. With this classification, both conditions (severe dysplasia short of in situ carcinoma and carcinoma in situ) are called CIN III and both are treated the same way. In CIN stage, no changes of cervix are visible to the naked eye, but cytological examination reveals atypical cells in most instances.

Cytology of dysplasia

Dysplasia usually develops in the cervical transformation zone (Fig. 37.2). Its development in an area of metaplasia is possible but less frequent.

General features

1. *Number of cells* : Scrapings from ectocervix usually contain more atypical cells than endocervical aspirations.

2. *Arrangement of cells* : Dysplastic cells shed singly (30%) and in small sheets or clusters (65%) and in small pearl formation (5%).

3. *Cell size* : Cytoplasmic maturation of dysplastic cells is unaffected and remains intact. Hence, all cell sizes found in normal squamous epithelium may be present in dysplasia. Dysplastic cells originating in mature squamous epithelium are largest in size and those arising from parabasal and metaplastic cells are represented by cells that gradually decrease in size.

4. *Cell shape and origin* : Dysplastic cells of mature squamous type are polygonal in shape and those of metaplasia are spherical or oval in shape.

Cell boundaries are distinct. Dysplastic cells stain deeply cyanophilic and cytoplasm contains single or multiple vacuoles.

5. *Nuclear morphology* : Nucleus shows marked enlargement with increased nuclear-cytoplasmic ratio. Nuclear membrane is prominent. Majority of cells are mononucleate and only 4–5% cells are binucleate or multinucleate. In most cells, nuclei are hyperchromatic and uniformly granular.

Mild dysplasia

(a) *Mild metaplastic dysplasia* (CIN I) (Fig. 37.24) : Pap. smear shows polygonal mononucleate and binucleate dysplastic cells with cyanophilic and finely vacuolated cytoplasm.

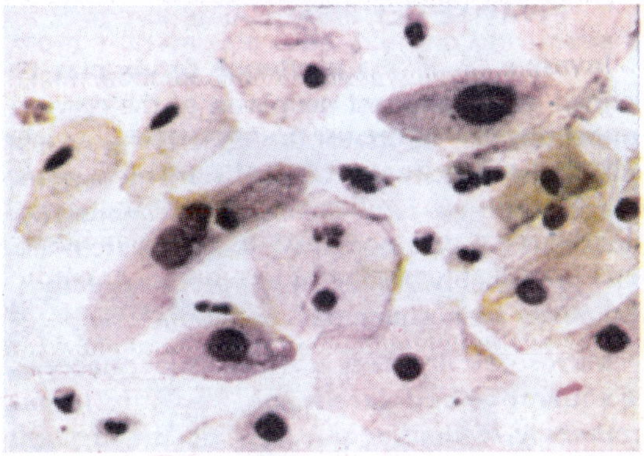

Fig. 37.24. Mild metaplastic dysplasia : Two mononucleate and one binucleate dysplastic cells with dense cyanophilic vacuolated cytoplasm. Nuclei are hyperchromatic and slightly irregular

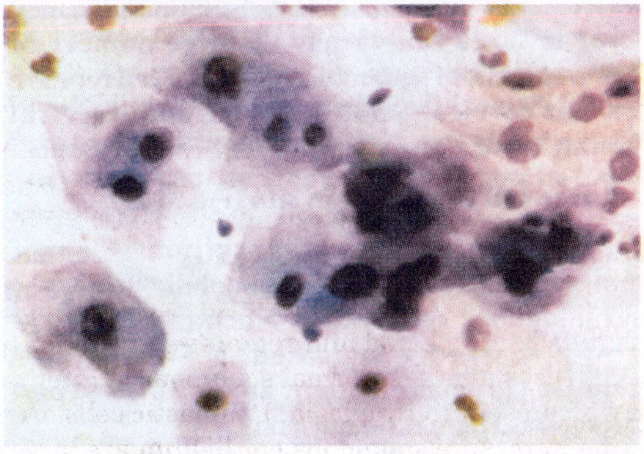

Fig. 37.25. Mild keratinising dysplasia : cells are polygonal, eosinophilic cytoplasm and hyperchromatic nuclei

The nuclei are hyperchromatic and slightly enlarged.

(b) *Mild keratinising dysplasia* (CIN II) (Fig. 37.25) : Pap. smear shows several dysplastic cells with eosinophilic cytoplasm and mild hyperchromasia of nuclei. There is anisokaryosis.

Moderate dysplasia (CIN II)

Pap. smear (Fig. 37.26) shows eosinophilic moderately dysplastic cells, one of which is binucleate, and several parabasal and small intermediate cells with cyanophilic cytoplasm. There is anisokaryosis and hyperchromasia of nuclei.

Severe dysplasia (CIN III)

Pap. smear (Fig. 37.27) shows clean background, normal superficial and intermediate cells; several dysplastic cells with anisocytosis, anisokaryosis, hyperchromasia and uniformly granular chromatin.

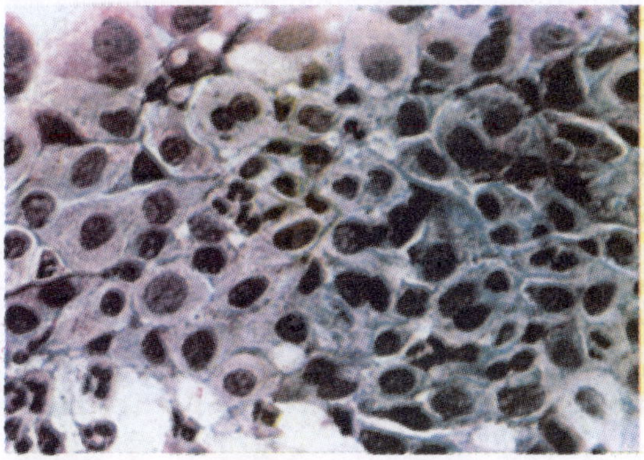

Fig. 37.26. Moderate dysplasia. A sheet of moderately dysplastic parabasal and small intermediate cells with cyanophilic cytoplasm. Nuclei are enlarged with anisokaryosis and hyperchromasia

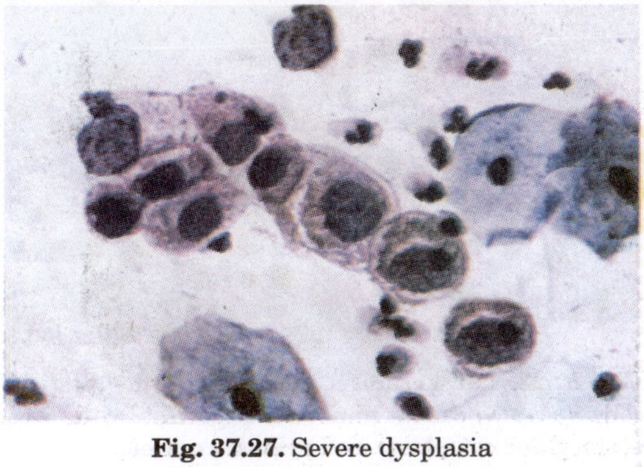

Fig. 37.27. Severe dysplasia

SQUAMOUS CELL CARCINOMA IN SITU OF CERVIX

The neoplasm may be multifocal and usually arises from transformation zone where dysplasia or squamous metaplasia pre-existed.

In *carcinoma in situ*, entire thickness of the epithelium is involved (Fig. 37.28). Stratification is totally lost. Cells are highly atypical and cell borders are invisible in histological section. There is no infiltration of the underlying stroma and basement membrane remains intact. The *in situ* carcinoma expands only towards the surface of squamous epithelium or towards the lumen of gland and the cells are exfoliated. The cytologic diagnosis has to be confirmed by examination of a tissue biopsy. Based on cellular size, carcinoma in situ may be differentiated into : (a) *large cell* well-differentiated carcinoma in situ and, (b) *small cell* or poorly differentiated carcinoma in situ. Keratinisation may occur in large cell variety. A large number of abnormal cells of squamous or reserve cell type are seen in cervical scrapings and endocervical aspiration of a case of *in situ* cervical carcinoma.

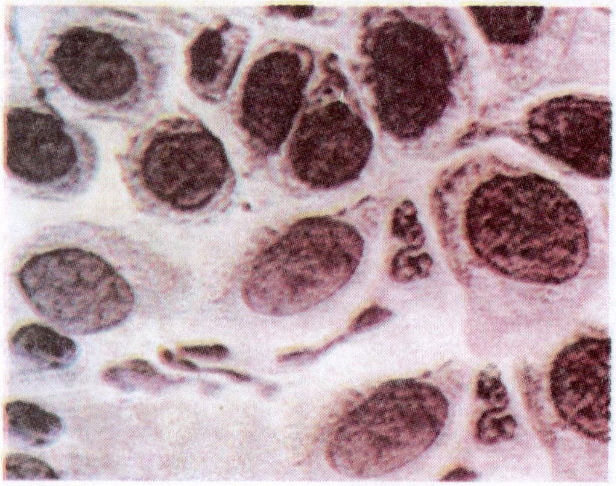

Fig. 37.28. Large cell carcinoma in situ

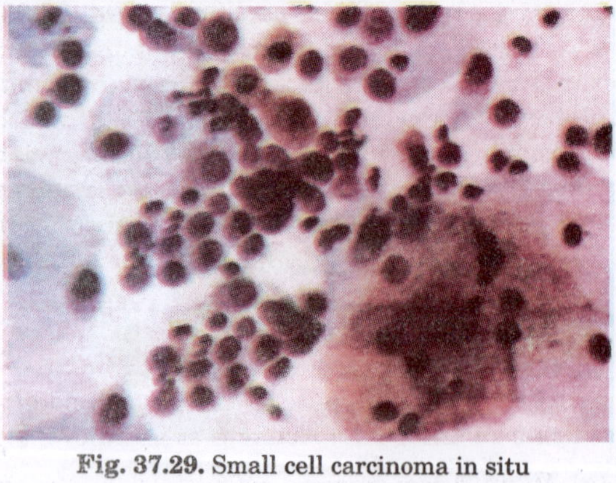

Fig. 37.29. Small cell carcinoma in situ

Large cell carcinoma in situ (Fig. 37.28)

Pap. staining shows syncytium of small immature cells with scant cyanophilic cytoplasm and ill-defined cell borders. Nuclear cytoplasmic ratio is markedly increased. Nucleus shows granular chromatin pattern and marked hyperchromasia. There is no nucleoli.

Small cell carcinoma in situ (Fig. 37.29)

Pap. staining shows clean background. Predominantly small cells of the carcinoma *in situ* type occur singly or in syncytium which have a tiny rim of cytoplasm and hyperchromatic nuclei. Chromatin structure is coarse.

INVASIVE CERVICAL CARCINOMA

Invasive carcinoma of uterine cervix may be defined as a malignant neoplasm of the cervical epithelium that infiltrates the underlying stroma and has the capacity to produce distant metastases. Histologically cervical carcinoma is classified as squamous cell carcinoma (90%), adenocarcinoma (5%) presumably arising in endocervical glands, and mixed adenosquamous carcinoma (5%).

Squamous cell carcinoma : Microscopically, there are three major categories of squamous cell carcinoma : *large cell non-keratinising, keratinising* and *small cell.* The large cell non-keratinising type has the best prognosis and the small cell type is the most aggressive neoplasm.

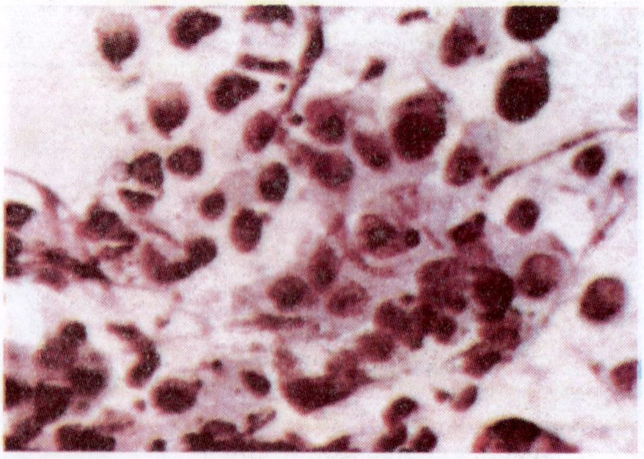

Fig. 37.30. Large cell undifferentiated squamous cell carcinoma

Non-keratinising infiltrating large cell squamous carcinoma

This cancer probably originates from a large cell type in situ carcinoma, also called large cell undifferentiated carcinoma.

Microscopic examination (Fig. 37.30)

The malignant cells are large and show marked anisocytosis. They occur either singly (70%) or in syncytial formation. Cytoplasm is usually cyanophilic and does not contain keratin. Cytoplasm is fragile and often lysed. There are naked nuclei. Nucleus is hyperchromatic with coarse chromatin pattern.

Well differentiated keratinising squamous cell carcinoma

The cancer cells show marked anisocytosis. They are pleomorphic in shape — flat, round, polygonal (70%), tadpole-like (10%), spindle or pearl formation (10%) or irregular (10%) depending on the maturation of the tumour. Pearl formations are cluster of malignant cells in concentric arrangement.

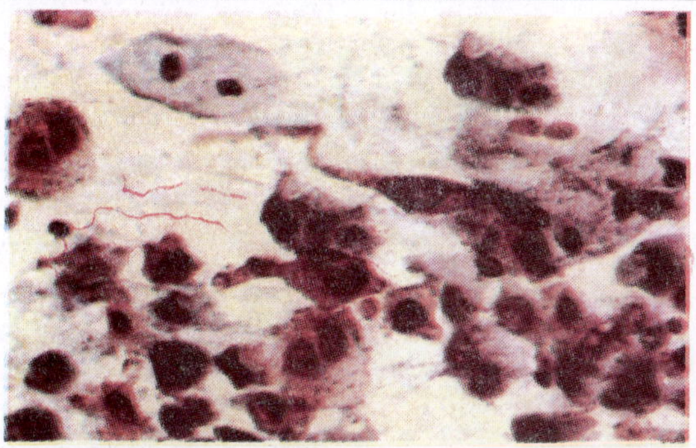

Fig. 37.31. Keratinising squamous cell carcinoma

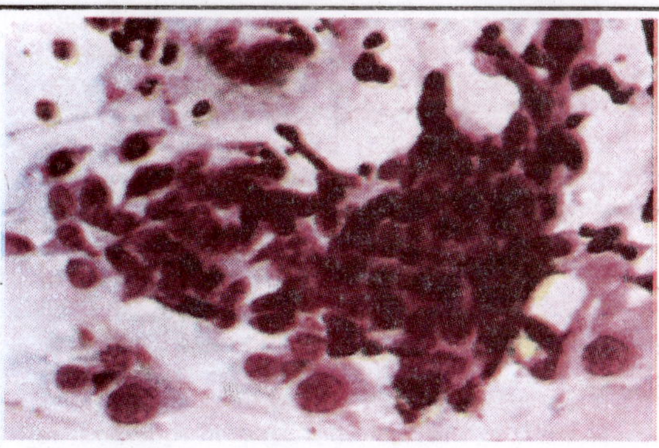

Fig. 37.32. Squamous cell carcinoma — small cell undifferentiated

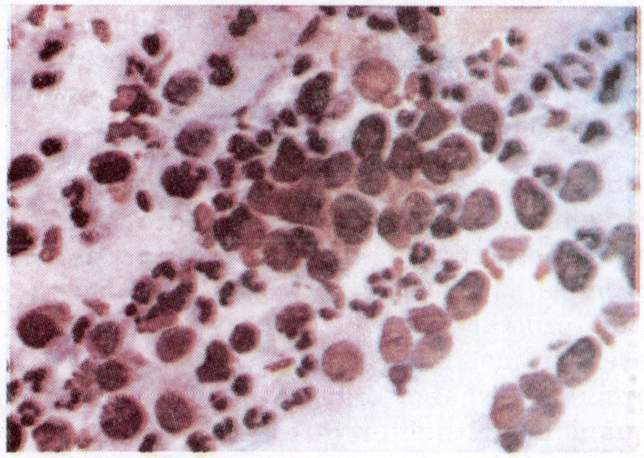

Fig. 37.33. Microcarcinoma. Background consists of exudate, leucocytes and debris, syncytium of small immature cells with severely nuclear-cytoplasmic ratio. There is hyperchromasia and mild anisokaryosis

Microscopic examination

Section (Fig. 37.31) shows large number of pleomorphic tumour cells, several squamous cells with eosinophilic (keratinising) cytoplasm, and groups of spindle cells. Nuclear chromatin is hyperchromatic and coarsely granular.

Small cell poorly differentiated squamous carcinoma

There are numerous oval and round cells with cyanophilic cytoplasm; oval, hyperchromatic and coarsely granular nuclei (Fig. 37.32). There is extreme increase in nuclear cytoplasmic ratio. They occur usually singly (80%) and may be found in loose syncytia or clusters (30%).

Microinvasive squamous cell carcinoma of cervix

Invasive squamous cell carcinoma (Fig. 37.33) in which the depth of invasion is no more than 5 mm in cervical stroma is called *microcarcinoma.* There are numerous atypical cells, 90% of which are round or oval and 10% polygonal, with cyanophilic cytoplasm. Atypical cells are arranged in syncytia (60%), sheets (15%) and singly (25%)). Cytological character is prominent in the depth of invasion.

ADENOCARCINOMA

The average detection rates of endometrial adenocarcinoma in different specimens is as follows :

(a) Vaginal pool smear — 40%

(b) Cervical scraping out — 15%

(c) Endocervical aspirations and vaginal pool smears — 65%

(d) Intrauterine and endocervical aspiration and lavage — 90%.

Desquamated endometrial cells get blocked by endocervical mucus plug which results in delay to reach vagina.

The exfoliated cells are larger than normal and imitate somewhat the benign columnar cells of their origin. Malignant cells are scanty in number. The cells are shed in tight clumps or clusters (Fig. 37.34).

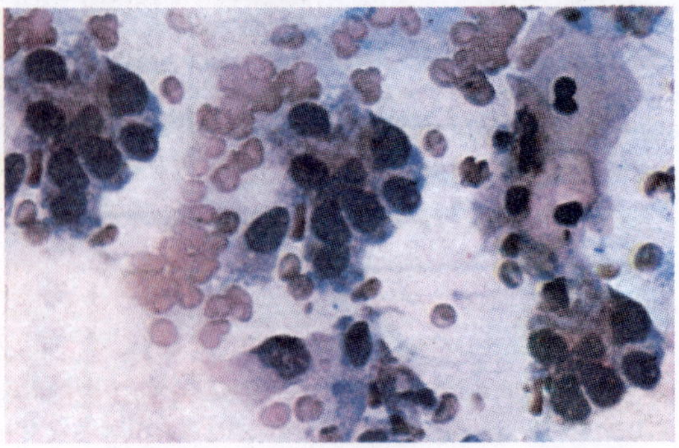

Fig. 37.34. Adenocarcinoma of endocervix

Chapter 38

Cytology of Body Cavity Fluids (Effusions)

The cellular composition of different body fluids – pleural, pericardial or abdominal cavities is identical and normally contain only a few ml of lubricating serous fluid and 0-2 lymphocytes/cu.mm fluid. These body cavities are normally lined by a single layer of flattened cuboidal epithelium made of mesothelial cells.

Pathological changes

Accumulation of fluid in body cavities in appreciable amount is an indication of disease. Accumulated fluid (plasma filtration) serves as a good culture medium for microbial agents and exfoliated benign or malignant cellls. This is why mitosis of tumour cells are often seen in effusion fluid. The single layer of flattened cells of mesothelium become stratified and cuboidal in response to an injury (e.g., accumulation of fluid).

The aspirated material is centrifuged and the deposit is smeared on albuminised glass slides and stained with Papanicolaou's stain and examined.

Neoplasms of serosal membrane

I. *Primary tumours* : Rare; except primary-mesothelioma and few sarcomas.

II. *Secondary carcinoma* : Most tumours of serosal membranes are secondary in type.

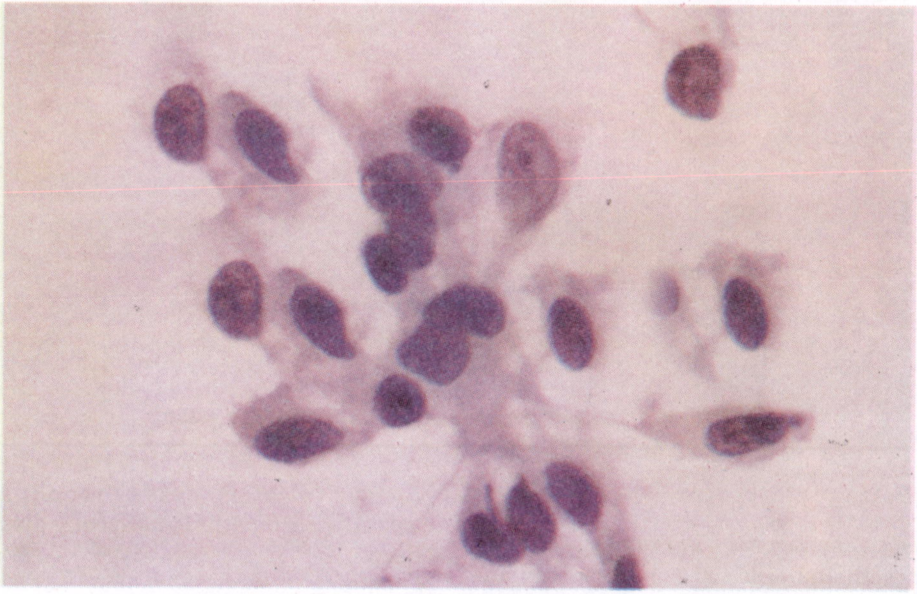

Fig. 38.1. Normal mesothelial cell of peritoneum *(Pap. staining)*, × 400

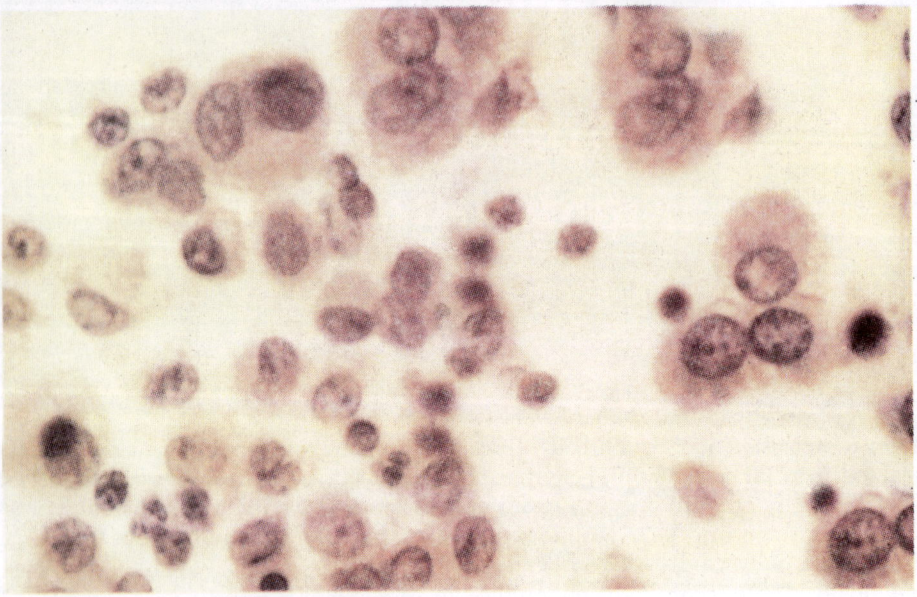

Fig. 38.2. Reactive mesothelial cell, Pap. × 320

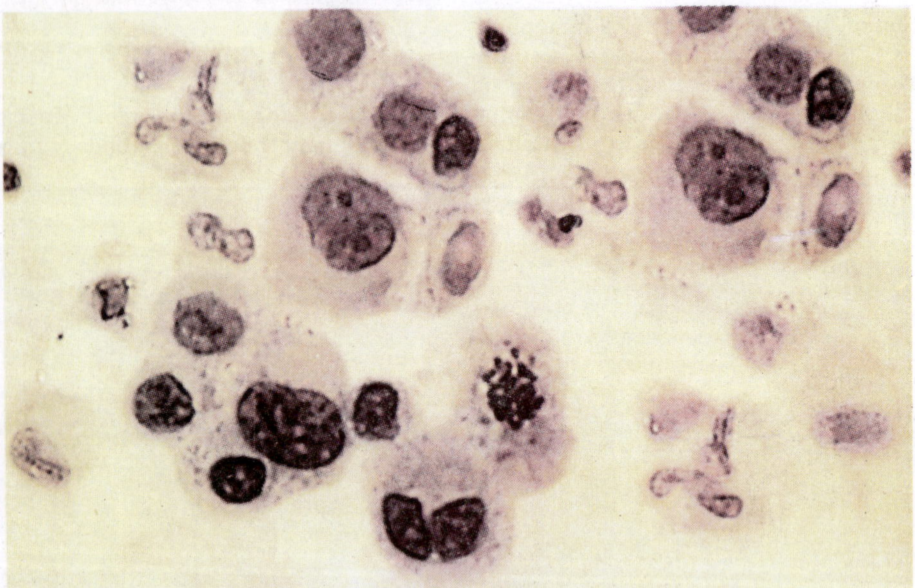

Fig. 38.3. Malignant mesothelioma of pleura, Pap. × 450

Non-reactive mesothelial cell (Normal) (Fig. 38.1)

Pap. staining of peritoneal scraping shows young cuboidal mesothelial cells (15 ± 5 μm) singly and in small clusters. Some cells are round while others are oval in shape. Cytoplasm on an average is foamy and pink and basophilic in few cells. Nucleus is single, oval or round, and located centrally; chromatin is uniformly distributed and sharp.

Reactive mesothelial cells (Fig. 38.2)

Pap. staining of sediment of pleural fluid shows round to oval mesothelial cells (60 ± 30 μm)

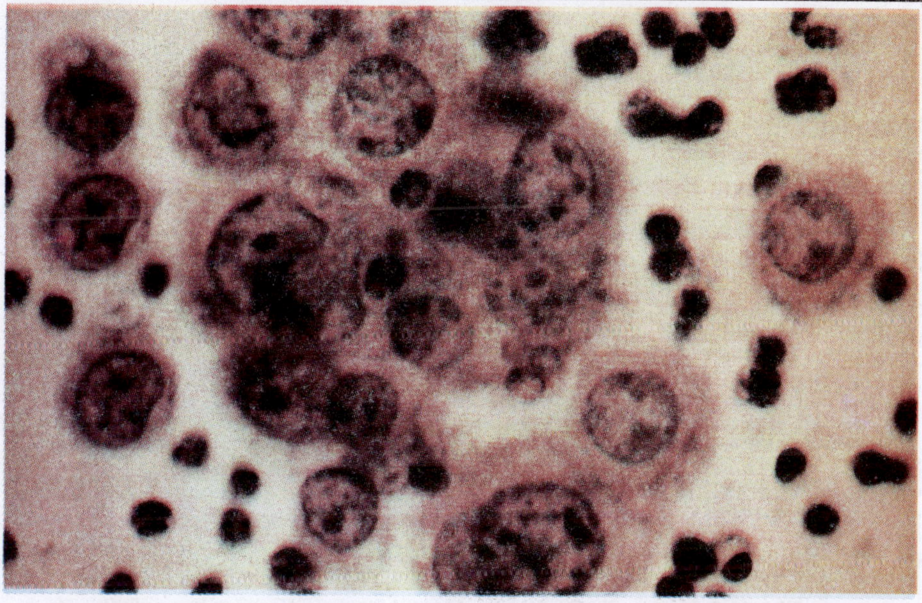

Fig. 38.4. Metastatic squamous cell carcinoma of lung in pleural cavity, Pap. × 450

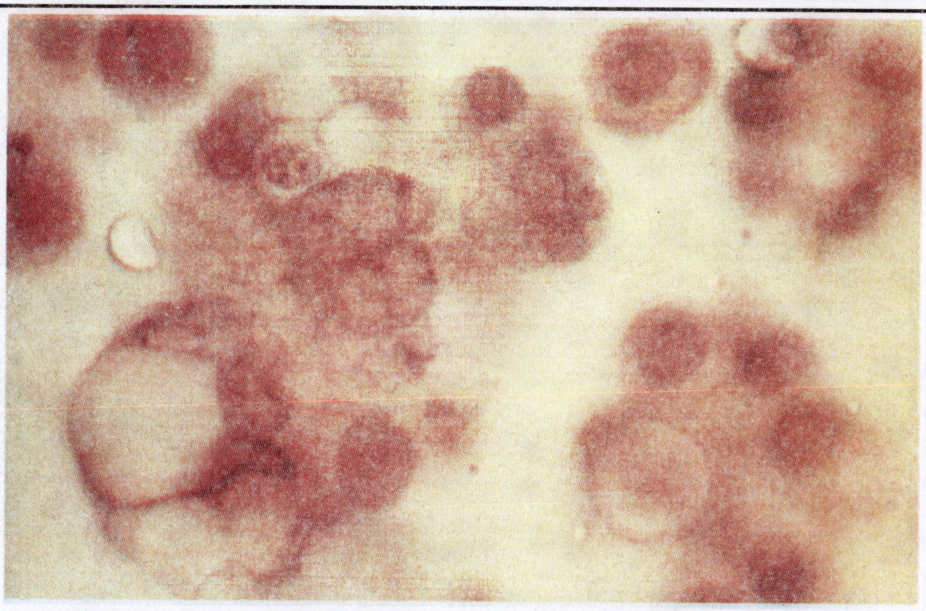

Fig. 38.5. Metastatic mucinous adenocarcinoma of ovary in peritoneum × 400

arranged in small clusters with variation in size. There are several binucleated cells and several lymphocytes. Cytoplasm is scanty to abundant and purple.

Malignant mesothelioma (Fig. 38.3)

Pap. staining of sediment of pleural fluid shows neoplastic cells resembling large, reactive mesothelial cells except that they are larger with more hyperchromatic nuclei which show an irregular chromatin.

Metastatic squamous cell carcinoma of lung (Fig. 38.4)

Pap. staining of pleural fluid shows cluster of pleomorphic poorly differentiated cells of primary

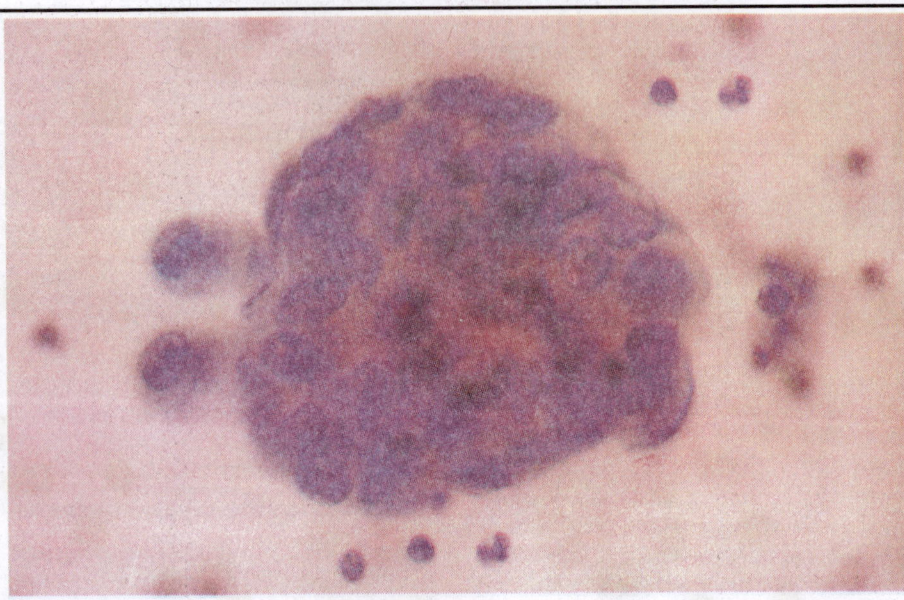

Fig. 38.6. Metastatic carcinoma of breast in pleural cavity, Pap. × 500

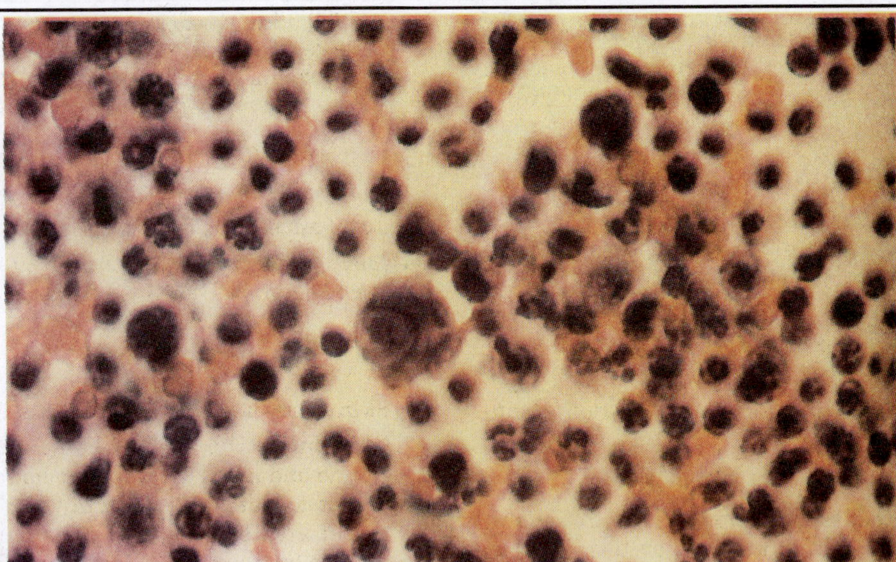

Fig. 38.7. Metastatic oat cell (Pleural fluid) × 250

bronchogenic carcinoma (squamous cell type) with expansion into pleural serous membrane.

Metastatic mucinous adenocarcinoma of ovary (Fig. 38.5)

Pap. staining of peritoneal fluid shows large number of malignant cells embedded in thick mucinous material. Tumour cells are distended by large mucous containing vacuoles pushing the nucleus to the periphery.

Metastatic carcinoma breast (Figs 38.6 and 38.7)

Pap. staining of pleural fluid shows malignant cells in ball-like nests. The malignant cells are oval, fairly uniform in size and shape. Cytoplasm is scanty and stained pink to purple, and nuclei are moderately hyperchromatic.

Chapter 39

Fine Needle Aspiration Cytology (FNAC)

Cells from any site of the body can be obtained by fine needle aspiration. Fine needle aspiration cytology (FNAC) of superficial nodule and thyroid lesions has become a routine diagnostic procedure. FNAC is being increasingly used in the recent years in the diagnosis of bone lesions, breast lesions and in lesions of internal organs (pancreas, prostate, salivary glands, etc). The aspirated material is smeared on glass slides and stained by Leishman-Giemsa, May-Grunwald-Giemsa or Papanicolaou's stain and also by H.E. stain.

Advantages of FNAC

1. Eliminates the need for more complicated diagnostic tests.
2. Less traumatic than usual knife biopsy.
3. Rapid and accurate, permits early treatment.
4. Investigation of a mass is possible without excision.
5. Provides preoperative knowledge of deep-seated lesions.

Disadvantages

1. Danger of dissemination of tumour cells in the needle tract or natural cavities.
2. It may cause internal bleeding and complications like air emboli, pneumothorax.
3. Accuracy of the method has been questioned—the point of the needle may miss the target.

Indications

(a) *When surgery is not possible* :

(i) Patient refuses surgery or tolerates anaesthesia poorly.

(ii) Exploratory mass in a poor risk patient.

(iii) Difficult or dangerous site of location of mass.

(b) *When surgery is contraindicated* :

(i) Clinically an obvious malignant mass.

(ii) Clinically the mass is a cyst or obviously benign.

(iii) Age of patient and other factors, e.g., pregnancy.

Materials

1. Disposable 20 ml syringe.
2. Disposable fine needle (18-23 gauge).
3. Local anaesthesia is not necessary.
4. Slide, saline, antiseptic, fixative (equal volume of ether and absolute alcohol).

Technique (Figs. 39.1A-L, 39.1M)

The biopsy procedure

1. Skin is cleaned with antiseptic solution.
2. Immobilise the area to be aspirated with thumb and index finger of one hand and then insert a sterile needle (22 G/23 G) in the target area by supporting the barrel of the syringe by free hand (Fig. 39.1M). The needle of the 20 ml syringe is preferably fixed in Franzen's syringe holder before introducing the needle in the target area.
3. Once the needle in the mass (39.1A), retract the piston to maintain a negative pressure (Fig. 39.1B).
4. Move the needle back and forth several times in different directions to obtain cells from the different areas of the mass to be investigated (Fig. 39.1C).

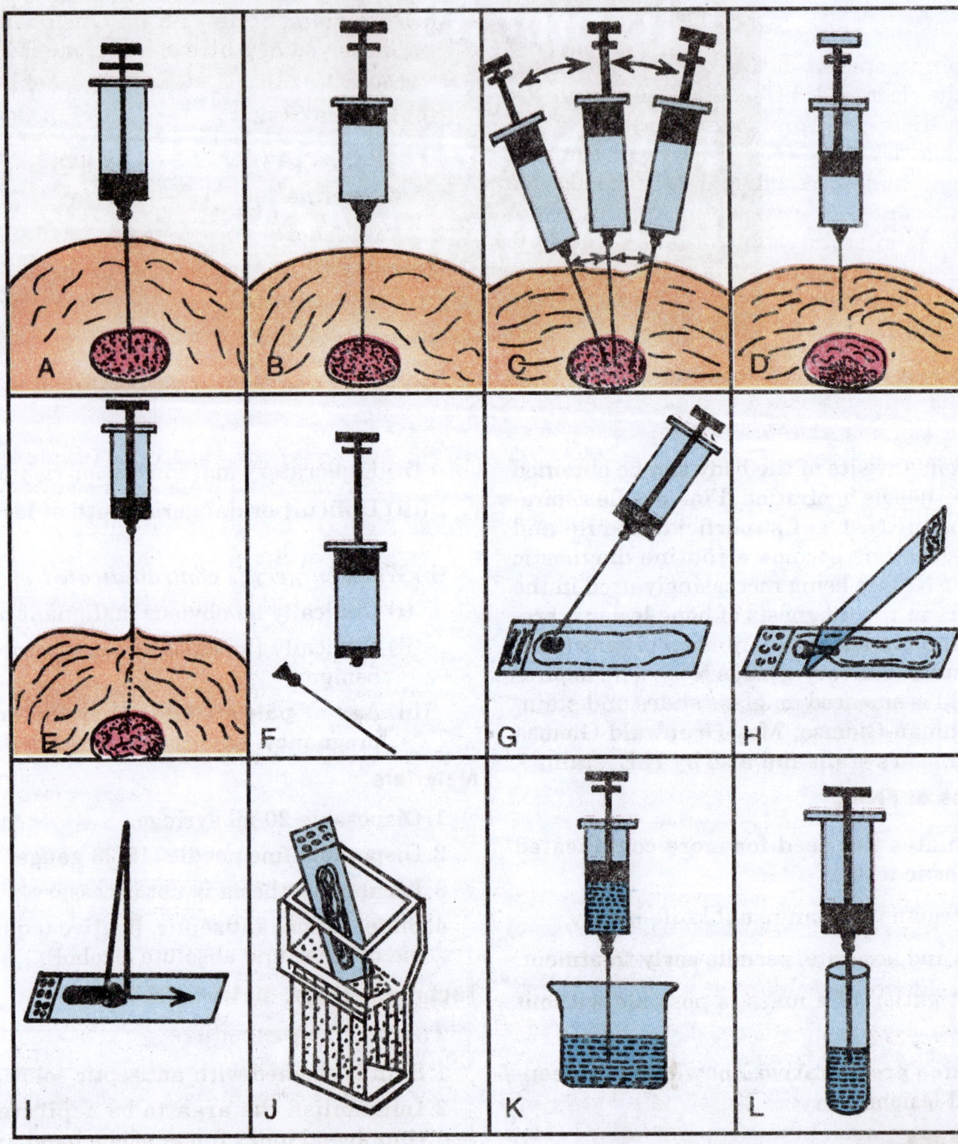

Fig. 39.1 (A to L). Technique of fine needle aspiration

5. Withdraw the needle slowly while maintaining a negative pressure until the subcutaneous tissue is reached (Fig. 39.1D). Then the piston of the syringe is released to equalise the pressure (Fig. 39.1E).
6. Withdraw the needle completely and disconnect from the syringe (Fig. 39.1F).
7. Fill the syringe with air and reconnect to the needle (Fig. 39.1F).

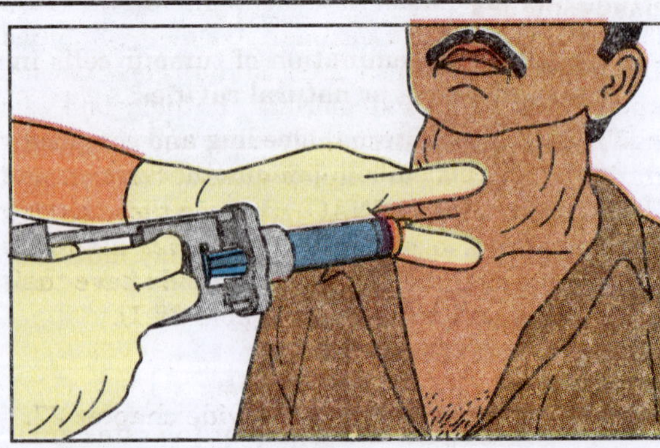

Fig. 39.1 (M). Technique of FNAC with the aid of Franzen's syringe holder

Preparing the aspirate

Direct smearing

The aspirate present in the core of the needle is blown on the clean slides (Fig. 39.1G) . Smears are made immediately by applying a gentle pressure with another dry slide (Fig. 39.1H, I). For Pap. staining both slides are immediately placed in a Couplin jar containing fixative (Fig. 39.1J). A small amount of saline solution is aspirated to rinse the needle core and syringe. The saline is then passed through a membrane filter and processed (Fig. 39.1 K, L).

The aspirate is referred to as 'dry' if it consists of numerous cells suspended in a small amount of tissue fluid and has a creamy consistency. Such a dry smear represents the perfect sample for most malignant tumours.

Indirect smearing

A 'wet' aspirate consists of a small number of cells suspended in fluid or blood. The process of centrifugation and preparation of smear from deposit is called *indirect smearing*.

When aspirated cellular material is abundant, then even paraffin cell block can be prepared. Moreover, material from the aspirate can be utilised for special stainings, immuno-biochemisty, cell marker studies, chromosomal analysis and tumour marker.

The smears prepared from the aspirate are ready for staining in dry state by haematological stains, while these are immediately fixed in alcohol-ether solution in Couplin jar for Pap staining.

Fixation and Staining

Different methods of fixation and staining are used in FNAC; air drying followed by staining with a haematological stain such as MGG (May Grunwald Giemsa), Leishman, Giemsa, combined Leishman and Giemsa (LG); and alcohol fixation and staining with Pap or H&E. Pathologists who had their basic training in gynaecological cytology find it convenient to employ alcohol fixation and Pap staining also in FNAC, whereas those having a background in haematology prefer air-dried Giemsa stained smears. Both methods have their advantages and deficiencies (Table 39.1).

Stains

1. *Papanicolau's staining* — vide chapter 37.
2. *Leishman–Giemsa Stain* (LG).

Preparation

(a) Leishman Stain : 1.5 gm Leishman powder dissolved in 1 litre of a acetone-free methanol.

(b) Giemsa Stain :

Giemsa powder	—	1.0 gm
Glycerine	—	66 ml
Methanol	—	66 ml

Dissolve all three to form concentrated Giemsa stain (stock solution).

Procedure

(a) Cover the slide with Leishman stain — 1 mm.

(b) Add equal volume 1 in 20 (diluted) Giemsa stain prepared from stock solution.

(c) Keep it for 10-15 minutes and wash in running tap water.

(d) Dry the smear and mount with coverslip.

SUPERFICIAL NODULE ASPIRATE

LYMPH NODE

Benign reactive hyperplasia

Microscopy (Fig. 39.2) : There are a large number of mature small lymphocytes mixed with scattered large immature lymphocytes that have originated from germinal centres of follicles. There are several macrophages (histiocytes).

Table 39.1
Comparison of air-dried and wet-fixed smears

Properties	Air-dried LG	Wet-fixed Pap
'Dry' smear	Good fixation	Drying artefact common
'Wet' smear	Artefacts common	Good fixation
Cell and nuclear size	Exaggerated, differences enhanced	Comparable to tissue sections
Cytoplasmic detail	Well demonstrated	Poorly demonstrated
Nucleoli	Not always discernible	Well demonstrated
Stromal components	Well shown, often differentially stained	Poorly demonstrated
Partially necrotic tissue	Poorly defined cell details	Well defined single intact cells

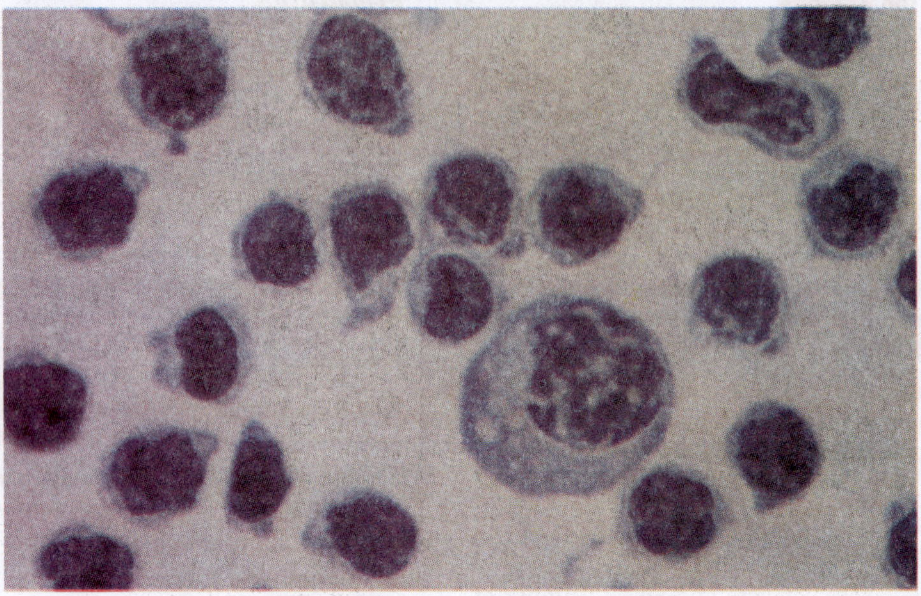

Fig. 39.2. Benign reactive hyperplasia lymph node (Pap. × 500)

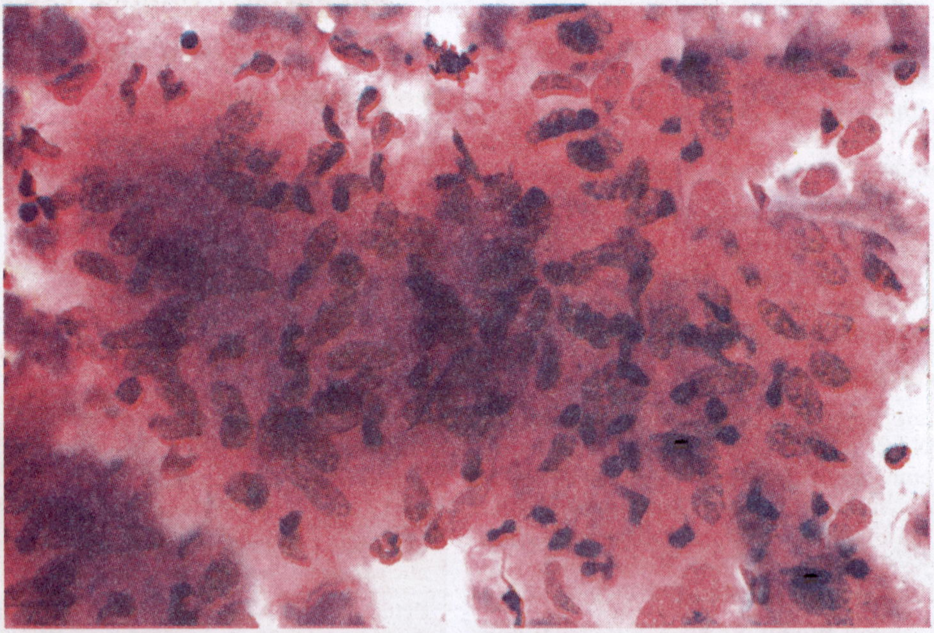

Fig. 39.3. Tuberculous lymphadenitis showing cohesive epitheloid granuloma (MG × 500)

Lymphadenitis : In addition to large number of mature small lymphocytes, there are scattered larger immature lymphocytes, monocytes and plasma cells and leucocytes.

In tuberculous lymphadenitis (Fig. 39.3), there are variable numbers of epitheloid cells, histiocytes and giant cells (Langhans' giant cell). The background of the smear often shows necrotic debris.

Immunoblastic reaction

Immunoblastic reaction such as *angioimmuno-*

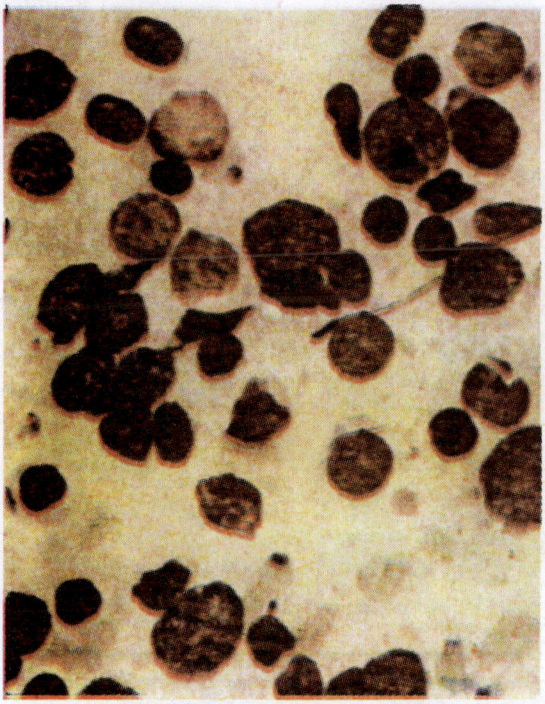

Fig. 39.4. Immunoblastic lymphadenopathy showing transformed lymphocytes, immunoblasts, histiocytes (MG × 250)

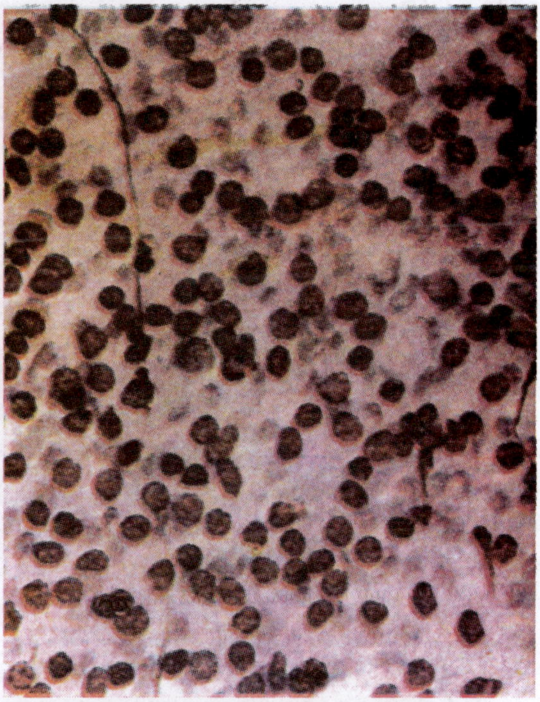

Fig. 39.6. Poorly differentiated lymphocytic lymphoma. Showing predominantly medium-sized cells with cleaved nuclei (MG × 200)

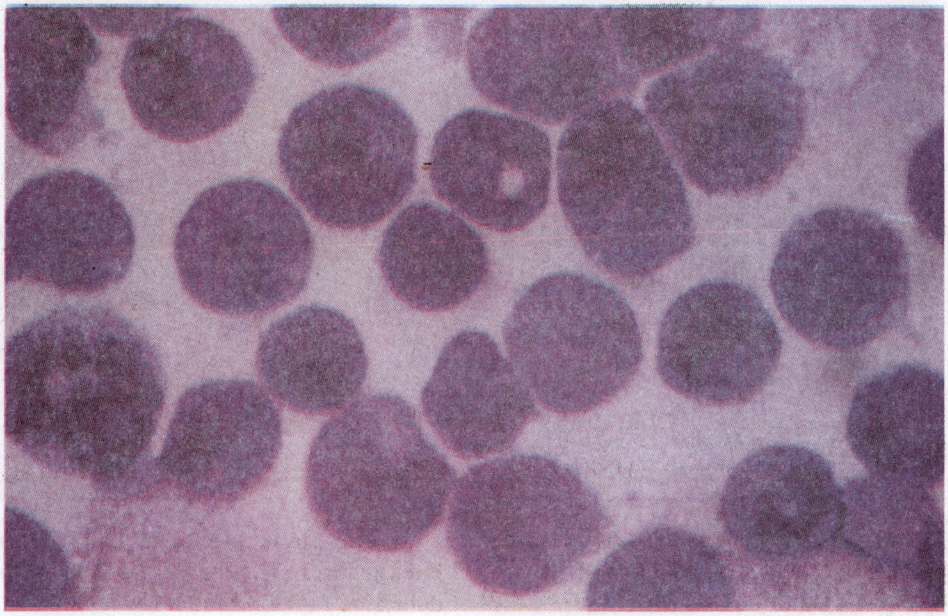

Fig. 39.5. Malignant lymphoma, T lymphoblastic. Papanicolaou's stain (× 500) of FNAC. Mixture of small and large lymphoid cells, majority of which show markedly irregular nuclei

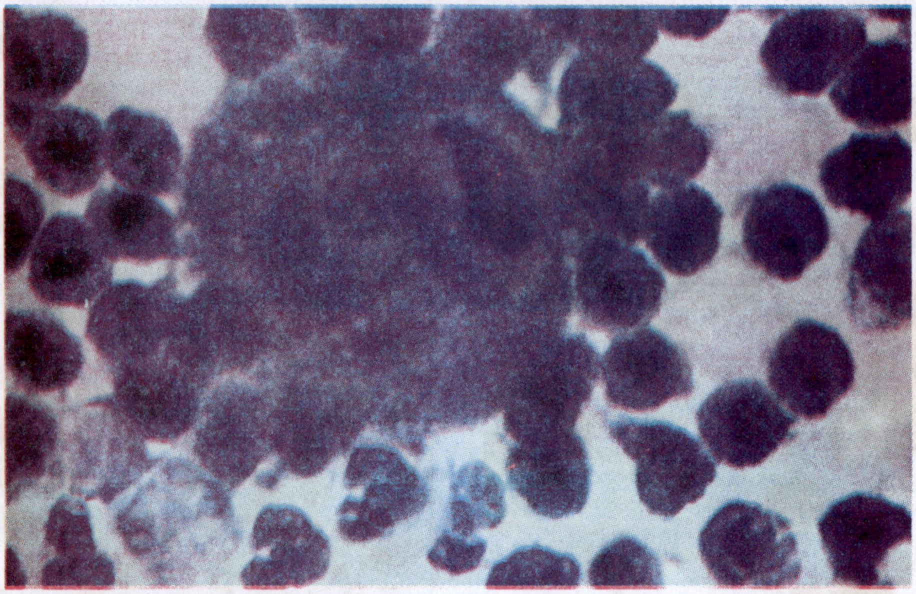

Fig. 39.7. Hodgkin's disease, FNAC. MG staining : There are small lymphocytes and a classical Reed-Sternberg cell (× 500)

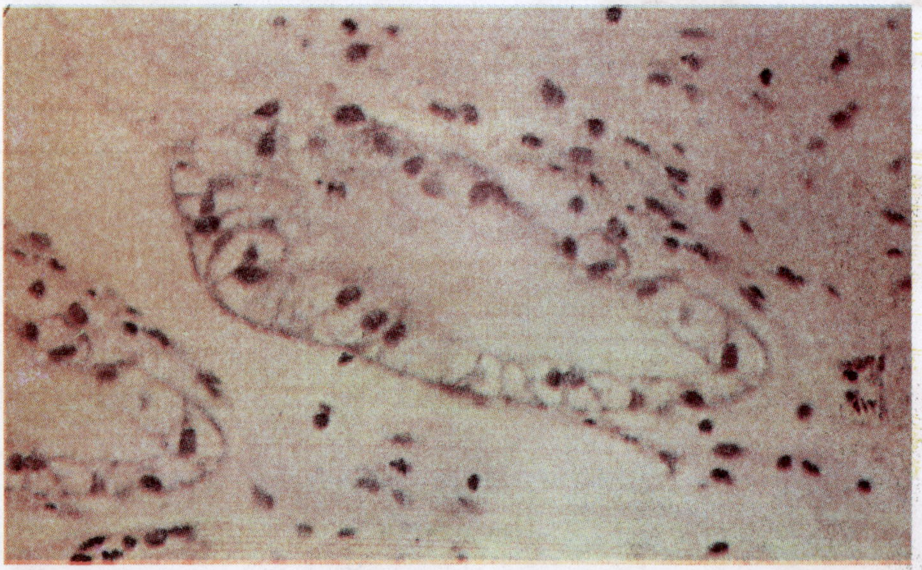

Fig. 39.8. H.E. Section of FNAC of superficial nodule showing metastatic clear cell adenocarcinoma (HE × 500)

blastic lymphadenopathy (AILD) are difficult to differentiate from T cell lymphoma and in some cases they progress to lymphoma. Aspirate shows transformed lymphocytes, immunoblasts and histiocytes. The diagnosis has to be established by histological examination of excised lymph node (Fig. 39.4).

Lymphoma

Non-Hodgkin's lymphoma

(Poorly differentiated lymphoblastoma)

Microscopy

There are small atypical lymphocytes with scanty cytoplasm and prominent nucleoli. No indication of lymphocytic differentiation is observed (Figs 39.5 and 39.6).

Hodgkin's disease

Microscopy : Needle aspirate shows scattered Reed-Sternberg cells in the midst of variable numbers of reactive lymphocytes, histiocytes, eosinophils and plasma cells (Fig. 39.7).

Metastatic Carcinoma

Microscopy : Sections from cell block of a superficial nodule (HE Stain) shows clear cell adenocarcinoma (Fig. 39.8).

THYROID GLAND

Confirmation of cellular nature of most thyroid nodule is necessary. Aspirates from benign lesions of thyroid contain few thyroid cells. Moreover, diagnosis of thyroiditis can also be made by examining the aspirate.

Aspiration cytology on tumours of thyroid is described here and routine histopathological features of the same are described in chapter 35.

Follicular adenoma

In the majority of the follicular adenomas, there are large number of benign follicular cells of uniform size, shape and texture (Fig. 39.9).

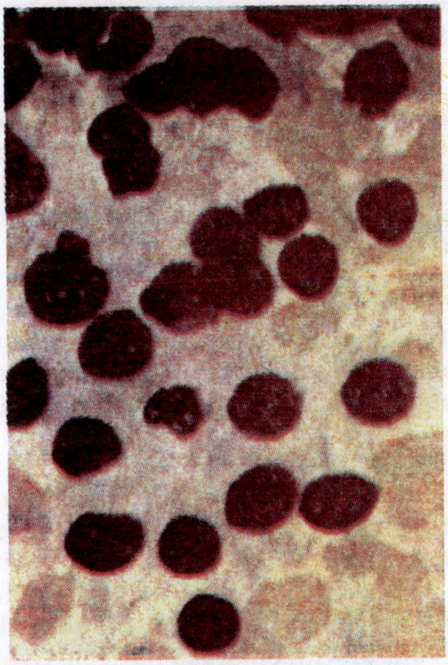

Fig. 39.9. Follicular adenoma thyroid. Cells are of uniform size arranged in clusters, forming micro-follicles (MG × 200)

Atypical adenoma (less than 5% of adenomas) : Aspirate materials show moderate variation in size and shape of benign follicular cells. Nucleus is hyperchromatic and cell contains scanty cytoplasm. Differential diagnosis with early carcinoma is difficult.

Papillary Adenocarcinoma

Microscopy : There is increase in number of follicular cells with tight clusters or papillary structures. Malignant cells show variable degree of polymorphism (Fig. 39.10).

OTHER USES OF FNAC

(a) Salivary gland lesions

(b) Breast

(c) Bone

(d) Transthoracic : Lung tumours

(e) Transabdominal : Liver, pancreas, kidneys, adrenal glands

(f) Miscellaneous use : Prostate, ovary, etc.

FNAC is becoming widely recognised as a practical and useful technique in the diagnosis of salivary, prostatic, breast, bone and space-occupying lesions.

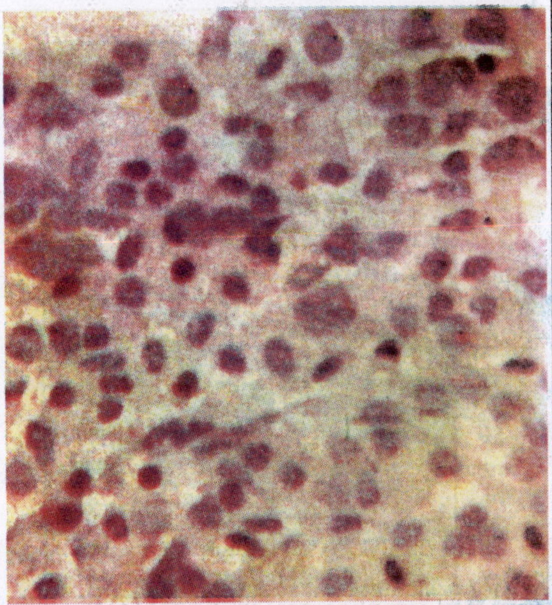

Fig. 39.10. Papillary carcinoma thyroid showing malignant cells having pale nuclei with irregular outline (MG × 200)

SALIVARY GLAND

Benign tumours

1. *Lymphoepithelioma* : Predominance of mature and immature lymphocytes mixed with various numbers of benign, small, epithelial ductal cells and serous cells and histiocytes is diagnostic.

2. *Pleomorphic adenoma* : Clusters, acini or sheets of epithelial cells mixed with mucoid substance and stromal cells of mesenchymal origin are found (Fig. 39.11).

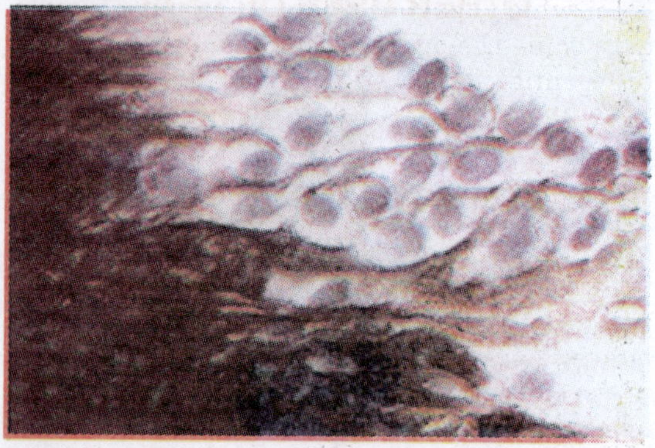

Fig. 39.11. Pleomorphic adenoma salivary gland (parotid) showing mixture of epithelial cells and chondromyxoid stroma obscuring the epithelial cells on one side (MG × 200)

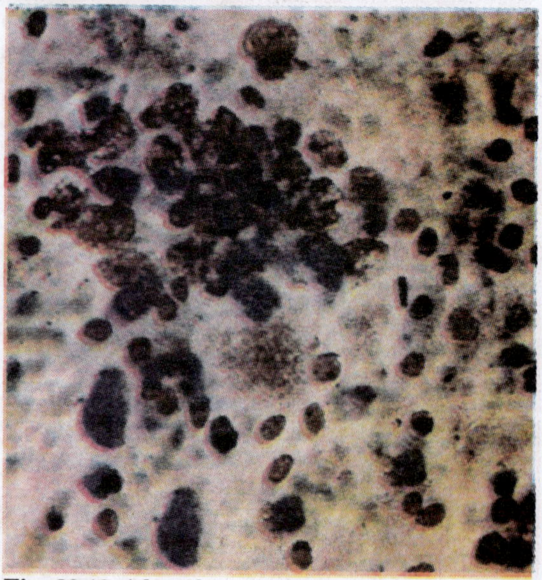

Fig. 39.12. Adenoid cystic carcinoma showing malignant cells arranged in small clump and dispersed throughout the field (MG × 200)

3. *Papillary cystadenoma lymphomatosum* : Variable number of cuboidal or columnar epithelial cells (oncocytes) are found in loose clusters, sheets, or palisade formation, which are often surrounded by numerous mature lymphocytes.

Malignant tumours

1. *Adenoid cystic carcinoma* : Presence of tight clusters or globules of small cuboidal epithelial cells with scanty cytoplasm and round or oval nuclei is diagnostic (Fig. 39.12).

2. *Mucoepidermoid carcinoma* : There are variable numbers of malignant squamous cells mixed with mucus-secreting, benign-appearing columnar cells. Squamous cancer cells are moderately differentiated and contain increased cytoplasmic keratin and bizarre pleomorphic nuclei.

3. *Mixed carcinoma* : A mixture of malignant squamous and columnar cells, and in rare instances, there are also stromal, mesodermal, sarcomatous cells. Preponderance of cell type depends on the nature of the tumour and the part sampled.

BONE

Benign lesions

1. *Osteomyelites* : Large numbers of neutrophils mixed with cellular debris and other necrotic precipitate are seen. Epitheloid and Langhans' giant cells when present, indicates tuberculous lesion. Smear may be stained for acid-fast organisms.

2. *Bone cysts* : Number of cells are scanty. A scattering of histiocytes, lymphocytes and other monocytes are found mixed with a few epithelial-appearing flattened cells (transparent cytoplasm with benign vesicular nuclei).

Giant cell tumour of bones

Aspirate shows multi-nucleate osteoclast-like giant cells and cluster of cohesive clump of spindle cells, some of which are vacuolated (Fig. 39.13).

Malignant tumours

1. *Osteogenic sarcoma* : Scattering of normal osteoid proliferating cells, elongated benign stromal cells, and variable numbers of scattered, bizarre, large, malignant cells are seen. The cells often contain abnormal, irregularly shaped, often multiple nuclei with enlarged nucleoli. Cytoplasm of these cancer cells are eosinophilic and abundant which makes them resemble keratinising squamous carcinoma cells (Fig. 39.14).

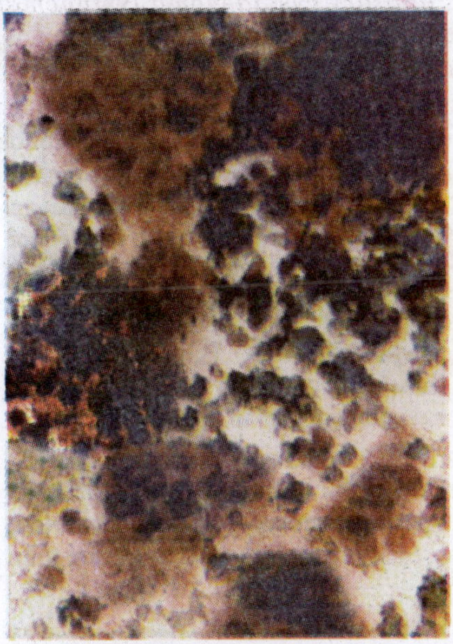

Fig. 39.13. Giant cell tumour of bone showing 2 multinucleate osteoclast like giant cells and cohesive cluster of spindle cells (MG × 200)

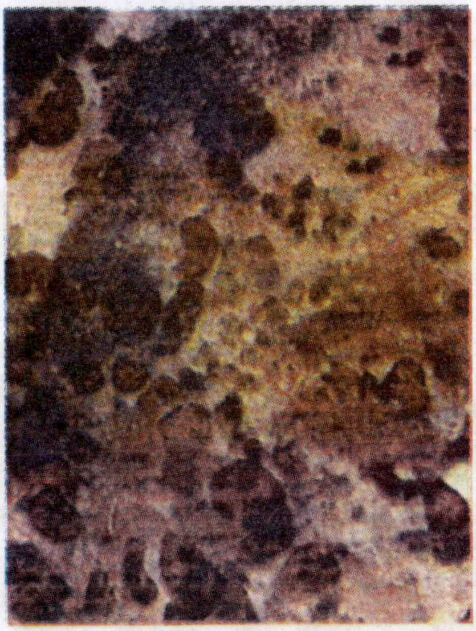

Fig. 39.14. Osteosarcoma (fibroblastic) : Pleomorphic spindle cell sarcoma with fragments of pink amorphous osteoid material (MG × 200)

2. *Chondrosarcoma* : Mixture of stromal and single cartilaginous cells. Cartilaginous cells are round or oval with abundant cytoplasm and large, often double nuclei, which are surrounded by large prominent halos. The tumour cells appear benign or obviously malignant with extremely bizarre features depending on the differentiation of the tumour.

3. *Ewing's sarcoma* : Uniformly small, poorly differentiated, malignant cells are mainly scattered singly but may be found in clusters or sheets or rosettes. Cytoplasm is very scanty. It is difficult to differentiate the cells from similar lymphoblastic cells of a lymphoma, but the small nucleoli and rosette pattern help in their identification.

4. *Metastatic carcinoma* : Metastatic tumour cells are easy to recognise. Their morphology varies depending on the nature of primary cancer from which they originate. It is not possible to determine the origin of malignant cells in poorly differentiated metastatic carcinoma by cytology.

BREAST

Benign lesions

1. ***Acute mastitis*** : Large amount of inflammatory cells, with a predominance of polymorphonuclear leucocytes in a background of cellular debris, microorganisms and protein precipitates are seen. Smear may contain degenerate, normal or reactive duct cells.

In acute mastitis in lactating breast, there are large number of inflammatory cells and cyst macrophages in a background of lipid secretions (Fig. 39.15).

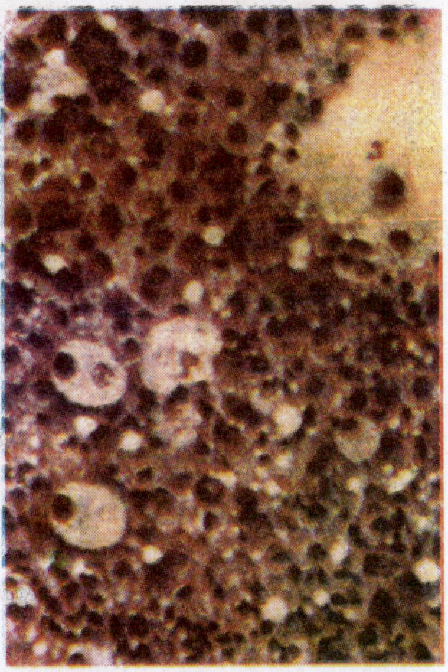

Fig. 39.15. Acute mastitis in lactating breast showing large number of inflammatory cells and cyst macrophages in a background of lipid secretions (MG × 200)

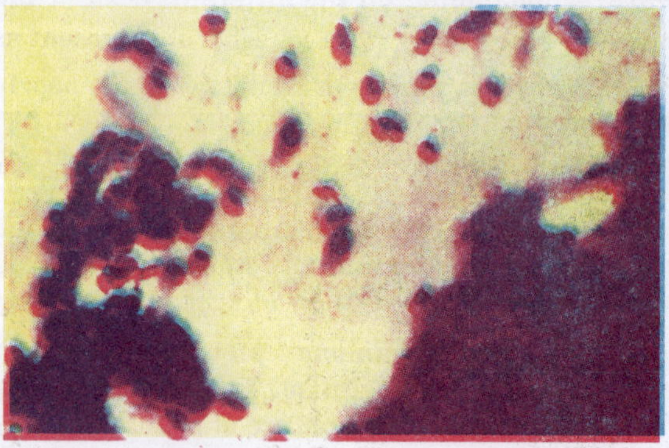

Fig. 39.16. Fibroadenoma breast : Cluster of highly cellular ductal cells of usual type; some bare nuclei and myxoid connective tissue are present (HE × 265)

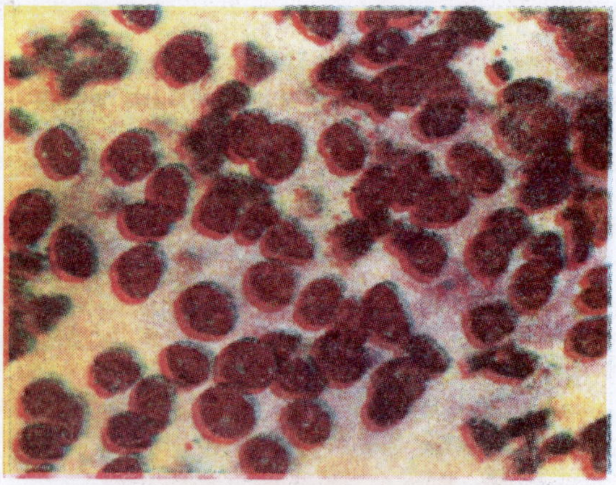

Fig. 39.17. Benign epithelial hyperplasia of breast : Large slightly disorganised cluster of ductal cells with some bare nuclei (MG × 200)

2. ***Fibroadenoma*** : Smears are highly cellular showing cuboidal, ovoid, and spindle epithelial cells often without cytoplasm. Cells are arranged in tight clusters or large sheets in honeycomb appearance (Fig. 39.16).

3. ***Benign epithelial hyperplasia*** : A localised or diffused intraductal hyperplasia may produce a bloody or lemon yellow discharge particularly when present in terminal excretory ducts. The discharge requires to be differentiated from that of intraductal carcinoma and that occurring during pregnancy.

Microscopy (Fig. 39.17) : Loose clumps of ductal cells with acinus-like structure and dispersed bare nuclei are found. Some variations in nuclear size is seen.

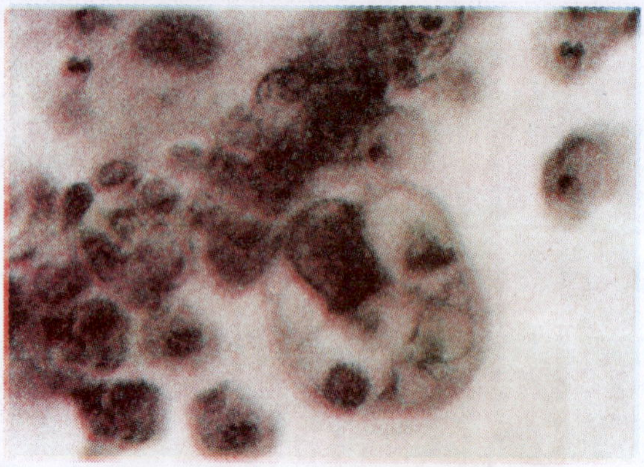

Fig. 39.18. Comedocarcinoma : Pleomorphic malignant cells with a background of necrotic debris (MG × 200)

Malignant tumours

1. ***Comedocarcinoma***

Worm-like plugs of a mixture of cancer cells and necrotic material may be expressed by nipple massage. *Microscopy* shows variable number of hypertrophic cells, usually single (70%) or in sheets, papillae or clusters in the background of abundant necrotic debris. The cell types are large, pleomorphic and show all the usual criteria of malignancy (Fig. 39.18).

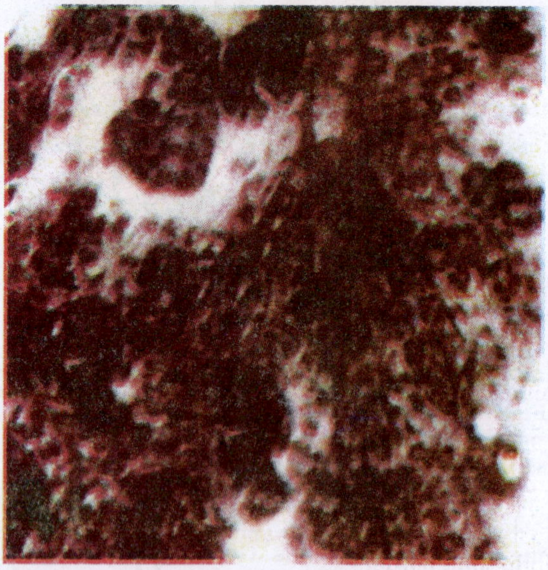

Fig. 39.19. Papillary carcinoma of breast : Smear is highly cellular. There are papillary aggregates with central fibrovascular core, × 150

2. *Infiltrating ductal adenocarcinoma*

ME. Smear shows large number of sheets, irregular papillary projections and clusters of single cells. Cohesion of cell is poor and the tumour cells form loose clusters.

In papillary duct carcinoma, clusters of hyperchromatic cells form papillary structures (Fig. 39.19).

TRANSTHORACIC ASPIRATION

1. Mediastinum

Fine needle aspiration directed by TV-fluorography or CT scan is useful in the diagnosis of aetiology of the most anterior and posterior mediastinal disease. The main complication is the production of a limited pneumothorax (20% patients). Diagnosis of a metastatic carcinoma may prevent an unecessary exploratory thoracotomy.

Transthoracic, percutaneous, fine needle aspiration of enlarged mediastinum, lung tumour, mass in lung as seen by X-ray is also done directly.

2. Lung

Indication of FNAC

(a) Patient is unable to cough and produce an adequate sputum or when bronchoscopy or bronchial washings cannot be done.

(b) Sputum, bronchial washings and brushings have repeatedly remained negative inspite of a persistent clinically suspected cancer.

(c) The lesion is a peripheral primary or metastatic tumour.

(d) Lesion is cavitary and a sample of fluid is required for culture.

(e) Lesion is inoperable.

Benign and malignant cells in FNAC are very similar to those seen in sputum, bronchial washing or brushing specimens.

Tuberculosis lung (Fig. 39.20)

Smear shows epitheloid cells with elongated footprint-shaped nuclei and pale cytoplasm with indistinct borders.

Squamous cell carcinoma

The tumour may be keratinising or non-keratinising, the former shows bizarre cell shapes with dispersion of malignant cells. Non-keratinising tumours are usually more cohesive and present as multi-layered fragments (Fig. 39.21).

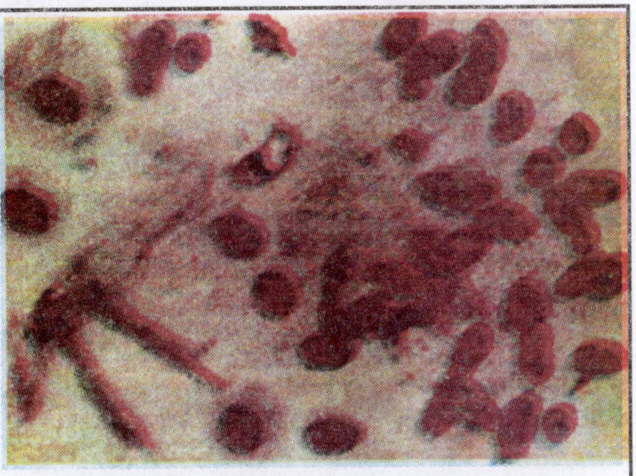

Fig. 39.20. Tuberculosis lung showing clustered epitheloid histiocytes (MG × 200)

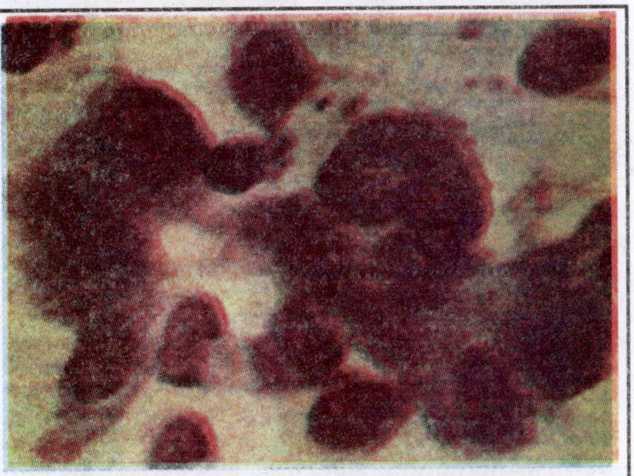

Fig. 39.21. Bronchogenic carcinoma : Squamous cell carcinoma : Irregular clumps of relatively cohesive non-keratinising malignant squamous cells, slightly larger than lymphocytes (MG × 200)

TRANSABDOMINAL ASPIRATION

Ultrasonic, fluoroscopic, or computerised tomography guidance, have made deep organs and tissues of abdominal cavity and the retroperitoneum readily accessible to percutaneous, fine needle aspiration.

FNAC is also performed directly by palpation of palpable abdominal mass and the result is satisfactory.

Liver

(a) *Non-neoplastic lesions*

In cases of *hepatitis, abscess* and other *infections,* there are various amounts of inflammatory cells and debris mixed with hepatocytes in varying degrees of degeneration.

(b) ***Neoplasia***

(i) *Primary hepatocarcinoma (hepatoma)* : The diagnosis is difficult from cytology especially when the tumour is well differentiated. The tumour is composed of poorly cohesive hepatocytic cells with some anisokaryosis and very large nucleoli. The tumour cells resemble reactive benign hepatocytes and difference from adenoma is difficult or impossible.

(ii) *Metastatic tumour* : The "alien" tumour cells are quite different from that of normal hepatic cells.

Pancreas

(a) ***Benign lesions***

In *acute pancreatitis,* there are various inflammatory cells in addition to necrotic cellular debris and a few regenerating atypical acinar cells. The inflammatory cells in *chronic pancreatitis* are mainly lymphocytes, plasma cells, and debris-laden histiocytes.

Pancreatic duct obstruction often leads to fibrosis and cyst formation *(pancreatic cyst,* dilated duct). Few sheets of fibroblasts and clusters of slightly atypical ductal cells are present in the aspiration.

(b) ***Malignant lesions***

Most pancreatic adenocarcinomas are of ductal type. The malignant cells may have a columnar or cuboidal shape with rounded or ovoid nuclei. The degree of pleomorphism depends on the degree of differentiation of tumour.

Kidney

1. **Benign lesions**

Aspirated fluid of *renal cyst* for inflammatory cells, histiocytes and scanty flattened epithelial cells.

2. **Malignant lesions**

(a) ***Renal carcinoma* (hypernephroma)**

Cluster of cells with small nuclei and large, abundant, pale blue vesicular cytoplasm are seen in aspirated fluid smear.

(b) ***Wilms' tumour* (nephroblastoma)**

Smear shows numerous small cells, single and in tight clusters. The cells have round or ovoid, hyperchromatic nuclei. Tubular structures, palisades or cords (epithelial cells) and cluster of spindle cells (mesenchymal cells) are found.

Retroperitoneal tumours

Liposarcoma, leiomyosarcoma and malignant fibrous histiocytomas are common malignant tumours of retroperitoneum, criteria for their diagnosis has not yet been clearly defined.

Adrenal glands

Phaeochromocytoma is diagnosed by the presence of loose cluster of larger cells with abundant, granular cytoplasm and central round to oval nuclei with coarse, but uniform chromatin pattern.

MISCELLANEOUS USE

Virtually any organ of the body can be aspirated (prostate, ovaries, eyes, nervous system and so on).

Section V

CLINICAL PATHOLOGY

Section V contains

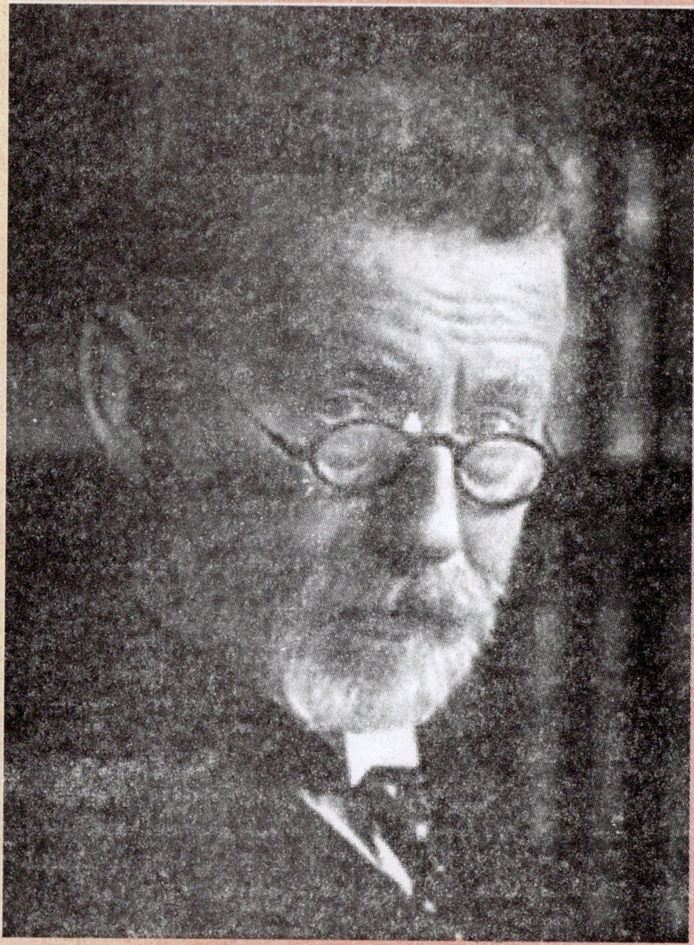

Paul Ehrlich (1884–1915)

Immunologist and Clinical Pathologist — *He was a German Physician and pioneer in different branches of pathology, haematology, and bacteriology. He is a winner of Nobel Prize for his work in immunology. He described Ehrlich's test for urobilinogen, staining techniques of cells and bacteria, and laid the foundations of haematology.*

Chapter 40

Examination of Urine

URINE REPORT OF NORMAL ADULT		
Physical examination		
Quantity	:	1,200–1,800 ml/24-hour sample
Odour	:	Faint aromatic odour
Colour	:	Amber yellow or pale yellow
Appearance	:	Clear, but may be cloudy due to phosphates
Sediment	:	Nil, but amorphous phosphates and urates may cause sedimentation
Specific gravity	:	1.001–1.035, estimated by 'Urinometer'.
Chemical examination		
Reaction	:	pH 6.0 to 6.8 (acidic)
Albumin	:	Nil or faint trace amount (< 150 mg/day)
Qualitative tests	:	Heat and acetic acid test, sulphosalicylic acid test, Heller's nitric acid test
Quantitative test	:	Esbach's test (Esbach's albuminometer)
Reducing substances	:	Nil, tested by glucose oxidase strips; Benedict's / Fehling's solution (50-300 mg/day)
Bile salt	:	Nil, detected by Hay's sulphur test
Bile pigment	:	Nil, tested by Fouchet's test
Excess of phosphates	:	Nil or traces; dissolved by dil. acetic acid
Bence-Jones protein	:	Absent, Heat test; Immunoelectrophoresis
Ketone bodies	:	Nil, tested by Ketostrip / Rothera's test
Urobilinogen	:	0.5–2.5 mg / 24 hr; Ehrlich's aldehyde test.
Microscopical examination (Fresh sample) (15 ml urine centrifuged for 5 minutes at 2,000 rpm)		
Unorganised deposits	:	Urates, uric acid, calcium oxalates normally present in acid urine, and phosphates and biurates in alkaline urine.
Abnormal constituents	:	Leucine, tyrosine, sulpha crystals.
Organised constituents	:	Occasionally hyaline casts seen in normal urine.
Abnormal constituents	:	Granular, cellular, fatty and waxy casts.
Epithelial cell	:	Squamous epithelium — 2 to 3/HPF in male, 8 to 10/HPF in female in normal urine.
Pus cell	:	May occur in normal urine, usually 0–2 but less than 5/HPF
RBCs	:	Occasional (0–2/HPF)
Microorganisms	:	Nil.

Examination of urine reflects the state of function of kidneys and urinary tract. Functions of kidney are described in chapter 47 (Renal function tests). Routine examination of urine is divided into four parts :

A. Adequacy of specimen

B. Physical/gross examination

C. Chemical examination

D. Microscopic examination.

Collection of urine (for routine and culture)

1. Clean-catch fresh mid-stream specimen collected at any time of the day, after proper cleansing of the glans penis in the male or vulva in the female, is suitable. However, morning sample is preferable because the early **morning sample** of urine is concentrated.

2. Container should be clean and dry for routine examination and sterile for cultural examiation.

Preservation of urine

The sample should be examined within 1–2 hours after voiding. If delay is anticipated, the specimen is best preserved when refrigerated at an acid pH (about 6.0) without any preservative.

Chemical preservatives used for urine collections usually prevent decomposition and contamination by bacteria and fungi. *Toluene* is an all-round good preservative which is to be added in sufficient quantity to form a thin layer on the surface of urine. However, the chemical interferes with protein examinations of urine by sulphosalicylic method.

1. **Boric acid (1%)** : Preservative for many hormones and other substances, 1 gm is added to 100 ml urine.

2. **Conc. HCl** : 10 ml per 24 hours sample (i.e., 1 ml in 150 ml urine).

3. **Formalin or chloroform** : It preserves cells and casts well, used in a proportion of 1 drop per 15 ml urine.

4. **Sodium fluoride** : It is useful for glucose test as it prevents glycolysis and is used in a concentration of 5 mg per 100 ml urine.

24-hour urine sample : After discarding the first morning sample of urine, all subsequent samples are collected in a clean/sterile bottle of 1.5-2 litre capacity. The last sample includes the morning sample of the following day. The total volume of urine is measured by a measuring cylinder and tests like quantitative analysis of proteins in nephrotic syndrome and VMA in phaeo-chromocytoma and other tests can be done.

PHYSICAL EXAMINATION

A. Volume

Normal range of 24 hours urine in adult is 1200 to 1800 ml. In infants, the volume of urine is 300-600 ml/day. Volume is measured by collecting 24-hour urine samples in a clean preferably sterile container and then measured by a measuring cylinder.

(i) *Polyuria* refers to increased quantity of urine (more than 2000 ml/24 hours).

(ii) *Oliguria* is the decreased quantity of urine (less than 500 ml/24 hours). Both polyuria and oliguria may be physiological depending on intake of quantity of fluid or on weather; both may also occur in certain diseases of kidney.

(iii) *Anuria* is complete absence of urine formation and always denotes disease.

Causes of polyuria

(i) Diabetes insipidus

(ii) Diabetes mellitus

(iii) Chronic glomerulonephritis

(iv) Chronic pyelonephritis

(v) Benign nephrosclerosis

(vi) Addison's disease

(vii) Hyperparathyroidism.

Causes of oliguria

(i) Acute glomerulonephritis

(ii) State of shock with renal ischaemia

(iii) Severe dehydration

(iv) Bilateral hydronephrosis

(v) Toxic or ischaemic nephrosis.

B. Odour

Normal fresh urine has a faint *aromatic* odour.

(i) *Pungent* : It gives a strong ammonical odour when allowed to stand due to decomposition of urea to ammonia (normal).

(ii) *Fruity* : Presence of ketone bodies produces fruity odour (diabetes mellitus).

(iii) *Putrid* : UTI due to *Proteus* spp., produces rotten fish smell.

(iv) *Mousy* : Mousy smell in phenylketonuria.

C. Colour

Normal urine is amber yellow or pale yellow in colour largely due to the pigment *urochrome* and to small amounts of *urobilins*. Certain foods and drugs also produce colour in urine. Some of the examples of a pathological change in colour of urine are described below :

(i) *Reddish brown* : Increased urobilinogen or porphyrins.

(ii) *Deep yellow / yellow green* : Bile pigments (bilirubin, biliverdin).

(iii) *Pink* : A small amount of fresh blood.

(iv) *Bright red* : Large amount of fresh blood.

(v) *Milky white* : Chyluria due to filaria, pyuria with many neutrophils.

D. Appearance

Fresh urine is normally clear but may be *cloudy* due to presence of :

(a) *Amorphous phosphates* in alkaline or neutral urine that disappears on addition of dilute acetic acid.

(b) *Amorphous* urates in acid urine disappearing on heating.

(c) *Cloudy urine* — Some of the diseases producing cloudy urine include :

(i) Turbidity caused by presence of pus (*pyuria*) which clears on centrifugation or filtration;

(ii) Fat or chyle in urine which cannot be got rid off by filtration/ centrifugation.

E. Specific gravity (sp. gr.)

Normal adults produce a urine of sp.gr. 1015 to 1026 in a 24-hour urine (sp. gr. of distilled water 1000). Substances that influence sp. gr. of urine are urea, mucous and phosphates, and abnormally due to albumin and sugar.

(a) *Low specific gravity (less than 1007). Kidney disease (hyposthenuria).*

(b) *Low fixed specific gravity* : It is observed in end stage kidney, chronic renal failure, due to loss of concentration power of kindey. (At 1010) : Isosthenuria.

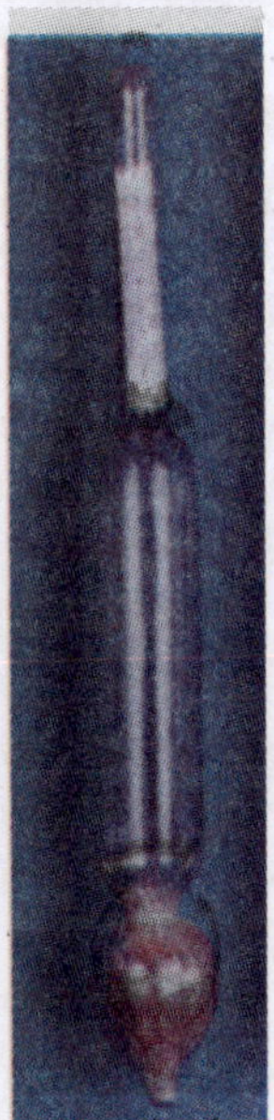

Fig.40.1A. Urinometer for testing specific gravity of urine

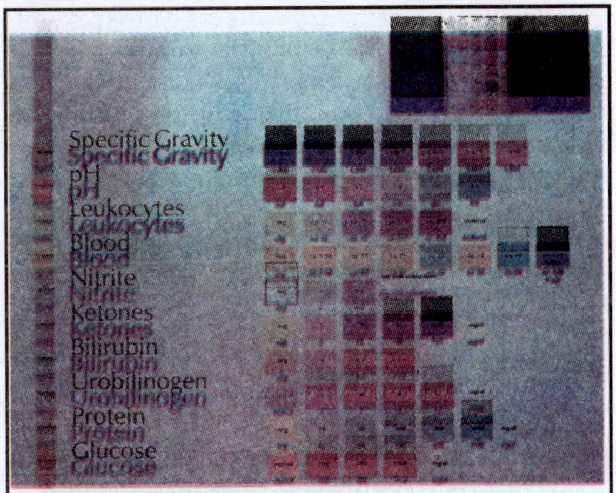

Fig. 40.1B. Dipstick (multistix) for 10 parameters

Determination of Sp. Gr.

It can be done by :

- Urinometer
- Refractometer
- Dipstick method

Urinometer (Fig. 40.1A) : It is a hydrometer adapted to measure the sp. gr. of urine at room temperature. Urinometer vessel (glass cylinder) is filled three-fourths full with urine. Then the urinometer is gently floated in the urine so that it does not touch the sides or bottom of the cylinder. The bottom of the meniscus is read. Some correction of the reading is made based on temperature and albumin present in urine.

Refractometer : The test measures refractive index of urine and requires only a few drops of urine but it should be clear.

Procedure : A few drops of urine is placed on glass surface of the refractometer and looked through the meter towards the light source. Now S.G. of urine is recorded.

Dipstick method (Fig. 40.1B) : Commercially available chemical reagent strip is dipped in urine. The strip area contains polyelectrolyte and indicator bromothymol blue.

Reading : SG is recorded by change of colour on the strip and the same is compared with the colour chart on the multidisc bottle.

Principle : Colour changes result from displacement of H^+ by Na^+/K^+ ion. Na^+/K^+ ion concentration is higher than H^+ in the concentrated urine with a high SG.

Increased specific gravity of urine is observed in dehydration, diarrhoea, restricted fluid intake,vomiting, fever, excessive sweating, diabetes mellitus, albuminuria and acute glomerulonephritis.

Decreased specific gravity of urine is observed in excessive fluid intake, diabetes insipidus and **end stage kidney disease** — chronic glomerulonephritis, other renal diseases such as bilateral polycystic kidneys, chronic pyelonephritis and hypertension when concentration power of kidney is severally reduced to a low and fixed specific gravity of 1.008-1.010.

Urine Concentration Test : This test is useful in detecting the ability of kidneys to concentrate urine.

Procedure :

(1) The patient gets an early dinner at 6 p.m. and no food or water is given after 7 p.m.
(2) The urine samples voided during the night is discarded.
(3) The first morning sample voided at 7 a.m. is discarded and bladder is emptied completely.
(4) A second specimen of urine is collected at 8 a.m. i.e., 14 hours of deprivation of water.
(5) The S.G. of this sample collected at 8 a.m. checked; S.G. of which should be > 1.022.
(6) When the S.G. of the sample is less than 1.022, another (second) sample is collected at 9 a.m.
(7) When S.G. of this sample is less than 1.022 concentrating ability of kidney is decreased.

Interpretation :

(1) When S.G. is < 1.022, concentrating ability of kidney is impaired.
(2) Normal value : 1.001–1.035.
(3) When S.G. is **low** and **fixed** at 1.010, it signifies total loss of concentrating power of kidney.

Note : The test is contraindicated in uraemia (vide ch. 46, p. 414).

CHEMICAL EXAMINATION

Common chemical substances of urine that are examined routinely include *protein* (albumin), *sugar blood, ketone bodies* and *bile pigments; tests* for other chemical substances, such as *urobilinogen, porphyrins, Bence-Jones protein,* etc. are also required to be done. Commercial reagent strips and multiple reagents strips are now widely used for mass screening which have got some limitations because of interference problems. The standard chemical tests are still preferred by many laboratories.

A. Reaction

In normal health, pH of urine varies from 6 to 6.8. The pH of urine of vegetarians are usually higher than 6.2. The reaction of urine becomes less acidic after meal which is called *alkaline tide*. The reaction of urine is somewhat altered in urinary tract infection, such as highly acidic in *E. coli* infection and alkaline in *Proteus* spp. infection. The pH of urine is increased in metabolic acidosis and decreased in alkalosis. A rough estimate of pH is made by indicator paper, blue litmus or wide range indicator paper.

1. *Reagent strip* : Litmus paper indicates whether the urine is acidic or alkaline. But by the use of pH indicator paper, pH of urine is determined. The strip is dipped in urine and colour produced is compared with a standard chart.

2. *By the use of pH meter* than gives exact pH of sample of urine.

B. Protein

About 20 mg of protein (albumin) is normally excreted in 24-hour urine which is not usually detected by routine test. The testing of urine for proteins — of which albumin is the chief — is one of the commonest laboratory tests. Detection of an abnormal amount of protein in urine is a reliable indicator of renal disease.

Nature of proteins

The following types of chief proteins may be present in urine :

(i) *Serum or plasma albumin* : Commonest urinary protein, hence the term albuminuria is used (*proteinuria* is a more scientific term).
(ii) *Serum or plasma globulin* : This is usually found together with serum albumin in urine. These two proteins constitute what is usually known as urinary albumin. When equal volumes of urine and saturated solution of ammonium sulphate are mixed, globulin gets precipitated.
(iii) *Mucus or mucin* may be present in traces. It is precipitated by dilute (10%) acetic acid without heating.

(iv) *Haemoglobin* appears in urine only after haemolysis of red cells.

(v) *Bence-Jones protein* is found in plasma cell myeloma.

Qualitative tests for protein

When urine is alkaline, it is made acidic because phosphates get precipitated in alkaline urine but in acidic urine the proteins get precipitated readily either by heat test or by other chemical test.

(a) **Heat and acetic acid test** : The urine should be acidic; a few drops of 3% acetic acid is added to an alkaline urine to make it slightly acidic. Urine should be clear, turbid urine is centrifuged in tube first and then supernatant portion is taken out for examination.

Technique :

Take urine in a clean test tube filling two-third portion and boil upper half inch (1.25 cm) or inch (2.5 cm) of the column of urine holding at the bottom. A white cloud appears in the heated portion if proteins or phosphates are present. Add two to three drops of 3% glacial acetic acid. If the cloudiness disappears, it is due to phosphates; if it persists, it is *albumin*.

If the cloudiness appears while the tube is heated and disappears at boiling point, it may be *Bence-Jones* protein. Both albumin and BJ proteins are present in multiple myeloma.

Recording results (approx. protein conc. in %)

(i) Negative	: No cloudiness
(ii) Trace	: Barely visible cloudiness
(iii) 1 + (< 0.10%)	: Definite cloud without granular flocculation.
(iv) 2 + (0.10-0.25%)	: Heavy and granular cloud without flocculation.
(v) 3 + (0.25-0.50%)	: Dense cloud with flocculation.
(vi) 4 + (> 0.5%)	: Thick, curdy precipitate and coagulation.

(b) **Sulphosalicylic acid test** : Specimens are to be centrifuged and clear supernatant is used.

Technique : Take 2 ml of clear urine in a test tube and add equal volume of 3% sulphosalicylic acid solution. Invert to mix and let stand for 10 minutes.

Recording result : Almost similar as in heat test, but the test in addition gives an idea of amount of protein present in the sample. Thus, trace amount suggests less than 0.01 gm%, 1 plus = 0.01 to 0.05 gm%, 2 plus = 0.05 to 0.2 gm%, 3 plus = 0.2 to 0.5 gm% and 4 plus = more than 0.5 gm%.

(c) **Heller's nitric acid test** : Take 1 ml concentrated (fuming) nitric acid in a test tube and add 2 ml of urine by means of a pipette by the side of the test tube and layer on top of the acid. A whitish ring of precipitate forms at the junction of the two fluids due to formation of metaprotein when albumin is present.

(d) **Dipstick method** : Sensitive strip tests are now commercially available that can detect a minute amount (a few mg) of albumin in urine. This method is useful in detecting causes of early kidney disease such as diabetes mellitus.

Testing : When the medicated strip is dipped in urine there is a development of colour of the strip which is compared with the colour chart for proteins provided on the container.

Advantage : It can detect as low as 20 mg% of albumin in urine. Thus by medicated strips presence of very little amount (a few mg) of albumin (known as microuria) can be detected (Fig. 40.1B).

Quantitative estimation of albumin

Sometimes it becomes necessary to quantitatively analyse the amount of protein lost in 24-hour urine which provides useful information for diagnosis of kidney disease.

Esbach's method

Esbach's (1874) method of protein precipitation in which picric acid is used to precipitate the protein and the amount of protein precipitate is measured by volume. However, it is not a very accurate method.

Materials

(i) *Esbach's albuminometer* (Fig. 40.2) : It is a thick-walled glass tube graduated in grams of dried albumin per 1000 ml of urine. There is a mark "R" above and "U" near the middle.

(ii) *Esbach's reagent* :

Picric acid – 10 gm (precipitates albumin)

Citric acid – 20 gm (disssolves phosphates)

Distilled water to – 1,000 ml.

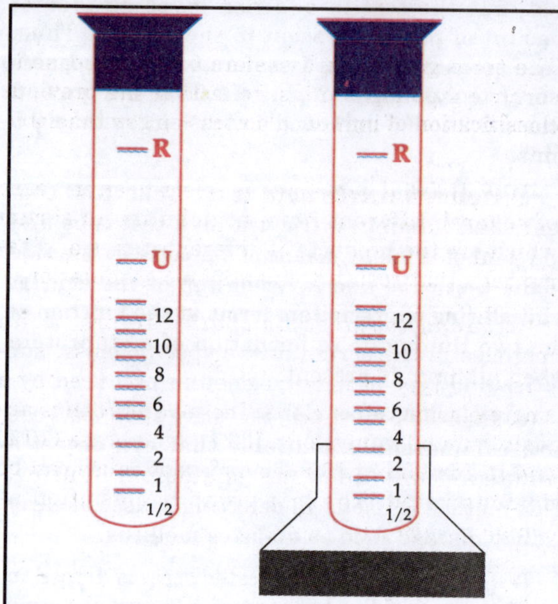

Fig. 40.2. Esbach's albuminometer

(iii) 24 *hour urine sample* : Urine is rendered clear by filtering and acidifying with 10% acetic acid. If the sp. gr. of urine exceeds 1025, it should be diluted 1 : 2 or 1 : 4, otherwise albumin precipitate will float.

Method

(i) The albuminometer is filled with filtered acidified urine of correct specificity up to the mark 'U'.

(ii) Esbach's reagent is added up to the mark 'R' and mixed well.

(iii) The tube is corked and kept vertically in the stand for 24 hours.

Recording result : The level of precipitate is measured against the graduation on the tube. The reading at the level of precipitation in the albuminometer tube is given in gm per litre. The result should be divided by 10 to get gm %. If the urine has been diluted, multiply the result by dilution factor.

Thus, 24 hours urine excretion

$\frac{x \text{ gm}}{10}$ % when urine is diluted, multiply the result by dilution factor.

Normal value = 100 to 150 mg / 24 hours.

Albuminuria

I. **Asymptomatic (functional)**

(a) Exercise induced

(b) Orthostatic, albuminuria when the individual in upright position.

(c) Pregnancy

II. **Massive proteinuria (> 3 g/day)**

(a) *Post-streptococcal glomerulonephritis*

(b) *Nephrotic syndrome*

Glomerular lesions associated with nephrotic syndrome :

(i) *Primary-renal disease*

Minimal change glomerulonephritis

Membranous glomerulonephritis

Membranous proliferative glomerulonephritis.

Focal glomerulonephritis

(ii) *Associated with systemic diseases*

Systemic lupus erythematosus

Amyloid nephrosis

Diabetic nephrosis

Rheumatoid nephrosis

Polyarteritis

III. **Moderate proteinuria (1–3 g/day)**

(a) Chronic glomerulonephritis

(b) Nephrosclerosis (c) Multiple myeloma

(d) Pyelonephritis

IV. **Mild proteinuria (< 1.0 g/day)**

(a) Hypertension (b) Polycystic kidney

(c) Chronic pyelonephritis (d) UTI (e) Fever

Nephrotic syndrome

It is a clinical syndrome complex characterised by massive proteinuria, hypoproteinaemia, lipidaemia (hypercholesterolaemia) generalised oedema and lipiduria. The list of diseases that produce nephrotic syndrome includes virtually every disorder that affects glomerulus resulting in increased glomerular membrane permeability evidenced by albuminuria. Some important causes are mentioned above.

Bence-Jones proteinuria

Bence-Jones proteins represent either the *kappa* or *lambda* light chains of immunoglobulins. About 70% of patients with multiple myeloma and other proteinaemias excrete light chains of immunoglobulin in their urine.

Tests for B-J protein in urine

It is best identified by immunoelectrophoresis of urine and blood. However, the protein can also be detected in urine by chemical method. Strip test is also done.

(a) *Heat test* : A volume of 5 ml urine is taken in a test tube with a thermometer inside. A white coagulum of B-J protein develops on heating at 56°C (40-60°C) and redissolved on heating above 90°C (90-100°C). On cooling again, the precipitate reappears at 40-60°C.

(b) *Protein electrophoresis* : A homogeneous band of Bence-Jones protein is formed on electrophoresis of urine/blood. This is followed by immune electrophoresis for identification of light chain. Urine is to be concentrated before electrophoretic study.

Cause of B-J proteinuria

(i) Multiple myeloma,

(ii) Malignant lymphoma,

(iii) Chronic myeloid leukaemia,

(iv) Osteosarcoma,

(v) Osteomalacia,

(vi) Generalised carcinomatosis.

Plasma cell tumours

Plasma cell neoplasms comprise of a group of disorders in which there is a neoplastic proliferation of plasma cells resulting in :

(a) multiple nodules of tumour deposits in the bone marrow *(multiple myeloma);*

(b) a single tumour mass, which is most frequently extra-medullary *(plasmacytoma);* or

(c) diffuse infiltration of bone marrow, lymph nodes and spleen (*Waldenstrom's macroglobulinaemia* and other syndromes).

Plasma cells are derived from B cells and secrete immunoglobulins. Proliferation of a single clone of plasma cells occur in myeloma which produce a monoclonal immunoglobulin of a single class, IgG is the commonest (50%), followed by IgA and IgM; IgD and IgE are rare. These patients have increased serum globulins. In each of these groups of myeloma, some patients secrete light chains, *kappa* or *lambda* (Bence-Jones protein) in addition to whole immunoglobulin molecule, which are excreted in the urine because of their low molecular weight (25 KDa).

Gammopathy

The term gammopathy refers to an increase in serum immunoglobulins, reflecting the previous classification of immunoglobulins as gammaglobulins.

(i) *Polyclonal gammopathy* refers to an increase of several different immunoglobulins in serum which are the products of different clones of plasma cells that result from antigenic stimulation.

(ii) *Monoclonal gammopathy* refers to an increase in the serum of one specific class, subclass and type of immunoglobulin produced by a single plasma cell or clone. These *paraproteins* are mainly found in myeloma (80%), lymphoma (10%) and in remaining 10%, no apparent cause can be demonstrated. The last group is classified as *benign gammopathy*.

C. Sugar tests

Reducing substances are those compounds which on reaction with cupric oxide of Benedict's reagent reduce cupric oxide to cuprous oxide. These include :

Sugars : Glucose, fructose, pentose, lactose, galactose and L-xylulose.

Non-sugars : Uric acid, urates, creatinine, glucoronides, salicylates, phenol, PAS, ascorbic acid.

Glucose and other reducing substances in urine are detected by :

(a) *Copper reduction tests* : (i) Fehling's test, (ii) Benedict's test.

(b) *Reagent strip or enzymatic test* : Glucose oxidase reagent strip test (glucostix or clinistix) — reliable method. The test-end of the strip is dipped into the specimen and kept for 10 to 30 seconds and then taken out. Excess of urine is drained out. The colour of the reagent area of the strip is compared with the colour chart supplied by the manufacturer. The result is reported as indicated on the chart.

(c) *Osazone test* : There forms glucose osazone crystal which is identified under the microscope.

Glucose oxidase reagent strips are widely used in busy clinics

Principle : Glucose reagent strip (diastix/multistix/dipstix) contains : (i) glucose oxidase, (ii) peroxidase, (iii) chromogen-o-toluidine and potassium iodide. Following reaction occurs when glucose is present in urine :

(a) Glucose + H_2O + O_2 $\xrightarrow[\text{oxidase}]{\text{Glucose}}$
(urine) (atmospheric)
= gluconic acid + H_2O_2

(b) H_2O_2 + chromogen $\xrightarrow{\text{Peroxidase}}$
(colourless in reduced state)
= H_2O + Oxidised chromogen
(coloured substance)

Enzymatic tests **specifically** detect glucose. However, *Benedict's* and *Fehling's tests* are commonly done in many laboratories. Some non-glucose sugars such as fructose, lactose, galactose, L-xylulose and non-carbohydrates, e.g., uric acid, creatinine, salicylic acid and homogentisic acid cause positive copper reduction tests in urine while the glucose oxidase test is negative. The examination of urine for sugar is primarily done for detection of diabetes mellitus.

Causes of glycosuria : Appearance of glucose in urine is called glucosuria or glycosuria.

(a) **Due to hyperglycaemia** :

(i) Diabetes mellitus; (ii) Hyperpituitarism; (iii) Hyperthyroidism; (iv) Cushing's syndrome; (v) Intracranial injury; (vi) Functioning alpha and beta cell pancreatic tumours.

(b) **Other causes** :

(i) Renal glycosuria; (ii) Alimentary glycosuria; (iii) Fanconi syndrome.

Qualitative tests for sugar in urine

(a) **Benedict's test (Benedict, 1909)**

Take 5 ml Benedict's qualitative reagent in a test tube (150 × 18 mm) and boil for a minute. Then add 0.5 ml (8 drops) urine drop by drop and boil 2–4 minutes and cool.

Result :

(i) Negative	:	No change in colour
(ii) Trace	:	Pale green with slide cloudiness (0.5 g%)
(iii) 1 +	:	Green deposit (1.0 g%)
(iv) 2 +	:	Yellow deposit (1–1.5 g%)
(v) 3 +	:	Orange to red precipitate (1.5–2.0 g%)
(vi) 4 +	:	Brick red precipitate (> 2 g%)

Composition of reagent :

(Benedict's qualitative reagent)

Cupric sulphate	17.3 gm
Sodium carbonate (anhydrous)	100 gm
Sodium citrate	173 gm
Distilled water to	1000 ml

Dissolve with heat, 173 gm sodium citrate and 100 gm anhydrous sodium carbonate in about 600 ml water in a beaker. Then run slowly by constant stirring, about 100 ml of copper sulphate solution containing 17.3 gm $CuSO_4, 5H_2O$. The solution is cooled and made to a litre with water.

Principle : Sodium carbonate and sodium citrate ionise forming strong alkali ions (Na^+ OH^-) and weak acid ions (H^+ and citrate). Copper sulphate reacts with reducing substances converting cupric sulphate into insoluble cuprous oxide of yellow or red colour.

$$Cu^{++} \xrightarrow{\text{hot alkaline solution}} Cu^{+}$$
$$Cu^{+} + OH \longrightarrow CuOH\ (\text{yellow})$$
$$2\ CuOH \xrightarrow{\text{heat}} Cu_2O\ (\text{red}) + H_2O$$

(b) **Fehling's test**

Fehling's reagent

Solution A	Solution B
Copper sulphate – 34.65 gm	Sodium hydroxide – 125 gm
Distilled water – 500 ml	Sodium pot. tartarate – 173 gm
	Dist. water – 500 ml

Test : Take equal volumes (2.5 ml) each of Fehling's solution A and solution B in a test tube, mix and boil. Add 0.5 ml (8 drops) of urine and boil again for 3-5 minutes. When sugar is present, the Fehling's solution shows same type of colour changes as in the Benedict's test.

Quantitative test for sugar

Benedict's test : *Reagent* (quantitative)

Anhydrous Sod. carbonate	100 gm
Sod. or Pot. citrate	200 gm
Pot. thiocyanate	125 gm
Copper sulphate	18 gm
5% Potassium ferrocyanide	5 ml
Distilled water to	1,000 ml

Method

The urine is first tested by Benedict's qualitative reagent. If it is strongly positive, urine is diluted to 1 in 10. If it is weakly positive, then undiluted urine is used. Take 25 ml Benedict's quantitative reagent in a conical flask and add 15 gm of crystalline sod. carbonate and boil. Add sample of urine drop by drop from a graduated burette till a chalky white precipitate develops with complete disappearance of blue colour. It indicates end point.

Calculation : 25 ml Benedict's reagent requires 0.05 gm of sugar for reduction.

Let 15 ml (1 : 10 dil) urine required for reduction. Hence, 15 ml (x) urine contains = 0.05 gm × dilution factor.

∴ 100 ml urine contains

$$= \frac{0.05}{15} \times 10 \times 100 \text{ gm}$$

= 3.33 gm glucose

$$\text{or, } \frac{0.05}{X} \times 100 \times \text{dilution factor gm \%}$$

Normal findings

Qualitative test for glucose is negative. Normally, an amount of 50–300 mg is excreted in urine in 24 hours and such minute quantity is not detected in qualitative test.

False positive results

Apart from glucose, other substances reducing Benedict's reagent belong to two categories :

(a) *Carbohydrates* : Fructose, Lactose, Galactose and L-xylulose.

(b) *Non-carbohydrates* : Uric acid and creatinine, salicylic acid, homogentisic acid and melanogen.

Lactose may appear in urine late in normal pregnancy or during lactation; fructose during parenteral feeding with fructose; galactose as inherited enzyme deficiencies and sucrose after ingestion of sugar cane. Similarly, non-carbohydrate substances appear in various clinical states. Elaborate test procedure are necessary for their identification. In such cases, if urine is tested with glucose oxidase reagent strip, the test will be negative for non-glucose substances.

D. Ketone bodies in urine (Ketonuria)

Ketone bodies are the intermediate products for fat metabolism which comprise of *acetoacetic acid, acetone* and *β-hydroxybutyric acid*.

Ketosis (keto-acidosis) is the consequence of the increased metabolism of fat in the diabetics and in a few other conditions resulting in accumulation of ketone bodies in blood and their excretion in urine (ketonuria). In addition to ketosis of diabetes, ketosis in starvation arises in the same way. Unless adequate glucose is available, the liver is forced to use an increased amount of fat producing excess quantities of fatty acids that are too great for the tissues to metabolise.

$$\text{Acetoacetic acid} \xrightarrow{-CO_2} \text{Acetone}$$

$$\text{Acetoacetic acid} \underset{-\,2H}{\overset{+\,2H}{\rightleftharpoons}} \text{Beta hydroxybutyric acid}$$

When urine is left at room temperature, acetoacetic acid slowly converts into acetone.

Causes of ketonuria

(i) Uncontrolled diabetes mellitus.

(ii) Chronic starvation.

(iii) Pregnancy toxaemia with vomiting.

(iv) Clinical condition with severe vomiting and toxaemia.

(v) Glycogen storage disease.

Tests for Ketone bodies

(a) **Dipstick tests** : Ketostix, acetotest and other commercial plastic strips with one end impregnated with a buffered mixture of sodium nitroprusside and glycine are now widely used. The strip is dipped into a fresh urine, serum or plasma and removed immediately, then compared with the colour chart of manufacturer. They detect both acetoacetic acid and acetone. The dip strip method is based on Rothera's test.

(b) **Rothera's test** : It is highly sensitive for both acetoacetic acid and acetone and is routinely done in many laboratories.

Principle : Acetoacetic acid and acetone produce a purple coloured complex with sodium nitroprusside in an alkaline environment.

Procedure

1. Take about 5 ml urine in a test tube and saturate with ammonium sulphate and add a crystal (or about 0.5 ml of 20% aqueous solution) of sodium nitroprusside. If a solid crystal of sodium nitroprusside has been addeed, shake the tube and allow to stand for about 10 minutes till it dissolves.

2. About 2 to 3 ml concentrated ammonia (liquor ammonia) is carefully poured down the side of the tube so that it forms a layer on the top of saturated urine.

Result : Presence acetoacetic acid and acetone is indicated by formation of a purple colour ring at the junction.

(c) **Gerhardt's test** : The test is not very sensitive.

Procedure :

(1) Take 5 ml of urine in a test tube.

(2) Add 10% ferric chloride solution drop by drop till a precipitate occurs.

(3) Filter it.

(4) Add excess of $FeCl_2$ solution to the filtrate.

Finding :

A red colour indicates presence of ketone bodies.

Detection of β-hydroxybutyric acid

There is no test in every day routine use. However, the three ketone bodies almost always occur together. For detection, if desired, it has to be oxidised by adding H_2O_2 to acetoacetic acid.

Add 2-3 drops of acetic acid to 5-6 ml 1 : 10 diluted urine. Boil for 3-4 minutes to drive away acetone and acetoacetic acid present in urine. Then add 1 ml of hydrogen peroxide, warm gently, cool and perform Rothera's test.

E. Bile derivatives in urine

Of the three bile derivatives—urobilinogen, bile salts and bile pigment, only urobilinogen is normally excreted in the urine in small amounts, but bile salts and bile pigments appear in urine in liver diseases only.

Unconjugated bilirubin of blood cannot pass through the glomerulus in urine, but conjugated bilirubin (water soluble) is liable to pass through glomerulus in urine.

I. Tests for bilirubin (bile pigment)

(a) Fouchet's test

Principle : Bilirubin is initially concentrated on insoluble barium salts by absorption. It is then oxidised to a greenish blue product by adding Fouchet's reagent.

Reagents :

(i) 10% barium chloride solution.

(ii) Fouchet's reagent

Trichloroacetic acid	25 gm
Distilled water	100 ml
10% $FeCl_2$	10 ml

Dissolve 25 gm trichloroacetic acid in 50 ml distilled water, and add 10 ml ferric chloride solution (10%) and make to 100 ml with water.

Test :

1. Take 10 ml of urine in a test tube and add 2-5 ml of 10% barium chloride, mix, allow to stand for a few minutes and filter.

2. Unfold the filter paper and spread it on another dry paper. Add a drop or two of Fouchet's reagent on the precipitate.

Alternatively, the urine and barium chloride mixture is centrifuged for 5 min at 2000 RPM. The supernatant is thrown out. Add a drop or two of Fouchet's reagent on the deposit.

Result : A greenish blue colour indicates the presence of bilirubin. The intensity of colour depends on the amount of bile pigment present in urine.

Fouchet's test can also be done by a filter paper strip soaked in saturated solution of barium chloride and then dried.

(b) **Gmelin's test**

In this test, slightly yellow nitric acid is brought in contact with urine. Five ml of urine is filtered and then the filter paper is dried. Add a few drops of fuming nitric acid at the centre of the filter paper. A play of colourings develop, the most prominent being green — indicates the presence of bile pigment.

(c) **Reagent strip test**

Reagent strips of commercial houses are also available with different modifications. The test is based on a coupling reaction of bilirubin with diazolium salt. Dip the strip in urine. The strip changes to blue colour if bilirubin is present.

All these tests should be done with *fresh urine* as bilirubin is destroyed on standing, particularly when exposed to light. The chemical methods are most sensitive, while reagent strips have the advantage of convenience for tests performed outside the laboratory.

Interpretation

Normally bilirubin (bile pigment) is not passed in urine. Bilirubin is a breakdown product of haemoglobin. Bile pigment (bilirubin) in urine is an indicator of regurgitation of conjugated bilirubin which is water soluble and loosely attached to plasma albumin. The causes include :

(i) Extra-hepatic obstruction jaundice.

(ii) Hepatic jaundice caused by cholestasis.

II. Tests for bile salts in urine

There is only a trace of bile salt in normal urine. Bile salt (sod. taurocholate, sod. glycocholate) concentrations is increased in blood in obstruction of common bile duct and in drug-induced cholestasis which leads to excretion of considerable amount in urine.

(a) *Hay's sulphur test*

1. Take 10 ml urine in a test tube, or 50 to 100 ml urine in a beaker.

2. Sprinkle a pinch of finely divided flowers of sulphur on to the surface of urine cooled below 15°C.

Result : Bile salt reduces the surface tension so that the sulphur particles sink to the bottom of the test tube.

(b) *Strip method*

Commercially available reagent-coated strips can be used in detection of bile salt as for other constituents in urine.

III. Tests for urobilinogen in urine

Freshly voided urine should be examined for urobilinogen because urobilinogen in urine becomes converted into urobilin within short time when exposed to air.

(a) *Ehrlich's qualitative test*

Principle : Ehrlich's reagent, paradimethylaminobenzaldehyde in concentrated hydrochloric acid, reacts with urobilinogen and porphobilinogen to form aldehyde.

Ehrlich's aldehyde reagent

Paradimethylaminobenzaldehyde	–	2.0 gm
Concentrated hydrochloric acid	–	48 ml
Distilled water	–	50 ml

Dissolve the reagent in 48 ml HCl and then make to 100 ml with water.

When stored in brown bottle, it is stable for six months.

Method

1. Take 10 ml of freshly voided urine in a test tube and add 1 ml of Ehrlich's aldehyde reagent and mix well.

2. Allow to stand for 3 to 5 minutes and note any colour produced.

Result

1. Normal urine gives only a pink colour but a distinct red colour suggests the presence of increased amounts of urobilinogen. Urobilinogen has to be distinguished from porphobilinogen by differential extraction procedure (see below).

2. For a semiquantitive assessment of urobilinogen, repeat the test with 1:10, 1:20, 1:40, 1: 80, 1:160 dilutions of urine and report in terms of highest dilution showing a positive reaction. With normal urine, no pink colour usually appears at 1:20 dilution.

Interpretation :

(i) Normal adult urine contains 0.5 to 2.5 mg urobilinogen in 24 hours.

(ii) Urine urobilinogen is *increased* in haemolytic jaundice (e.g.,thalassaemia, sickle cell anaemia, hereditary spherocytosis) and in preicteric phase of infective hepatitis.

(iii) It is *absent* or *diminished* in extra-hepatic obstructive jaundice.

(iv) The amount is *variable* in hepato-cellular jaundice.

(v) In obstructive jaundice bilirubin cannot reach the intestine and hence is not converted into urobilinogen.

(b) *Reagent strip test*

Strips are coated with para-dimethyl-aminobenzaldehyde. When the dried strip is dipped in urine it turns reddish brown if urobilinogen is present in the sample.

F. Porphyrins in urine

Haemoglobin of blood is a conjugated protein in which haem is attached to the apoprotein globin. The haem molecule is made up of a porphyrin ring, in the centre of which there is an atom of iron (vide chapter 4).

Porphyrins are synthesised in the liver and bone marrow. The initial step is the formation of δ-aminolevulinic acid (ALA) by condensation of succinyl-coenzyme A with glycine (Fig. 40.3).

Porphyrias : The porphyrias mainly comprise of a group of inherited autosomal disorders characterised by aberrations in the activities of the

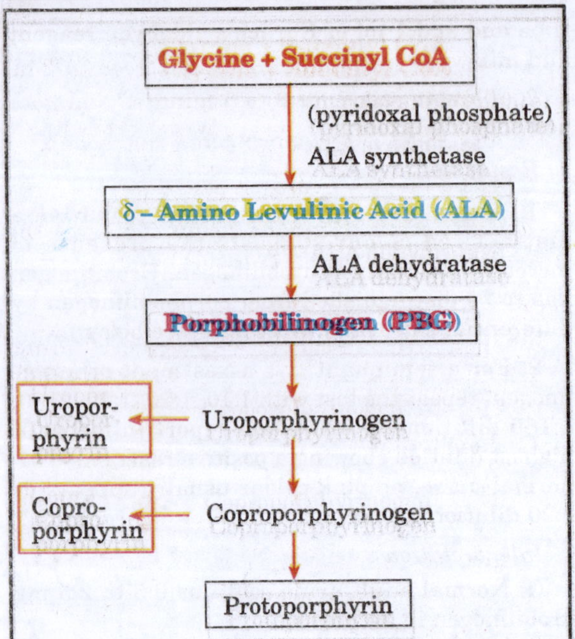

Fig. 40.3. Initial step in formation of ALA

specific enzymes of the haem biosynthetic pathway. The principal control lies at the level of ALA synthetase and decreased level of this enzyme leads to accumulation of ALA and PBG, while increased levels bring about excessive production of free porphyrins. The defective metabolism of porphyrin results in accumulation of the intermediate products in blood and excretion in urine.

Porphyrinuria : Porphyrins in the urine may be found in the form of δ-aminolevulinic acid (ALA), porphobilinogen, uroporphyrin or coproporphyrin. Diagnosis generally begins with screening tests for porphyrins or their precursors — ALA and PBG. PBG and uroporphyrins are mainly excreted in urine, while protoporphyrins are mainly excreted in the bile. Coproporphyrin is excreted in bile and also in urine.

Test for porphobilinogen in urine

(Ehrlich's differential extraction test)

Ehrlich's reagent

p-dimethyl-aminobenzaldehyde	..	2.0 gm
Concentrated hydrochloric acid	..	38 ml
Distilled water	..	50 ml

Test

1. Mix 5 ml of urine and 5 ml of Ehrlich's reagent in a test tube and mix well. Allow to stand for 3 minutes.

2. Add 5 ml of saturated aqueous solution of sodium acetate and shake well and leave for 3 minutes.

3. Development of pink colour indicates presence of either porphobilinogen or urobilinogen.

4. Add 3-4 ml of chloroform to one portion of coloured solution and shake thoroughly.

Result

(i) Pink colour formed by urobilinogen is extracted by chloroform.

(ii) So any red colour remaining in aqueous phase after addition of chloroform constitutes a positive test for porphobilinogen.

Types of porphyrias

About 80% of haem synthesis occurs in erythroid cells in bone marrow and 20% in liver.

(a) *Erythropoietic porphyrias*

(i) X-linked sideroblastic anaemia (deficiency of ALA synthetase).

(ii) Congenital erythropoietic purpura (deficiency of URO synthetase).

(iii) Erythropoietic protoporphyria (deficiency of ferrochelatase).

(b) *Hepatic porphyrias.*

(i) ALA dehydrogenase deficiency.

(ii) Acute intermittent porphyria (deficiency of HMB synthetase).

(iii) Hereditary coproporphyria (deficiency of coprooxidase).

(iv) Variegate porphyria (deficiency of protooxidase).

(v) Porphyria cutanea tarda (deficiency of urodecarboxylase).

G. Blood in urine

Normally an occasional red cell may be found on microscopic examination in urine except during menstruation when urine may get contaminated with menstrual blood.

Haematuria : Presence of abnormal number of red cells in urine is called *haematuria.*

Haemoglobinuria : Presence of haemoglobin or blood pigments in urine without any associated presence of RBCs is called *haemoglobinuria.* In haemoglobinuria, the colour of urine is dark brown because of conversion of Hb to acid haematin (in acidic urine). When the colour is very dark, it resembles a cola colour.

Both blood and haemoglobin show positive reactions to chemical tests. Because of the diagnostic importance of small amounts of haematuria, and the tendency of red cells to undergo lysis in urine, a screening test for haem is a useful adjunct to microscopical examination. Since haemoglobinuria is uncommon, a fresh sample of urine should be examined microscopically for presence of red cells. Haemoglobinuria can be detected by commercial Haemastrip test and by chemical tests.

Benzidine test was most commonly used for many years until it was realised that benzidine is carcinogenic and persons were warned to avoid handling or inhaling it. Then benzidine was replaced by orthotoluidine but the latter was also proved to be carcinogenic and warned to handle carefully. Other aromatic amine, orthodianisidine has been used in many laboratories in place of benzidine and orthotoluidine.

In general, methods of detection of occult blood rely on catalytic splitting of a peroxide (e.g., H_2O_2) by haemoglobin and its derivatives. The oxygen thus released oxidises a colourless substance to a coloured form.

(a) **Benzidine test**

Reagent :

A. Saturated solution of benzidine in glacial acetic acid.

B. Hydrogen peroxide (10 volumes per cent).

Method :

1. Mix equal parts of A and B in a test tube.
2. Take 4 ml urine in a test tube, and add 4 ml of the mixed reagent.

Result : Development of blue colour indicates presence of occult blood or haemoglobin. It is a very sensitive test.

(b) **Orthotoluidine test**

Principle : Glacial actic acid leads to lysis of red cells and haemoglobin is released by the lysed red cells. Orthotoluidine acts as chromogen.

H_2O_2 + Peroxidase (released from Hb) → H_2O + O

O + Benzidine (chromogen) → Blue colour

1. Pinch of orthotoluidine is dissolved in 2 ml glacial acetic acid in a test tube.
2. Add 10-15 drops of urine and shake well.
3. Add 4 ml 30% hydrogen peroxide.

Result : A greenish blue colour indicates the presence of haemoglobin or occult blood.

(c) **Reagent strip test**

Reagent strip is coated with orthotoluidine. When dipped in urine, it changes blue colour indicating presence of blood in the sample.

Orthotoluidine acts as chronogen.

Procedure :

1. Before the test, urine is thoroughly mixed so as to mix the sedimented RBCs.
2. Dipstick is dipped in urine for the time given.
3. Colour developed is matched.

Causes of haemoglobinuria :

1. Paroxysmal nocturnal haemoglobinuria (PNH)
2. Extensive burns
3. Marching haemoglobinuria
4. Cold haemoglobinuria
5. Autoimmune haemolytic anaemia
6. Blackwater fever
7. Snake venom poisoning
8. Mismatched blood transfusion
9. Gas gangrene
10. Drug sensitivity with quinine, sulphonamides.

Causes of haematuria :

(a) *Prerenal causes*

1. Acute febrile conditions

*2. Subacute bacterial endocarditis

*3. Malignant hypertension

*4. Blood dyscrasias, e.g., haemophilia, purpura, leukaemia

5. Anticoagulant therapy

6. Drug reaction with sulphonamide, salicylates.

(b) *Renal causes*

*1. Glomerulonephritis

2. Acute pyelonephritis

*3. Stone in kidney

*4. Tuberculosis of kidney

5. Hydronephrosis

*6. Papilloma pelvis

*7. Clear cell carcinoma kidney

8. Wilms' tumour

9. Renal vein thrombosis.

(c) *Post renal causes*

1. Haemorrhagic cystitis

2. Carcinoma prostate

3. Enlarged prostate

*4. Carcinoma bladder

5. Salpingitis.

Myoglobinuria : Presence of myoglobin in urine is called myoglobinuria. During acute destruction of muscle fibres (rhabdomyolysis), myoglobin is released in the blood which is rapidly excreted in the urine. It is a red brown pigment.

Detection : It can be detected by spectroscopic and electrophoretic study. It is difficult to distinguish haemoglobin from myoglobin.

H. 5-Hydroxy Indole Acetic Acid (5-HIAA)

Most patients with metastasising carcinoid tumour excrete a large amount of 5-HIAA. It is a metabolic derivative of 5-hydroxytryptamine (5-HT or serotonin) synthesised by the argentaffin cells of submucous coat of intestine. The 5-hydroxyindoles are formed from tryptophan as shown in Fig. 40.4.

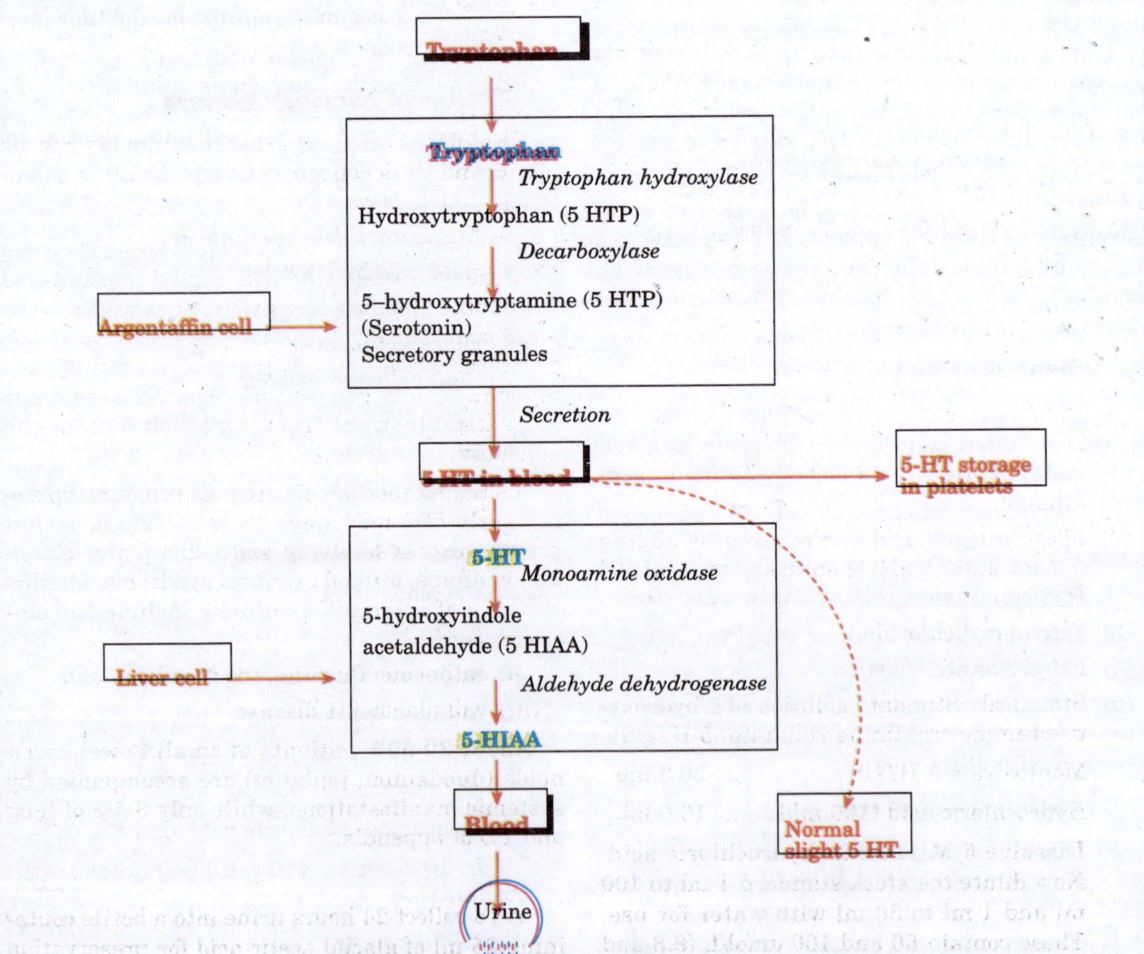

Fig. 40.4. Steps of formation of 5-Hydroxyindoles

Normal level

Less than 5 mg is passed in urine in 24 hours. In about 75% of patients, the level is highly increased in carcinoid syndrome, up to 350 mg / 24 hours.

Qualitative test

Reagent :

(1) 0.1%, 1-nitroso-2-naphthol solution in 95% ethanol.

(2) Fresh nitrous acid — Prepared by adding 0.2 ml 2.5% $NaNO_2$ solution to 5 ml 2N H_2SO_4.

(3) Ethylene dichloride.

Method :

(i) Take 0.2 ml urine in a test tube and add 0.8 ml distilled water and 0.5 ml 1-nitroso-2-naphthol solution and mix well.

(ii) Add 0.5 ml freshly prepared nitrous acid. Mix well and leave at room temperature for 10 minutes.

(iii) Add 5.0 ml ethylene dichloride. Shake well and allow to separate into two layers.

Result :

Note the colour of the upper aqueous layer :

(i) Normal urine : Not more than a faint pinkish colour.

(ii) Urine of carcinoid syndrome : Shows marked purple colours in carcinoid syndrome.

Semiquantitative test

Reagent :

(1) 0.1%, 1-nitroso-2-naphthol solution in 95% ethanol.

(2) Fresh nitrous acid — Prepared by adding 0.2 ml 2.5% $NaNO_2$ solution to 5 ml 2N H_2SO_4.

(3) Ethylene dichloride.

(4) Ethyl acetate.

(5) Standard : Standard solution of 5 hydroxytryptamine creatinine sulphate (5 HTCS).

Monhydrate 5 HTCS ... 20.3 mg

Hydrochloric acid (100 ml/L) ... 10.0 ml

Dissolve 5 MHTCS in hydrochloric acid. Now dilute the stock standard 1 ml to 100 ml and 1 ml to 50 ml with water for use. These contain 50 and 100 µmol/L (8.8 and 17.6 mg/L) as 5-hydroxytryptamine respectively.

Method :

(1) Two *standards* are put up by taking 1 ml of the above dilute standards to each of which 1 ml of urine is added. Then proceed as described in test below.

2. *Test* : To 1 ml fresh overnight specimen of urine, add 1 ml water and 1 ml nitroso-naphthol. Mix and add 1 ml nitrous acid reagent. Allow to stand for 10 minutes. Shake the tube twice with 5 ml ethyl acetate. Now remove and discard the ethyl acetate layers. In normal urine a faint pink colour is obscrvable.

3. *Blank* : As blank take 1 ml distilled water instead of urine and repeat the procedure as in test. Read test and standards against blank at 540 mm or using a yellow-green filter.

Calculation :

$$\frac{\text{Test}}{\text{Standard}} \times 50 \text{ or } 100 \ \mu\text{mol/L depending on high or low standard.}$$

After subtracting the reading of unknown from that of the two standards, the readings for 50 and 100 µmol/litre of total 5-hydroxyindoles can be found and thus concentration in urine is calculated.

Carcinoid tumours : Carcinoid tumours arise from the neuroendocrine cells and have infiltrative and metastasising potentialities but are of a low grade malignancy. They are most prevalent in the gastrointestinal tract, pancreas and pulmonary bronchi. Ninety per cent of these tumours occur in gastrointestinal tract, of which 60% in the appendix.

A small proportion of carcinoid tumours (approximately 5%) may have liver metastases that produce excess serotonin and a distinctive classical syndrome, termed carcinoid syndrome. Manifestations of *carcinoid syndrome* include the *classical triad* :

(i) cutaneous flushing, (ii) diarrhoea and

(iii) valvular heart disease.

About 30-60% patients of small bowel carcinoids (duodenum, jejunum) are accompanied by systemic manifestations, while only 3-5% of lung and 1% of appendix.

Precaution

(i) To collect 24 hours urine into a bottle containing 25 ml of glacial acetic acid for preservation of 5-HIAA as it decomposes quickly on keeping in urine.

(ii) Patient should not take any drug 72 hours before test.

(iii) Certain foods known to elevate 5-HIAA levels such as bananas, plantain, pineapple, Kiwi fruits, walnuts, plums, pecans, avocados, gwaifensein and acetaminophen should be excluded from diet at least for 3 days before the test.

I. Melanin in urine

Melanin is never found in normal urine but occurs in patients with a malignant melanoma, usually when there is metastasis in the liver. Freshly voided urine of patient contains a colourless precursor melanogen. Melanogen is oxidised to melanin within 24 hours when the urine is allowed to stand in contact with air.

Test

1. *Ferric chloride method* : To 5 ml fresh urine add 1 ml of 10% $FeCl_2$ prepared in 10% HCl. Melanogen is oxidised to black coloured melanin.

2. *Nitroprusside test* : To 2 ml fresh urine add 3-4 drops of freshly prepared aqueous solution of sodium nitroprusside and then add 2 drops of 10% NaOH solution. A red colour develops which indicates presence of acetone, creatinine or melanin. Add 2 ml glacial acetic acid :

blue to black	–	melanin
purple colour	–	acetone
amber colour	–	creatinine

MICROSCOPIC EXAMINATION OF URINE

1. Random mid-stream specimen of urine is satisfactory for screening purposes. For better morphology, it is preferable to collect a two-hour voided urine, after the first morning voiding has been discarded.

2. Urine must be examined while fresh, since cells and casts begin to lyse within 1-3 hours. If it cannot be examined within an hour of voiding, it should be refrigerated at 2-8°C before and after transportation or a preservative should be added.

Centrifugation of urine

Mix the specimen well and take 15 ml of urine into a conical centrifuge tube. If the deposit cannot be examined immediately, a drop of concentrated formalin is added to the tube, which will inhibit the growth of contaminants. Centrifuge the tube at 2000 rpm for 5 minutes. Remove the supernatant by decanting in another test tube. The fluid clinging to the sides of the tube is allowed to run down and mix with the centrifuged deposit. The sediment is resuspended and a drop is placed on one area of a slide and covered with a 18 mm square coverslip, avoiding bubbles. Excess fluid should be avoided as it causes the coverslip to float.

Microscopy

Examine first under the low power objective with subdued light and then under high power objective :

1. *Red cells, Pus cells (leucocytes)* and *renal* epithelial cells are identified under HP objective and counted in 10 representative high power fields.

2. *Casts* are identified under low power objective but the finer structures are viewed under high power (HP) objective.

3. *Crystals* are examined under low power, abnormal crystals should be confirmed chemically.

4. *Others* : Bacteria, yeast cells and trichomonas are reported in terms of number per high power field (HPF) and identified under HP objective.

Urinary sediments are divided into two broad classes :

1. *Unorganised sediment;*
2. *Organised sediment.*

A. Unorganised sediment

Crystals (Fig. 40.5) are found in normal as well as in abnormal condition in urine. Oxalates, urates and phosphates are specially common and occur in normal urine. Hence crystals in the urine are of limited clinical significance.

Crystals in urine are mostly developed in relation with reaction of urine and hence a knowledge of urinary pH is necessary for their preliminary separation.

Excretion of excess crystals : Their presence in urine suggests excessive excretion of that substance in the urine. When crystals are associated with stone in urinary tract, it gives the idea of possible type of stone. In addition, uric acid crystals/urates are excreted in gout and triple phosphate in urinary tract infection due to urea splitting organisms making alkaline urine.

I. *Crystals found in normal acid urine* (Fig. 40.5A, B, C, D)

1. Amorphous urates

(Calcium, magnesium, sodium and *potassium urates)*

Amorphous urates precipitate in concentrated urine of a slight acid pH as reddish yellow granules. They are dissolved by heat (60 °C) and by sodium hydroxide but not by acetic acid. They are converted to uric acid crystals when treated with acetic acid.

2. Crystalline urates

(Sodium, potassium and *ammonium urates)*

These are small brown needles or colourless needles in slightly acidic urine or in spheres and triplets (Fig. 40.5D). On addition of acetic acid, they revert to uric acid on the microscope slide.

3. Crystalline uric acid

They have got variety of shapes and usually coloured. Typical crystals are four-sided, flat, yellow or reddish brown; rhombic plates or prisms are the other shapes (Figs. 40.5A, D).

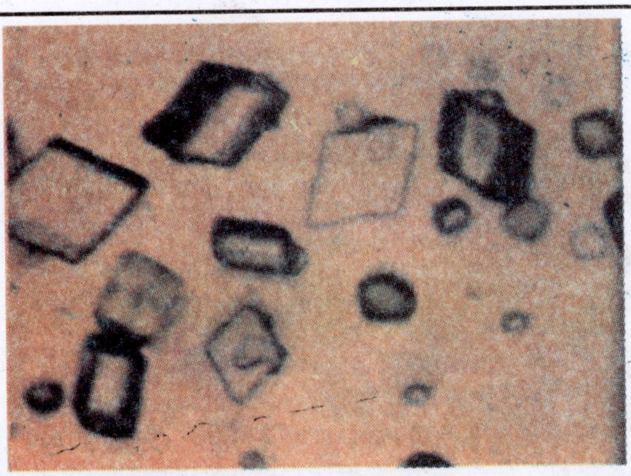

Fig. 40.5A. Uric acid crystals

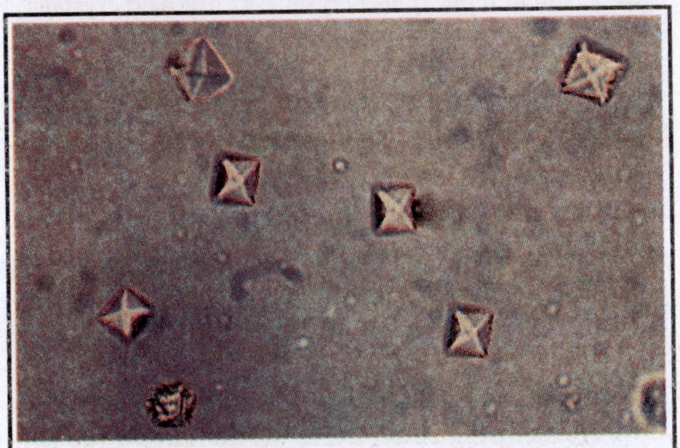

Fig. 40.5B. Calcium oxalated crystals (envelope-shaped)

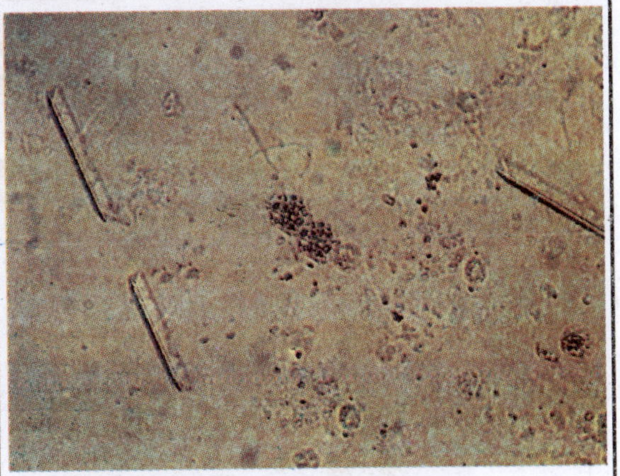

Fig. 40.5C. Triple phosphate crystals *(prism-shaped)*

4. Calcium oxalate

These have the typical envelope shape and may appear as dumb-bells. They occur at pH 6 or in neutral or slightly alkaline urine (Figs. 40.5B, D). They are often associated with food like tomatoes, spinach, etc.

II. *Crystals found in normal alkaline urine*

1. Amorphous phosphates

(Calcium and magnesium)

These are colourless amorphous granular precipitates found in an urine of alkaline or slightly acidic pH. They get dissolved in acetic acid.

2. Crystalline phosphate

(Triple phosphate)

Triple phosphates (ammonium, magnesium and calcium) are colourless, refractile, six-sided prisms (Figs. 40.5C, D) with oblique ends referred to as coffin lids or less often as feathery or leaf-like forms. They occur in alkaline pH, often with infection present. Their presence in fresh urine may indicate stones in the kidney. Larger stones of renal pelvis (staghorn calculi) and of bladder contain large amount of triple phosphate.

3. Calcium carbonate

They are small granular or colourless spheres

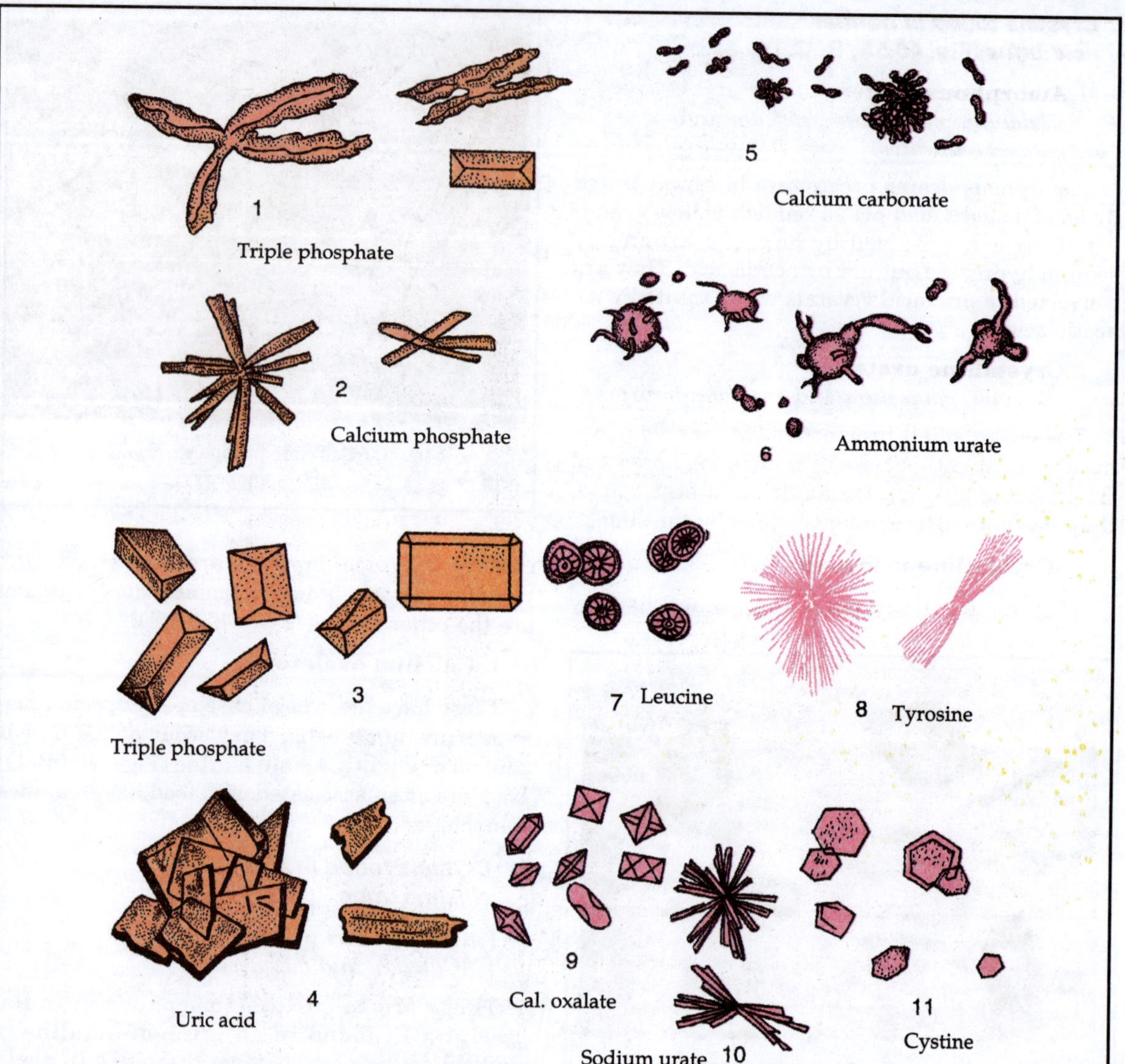

Fig. 40.5D : Urinary crystals — 1 and 3 : triple phosphate crystals; 2 : calcium phosphate crystals; 4 : uric acid crystals; 5 : calcium carbonate crystals; 6 : ammonium urate crystals; 7 : leucine spheres; 8 : tyrosine needles; 9 : calcium oxalate crystals; 10 : sodium urate crystals; 11 : cystine crystals.

and soluble in acetic acid with gas formation. It is rare in man.

4. **Ammonium biurate**

These crystalline urates form in an alkaline, neutral or occasionally in slightly acid urine. They are generally found with phosphate crystals and amorphous phosphates in decomposing urine when free ammonia is present. These are yellow brown spheres showing concentric striations. They dissolve with acetic acid and by heating at 60°C.

III. *Crystals found in abnormal urine* (Fig. 40.5)

1. **Leucine and tyrosine**

They usually occur together (Fig. 40.5D) and are occasionally seen in association with severe liver disease. Both are uncommon.

Leucine crystals are oily appearing spheres with radial and concentric striations. *Tyrosine* crystals look like fine silky needles arranged in clumps. They may appear black.

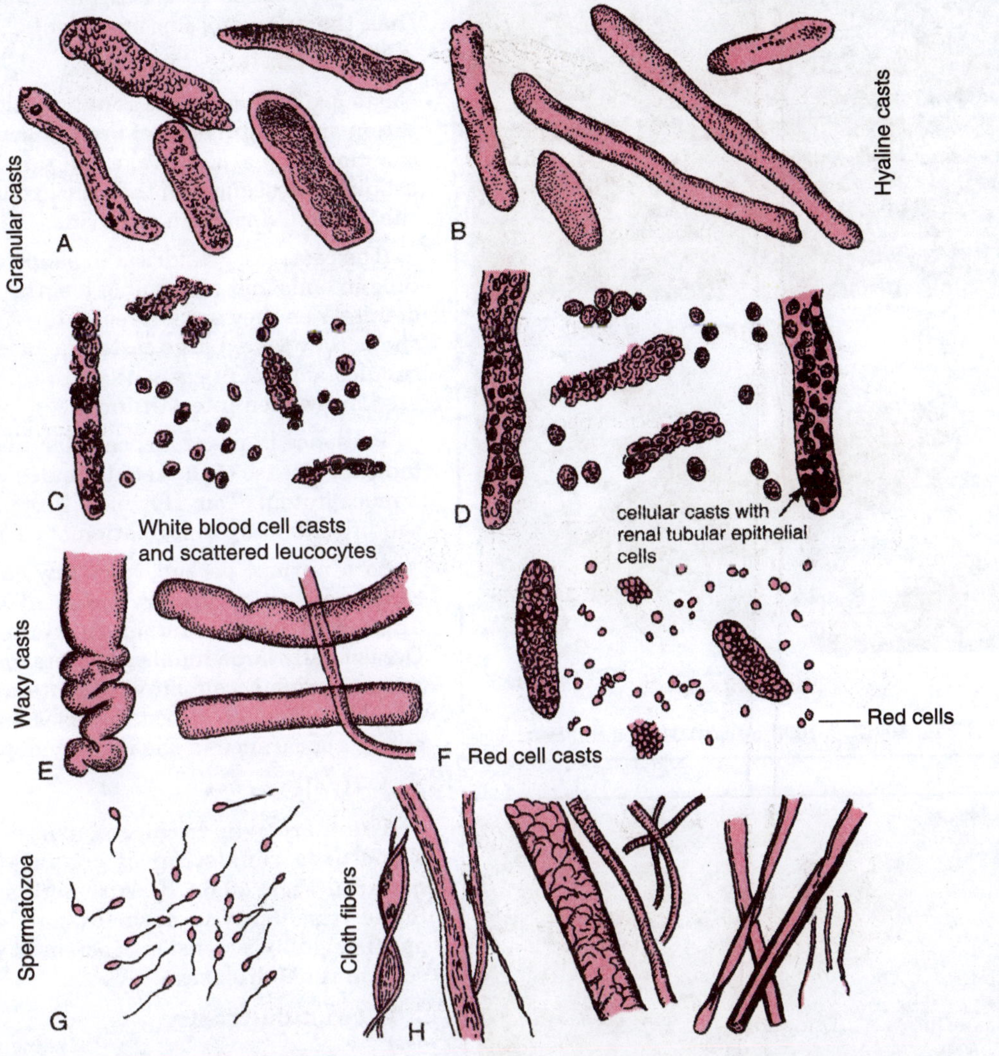

Fig. 40.6A : Casts, red blood cells, and other findings in urine — A : fine and coarse granular casts; B : hyaline casts with fine granules; C : white blood cell casts and scattered leukocytes; D : cellular casts with renal tubular epithelial cells; E : waxy casts; F : red blood cell casts (erythrocyte casts) and scattered red cells; G : spermatozoa; H : cloth fibers; from left to right, cotton, wool, and silk, (Original drawing adapted from *Atlas Urinary Sediments* by Hermann Rieder, translated by A. Sheridan Delepine)

2. **Cystine**

These hexagonal, colourless, refractile plates (Fig.40.5D) form in acidic pH and resemble somewhat uric acid crystals. They are found in cystinuria, a congenital renal tubular defect.

3. **Drug crystals**

Sulphonamide (during therapy), ampicillin (high dose) and radiographic media (meglumine diatrizoate) may be found in urine.

B. Organised sediment (Fig. 40.6A, B, C)

The principal organised constituents in urinary sediment are :

(i) Tubular casts (ii) Epithelial cells
(iii) White blood cells (pus cells)
(iv) Red cell casts (v) Bacteria
(vi) Others—spermatozoa, parasites and yeast cells.

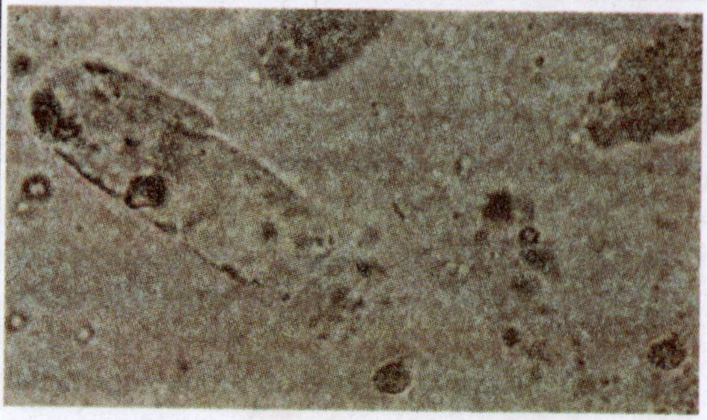

I. HYALINE CAST

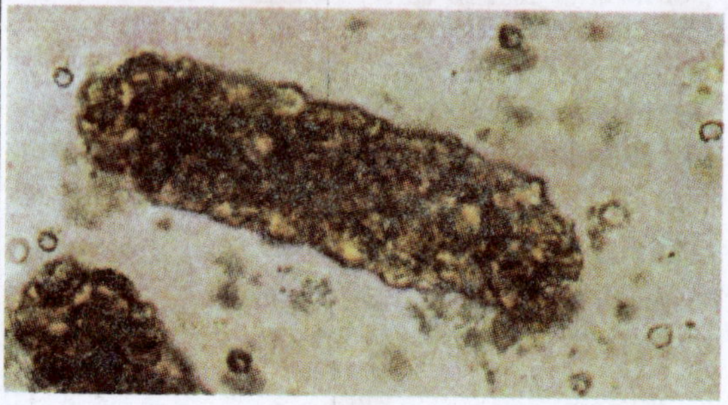

II. RED CELL CAST

Fig. 40.6B. I. Hyaline cast. II. Red cell cast

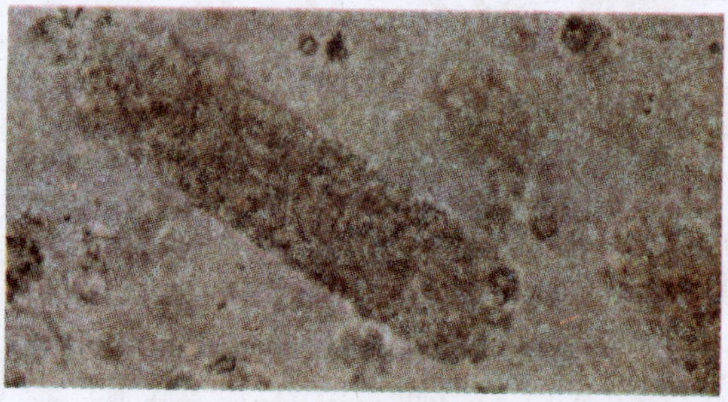

I. GRANULAR CAST

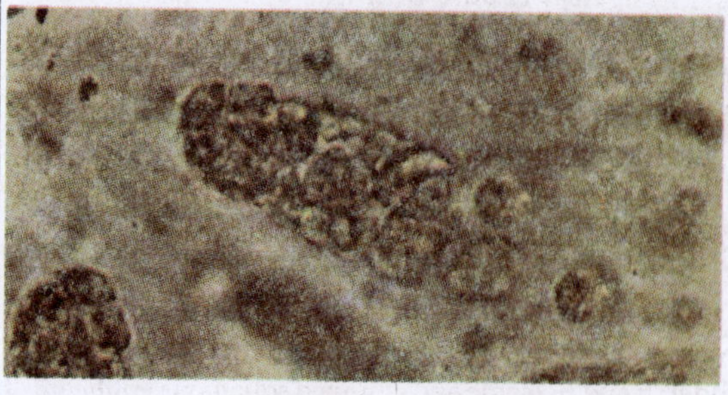

II. LEUCOCYTE CAST

Fig. 40.6C. I. Granular cast. II. Leucocyte cast

The organised structures are much important than the unorganised constituents.

A. Tube casts

Casts are formed in the renal tubules by precipitation and coagulation of protein leaking through the glomerulus. They take the tortuous shape of tubules. Subsequently, they are extruded from the tubules and appear in the urine.

The casts are cylindrical in shape with round or broken ends and of variable lengths, but note the diameter as they are formed in the tubules, whose shape they take. Large casts are formed in dilated tubules and small casts occur in tubules compressed by swollen interstitium.

Presence of granular, cellular and fatty casts indicate disease of the renal tubules which secrete a mucoprotein (Tom Horsefall Proteins) that gets solidified leading to formation of cast.

In a normal person, very few casts (hyaline casts) are seen in urinary sediment but they may appear in large number in kidney diseases. Occasionally large number of casts may be seen in normal urine accompanying proteinuria of exercise. Classification of casts is based on their microscopic appearance in the urinary deposit.

1. Hyaline cast

These are cylindrical, colourless, translucent structures consisting of coagulated protein material(Figs. 40.6A,B). Although a few may be found transiently in normal urine (exercise, old age, benign hypertension), increased numbers are seen in renal diseases.

2. Granular casts

These are casts containing large granules embedded in coagulated proteins (Figs. 40.6A, B). The granules are usually due to disintegration of epithelial cells or leucocytes. Granular casts appear with glomerular and tubular diseases, e.g., chronic glomerulonephritis, chronic pyelonephritis, long standing benign nephrosclerosis and chronic lead poisoning. These are not found in normal urine.

3. Cellular casts

Red blood cell and epithelial cell, pus cell casts (Figs. 40.6A, 40.6C) are also seen, containing, as their names suggest red bloood cells, leukocytes and epithelial cells, respectively. Most often small number of cells are entangled with casts.

(i) *Red cell casts* imply renal haematuria and

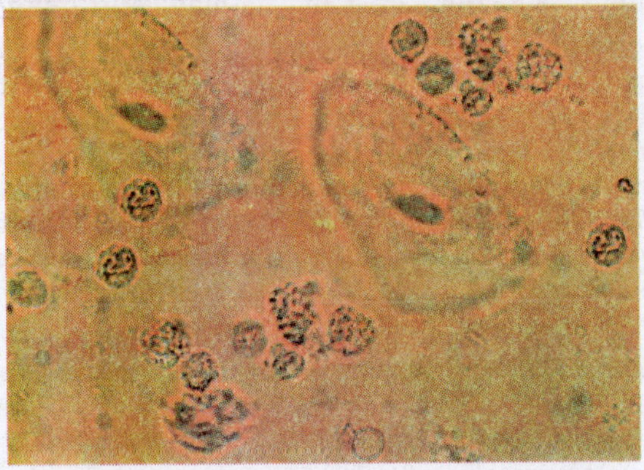

Fig. 40.7A. Squamous epithelial cells with pus cells

are found in acute glomerulonephritis, subacute bacterial endocarditis or other causes of renal infarction and in collagen disorders (SLE etc.). Red cell casts have a yellowish orange colour.

(ii) *Pus cell casts* (leucocyte casts) are suggestive of pyelonephritis, acute glomerulonephritis, nephrotic syndrome, SLE. Pus cell casts contain granular cells (WBCs) in a clear matrix.

(iii) *Epithelial cell casts* indicate acute and subacute glomerulonephritis and also pyelonephritis.

4. **Fatty (colloid) casts**

These are epithelial casts in which the cells show severe fatty degeneration. It contains refractile fat droplets with a certain amount of granular material. They are found when there is no heavy proteinuria and are a feature of the nephrotic syndrome.

5. **Waxy casts**

They somewhat resemble hyaline casts but are much more opaque with a yellowish tinge. They are mostly found in chronic renal failure. When the waxy casts are unusually broad, they are termed *renal failure casts*.

Cellular constituents

I. *Epithelial cells*

A small number of squamous epithelial cells originating from urethra, vagina and vulva may be found in the deposit from normal urines, there being more in the urine of women (8-10/HPF) than that of men (2-3/HPF). They have got no clinical significance and only large numbers are of patho-

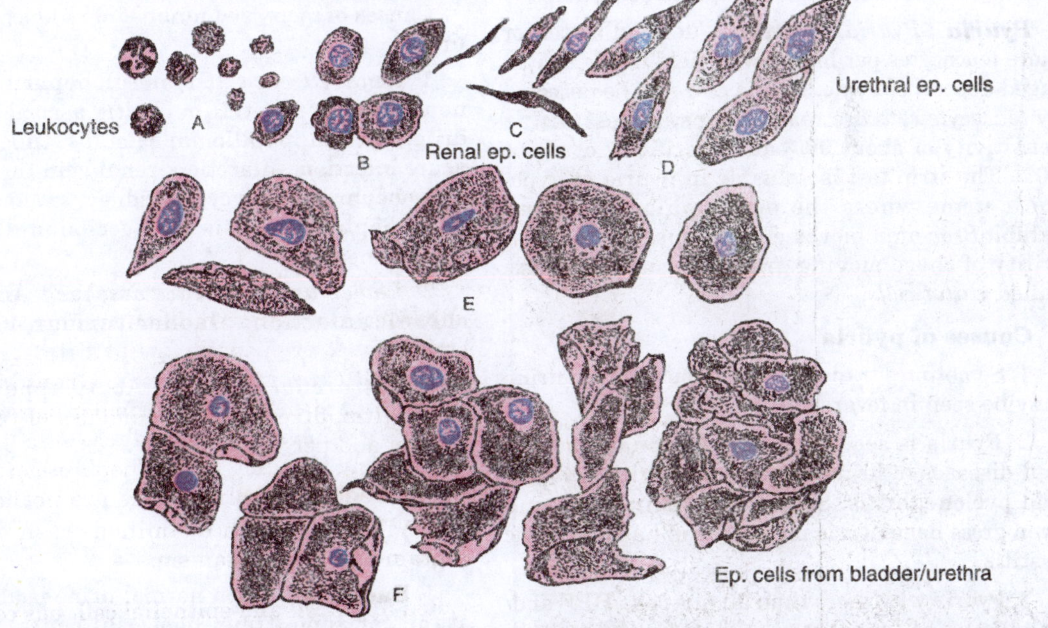

Fig. 40.7B. Types of cells found in urine — A : leukocytes, B : renal epithelial (transitional) cells; C : caudate epithelial cells from kidney pelvis; D : epithelial cells from urethra and bladder; E and F : single and clumped squamous epithelial cells from bladder, urethra, or vagina.

logical significance. The epithelial cells fall into 3 groups (Figs. 40.7A and 40.7B).

1. *Squamous cells* — from urethra and vagina.

2. *Transitional cells* with a tail-like process, 2-3 times the size of leucocyte—derived from bladder, prostate, ureters and pelvis of kidney, often seen after prostatic massage and ureteric catheterisation.

3. *Small round or polygonal cells*—originate from kidney tubules. These are rarely found in normal urine but occur in some renal diseases.

II. Pus cells (Leucocytes)

A few leucocytes, mainly polymorphonuclears, may occur in the morning urine (about 1 to 5/HPF). Pus cells are mainly neutrophils. They appear as granular spheres under high power about 12 µm in diameter. Nuclear segments are well-defined (small round discrete nuclei) in freshly voided urine. Nuclear details may be lost with onset of cellular degeneration (Fig. 40.7A). Pus cells are rapidly lysed by hypotonic or alkaline urine. About 50% pus cells are lysed following 2-3 hours of standing of urine at room temperature.

Increased number of pus cells in urine indicate some infection in the urinary tract; or in the female, contamination with vaginal secretions.

Pyuria : *Pyuria,* arbitrarily defined as ten or more leucocytes per high-power field in the centrifuged deposit of urine. Pyuria can also be detected by *leucocyte esterase* reagent dipstick test with a sensitivity of about 90% and specificity of about 80%. The strip test is valuable in pyuria of hypotonic urine where the neutrophils swell and exhibit *Brownian* movement. Because of the refractility of these moving granules, such cells are called *glitter cells.*

Causes of pyuria

1. Sometimes transient rise of pus cells in urine may be seen in fevers.

2. Pyuria is seen in almost all renal diseases and diseases of urinary tract : urethritis, cystitis and pyelonephritis. Some red cells in urine and even gross haematuria may occur in haemorrhagic cystitis.

3. Pyuria with more than 50 pus cells/HPF and/or clumps of leucocytes in sediment strongly suggests acute infection (pyogenic or tuberculous) of kidney and urinary tract. If repeated sterile cultures are obtained, it may be tuberculosis or lupus nephritis. Gross pyuria may occur due to rupture of a renal or urinary tract abscess.

4. Moderate number of pus cells along with leucocyte casts may be due to bacterial infection (chronic pyelonephritis) or non-bacterial renal disease (acute glomerulonephritis, lupus nephritis). There will be some amount of red cells in urine along with significant proteinuria in acute nephritis.

5. STD : There is increase in pus cells, more than 5 neutrophils per HPF in gonococcal and non-gonococcal (*C. trachomatis*) urethritis although large number of neutrophils (more than 50/HPF) may be seen in urine in gonococcal urethritis.

III. Red blood cells

The red cells appear as pale discs under high power (Fig. 40.6A). They may become crenated in hypertonic urine. Red cells require to be carefully distinguished from yeast cells. Yeast cells (e.g., *C. albicans*) are spherical or ovoid budding cells. Normally, occasional red cells (0 to 2 / HPF or 3 to 12 / µl) may be found in the sediment of urine.

Increased number of red cells with red cell casts reflect renal disease. In absence of proteinuria and casts, the presence of red cells in urine suggests a bleeding site distal to kidney.

Causes of increased number of red blood cells in urine :

1. *Renal disease* : Glomerulonephritis, lupus nephritis, interstitial nephritis associated with drug reaction, papilloma, calculus, tuberculosis, acute infection, infarction, renal vein thrombosis, hydronephrosis, polycystic kidney, trauma, malignant nephrosclerosis and occasionally acute tubular necrosis.

2. *Lower urinary tract disease* : Acute and chronic infection, bladder tumour, calculus, stricture.

3. *Extrarenal disease* : Acute appendicitis, salpingitis, diverticulitis, tumours of the colon, rectum and pelvis, chyluria.

IV. Microorganisms

Normal urine when examined fresh does not contain any microorganism.

1. **Bacteria** : When normal urine is allowed to stand for some time, bacterial contamination occurs. In bacterial infection of kidney and urinary tract, the urine may show bacteria which include :

(a) *Bacteria* causing UTI.

(b) *Tubercle bacilli* — Concentrated deposit is stained by acid-alcohol fast strain.

(c) *Gonococcus*—Centrifuged deposit is stained by Gram's stain.

2. **Candida albicans** : Sometimes yeast cells may be found in deposit of urine which is mostly a genital contamination in women.

3. **Parasites** : (a) *Trichomonas* : Trichomonas is sometimes found in cases of urethritis, more common among the women. In women, genital contamination of urine may also be responsible for the presence of *Trichomonas vaginalis* in urine. These are most often motile protozoa with visible axostyle, about 20-25 μm in diameter.

(b) *Schistosoma haematobium* : The eggs are found in urine accompanied by pus. *S. haematobium* infection is endemic in Africa, South-East Asia and in North-Eastern India. The egg is long, oval with terminal spine.

(c) *Microfilaria* : In chyluria, the centrifuged deposit may contain microfilaria.

V. Spermatozoa

Spermatozoa may be present in urine in the following conditions :

(i) In urine of men after epileptic convulsions

(ii) Noctural emissions (iii) Spermatorrhoea

(iv) In urine of both sexes after coitus.

VI. Malignant cells

Take the urinary deposit preferably on albuminised glass slide. Spread the deposit on the slide.

1. The smear is fixed in methanol for Giemsa, alcohol-ether mixture for Pap stain. After staining the slide is examined microscopically for malignant cells.

2. Cytospin preparation stained by Pap staining provides a better method for detection of malignant cells.

3. When cellular material is adequate, paraffin block and HE staining of section may be examined.

MULTISTIX

Reagent strips of 10 cm long and 5-8 mm wide with single/multiple discrete cellulose squares impregnated with reagents for testing pH, Sp. Gr., protein, glucose, haemoglobin, ketone bodies, bilirubin and urobilinogen are commercially available. There are strips for single test, eg., diastix for glucose and multistix for multiple tests.

CHYLURIA

The term chyluria is applied to milky urine resulting from ruptured lymphatics in the wall of bladder or kidneys. The lymph with its fat droplets escapes into the urine which also contains red blood cells. In some cases there may be enough fibrinogen to clot.

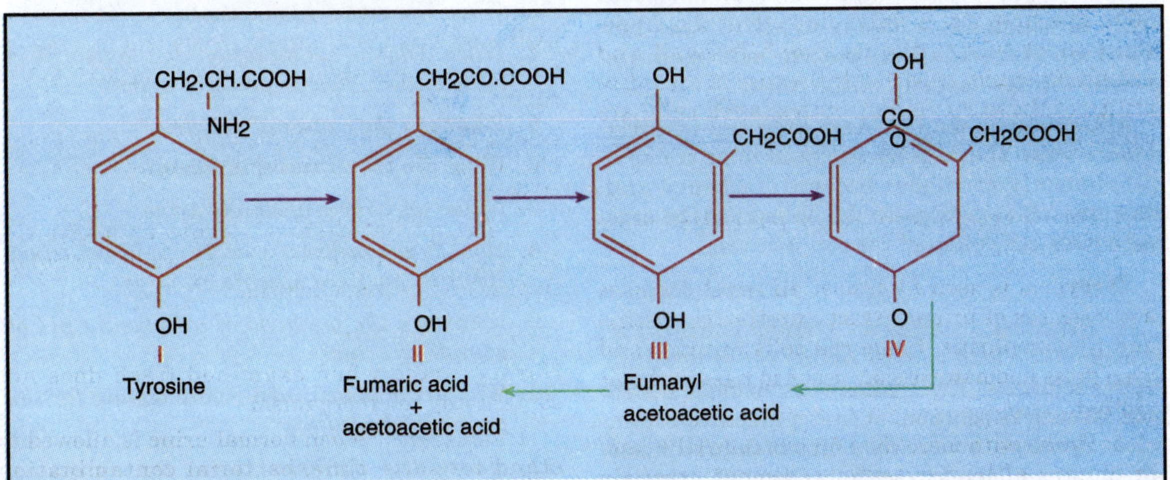

Fig. 40.8. Metabolism of tyrosine : I — tyrosine. II — parahydroxyphenylpyruvic acid. III — homogentisic acid. IV — maleylacetoacetic acid.

Composition :

(a) *Fat* : Content varies with changes in fat absorption, average 2-3 gms %, finely dispersed. Presence of fat is determined by :

(i) Staining with Sudan III.

(ii) By adding equal volume of chloroform and ether that dissolve the fat.

(b) *Protein* : Present in variable extent.

(c) *Deposit* : Contains leucocytes and red cells. Microfilaria may be found in filarial disease.

Causes of chyluria :

(i) Filariasis in the late stage.

(ii) Abdominal lymph node enlargement.

(iii) Abdominal tumours.

HOMOGENTISIC ACID IN URINE, ALKAPTONURIA

Metabolism of tyrosine (I) is defective in alkaptonuria because of congenital absence of homogentisate 1-2-dioxygenase. Normal metabolic pathway is shown in Fig. 40.8.

As a result homogentisate accumulates in body fluids which is excreted in the urine causing the urine to darken on standing. Homogentisate undergoes conversion to dark polymeric products of unknown composition. The colour of the product is similar to that of melanin which appears in the surface layer. Colour development occurs within a few seconds when the urine is made alkaline. Thus homogentisate differs from melanogen in urine in which the addition of alkali does not speed up the oxidation, but an acid medium favours the development of the colour.

Alkaptonuria may be first detected in early infancy when the napkins are seen to be stained. Subsequently cartilages become blackened and may give a bluish tinge to the hollows of the ears and brown coloration of the conjunctivae.

Tests

(i) *Benedict's solution* : Urines containing homogentisic acid causes reduction of alkaline copper solutions. Thus, when such urine is boiled with Benedict's solution, at first a greenish-brown colour develops, producing a brownish precipitate which when allowed to settle is seen to be similar to the cuprous oxide formed with other reducing substances. Urine containing melanogen may give a greenish-black precipitate with Benedict's solution if an appreciable amount is present but otherwise there is little or no change.

(ii) *Ammoniacal silver nitrate* : When a few drops of ammonia (100 ml sp. gr. 0.88/1 in water) are added to a mixture of 0.5 ml urine and 5 ml silver nitrate solution (30 g/l) in a test tube, a black colour develops. Black colour is often produced without the addition of ammonia in alkaptonuria. The mixture should not be exposed to direct sunlight.

(iii) *Ferric chloride* : On addition of a few drops of ferric chloride solution (100 g/l) to a few ml of urine, in addition to the formation of ferric phosphate a transient blue or green colour develops in alkaptonuria.

It should be remembered that ferric chloride gives a brown to black colour with melanogen.

Nitroprusside test for melanogen is not positive with the urine in alkaptonuria.

QUESTIONS

(For questions on diabetes mellitus, renal and alimentary glycosuria — refer to Chapter 48 : Estimation of Blood Glucose)

1. *What is the normal volume of urine in an adult in 24 hours?*
2. *What type of urine sample is suitable for routine examinations?*
3. *When the urine is to be tested?*
4. *When delay of examination due to transport is inevitable, how to preserve urine?*
5. *What are the causes of polyuria?*
6. *What are the causes of oliguria?*
7. *Name the causes of cloudy urine.*
8. *How do you measure specific gravity of urine? What is low fixed specific gravity?*
9. *What are the methods of measuring pH of sample of urine?*
10. *Why urine is acidified before testing for the presence of albumin?*
11. *Name the different tests for detecting albumin in urine.*
12. *Why only upper part of urine in test tube is heated for testing albumin?*

13. *Name the condition in which both albumin and Bence-Jones protein are present in urine.*
14. *What are the causes of albuminuria?*
15. *What is microuria? How do you detect it?*
16. *What are the causes of B-J proteinuria?*
17. *What is gammopathy?*
18. *What is the composition of Benedict's qualitative reagent?*
19. *What is the composition of Benedict's quantitative reagent?*
20. *Name the ketone bodies. How are they formed?*
21. *How do you test for ketone bodies?*
22. *Which type of bilirubin is liable to pass in the urine? Name the causes of presence of bilirubin in urine.*
23. *When is the concentration of bile salts are increased in urine?*
24. *When is the concentration of urobilinogen is increased in urine?*
25. *How do you test for urobilinogen in urine?*
26. *What is porphyria? Deficiency of which enzyme causes porphyria?*
27. *How to differentiate urobilinogen from porphobilinogen?*
28. *How does the colour of urine in haemoglobinuria look and why?*
29. *How does haematuria differ from haemoglobinuria?*
30. *Name the causes of haematuria and haemoglobinuria.*
31. *Name the condition in which 5 HIAA is excreted in urine.*
32. *What are the carcinoid tumours?*
33. *Name the crystal that make the urine alkaline.*
34. *What is the significance of crystals in urine?*
35. *What precautions should be observed while examining urine for casts? What information is obtained by the presence of casts in urine?*
36. *How are malignant cells detected in urine?*
37. *What is the cause of alkaptonuria?*
38. *How do you detect alkaptonuria?*
39. *What is chyluria? How do you detect chyluria?*

Chapter 41

Body Cavity Fluids

NORMAL

The body cavities (peritoneal, pleural, myocardial) are normally lined by a single layer of flattened or cuboidal epithelium made of mesothelial cells. This epithelium is supported by a rich network of capillaries, lymphatic channels and loose connective tissue. The visceral and parietal surfaces are separated by a potential space which normally contains 10-50 ml fluid (pleural fluid 10-20 ml, pericardial fluid 10-50 ml, peritoneal fluid 10-50 ml). It is a pale yellow, clear serous fluid that serves as a friction lubricant. This small amount of fluid cannot normally be aspirated. This ultrafiltrate of plasma of the capillaries is reabsorbed continuously, but at various speeds, by the venules and lymphatic vessels. Normally, the net fluid movement from the body cavity into the plasma occurs at a rate of about 10 to 20 ml per hour.

Composition

(i) Normal serous fluid has a protein concentration of less than 2 gm% and a pH (7.0) and glucose concentration similar to those of blood.

(ii) The cellular content includes scanty mesothelial cells and occasional lymphocytes. The cellular composition of all the aspirated fluid is identical.

ABNORMALITIES

Any appreciable accumulation of fluid in the body cavities is an indication of disease. The basic mechanism leading to the collection of fluid in tissues and body cavities is explained below.

Transudate : Increased venous pressure or decreased oncotic pressure, usually from a disturbance of cardiac function, leads to a greater exit of fluid from the vascular system than is reabsorbed.

Composition : (i) The aspirated fluid is low in protein (less than 2 gm%), low specific gravity (1.005 to 1.015) and low cell count (scattered mesothelial cells of serosal origin). (ii) A few histiocyte or lymphocyte are also present. It has a little tendency to clot.

Exudate : Exudates are fluid accumulation that results from the break-down of the normal formation—resorption mechanism due to inflammation or toxic damage to the pleural, peritoneal or pericardial capillaries. Irritation of the serosal mucosa caused by various agents, such as cancer, inflammation, a foreign body or haemorrhage is associated with damage to the underlying wall of capillaries and venules of the mesothelial membrane.

Table 41.1
Different characteristics of effusions

Properties	Transudate	Exudate
Appearance	Clear and watery	Cloudy, may be clotted
Sp. Gr.	< 1.015	> 1.015
Protein	< 2 gm %	> 2 gm %
Fibrin	Poor	Rich
Glucose	High (15-30 mg %)	Low
Cell count	Few	Abundant

Composition : In pathological conditions : (i) The protein content is high, specific gravity is more than 1.015. It is rich in fibrin and clots readily. (ii) Abundant inflammatory cells (leucocytes), fresh and old red cells, single or clusters of mesothelial cells larger than usual are often found. (iii) Occasionally colonies of microorganisms may be found. When the effusion results from metastatic spread, cancer cells may be found. The difference between transudate and exudate is shown in Table 41.1. The causes of pleural, pericardial and peritoneal infections are listed in Table 41.2.

Suppurative or purulent pericarditis (Fig. 41.1) or lesions of other body cavities are almost due to invasions of these spaces by infective organisms.

Chylous effusion

Sometimes effusions may form due to escape of chyle from the thoracic duct as a result of interference with lymphatic flow by filarial worms (scar tissue formed around the dead filaria) or to obstruction by cancer. This is called chylous effusion. The chylous fluid resembles chyle of urine in chyluria (see urine analysis).

LABORATORY INVESTIGATIONS

Specimen : Specimen is collected aseptically in at least two sterile containers (test tubes) for physical, chemical, cytological, microbiological examinations and for Papanicolaou's smear preparation (for malignant cell).

When there is frank blood in the specimen, the total and differential leucocyte count and protein content of the specimen should be cautiously interpreted, because the finding will be exaggerated due to cellular contribution from blood. The various causes effusions are shown in Table 41.2.

I. Physical examination

1. **Volume** : Large amount of normal looking fluid is commonly seen with congestive cardiac failure or chronic liver abscess, e.g., hydrothorax.

2. **Appearance** : Turbid or cloudy fluid is usually due to the presence of large number of pus cells (leucocytes), associated inflammatory reaction of either septic (pyogenic, tuberculous) or non-septic (rheumatoid disease, rheumatoid fever).

Milky white fluid is often due to chyle but may also be pseudochylous in nature (cyst fluid, tuberculosis, fungus, rheumatoid disease). In pseudochylous effusion, chylomicrons are scanty or absent, and usually sterile on routine culture, but there occurs mixed cellular reaction.

3. **Colour** : Grossly haemorrhagic fluid must be distinguished from blood-tinged fluid due to traumatic tap. In traumatic tap, the blood is usually non-uniform in distribution and clears with continued aspiration when collected separately.

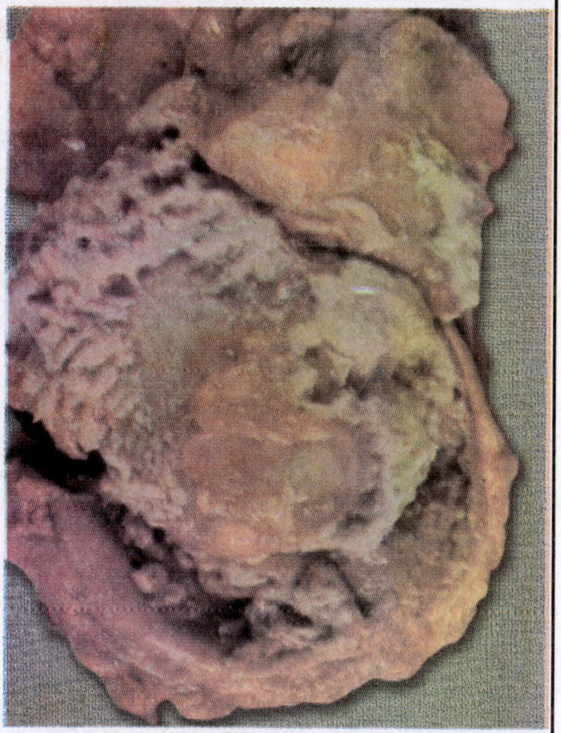

Fig. 41.1. Acute suppurative pericarditis, an extension from pneumonia. There is extensive purulent exudate

Haemorrhagic fluid may occur in a variety of conditions : intrapleural malignancy, pneumonia, closed chest trauma in pleural cavity; idiopathic haemorrhagic pericarditis, rheumatic and pyogenic pericarditis, post-myocardial infarction, tuberculous pericarditis, SLE, metastatic carcinoma, leaking aneurysm in pericardial sac; intra-abdominal injuries and metastatic carcinoma in peritoneal cavity.

II. Microscopical examination

(a) **Leucocytes** : Generally undiluted fluid is used for examination; but if it is grossly bloody a part of the fluid may be diluted with 3% acetic acid to haemolyse red cells. For differential count, centrifuged deposit is used which provides concentration of leucocytes. Film is stained by 1% aqueous methylene blue or by Leishman stain.

1. *Total cell count* : Total count is done in Neubauer's modified counting chamber. If the

Table 41.2
Causes of pleural, pericardial and peritoneal effusions

	Pleural	Pericardial	Peritoneal
Transudate	Congestive heart failure Hepatic cirrhosis Hypoproteinaemia (e.g. nephrotic syndromes)	—	Congestive heart failure Hepatic cirrhosis Hypoproteinaemia (e.g., nephrotic syndromes)
Exudate	*Neoplasm* Bronchogenic carcinoma Metastatic carcinoma Lymphoma Mesothelioma	*Neoplasm* Metastatic carcinoma Lymphoma	*Neoplasm* Hepatoma Metastatic carcinoma Lymphoma Mesothelioma
	Infections Tuberculosis Bacterial pneumonia	*Infections* Bacterial pericarditis Tuberculosis Fungal pericarditis	*Infections* Tuberculosis Primary bacterial peritonitis (may be superimposed on exudate)
	Viral or mycoplasmal pneumonia	Viral or mycoplasmal pericarditis	Secondary bacterial peritonitis (e.g., appendicitis, intestinal infarct)
	Trauma *Pulmonary infarct* } Haemorrhagic effusion ±	*Trauma* *Myocardial infarct*	*Trauma* *Pancreatitis*
	Rheumatoid disease *SLE* *Pancreatitis* *Chylous effusion*	*Haemorrhagic effusion* Secondary to anti-coagulant therapy, Leakage of aortic aneurysm	*Bile peritonitis* (Secondary to ruptured gall bladder or needle perforation of bile duct) *Chylous effusion*
	Obstruction or damage to thoracic duct by trauma, carcinoma, lymphoma, tuberculosis.	*Rheumatoid disease* *SLE*	Obstruction or damage to thoracic duct by lymphoma, carcinoma, tuberculosis, parasitic infestation.

fluid is turbid, it is diluted as in WBC/RBC count. Both leucocytes and erythrocytes are counted.

2. *Differential cell count* : Leishman's stained film of the deposit is examined to identify the predominant cell type : polymorphonuclear leucocyte, lymphocyte, mesothelial cell and atypical cells suggestive of cancer cells.

Observation

(i) Total leucocytes, more than 100 and usually 1000–10000/cu mm with 75-80% polymorphonuclear leucocytes suggest acute inflammation of bacterial origin such as pneumonia in lung, bacterial pericarditis in pericardium and bacterial peritonitis in peritoneum.

(ii) An absolute granulocyte count over 300/µl in undiluted ascitic fluid is suggestive of acute bacterial peritonitis.

(iii) A high percentage of lymphocytes indicate tuberculous infection.

(b) **Mesothelial cells** : The mesothelial cells are reported as percentage of leucocytes which has clinical significance in pleural fluid. The underlying disease stimulates hyperplasia of mesothelium. The cells are larger than normal and vary in size and some show binucleation (see chapter 38 : Cytology on body cavity fluids). They stain well by 1% aqueous methylene blue but better morphology of cell can be seen when stained by Papanicolaou's method.

(c) **Tumour cells** : Metastatic malignant cells vary in size, shape and number enormously. The background is bloody in at least one-third of cases. The cells may be found singly, in sheets, and in acini or papillary formation. Nuclear cytoplasmic ratio of the cells is increased and the enlarged nuclei show malignant features. These cells are identified by Papanicolaou's staining of deposit of effusion fluid.

III. Chemical examination

Proteins, sugar and chlorides are estimated by same methods as in CSF.

(a) **Protein**: Protein content less than 2 gm% is described as transudate. Exudates have higher values, more than 2 gm %. When fibrinogen enters the fluid, the sample clots after collection and is called fibrinous exudate.

(b) **Glucose** : Most infective exudates contain low glucose as glucose is utilised by bacteria during growth cycle.

IV. Microbiologic examination

(a) **Smear examination** : Smear prepared from centrifuged deposit is examined by Gram and by Ziehl-Neelsen staining. These give 25-50% positive result in infective cases.

(b) **Culture** : Routine culture and culture for tubercle bacilli increase the incidence of positive results. Concentrate of the specimen is prepared by Petroff's method for culture for tubercle bacilli.

SYNOVIAL FLUID

The synovial membrane lines joints, bursae and synovial tendon sheaths but not the articular cartilage or menisci. The synovial round cells are loosely arranged in a layer one to three cells thick, over a mucopolysaccharide complex. Synovial fluid (SF) is a plasma ultrafiltrate to which a hyaluronate-protein complex secreted by synovial membrane has been added. SF serves as a lubricant and nutrient for articular cartilage. Analysis of synovial fluid in a case of joint effusion is an important diagnostic procedure to ascertain whether it is caused by a non-inflammatory or inflammatory process. See table 41.3.

Investigation of synovial fluid

Synovial fluid is examined for appearance, *viscosity, glucose, leucocyte count, microscopy, Gram-stain, serology* and *culture*.

(a) **Non-inflammatory fluid** : Clear, viscous, amber-coloured, leucocyte < 300 cells/cu mm with a mononuclear cell predominance, glucose level is normal. Such finding is typical of *osteoarthritis* and *trauma*.

Red cells : Few red blood cells are usually the result of traumatic tap, but when present in large numbers, they should be differentiated from *haemarthrosis,* which gives a red brown hue to the supernatant fluid.

(b) **Inflammatory fluid** : Turbid, yellow, cell count – 3,000 to 5,000/cu mm; protein elevated, glucose normal or low, viscosity diminished. Such effusions are seen in *rheumatoid arthritis, gout,* other inflammatory arthritides, and occasionally septic arthritis.

In rheumatoid arthritis, SF also contains large number of plasma cells (more than 500/cu mm), whereas the polymorphonuclear leucocytes may exceed 50,000/cu mm in septic arthritis.

Table 41.3: Composition synovial fluid (normal)

Volume in a joint	0.1 to 2.0 ml, transparent straw coloured droplets.
Content per 100 ml	Protein 1-3 gm% Hyaluronate 0.3-0.4 gm% Glucose 70-110 mg% Uric acid 2-8 mg% Lactate 10-20 mg%
Cytology	*Leucocyte* 20/cu mm, upper limit of normal, usually 1-2.0 cells/cu mm; these are mainly lymphocytes/histiocytes. *Synovial cells* — Occasional/few

Polarised microscopy : Cellularity and crystals are analysed by polarised microscope. Needle-shaped crystals of monosodium urate, usually intracellular crystals, are seen in gouty effusions. Rhomboid shaped crystals are seen in SF of chondrocalcinosis and pseudogout.

Gram-film : Gonococcus or other bacteria may be detected in deposit.

Culture : SF is to be cultured, particularly when gonococcal arthritis is suspected.

Serological test : Serological tests for rheumatoid factor (anti-IgG), antinuclear antibodies, complement levels, or antistreptolysin O titres should be done when clinical evidence suggests a specific diagnosis.

QUESTIONS

1. *What are the differences between exudates and transudates?*
2. *When are the causes of milky-white body fluid?*
3. *How do you diagnose metastatic tumour cells in pleural/peritoneal fluid?*
4. *Name the causes of haemorrhagic fluid in pleural cavity.*
5. *Which serological test in synovial fluid is useful?*
6. *What is the composition of normal body cavity fluid?*
7. *What are the causes of peritoneal and pleural effusions?*
8. *What is the composition of synovial fluid in rheumatoid arthritis?*

Chapter 42

Cerebrospinal Fluid (CSF)

Lumbar Puncture Needle

LUMBAR PUNCTURE (LP) NEEDLE

It is a slender needle about 10 cm long and a bore of 1 to 1.5 mm. The needle is provided with a stilette (Fig. 42.1).

Use of LP needle

1. **Lumbar puncture** : It is mainly used for collection of CSF.

2. **Other sites of puncture**

(a) *Cisternal puncture* : It is done in spinal canal block, a vertebral deformity or an infection of tissues of the back. Contraindicated when tumours or adhesions are present at the base of the brain.

(b) *Ventricular puncture* is often done in infants who have open fontanelles.

(c) *Combined spinal-cisternal* and *spinal-ventricular or double spinal punctures* are done sometimes to establish the level of spinal canal block or compression.

3. **Other uses** : LP needle may be used for aspiration of fluid from a closed sac like peritoneal cavity, pleural cavity, joint space, etc.

FORMATION, CIRCULATION AND COMPOSITION OF CSF

The volume of CSF is about 150 ml. In experiments on animals, about 50-70% of the CSF is formed in the choroid plexuses and the remainder is formed around the blood vessels and along the ventricular walls. Presumably, the situation is similar in humans. The fluid in the ventricles flows through the foramens of Lushka and Magendie in the fourth ventricle and then subarachnoid space. It is then absorbed through the arachnoid villi into the veins, primarily the cerebral venous sinuses.

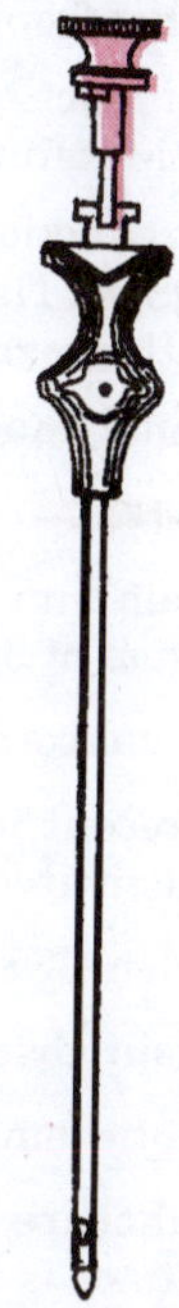

Fig. 42.1. Lumbar puncture needle with stilette

Cisternal, ventricular and lumbar CSF show some minor difference in composition. The lumbar region is principally tapped and the fluid is normally clear, colourless, sp. gr. 1.003-1.006, lymphocytes 2-5 cu.mm, glucose 40 to 80 mg %, protein 20 to 45 mg % and chloride 700 to 760 mg %.

Blood-brain barrier : Injected trypan blue (dye) in living animal, results in staining of all tissues except brain and spinal cord. This was explained by postulation of an existence of a *blood-brain barrier*. Anatomically blood-brain barrier represents the barrier in the capillary endothelium in contact with astrocyte foot processes. *Blood-CSF barrier*, on the other hand, is represented by the choroid plexus epithelium and the endothelium of all cerebral capillaries in contact with CSF which accounts for different concentrations of solutes in plasma and CSF. Water, chloride, CO_2 and O_2 diffuse rapidly through the barriers at ease, and the exchange of other substances between blood and brain is slow.

INDICATIONS FOR COLLECTION OF CSF

A. **Diagnostic**

1. Meningitis.
2. Meningoencephalitis.
3. Encephalitis.
4. Subarachnoid haemorrhage.
5. Intracranial haemorrhage due to injury.
6. Intracranial space occupying lesion.
7. To look for lymphoblasts to evaluate relapse of ALL in meninges.

B. **Therapeutic**

1. Relief from intracranial pressure.
2. Introduction of serum : Anti-meningococcus, anti-tetanus.
3. Introduction of drugs : Hypertonic solution of $MgSO_4$, NaCl, lipoidal ventriculography and methotrexate in acute lymphatic leukaemia.
4. Spinal anaesthesia : Novocaine, eucaine, etc.

CONTRAINDICATION

1. Brain tumour at cerebello-pontine angle or in region of 3rd ventricle associated.
2. Spinal cord tumour.
3. A recent intracranial haemorrhage may be reactivated by the disturbance of the clot.
4. When CSF pressure is very high.
5. Brain abscess may possibly spread.
6. Septicaemias.
7. Puncture should never be done when the patient is in convulsion.
8. Advanced cardiovascular disease including that of arteries.

COLLECTION OF CSF

CSF is usually obtained by lumbar puncture at the space between L_3 and L_4 vertebra or below to avoid injury to spinal cord.

1. Position : Patient on stool (or bed lying on right or left lateral position) with forward bending as much as possible with neck and legs flexed, and with knees and chin approximated. Back of the patient should be at the edge of the bed.

2. Overlying skin is prepared with antiseptics. The skin and fascia of the lumbar space selected for puncture are infiltrated with a small amount of anaesthetic agent (1% solution of novocaine).

3. A line is drawn from the highest points of the iliac crest down across the back. This line crosses the space between third and fourth lumbar spines or the fourth lumbar spine. Mark the area between L_3 and L_4 spines.

4. The LP needle stilette *in situ* is pushed forward and slightly upward in midline between L_3 and L_4 vertebrae till a peculiar 'give-way' sensation to the needle is felt. Now the stilette is removed, then the pressure is measured by fitting a manometer to the needle or by drop counting method (normally, 60 drops per minute).

When no CSF comes out, the stillete is reinserted and the needle is turned around. Then the stillete is removed for CSF to flow. If still no CSF comes out, the patient is asked to strain which raises the pressure of CSF. In case the needle hits bone, it is pulled out a little. Even if the CSF does not come out, lumbar puncture is tried elsewhere.

5. The CSF is then collected in three sterile tubes in 3-5 ml amount, total quantity of 10-12 ml is sufficient. One of 3 tubes is used for cytological, second for biochemical and the third for microbiological examination.

Pressure of CSF

Normal pressure

Adult : It is 70-180 mm of H_2O (17.15 mm of Hg) with the patient lying on his side; and 190-300 mm of H_2O (15.22 mm of Hg) when sitting up.

Children : It is 20-100 mm of H_2O when child is lying on the side. Absence of CSF indicates incorrect placement of needle.

Regulation of pressure

Pressure of CSF is normally regulated by rate of secretion, rate of absorption, arterial and venous pressures (jugular and vertebral veins), patency of cerebrospinal canal, thickness of dura and the intracranial bulk of fluid.

Decreased CSF pressure is found in : (1) circulatory collapse (shock, fainting), (2) spinal canal block (below the level of block), (3) dehydration, and (4) vomiting.

Increased CSF pressure is found in : (1) meningitis, (2) encephalitis, (3) meningoencephalitis, cerebral tumour, (4) cerebral abscess, (5) cerebral oedema, and (6) cerebral haemorrhage.

Note : LP is contraindicated when the pressure of CSF is very high as the procedure may lead to herniation of cerebellum and coning of medulla that can be fatal. To avoid complication in such cases, the stillete is partially and slowly withdrawn so that CSF flow drop by drop and not in a spurt.

Queckenstedt or Jugular sign

Normally, compression of jugular veins increases CSF pressure, which rapidly rises over 300 mm H_2O, and rapidly returns to normal when compression ceases, since jugular and vertebral veins communicate with intracranial venous sinuses. Absence or delay in the rise of CSF tension (positive *Queckenstedt test*) indicates sinus thrombosis, obstruction at the foramen of magnum, or a massive lesion in the spinal cord. The test is dangerous in increased intracranial pressure. It should be done only in selected cases.

MENINGITIS

A. **Meningitis in neonates**

Purulent : Causative agents include Gram-negative bacilli (*E. coli, Proteus* spp, etc.) and Gm +ve Group B streptococci.

Non-purulent : The most important pathogen is *Mycobacterium tuberculosis.*

B. **Meningitis in adults**

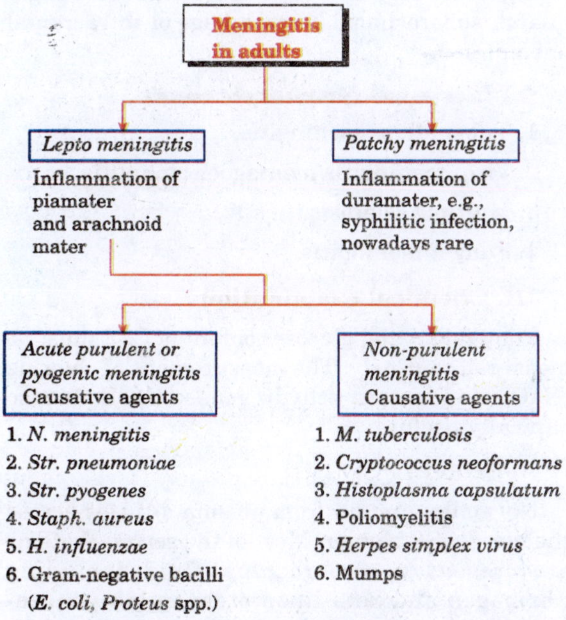

Common types of meningitis

The common types of meningitis in India include : (a) *Pyogenic meningitis* : Meningococcal and pneumococcal meningitis. (b) Tuberculous meningitis.

Fungal meningitis

Cryptococcal and other fungal meningitis are common in immunocompromised patients and AIDS, steroid or cancer therapy.

EXAMINATION OF CSF

CSF must be examined immediately or latest within half an hour.

I. Physical examination

Normal CSF is crystal clear and colourless and does not clot on standing. It has a specific gravity of 1.003-1.006. Normal volume is 120-150 ml and the pressure is 60-150 mm water. Normally 2-5 lymphocytes per cu. mm are found and there is no red cell (Table 42.1).

A. Colour

Any colour of CSF is abnormal. Presence of blood is the main cause of an abnormal colour of CSF.

Causes of coloured CSF :

1. Spontaneous *subarchnoid haemorrhage.*
2. Intracerebral haemorrhage.
3. Traumatic haemorrrhage.
4. Associated obstructive jaundice.
5. Spinal tumour.

Traumatic tap must be distinguished from the pathologic bleeding. Fresh blood due to traumatic tap renders the CSF bright red, whereas old blood pigments leave a trace of colour in the form of *xanthochromia* or yellow colour due to bilirubin.

A traumatic tap will show gradual clearing as several samples are taken, the second tube will be paler than the first and the third may be almost clear. When centrifuged, the supernatant of traumatic sample becomes crystal clear. Pure blood clots quite quickly, but that admixed with CSF (subarachnoid haemorrhage) does not clot.

Xanthochromia refers to a pale pink to orange or yellow colour in the supernatant of centrifuged cerebrospinal fluid, e.g., subarachnoid haemorrhage. For xanthochromia, the blood must be present in CSF sufficiently long to cause lysis, i.e., more than 4 hours. The lysis of red cells is probably due to lack of plasma proteins and lipids which are necessary to stabilise the erythrocyte membrane. Haemolysis causes liberation of haemoglobin which is slowly converted into bilirubin. Bilirubin is the cause of xanthochromia. Other haemoglobin derivatives lending colour to CSF include oxyhaemoglobin (red tint) and methaemoglobin (brown tint).

Jaundice also produces an increased CSF bilirubin content, in the unconjugated form. When the spinal cord is blocked by a spinal tumour, the CSF appears as xanthochromic due probably to a great increase in the protein level.

B. Appearance

Turbidity of CSF is due to presence of lucocytes, more than 200 polymorphs/mm^3 and micro organisms. Smaller number of red cells cause a smoky appearance and moderate number of lymphocytes (> 100 lymphocytes/cu. mm produce opalescent appearance).

C. Coagulum

Fibrin clots may form on standing when protein content is very high (over 1000 mg %). A fine *cobweb* coagulum is often formed in the fluid of tuberculous meningitis when it is allowed to stand overnight. The cobweb may take up tubercle bacilli that may be seen after staining with Z.N. Stain.

II. Cytological examination

A. Total count

If the CSF is almost clear or slightly opalescent, Undiluted fluid is used for total cell count. In case of turbid sample, it is diluted 1 : 10 in a test tube/ WBC pipette with WBC fluid.

It is better to examine as large a volume of CSF as possible. The *Fuchs-Rosenthal* chamber is specially meant for CSF cell count, which has a ruled area of 16 sq. mm and depth of 0.2 mm. Using all the 16 squares of the chamber, a total area of 16 × 0.2 cu. mm (µl), i.e. 3.2 µl of fluid is examined. If the number of cells counted in 3.2 µl of 1:10 diluted sample is x, then total count per µl

$$= x \times \frac{10}{3.2}.$$

When an improved, Neubauer chamber is used (0.1 mm depth), cells in 4 big square (1 mm^2) areas of corners are counted and calculated as follows :

$$\text{Total area examined} = 4 \times 1 \times \frac{1}{10} = \frac{2}{5} = \text{mm}^3.$$

Let x be the number of cells counted, and dilution factor is 10, then total count per mm^3 (µl)

$$= \frac{x \times 5}{2} \times 10 = x \times 25.$$

Erythrocyte count in bloody fluid is sometimes used to correct leucocyte count and CSF protein estimation for contamination of CSF by peripheral blood associated with traumatic tap. Approximately 700 red cells are responsible for 1 white cell and for 1 mg of protein.

B. Differential count

Leishman stained smear prepared from centrifuged deposit is examined and differential count of lymphocytes and neutrophils are made.

Tumour cells, when suspected, a part of CSF (4-5 ml) is diluted with alcohol and centrifuged; one or two thick smears are made from the sediment on albumin-covered glass slide and examined after Papanicolaou's staining.

Interpretation

Total and differential leucocyte count of CSF in some important meningovascular disease are shown in Table 42.1.

(a) *Increased neutrophil count*

1. *Infections* : Pyogenic meningitis, early viral meningoencephalitis.

2. *Non-infections* : Reaction to CNS haemorrhage, usually 3-4 days after haemorrhagic infarct, subarachnoid haemorrhage or intracranial haematoma.

(b) *Increased lymphocyte count*

1. Tuberculous meningitis.
2. Viral meningitis/meningoencephalitis.
3. Multiple sclerosis.
4. Fungal meningitis.

III. Chemical examination

The protein and glucose content of CSF must be measured routinely. The measurement of chloride (NaCl) and lactase dehydrogenase (LDH) is also clinically useful.

A. Protein

Normally, protein from plasma diffuses across the blood-CSF barrier. Most of the serum proteins are present in cerebrospinal fluid, including fibrinogen and beta-lipoprotein in low concentrations. Normal CSF contains 20-45 mg % protein and the ratio of albumin to globulin is 8 : 1 (approximately). An increase in total protein is the

Table 42.1 : CSF parameters in health and some common disorders

	Normal	*Subarachnoid haemorrhage*	*Pyogenic meningitis*	*Tuberculous meningitis*	*Viral meningitis*	*Multiple sclerosis*
Pressure	50–180 mm H_2O	Increased	Highly increased	Moderately increased	Normal/slightly increased	Normal
Physical examination Colour	Crystal clear colourless	Blood stained xanthochromic	Cloudy	Clear/slightly turbid	Clear	Clear
Coagulum of protein	Nil	Nil	Big protein clot develops within a few minutes	Fine, thread-like spider web coagulum develops after a few hours	Nil	Nil
Chemical examination Protein (lumbar)	15-50 mg%	Increased	Highly increased (100-600 mg%)	Slightly increased (80-120 mg%)	Slightly increased (60-80 mg%)	Normal/slightly increased
Glucose	40-80 mg%	Normal	Decreased (10-20 mg%)	Decreased (30-50 mg%)	Normal/ increased	Normal/ increased
Chloride	720-760 mg%	Normal/ slightly increased	Decreased	Extremely diminished	Decreased	Normal/ decreased
Cell count Total cell (per cu. mm)	0–4	Increased red blood cells	1000-20000	50-2000	20-200	1-100
Type of cell	Lymphocytes	Red cells	Neutrophils – 98% Lymphocytes – 2%	Lymphocytes – 90% Neutrophils – 10%	Lymphocytes	Lymphocytes + Plasma cells
Bacterio-logical examination Gram-film	Nil	—	Gram-negative or positive cocci or bacilli found	—	—	—
Acid-fast film	Nil	—	—	Acid-fast bacilli often found	—	—

commonest abnormality in inflammatory disease. Normally, albumin is the predominant protein, but depending on the abnormality, globulins appear in varying amount. However, globulin appears in abnormally high concentration in CSF in most pathological conditions.

Estimation of total protein
(Sulphosalicylic acid method)

In this method, proteins are precipitated by sulphosalicylic acid.

Reagents

1. *Sulphosalicylic acid — sodium sulphate solution :*

Sulphosalicylic acid	...	3.0 gm
Sodium sulphate (anhydrous)	...	7.0 gm
Distilled water	...	100 ml.

Dissolve in water, filter and store in a dark bottle. Discard when turbidity or colour develops.

2. *Sodium chloride solution* ... 0.85%

Technique

In a standard bore test tube, add 0.5 ml of clear supernatant of CSF after centrifugation to 3.0 ml of sulphosalicylicc acid reagent. Mix gently and leave for 5 minutes.

Reading : The content of tube is mixed by inversion and read against an acid blank and a known standard at 660 nm or using a red filter. Alternatively, the test is compared in a visual colorimeter with a set of turbidity standards, matching the tube with that standard which shows the same amount of turbidity.

Preparation of standards : Standards are prepared by diluting serum of known protein content with saline so as to obtain a solution of 200 mg%. A series of tubes is set up as shown in Scheme I.

When visual comparator is to be used, the tubes are stoppered with waxed corks and stored in dark. Fresh standards are to be prepared when there is contamination.

Interpretation : Protein content increases in :

1. Pyogenic meningitis,
2. Tuberculous meningitis,
3. Viral meningoencephalitis,
4. Syphilitic meningoencephalitis,
5. Fungal meningoencephalitis,
6. Poliomyelitis,
7. Brain tumour,
8. Diabetic neuropathy.

Globulin (Pandy test)

Principle : Globulins are precipitated by a saturated solution of phenol in water (10 gm phenol in 150 ml water).

Technique : Two drops of CSF are added to 2 ml phenol reagent. Normal CSF produces no precipitate or else just a very faint opalescence. When there is an excess of globulin in CSF, a bluish white streak of precipitated globulin will follow the CSF drops through the reagent. When mixed, the precipitate will dissipate and produce opalescence or turbidity of the reagent.

Result : The result is reported as : (i) Showing no opalescence. (ii) Slight opalescence. (iii) Opalescence. (iv) Marked opalescence or turbidity.

Interpretation : The test provides an approximate comparison between γ-globulin increase and that of total protein of CSF. The γ-globulin is disproportionately increased in :

(i) multiple sclerosis, (ii) neurosyphilis.

The Pandy test has become obsolete, replaced by protein electrophoresis. The colloidal gold test, formerly used to measure the γ-globulin content, is also obsolete and is no longer performed by many laboratories.

B. Glucose

The estimation of glucose is done either by glucose oxidase method or by Folin-Wu method.

Interpretation : Glucose content of normal lumbar fluid varies between 50-80 mg%. Glucose content is usually diminished in CSF in all cases of meningitis and meningoencephalitis.

1. *Pyogenic meningitis* : Very low or may disappear completely.
2. *Tuberculous meningitis* : Usually between 10-40 mg%.
3. Hypoglycaemia.

Cause of decreased glucose level

The reduction of glucose content is probably due to :

1. Increased utilisation by microorganisms and inflammatory cells.

Scheme I

Tubes	1	2	3	4	5	6	7	8	9	10	11
Mg protein per 100 ml CSF	0	20	40	60	80	100	120	140	160	180	200
Diluted serum (ml)	0	0.1	0.2	0.3	0.4	0.5	0.6	0.7	0.8	0.9	1.0
Saline (ml)	1	0.9	0.8	0.7	0.6	0.5	0.4	0.3	0.2	0.1	0

Add 0.5 ml of CSF to 3.0 ml sulphosalicylic acid reagent and read as above.

2. Increased utilisation by brain tissue.
3. Impaired mechanism of glucose transfer from blood to CSF.

C. Chloride

The chloride level of normal CSF is 720-760 mg% (120-130 m mol/l), which is appreciably higher than that of normal serum (98-106 m mol/1). The measurement of content of chloride of CSF is also not much done nowadays and is almost obsolete.

Technique

1. Take accurately 1 ml of CSF into a 150 × 25 mm test tube containing 2-3 ml distilled water. Add 1-2 drop(s) of 10% potassium chromate solution. Then titrate with silver nitrate solution (30 m mol/1 or 5.10 gm per litre) adding drop by drop from a 25 ml burette. When the end point is reached (sudden change to orange colour), note the volume of $AgNO_3$ added.

Normal CSF requires 4 to 4.85 ml reagent.

Calculation : Mg chloride % (as NaCl) = ml $AgNO_3$ required × 200.

Interpretation : The difference in the chloride content of blood and CSF is mainly a consequence of active secretion at the choroid plexuses. The difference becomes less if the meninges are inflamed. CSF chloride decreases in meningitis when there is much vomiting, particularly in tuberculous meningitis (600-700 mg%).

D. Other constituents

1. *Bicarbonate* : Normal 1.8 m mol/l, is lower than plasma to compensate increased chloride content.

2. pH : Normal pH of CSF is 7.31. Acidosis is found in acute meningitis and tuberculous meningitis.

3. *Urea* : Normal level is similar to that of plasma.

IV. Bacteriological examination

1. **Gram's staining of deposit** : Bacterial pathogens are found in 90% cases of pyogenic meningitis.

2. **Acid-fast staining of deposit** : Acid-fast bacilli may be detected in 60% cases of tuberculous meningitis.

3. **India-ink preparation of deposit**

Cryptococcus neoformans ... 50% positive

Str. pneumoniae ... 90% positive

4. **Culture** : For pyogenic organisms (blood agar in atmosphere of 10% CO_2), tubercle bacilli (Lowenstein Jensen medium) and fungus (Sabouraud's dextrose chloramphenicol agar) cultures are done as indicated by clinical and laboratory examinations.

V. Serological tests

1. **Tests for syphilis**: In patients with neurosyphilis, VDRL and FTA-ABS tests with CSF are useful. VDRL test may be negative in about 50% cases but FTA-ABS test is positive in 80-90% cases. FTA-ABS has also got much greater sensitivity.

2. **Latex agglutination test** : It is positive for cryptococcal antigen in about 80-90% cases.

3. IgG and IgM anti-tuberculous antibodies are increased (ELISA).

4. Viral inclusions may be detected by immunostains.

5. PCR is helpful for viral DNA detection.

QUESTIONS

1. *Describe a lumbar puncture (LP) needle.*

2. *What are the uses of LP needle?*
3. *What are the indications of LP?*
4. *What are the contraindications of LP?*
5. *What is the procedure of LP?*
6. *What are the common types of meningitis in India?*
7. *What is the role of LP in acute lymphatic leukaemia?*
8. *In which conditions cryptococcal and fungal meningitis are commonly observed?*
9. *What are the characteristic findings in CSF in pyogenic and tuberculous meningitis?*
10. *Why LP is contraindicated when CSF pressure is very high? How to avoid complication, when LP is unavoidable in such cases?*
11. *What are the causes of increased amount of protein in CSF?*
12. *How do you test CSF in cryptococcal meningitis and syphilis?*

Chapter 43

Semen Analysis

ROUTINE EXAMINATION OF SEMEN

Semen is a composite solution which consists basically of spermatozoa suspended in the seminal plasma.

(i) Routine examination of semen is often advised in relation to infertility.

(ii) It is also necessary at times to examine vaginal secretions or clothing stains for the presence of semen for alleged or suspected rape.

(iii) Semen analysis may sometimes be necessary to check the effectiveness of vasectomy.

(iv) Sometimes post-coital cervical mucous from the female partner is examined for viable spermatozoa.

In relationship to sterility the defect in the male partner constitutes about 50% cases. The cause of male infertility may be either in the *quality* or in the *quantity* of spermatozoa.

COLLECTION OF SPECIMEN

Abstinence : It is preferable to collect the specimen after 5 to 7 days abstinence.

Collection : Specimen is collected in a clean and dry wide-mouthed container, preferably in the pathology laboratory by masturbation. Less satisfactory method is to obtain the specimen in the patient's home by coitus interruption or masturbation and delivered soon thereafter to the laboratory.

The examination of semen should be done within 2 hours of ejaculation. It cannot be examined immediately as the highly viscous fluid must liquify, which takes usually 15 to 30 minutes.

EXAMINATION

Physical and chemical examination

1. Volume

Average normal volume is 1.5 to 4 ml. Volumes less than 1.5 ml is considered below normal. Greatly reduced semen volume can result in poor penetration of the cervical mucous by sperm.

2. Viscosity and colour

Freshly ejaculated specimen is a highly viscid, opaque, white or grey white coagulum. Self liquefaction takes place and should be completed within 15 to 30 minutes. The absence of liquefaction may inhibit the movement of spermatozoa in the vaginal canal and interfere with fertilisation.

The coagulation of semen is due to the action of a prostatic clotting enzyme on a fibrinogen like precursor formed by the seminal vesicles. The prostatic enzymes (fibrinolysin) initiate liquefaction.

3. Reaction

The reaction of semen is almost always on the alkaline side, varying between 7.2 to 8.5 with an average of about 7.7. Since the reaction does not vary greatly, abnormalities in relation to pH of semen is rare.

Microscopic examination

1. Sperm count : Following liquefaction of the semen (15 to 30 minutes after ejaculation), mix the semen sample thoroughly and dilute the semen 1 in 20 with semen diluting fluid.

Semen diluting fluid

Sodium bicarbonate	...	5 gm
Formalin (neutral)	...	1 ml
Distilled water to make	...	100 ml

Semen may be diluted in a test tube (0.1 ml semen + 1.9 ml diluting fluid) or in a WBC pipette (draw semen to the mark 0.5 and diluting fluid to the mark 11) and mixed well. After charging the improved Neubauer Counting Chamber, two minutes are allowed for the immobilised sperm to settle.

Calculation : Count spermatozoa in 2 sq mm (two large squares at two corners) and multiply by 100,000 (i.e., add 5 zeros) which gives the number of spermatozoa per ml of semen. Note that the count of spermatozoa is reported in terms of per ml instead of per cu.mm of WBC count.

Normal range : 60-150 million per ml, the count may go up to 300 million/ml in some persons. Sperm concentration increases with abstinence for 10 days with a daily average incremental increase of about 13 million/ml. Sperm count below 20 million/ml is considered abnormal, although still considered fertile.

2. Motility of spermatozoa

Spermatozoa should be actively motile in order to penetrate the cervical mucus and subsequent migration to fallopian tubes for fertilisation of ovum.

A small drop of liquefied semen is placed on a slide, covered by a cover slip and examined under a high power and low power objectives, respectively. The proportion of motile to non-motile forms is noted by observing at least 200 spermatozoa.

Observation : Normally 80-85% of sperm are found motile with a mean of 65%. Some prefer a qualitative estimate of motility of spermatozoa and grade as good, fair and sluggish.

Some investigators previously recommended motility study at intervals following ejaculation, e.g., 3 hours, 6 hours, 12 hours and 24 hours for estimation of degree of motility (Box-1). After 4 hours of collection of sample, the motile forms gradually decrease by about 5 per cent per hour. Since spermatozoa penetrate the cervical mucus within a few minutes after ejaculation (or become inactivated by the relatively low pH of secretions of vagina), and seminal fluid differs from the physiologic medium of the body, it is hardly useful to make a qualitative estimate of motility extending for a prolonged period.

Abnormalities

Certain abnormalities can be detected during microscopical examination of semen which include :

(a) *Aspermia* : Complete absence of spermatozoa in multiple slides.

(b) *Oligospermia* : On examining several fields, only a few motile spermatozoa are found.

(c) *Necrospermia* : Plenty of spermatozoa are found but all are non-motile. Addition of a drop of 1% aqueous eosin to the wet preparation assists to differentiate viable from non-viable spermatozoa. Non-viable forms stain red while viable forms remains unchanged.

(d) *Haemospermia* : When there are a large number of red blood cells and pus cells along with spermatozoa, it is called haemospermia. Such condition is usually associated with chronic gonococcal or tuberculous infections of prostate or seminal vesicle. If pus cells are found, report the same and examine a Gram stained smear for bacteria.

3. Sperm morphology

For evalution of normal and abnormal spermatozoa types, smears are prepared on clean glass slides with a drop of semen in a manner identical to blood films. The smear is best stained by Papanicolaou or haematoxylin methods. Other stains often used are basic fuchsin, methylene blue, Giemsa, and crystal violet, which give some poorer differentiation of sperm detail.

Basic fuchsin method of staining

(a) Make a thin smear of liquified semen on a slide, while still wet, the smear is fixed in 95 per cent alcohol for 5-10 min and then dried in the air.

The alcohol-fixed smear is washed with sodium-bicarbonate formalin solution (semen diluting fluid) to remove any mucus which may be present. Then the smear is rinsed with several changes of water.

(b) Stain the smear by dilute carbol fuchsin (1 in 10) for 3 minutes.

(c) Wash with water.

(d) Counterstain with Loeffler's methylene blue for 2 minutes.

(e) Wash in running tap water, dry in air and examine under oil immersion lens.

Methylene blue staining

Smear can also be stained by any other Romanowsky stain after fixation of smear in alcohol. Simple 1% aqueous methylene blue overlaid on smear, kept for 3 minutes, washed in water and examined.

Observation : Normal spermatozoa is 50-70 mm in length, with a large head (3-6 × 2-3 mm), a small neck and a slender long tail. The tail comprises 90% of total length (Fig. 43.1).

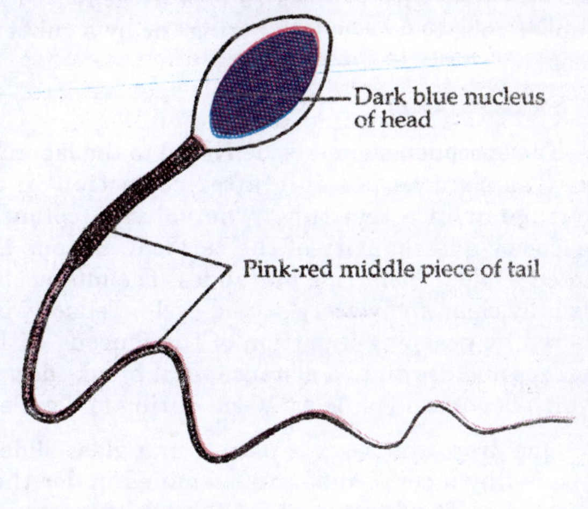

Fig. 43.1. Sperm stained with carbol fuchsin and Loeffler's methylene blue

Staining results :

Nucleus of head	...	Dark-blue
Cytoplasm of head	...	Pale-blue
Middle piece and tail	...	Pink-red

At least 200 spermatozoa are counted and the percentage of abnormal forms along with other cells are noted.

Abnormalities

(a) *Spermatozoa* (Fig. 43.2)

(i) abnormally shaped heads,

(ii) abnormally sized heads — giants and minute,

(iii) double heads,

(iv) middle piece or neck may be absent, bifurcated or swollen,

(v) tail may be double, curled, rudimentary or absent.

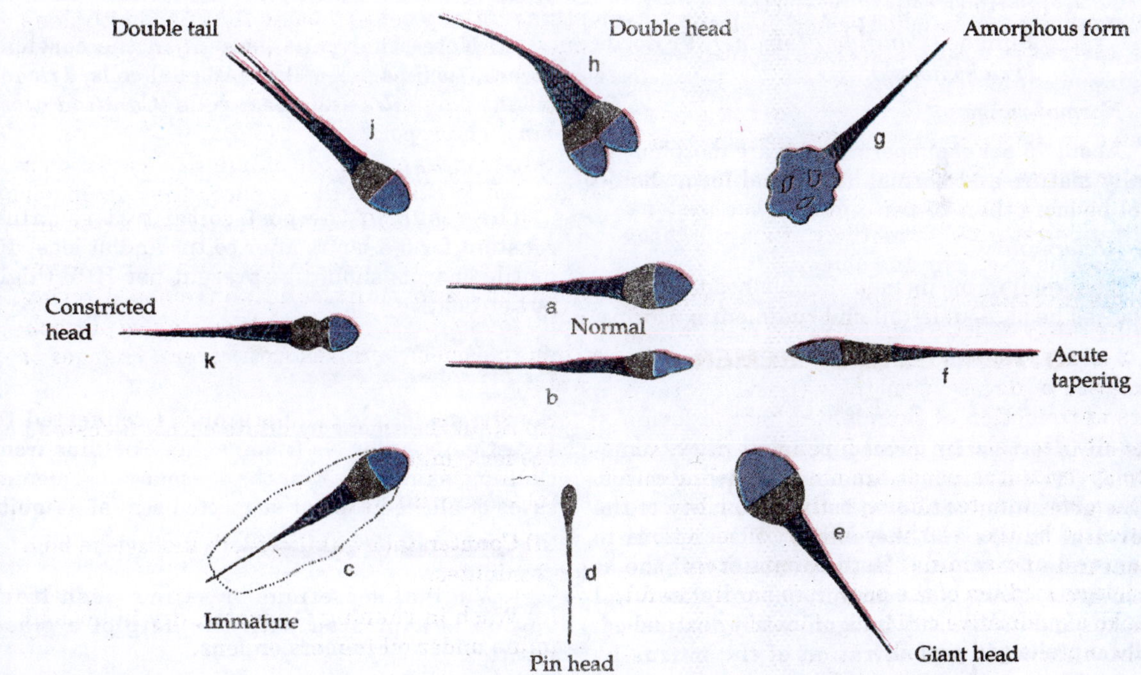

Fig. 43.2. Morphology of spermatozoa : Methylene blue staining — a = normal (frontal view); b = normal (lateral view); c = immature (spermatid). Abnormal types d-k; d = pin head; e = giant head; f = acute tapering form; g = amorphous form; h = double head; j = double tail; k = constricted head

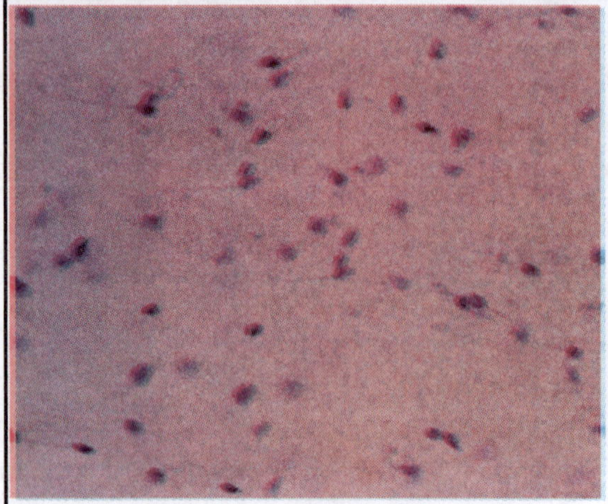

Fig. 43.3. Spermatozoa wet-stained by methylene blue

(b) *Others*

(i) Red cells,

(ii) Pus cells (leucocytes), suggestive of infection of genital tract and urethra,

(iii) Epithelial cells — germinal epithelium, squamous epithelium,

(iv) Sertoli's cells, (v) Bacteria,

(vi) Fungus (*Candida albicans),* Protozoa *(Trichomonas).*

Normal range

About 75 per cent spermatozoa are morphologically mature and normal. Abnormal form should not be more than 25 per cent.

Abnormality

Abnormal forms include : double-head, swollen, pointed head, double-tail and rudimentary forms.

OTHER TESTS OF SEMEN

Post coital test (Sims-Huhner test)

As an investigation procedure in sterility, sometimes cervical mucus is examined following coitus. This gives information on both the quality of the cervical mucus and the ability of the sperm to penetrate the mucus. In the ovulatory phase at mid-cycle, there is maximum amount of cervical mucus and its viscosity is significantly diminished, which facilitates penetration of the mucus by sperm. Increased viscosity of the mucous is caused by progesterone in the secretory phase.

Collection of material

The female partner is instructed to report to the gynaecologist/laboratory during ovulatory phase within a few hours of coitus. The ovulatory phase is determined by noting basal temperature. After 2-3 hours of coitus, the external cervical os is wiped clear with a cotton swab and cervical mucus is aspirated with a glass canula attached by a rubber tube to a Luer-lock syringe or by a rubber teat.

Examination

The specimen should be delivered to the laboratory as soon as possible after collection in a syringe or in a test tube. The volume, colour, viscosity and tenacity of the cervical mucous is noted while transferring into slides. The mucous is usually clear and watery at mid-cycle. Tenacity is tested by grasping a portion of the mucous with forceps and drawn to a distance till it breaks down which is normally at least 10 cm during mid-cycle.

One drop of mucous is placed on a glass slide, covered by a cover slip, and examined under the microscope for the presence of spermatozoa and their motility.

(i) Note the number of sperm per high power field with the percentage of motile sperms, and report.

(ii) Note other cells present in the cervical mucus, such as pus cells, epithelial cells, *Trichomonas vaginalis* and yeast cells (*Candida albicans*) and report.

Normal findings

The result of the post-coital test remains constant for 6-8 hours after coitus and at least 10 motile sperms should be present per HPF (high power field).

Medico-legal examination for presence of semen

Sometimes clinical laboratory is requested to investigate materials from vagina or stains from clothing, skin or hair for the presence of semen in cases of alleged rape or suspected sexual assault.

Collection of specimen

1. Vaginal secretions or saline wash from vagina is aspirated with the help of a glass pipette.

2. A saline wash is collected from the skin surface where necessary.

3. A 1 sq cm portion of stained piece of clothing is cut out and immersed in 1-2 ml of normal saline

and left for 1 hour and then fluid from the washing is collected.

Testing of material

The specimens collected as above are tested for the presence of semen.

1. *Examination for sperm* : It is desirable to collect direct vaginal smears for Papanicolaou's staining. The vaginal aspiration is examined by cover slip preparation as well as by stained smear examination. Smears prepared from washings of fabric is also stained by dilute carbol fuchsin for demonstration of sperms and their tails which are frequently broken off. The centrifuged deposits of washings provide concentrated material.

2. *Acid phosphatase test* : Acid phosphatase determination of vaginal aspirate or lavage or of the wash fluids of the stains provide higher values in presence of seminal fluid even in aspermic individual. Seminal fluid average about 2500 KÅ units of acid phosphatase per ml of semen, whereas other body fluids contain less than 5 units per ml.

3. *Determination of blood group substances* : About 80% individuals with secretory status secrete water soluble form of blood group substances (A, B or H) in body fluids including semen. As a result, the specific substance is identified on the basis of the ability of the semen to partially or completely neutralise the agglutinating ability of the specific antiserum.

4. *Immunofluoresence test* : It has largely replaced the acid phosphatase test and is usually performed on stains from clothing, other fabric and hair. The test depends on presence of high concentration of choline in seminal fluid. When a few drops of saline wash containing semen is mixed with an equal amount of iodine solution on a glass slide, semen forms rhombic or needle-shaped crystals of choline periodide within a few minutes. The test has limitation as high choline content is sometimes found in other tissue fluids of human or animal origin.

5. *Precipitin test* : High titre antiserum is raised in rabbit by immunising human seminal fluid. When the antiserum is overlaid on saline wash containing seminal fluid in a capillary tube, precipitation ring appears at the junction of two fluids.

6. Recently polymorphic semen antigens are detected with monoclonal bodies, or by DNA finger printing and DNA typing.

Specimen of report of a normal semen

1. **Physical examination** : Volume — 1.5 to 4 ml. It is greyish white, viscid. Liquefication occurs within 15-30 minutes.

2. **Agglutination** : Sperms do not show agglutination within half an hour of ejaculation.

3. **Reaction** : Alkaline, pH 7.2–7.5.

4. **Sperm count** : 60-150 millions/ml.

5. **Motility study** :

BOX – 1

Hours after ejaculation	1 hour	4 hours	8 hours
% of motility	80-85	75-80	60-70
Degree of motility	Excellent	Good	Good

6. **Morphology of sperm**

(a) Morphologically normal looking : 85-90%

(b) Others : Spermatids ... 8-12%
Amorphous ... 2-3%
Pin-head ... Occasional
Other form ... Occasional

7. **Smear examination**

(a) Pus cells : Nil/Occasional

(b) Squamous cell : Occasional

(c) Sertoli cell : Occasional.

QUESTIONS

1. *What are the reasons for semen analysis?*
2. *How is sperm counted?*
3. *What are the morphological abnormalities of spermatozoa?*
4. *What does the presence of pus cells in semen suggest?*
5. *What is the post-coital test?*
6. *What is the normal findings in post-coital test?*
7. *How do you collect specimen in a medicolegal case?*

Section VI

APPLIED CLINICAL CHEMISTRY

Section VI contains

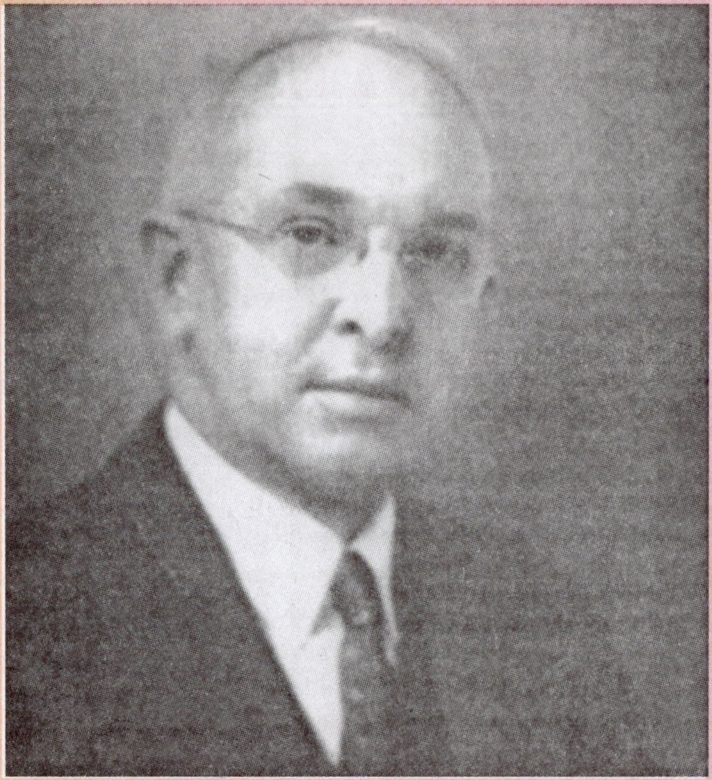

Dr Arthur H. Sanford (1882–1959)

Introducer of Clinical Pathology in medical practice *— In the preface to the 8th edition (1935) of Clinical diagnosis of Laboratory Methods Dr Sanford stated that "Clinical pathology has become a recognized speciality in medical practice". There was, for the first time, a separate 59-page chapter on "Clinical Chemistry". Other investigations included the Addis method for counting casts and cells in the urine and the heterophilic antibody test for infectious mononucleosis.*

Chapter 44

Exocrine Function of Pancreas

Pancreas has both endocrine and exocrine functions. Exocrine portion of the gland comprises of 80-85% of the pancreas. The endocrine pancreas, consist of about one million microscopic clusters of cells, called the islets of Langerhans. It is made of 4 main types of cells : β *cell* (secreting insulin), α *cell* (secreting glucagon), δ *cell* (contains somatostatin) and *PP* cell (contains pancreatic polypeptide). β and α cells induce hyperglycaemia and *PP* (pancreatic polypeptide) stimulates secretion of gastric and intestinal enzymes and inhibits intestinal motility. There are two other rare types of cells also : *DI* (enterochromaffin cells) producing serotonin and *VIP* cells (producing vasoactive intestinal polypeptide), a hormone that induces hyperglycemia and stimulates secretion of intestinal fluid causing secretory diarrhoea.

The exocrine pancreas produces major portions of all digestive enzymes which are important to digestion. Pancreatic juice is an alkaline secretion which is isotonic with plasma. The enzymes are formed in the acinar cells and discharged into the pancreatic duct which, in 90% of individuals, enters the duodenum forming a common channel with the biliary system (common bile duct) at the sphincter of Oddi; in about 10% cases the pancreatic juice directly reaches the duodenum.

Pancreas produces about 1200 ml of juice in 24 hours. This fluid is slightly alkaline and, besides water, contains mainly enzymes, Na^+, K^+, sodium bicarbonate, chloride and phosphate. The increased serum enzyme activity in acute pancreatitis presumably results from escape of enzyme into the interstitial tissue and peritoneal cavity, from where it is absorbed through lymphatics and veins.

Pancreatic Inflammation

1. *Acute pancreatitis* : Single episode.

2. *Relapsing acute pancreatitis* : Recurring episodes.

3. *Chronic relapsing pancreatitis* : Recurring episodes of acute pancreatitis.

4. *Chronic pancreatitis* : Persistent chemical and biochemical abnormalities.

Investigations (Table 44.1)

1. ***Amylase (α-amylase)*** : Determination of serum and urine amylase are most useful.

Acute pancreatitis : Serum amylase activity begins to appear 2-12 hours after onset, reaching a peak between 12-72 hours and thereafter falls rapidly because of renal clearance. Serum amylase activity returns to normal within 3-4 days. Values up to 600 Somogyi units/dl, or over 4 times the upper limit of normal (80-200 units/dl) are highly suggestive of diagnosis. Urinary amylase activity on a 24-hour urine sample may be helpful when the serum level is not diagnostic.

A persistently elevated level of serum enzyme activity is suggestive of continuing necrosis or possible pseudocyst formation.

The principle of amylase estimation is based on the hydrolysis of soluble starch at 38°C.

2. ***Serum lipase*** : Serum lipase activity tends to become elevated at about the same time as amylase.

3. ***Secretin test*** : Analysis of pancreatic juice (for bicarbonate and enzyme content) is done after stimulation of pancreas by secretin.

Procedure

(i) Patient is in a fasting state.

(ii) A metal tipped, double-lumen tube is introduced under fluoroscopic control into duodenum.

(iii) A basal sample is collected for 20 minutes (fasting sample).

(iv) Secretin 70 units (1 unit/kg body weight) is injected intravenously and then gastric contents are collected at 10-minute interval for 1 hour.

Results

(i) Volume of contents — 135-250 ml in an adult (normal) in a 60-minute period;

(ii) Bicarbonate — 90 mEg/1 or more;

(iii) Amylase — 80-200 somogyi units/dl;

(iv) Trypsin — 59 units in infants, and in children 39 units.

Interpretation : In duct obstruction (e.g., carcinoma of pancreas, pancreatic duct obstruction), volume of secretion and enzyme output are decreased with relatively normal bicarbonate level. In chronic parenchymal disease (e.g., chronic pancreatitis), all parameters are depressed.

Limitation

Such test has lost favour nowadays as it is not only unpopular with patients, but also because pancreatic disease is usually advanced before exocrine function is appreciably reduced. Hence, the test is of little help in distinguishing chronic pancreatitis and carcinoma.

4. ***Miscellaneous tests***

(a) Estimation of serum trypsin, chymotrypsin have been done to diagnose acute pancreatitis but the results have not generally been appreciated.

(b) There is leucocytosis in patients with acute pancreatitis, more than 20,000/cu. mm blood with neutrophilia.

Table 44.1
Investigations for chronic pancreatitis

Investigation or test	*Use of indication*
Radiographic	
Plain radiograph of the abdomen	Calcification of pancreas
Ultrasonography and computer tomography	To demonstrate atrophy and calcification, temporary enlargement in acute attacks and stricture of the common bile duct
ERCP	For planning surgery
Function tests	
N-benzoyl-tyrosyl-p-amino benzoic acid test	A normal test excludes pancreatic insufficiency
Secretin/CCK/stimulation test	To confirm pancreatic insufficiency
Glucose tolerance test	To demonstrate diabetes mellitus
5-day stool collection for fat excretion	To demonstrate steatorrhoea as the cause of diarrhoea and as a basis for monitoring treatment
Liver function tests	Raised serum alkaline phosphatase may indicate biliary obstruction

Chapter 45

Liver Function Tests, Jaundice

The liver performs a wide variety of functions. It is composed of complex circulatory system, biliary passages, reticuloendothelial tissue and hepatic cells.

FUNCTIONS OF LIVER

1. *Nutritional metabolism* : Carbohydrate, protein and fat.
2. *Protein synthesis* : Albumin, coagulation factors, complement factors, transferrin, haptoglobin, ceruloplasmin, protease inhibitors (α-antitrypsin), α-fetoprotein.
3. *Formation of bile.*
4. *Formation of urea.*
5. *Cholesterol metabolism.*
6. *Inactivation of some polypeptide hormones.*
7. *Reduction* and *conjugation* of adrenocortical and gonadal steroid hormones.
8. *Synthesis* of 25-hydroxycholecalciferol.
9. *Detoxication* of many drugs and toxins.

LIVER FUNCTION TESTS

A group of tests (Table 45.1) are done which are

Table 45.1
Liver function tests used in assessing disease of liver

Physical basis	Measurements	Assessment
1. **Bilirubin metabolism**	*Serum bilirubin, urine and stool*	Transport : bilirubin, urobilinogen
2. **Serum enzymes**	*Aminotransferases :* AST, ALT *Alkaline phosphatase,* *Gamma glutaryl transferase.*	Hepatocellular damage Biliary obstruction Enzyme induction
3. **Protein metabolism**	*Serum proteins :* Total protein, albumin, globulin *Clotting factors :* Fibrinogen (I), Prothrombin (II), (Factors — V, VII, IX, X).	Synthesis Synthesis
4. **Serum lipids and lipoproteins**	Triglycerides, cholesterol esters, abnormal lipoproteins.	Non-specific indicators
5. **Serological tests** (a) Autoantibodies	*Mitochondrial antibody* *Antinuclear and smooth muscle* antibody	Primary biliary cirrhosis Chronic active hepatitis
(b) Viral antigens and antibodies	*HBA, HBV — antigen and antibody, Delta virus and HCV.*	Viral hepatitis
6. **Liver biopsy**	*Percutaneous needle biopsy*	Diffuse or localised parenchymal disease

useful in revealing or confirming liver disease, in indicating whether hepatic cells or biliary tree is primarily involved, in giving an indication of the extent of liver damage, and in assessment of progress of disease.

BILIRUBIN

Metabolism

When red blood cells are destroyed in the tissue macrophage system, the globin portion is split off. The haem is converted into biliverdin, which is then converted to bilirubin (Fig. 45.1). The iron from the haem is rescued for haemoglobin synthesis. This unconjugated bilirubin is discharged into circulation where it gets bound to albumin; some of it is tightly bound, but most of it can dissociate in liver. Some 250-300 mg of bilirubin is produced daily, most of which are derived from haemoglobin breakdown by Kupffer cells in the liver and other macrophages in the spleen and bone marrow. Small amount is derived from catabolism of other haem-containing proteins, particularly myoglobin, cytochrome enzymes and free haem in liver, and ineffective erythropoiesis in the marrow. Bilirubin normally present in the blood is virtually all unconjugated, and does not pass into urine because it is albumin-bound and insoluble in water.

Bilirubin bound to albumin enters the liver and gets dissociated from albumin at the surface of the hepatocyte by a surface active enzyme (Fig. 45.2). Free bilirubin enters the cell where it is bound to cytoplasmic proteins. Bilirubin is next conjugated to glucuronic acid in a reaction catabolised by the enzyme *glucuronyl transferase* located in the smooth endoplasmic reticulum. Each bilirubin molecule reacts with 2 uridine diphosphoglucuronic acid (UDPGA) molecules to form bilirubin diglucuronide. This glucuronide is water soluble and excreted into the bile. Bilirubin diglucuronides predominate in human bile (70 to 80%), with the isomeric monoglucuronide in small amounts.

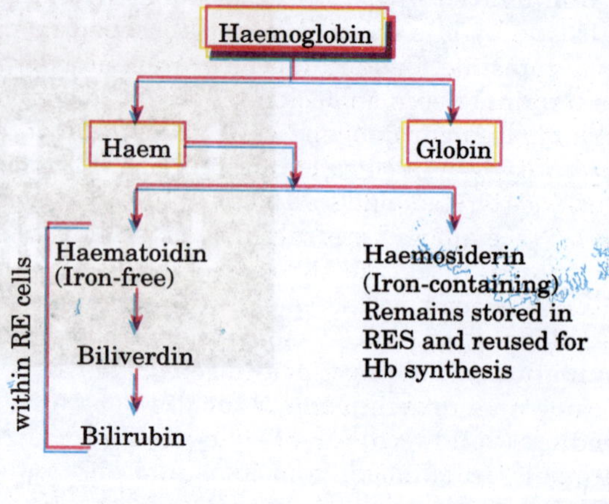

Fig. 45.1. Formation of bilirubin

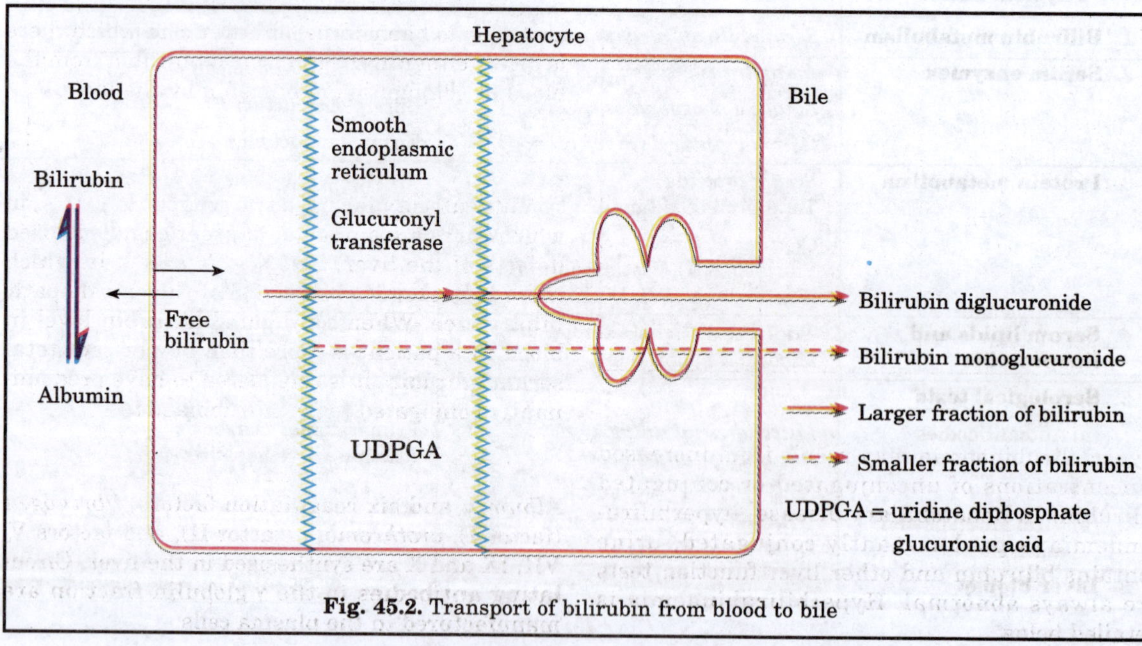

Fig. 45.2. Transport of bilirubin from blood to bile

Conjugated bilirubin is drained into small intestine by bile duct. It is not absorbed in the small intestine. Bacterial fermentation activity in the terminal ileum and colon reduces it to a group of colourless chromogens collectively known as *stercobilinogen* (also called urobilinogen), most of which is excreted along with stool (100 to 200 mg/day). Trace amount stercobilinogen is reabsorbed from large intestine through portal vain and enters the liver, where most are re-excreted in bile; a small amount (4 mg/day) enters systemic circulation and are excreted in the urine where it is known as urobilinogen, which is a colourless product (yellow colour of urine is due to urochrome). Urobilinogen and its oxidation product urobilin in the urine are identical, respectively, with stercobilinogen and its oxidation product, stercobilin, in the faeces. Thus, the total normal plasma bilirubin (less than 1 mg%) includes unconjugated bilirubin plus a small amount of conjugated bilirubin. Differential properties of unconjugated and conjugated bilirubin are shown in Table 45.2.

Table 45.2. Difference between unconjugated and conjugated bilirubin

	Unconjugated (indirect)	*Conjugated* (direct)
1. Structure	Bilirubin	Bilirubin diglucuronide
2. Solubility :		
Water	–	+
Alcohol	+	+
3. V.D.B. reaction	–	+
4. Presence in urine	–	+
5. Diffusibility in tissues	–	+
6. Associated with jaundice :		
Haemolytic	+	–
Obstructive and hepatocellular	+	+

Bilirubinaemia

Hyperbilirubinaemia may result from increased concentrations of unconjugated or conjugated bilirubin. In hepatobiliary disease, hyperbilirubinaemia is predominantly conjugated, urine contains bilirubin and other liver function tests are always abnormal. Hyperbilirubinaemia is detailed below.

JAUNDICE

Clinical jaundice refers to the yellow appearance of the skin, sclerae and mucous membranes resulting from an increased bilirubin concentration in the body fluids. It is detectable clinically when the bilirubin concentration in blood exceeds 2.5 mg/dl. Normal serum bilirubin level is < 1.0 mg%.

Latent jaundice

When the bilirubin level in hyperbilirubinaemia varies between 1.0 to 2.5 mg/100 ml serum, clinical jaundice does not appear, which is called latent jaundice.

Shunt hyperbilirubinaemia

It is a state of hyperbilirubinaemia which develops due to defective metabolism of haem associated with ineffective erythropoiesis in bone marrow as found in pernicious anaemia and thalassaemia.

Classification

Recent classification divides hyperbilirubinaemia into *unconjugated* hyperbilirubinaemia and *conjugated* hyperbilirubinaemia (Table 45.3).

1. Unconjugated hyperbilirubinaemia

The unconjugated category includes the forms of jaundice in which 80 to 85 per cent of total serum bilirubin is unconjugated (indirect). This may be prehepatic with excess bilirubin production due to haemolysis, or hepatic, in which there is defect either in the removal of bilirubin from the blood or conjugation of bilirubin by the liver.

2. Conjugated hyperbilirubinaemia

This category includes two groups : **hepatic**, in which there are a number of genetic and acquired defects of the liver, and **posthepatic**, in which there is anatomic obstruction of the extrahepatic biliary tree. When conjugated bilirubin level in blood in a patient is more than 50 per cent total serum bilirubin, it is considered to have predominantly conjugated hyperbilirubinaemia.

PLASMA PROTEINS

Albumin and six coagulation factors, *fibrinogen* (factor I), *prothrombin* (factor II), and factors V, VII, IX and X are synthesised in the liver. Circulating antibodies in the γ globulin fraction are manufactured in the plasma cells.

Table 45.3
Classification of Jaundice

Classification of hyperbilirubinaemia	*Physiologic defect*	*Etiology*	*Test of bilirubin metabolism*			
			Direct (% of total bilirubin)	Urine bilirubin	Urobilinogen	Faecal urobilinogen
Unconjugated						
Pre-hepatic	Excessive production of bilirubin	Haemolytic states	< 20	–	(↑)	↑
Hepatic	(a) Defective transport of bilirubin from sinusoidal blood into hepatocyte	1. Gilbert's disease 2. Certain toxins (Flavaspidic acid)	< 20	–	N	N/–
	(b) Inability to conjugate	1. Crigler-Najjar syndrome 2. Neonatal jaundice 3. Certain drugs (e.g., Novobiocin)	< 20	–	N	N/–
Conjugated						
Hepatic	(a) Hepatocellular : Hepatocyte injury	1. Viral or toxic hepatitis 2. Cirrhosis 3. Alcoholic hepatitis 4. Other causes of hepatocyte injury	> 40	+	N, ↑, or ↓	↓
	(b) Cholestatic : intrahepatic cirrhosis due to defective transport of bilirubin into canaliculus	1. Some drugs (e.g. chlorpromazine, anabolic steroids) 2. Viral hepatitis 3. Primary biliary cirrhosis 4. Some forms of family jaundice	> 50	+	N, ↑, or ↓	↓
Post–hepatic	Mechanical obstruction of biliary tree	1. Carcinoma of pancreas 2. Carcinoma of common bile duct 3. Gall stone 4. Other anatomic obstruction	> 50	+	↓	↓

Key: N = normal, ↑ = elevated, ↓ = depressed, + = positive

While interpreting serum protein levels, three important caveats should be kept in view :

1. They are neither early or sensitive indicators of disease of liver because of substantial hepatic reserve and their half-life.

2. They are not of much help in differential diagnosis of liver disease.

3. Decreases in serum levels of these proteins are not specific for liver disease.

(a) *Albumin*

Albumin is synthesised solely in the liver at a rate of 100 to 200 mg per kg body weight per day. Normal plasma/serum albumin level ranges from 3.5 to 5.5 gm/100 ml. Plasma albumin concentration is frequently low in chronic liver disease, especially cirrhosis. Synthesis of albumin is impaired by a variety of other non-hepatic factors such as malnutrition, hormonal factors, plasma osmotic pressure and toxins (ethanol, carbon tetrachloride). Nonetheless, hypoalbuminaemia usually detects patients with more severe liver damage and a falling concentration provides an excellent indication of the severity of chronic liver disease when there is no ascites. Albumin has a fairly long half-life (20-26 days) with less than 5% turnover daily. It is, therefore, not a good indicator of acute or mild liver injury. Thus, plasma albumin level remains normal even in severe acute hepatitis unless the illness continues for many weeks.

(b) *Globulin*

Plasma globulins are a heterogeneous group of proteins whose production in a variety of tissues is influenced by a number of factors. Plasma/serum globulins (normal 2 to 3.5 gm/100 ml) include α, β and γ globulins; they γ globulin is immunoglobulin. It is characteristic of chronic liver disease that hyperglobulinaemia occurs in addition to hypoalbuminaemia. Increase occurs most often of the γ globulins.

Mechanisms of hyperglobulinaemia

Hyperglobulinaemia may also be found in prolonged viral hepatitis or chronic hepatitis, irrespective of changes in plasma albumin concentration. The causes of hyperglobulinaemia in liver diseases are not fully understood; increases in γ globulin are prominent and probably is multifactorial reflecting an increased activity of the immune system.

Elevated plasma globulin states

1. *Mild to moderate rise* : Prolonged viral hepatitis or chronic hepatitis.
2. *Moderate rise* (3-5 gm/dl) : Alcoholic and biliary cirrhosis.
3. *Highly increased* (4-8 gm/dl) : Macronodular cirrhosis and chronic active hepatitis (CAH).

Immunoelectrophoresis

1. *IgG* is predominantly elevated in CAH, cryptogenic cirrhosis and subacute viral hepatitis.
2. *IgA* is elevated mainly in alcoholic cirrhosis, and
3. *IgM* in primary biliary cirrhosis.

Albumin-globulin ratio

Normal albumin : globulin ratio of 2-2.5 : 1 is altered to 0.75-1 : 1 in chronic liver diseases.

Coagulation factor

The liver synthesises six coagulation factors : I, II, V, VII, IX and X, and requires vitamin K to activate factors II, VII, IX and X.

Prothrombin time (PT)

Reduced concentration of coagulation factors occur in liver damage, which is detected by prolonged prothrombin time (PT) (Quick one stage method). The prothrombin conversion to thrombin in the presence of thromboplastin depends on most of the vitamin K-dependent clotting factors, and prothrombin time prolongs when the plasma concentration of any of these factors falls below 30% of normal. Deficiencies of active vitamin K results in increased PT. These processes can be differentiated from hepatic synthetic failure by demonstrating normal PT (within 24-48 hours) after parenteral injection of vitamin K.

Causes of increased PT

(i) Acute and chronic liver damage.

(ii) Prolonged biliary obstruction which reduces vitamin K absorption.

(iii) Poor dietary intake of vitamin K.

(iv) Antibiotic therapy.

(v) Use of warfarin type anticoagulants.

Importance

These proteins have a shorter half-life (5-72

hours) than that of albumin. Prothrombin is an earlier indicator than serum albumin level of severe liver damage. PT is a most valuable prognostic indicator in both acute (viral hepatitis) and chronic hepatitis. An increasing prothrombin time signifies a progressive disease with worse prognosis.

SERUM ENZYMES

A large number of serum enzymes are found in normal serum or plasma, which comes from the tissues. Liver cells also contain many enzymes which are released into the blood in various pathological states. They have been used to distinguish and assess hepatocellular injury and biliary tract dysfunction and obstruction (Table 45.4). However, they have inherent limitations in sensitivity and specificity as elevations of enzymes occur also in non-hepatic disorders. Nonetheless, with proper and careful interpretation, several serum enzymes provide important clinical tools.

Table 45.4
Abnormalities of tests of enzymes and proteins of liver function

Test	Type of liver disease	
	Obstructive	*Parenchymal*
AST and ALT (SGOT and SGPT)	+	++++
Alkaline phosphatase	+++	+
Albumin	Normal	Decreased
Prothrombin time	Normal, slightly increased	Markedly raised
Bilirubin	Normal or +++	Normal or +++
γ-Glutamyl transcriptase (GGT)	+++	Normal or +++
5'nucleotidase	++++	Normal or +

Aminotransferases (transaminases)

These enzymes catalyse the transfer of amino groups of alanine and aspartate to α-ketoglutarate. Alanine aminotransferase (ALT), a cytochrome enzyme, and aspartate aminotransferase (AST), present both in cytoplasm and mitochondria, are two important aminotransferases, and their activities have proven most useful. Based on the end products of reaction, oxaloacetic acid and pyruvic acid, ALT is also named as SGOT and AST as SGPT respectively.

(i) *Normal* serum contains low level of both ALT and AST (less than 30 U/L), but their source of origin is not clear.

(ii) Neither enzyme is specific to the liver, but ALT is found primarily in the liver and AST is present in many tissues, including heart, skeletal muscle, kidney and brain, and consequently increased serum ALT activity reflects liver damage more specifically.

Increased transaminase levels in blood is assumed to reflect leaking from the liver cells, and increased plasma enzyme activity is a very sensitive index of the hepatic damage.

(iii) *Striking elevations* (10-200-fold increase) of ALT and AST are found in extensive hepatic necrosis, such as viral hepatitis, carbon tetrachloride poisoning, drug-induced injury (Table 45.4). Abnormal levels of AST are also seen in myocardial and skeletal necrosis, but ALT elevations are absent or slight in diseases that do not involve liver.

(iv) In *viral hepatitis* the transaminase activity reaches maximal levels of 10 to 100 times the normal value usually early in the jaundiced phase after which activity falls rapidly. Hepatic damage due to paracetamol also causes high activities of 100 to 500 times the normal level.

(v) *Modest transaminase* elevations (10 to 50 fold) are seen in post-hepatic jaundice, intrahepatic cholestasis.

(vi) *Minimal elevations* occur in biliary tract obstruction; higher levels suggest the development of cholangitis. They are even lower (less than 10-fold) in most patients with metastatic carcinoma, cirrhosis or alcoholic hepatitis. In alcoholic hepatitis the AST/ALT ratio may be greater than 2; this is probably due to a reduction in the hepatic ALT content due to a deficiency in the cofactor pyridoxine-5-phosphate.

Alkaline phosphatase

This enzyme is situated principally in the plasma membranes of canalicular and sinusoidal liver cells. This enzyme of uncertain physiologic function hydrolyses synthetic phsophate esters at pH 9.0.

Normal level: Blood normally contains 4-11 KA (King and Armstrong) units/100 ml serum (20-130 U/L) alkaline phosphatase which is mainly derived from bone and liver, and to a lesser extent intestine; in pregnancy additional activity or placental origin is found.

Elevated level : In absence of bone disease and pregnancy, elevated levels of alkaline phosphate activity usually reflect the following :

(a) *Greatly increased in blood* : Biliary tract obstruction, where new alkaline phosphatase is synthesised by hepatocytes and biliary tract epithelium. Bile acids may be responsible in both by inducing synthesis and promoting solubilisation of the membrane associated enzyme activity.

A striking rise (3 to 10 times normal) of the enzyme occurs with extrahepatic biliary tract (mechanical) obstruction or with intra-hepatic functional cholestasis, as seen in drug-induced cholestasis or primary biliary cirrhosis (Table 45.4).

(b) *Slightly to moderate increase* : A 1-2 times normal enzyme activity is seen in many patients with acute or chronic hepatocellular disease. Transient rise may occur in all types of liver disease.

Gamma-glutamyl transferase (GGT)

GGT, a microsomal enzyme widely distributed in body tissue, catalyses the transfer of the γ-glutamyl group from peptides such as glutathione to other amino acids and may play a role in amino acid transport.

Increased level of GGT

Increased GGT level correlates with alkaline phosphatase levels :

1. GGT activity is highest in biliary obstruction.
2. Moderate rise is seen in alcoholic hepatitis.
3. It also rises in pancreatic, cardiac, renal and pulmonary disorders and diabetes.

OTHER LIVER FUNCTION TESTS

I. Special protein tests

1. ***Turbidity and flocculation tests*** : A large number of tests reflecting abnormality of plasma proteins have been developed, called flocculation tests (Table 45.5). These tests are rarely performed nowadays.

Comments : Abnormal result is seen in intrinsic hepatic disease, e.g., hepatitis, cirrhosis and normal in patients with obstructive jaundice.

Table 45.5
Flocculation test

Test	*Precipitating reagent*	*Protein responsible*
Cephalin flocculation	Cephalin cholesterol emulsion	γ-globulin
Thymol turbidity	Supersaturated solution thymol	γ (β)
Colloidal gold	Colloidal gold	γ
Zinc sulphate turbidity	$ZnSO_4$	γ

2. ***α-fetoprotein*** : α-fetoprotein is an α_1-globulin. It is present (2-3 μg/l) in an appreciable amount in the serum of the foetus, infant and normal pregnant female. In non-pregnant state, high values above 20 μg/l are found in association with a variety of tumours, especially 90% of hepatomas and 80% of teratomas. It can be determined by radioimmunoassay.

3. ***Ceruloplasmin*** : It is a copper binding protein present in low concentration (less than 100 mg/l) in the newborn and increases slowly to adult values of 150-600 mg/l by about the age of 12. It is of chief interest in differentiating Wilson's disease in which ceruloplasmin concentration is low, from chronic active liver disease in which it is increased.

II. Bromsulphthalein test

Several dyes including bromsulphthalein (BSP) and indocyanine green are taken up by the liver and excreted in the bile. Estimation of BSP clearance from the blood is a sensitive test for liver dysfunction but is rarely practised nowadays.

BSP in a dose of 2 mg dye/kg body weight is given intravenously and blood is collected from opposite arm after 25 and 45 minutes of injection. Normally, most of the BSP is excreted in 25 minutes, less than 15% being left at that time. In Dubin-Johnson syndrome, a higher value obtained at 120 minutes confirms the diagnosis.

III. Carbohydrate metabolism

Glucose tolerance test shows abnormality in cirrhosis liver with a rapid rise of plasma glucose to values above the upper normal limit with a slow return to normal.

IV. Lipid metabolism

1. *Cholesterol* : In general, the serum cholesterol

level is decreased or normal in hepatocellular jaundice and elevated in obstructive jaundice.

2. *Triglyceride* : Triglyceride level in plasma is increased in obstructive jaundice, fatty liver, alcoholic patients with haemolytic anaemia and hyperlipemia.

V. Serological tests

1. ***Hepatitis A virus*** : The virus HAV cannot be grown readily. Early in the disease (7-10 days), HAV can be demonstrated in the faeces by immuno-electron microscopy or by immuno-fluorescent techniques. This has got little clinical value since the virus has already disappeared from the faeces by the time hepatitis appears. However, antibody to HAV is found early in the clinical illness, and certainly by the time jaundice develops. Mere presence of anti-HAV is not enough for diagnosis since HAV infection being common to all communities and anti-HAV antibodies persists for years after primary infection. It is diagnostic only when anti-HAV of IgM type is detected, which indicates a primary immune response of recent infection. The titres of this antibody gradually fall to low levels after about 3 months. Measurements of anti-HAV (IgG) is required before administering immuno-globulins to travellers going abroad and to study incidence of HAV infection.

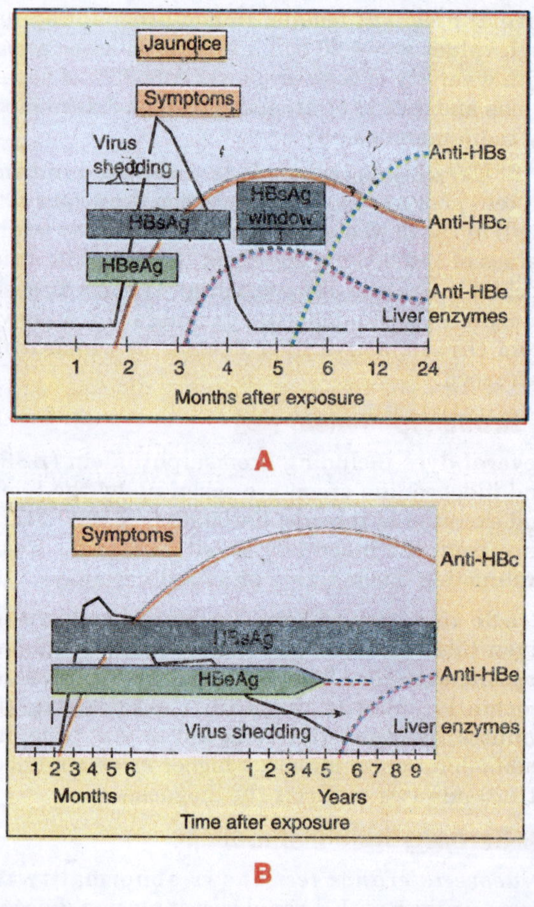

Fig. 45.3. Humoral responses in hepatitis B infections (see text). (A) With clinical recovery and viral elimination, (B) Chronic infection with continued viral replications. ALT, alanine aminotransferase. Units on the vertical axis are arbitrary

2. ***Hepatitis B virus*** : Hepatitis B virus (HBV) contains several antigens to which an infected individual can make immune responses. The important antigens and antibodies of HBV useful in identifying hepatitis B viral infection are shown in Table 45.6 and Fig. 45.3.

Table 45.6
Interpretation of serological tests used in the diagnosis of hepatitis B virus infection

Interpretation	*HBs Ag*	Anti-HBc *IgM*	Anti-HBc *IgG*	*Anti-HBs*
Incubation period	+	+	–	–
Acute hepatitis				
Early	+	+	–	–
Established	+	+	+	–
Established (occasional)	–	+	+	–
Convalescence	–	+	+	+
Post-infection				
> 1 year	–	–	+	+
Uncertain	–	–	+	–
Chronic infection				
Usual	+	±	+	–
Occasional	–	–	+	–
Immunisation				
Without infection	–	–	–	+

A. Acute infection

(i) *HBs Ag* : It is a reliable marker of HBV infection, a negative test makes hepatitis B virus infection very unlikely but not impossible. It appears in blood late in the incubation period and usually lasts for 3-4 weeks and may persist up to 3 months. However, HBs Ag may be present only for a few days, and may disappear even before jaundice has developed.

(ii) *Anti-HBs Ag* : Antibody to HBs Ag usually appears at the end of 3 months and persists for many years or perhaps permanently. Presence of anti-HBs Ag indicates that infection has occurred at some time (in which case anti-HBc is usually also present) or that the individual has been vaccinated.

(iii) *HBc Ag and anti-HBc* : Hepatitis B core antigen is not found in blood, but anti-HBc appears early in infection, which rapidly attains a high titre and then falls gradually and persists. Initially, anti-HBc is of IgM type and later it is of IgG type.

Sometimes anti-HBc can reveal an acute HBV infection when the HBs Ag antigen has disappeared and before the appearance of anti-HBs antibody, HBc Ag appears only transiently at the outset of the illness, which is followed by anti-HBc production. The presence of HBc Ag in serum reflects active replication of HBV.

B. Chronic infection

Chronic hepatitis B virus infection is marked by the presence of HBs Ag and anti-HBc (IgG) in the plasma. Anti-HBc (IgG) is rarely the sole evidence of chronic B hepatitis infection. Presence of anti-HBc in serum indicates that the replication of the virus is taking place at a much lower rate or that the DNA of the virus has become integrated into the hepatocyte DNA.

3. ***Delta virus*** : Hepatitis D virus contains a single antigen (delta antigen), which appears in the blood only transiently, and, in practice, HDV infection is diagnosed on the basis of presence of anti-delta antibody. Simultaneous infection (co-infection) of HBV and HDV followed by full recovery is associated with the appearance of low titres of anti-delta antibody of IgM type within a few days of the onset of the illness. IgM antibody disappears in about two months, but persists in a few patients.

Superinfection of HBV infected patient by HDV leads to production of high titres of anti-delta, initally IgM and later IgG. This type of patient may then develop chronic hepatitis with both the viruses, in such a case the titres of anti-delta reach high values.

4. ***Non-A, non-B virus (HCV, HEV)*** : Antibody to polypeptide component of HCV and HEV appears in the blood and can be detected in sophisticated laboratories.

VI. Autoantibodies

So far three autoantibodies in respect of liver disease have been detected in the serum :

1. *Antinuclear antibody*
2. *Anti-smooth muscle antibody*
3. *Antimitochondrial antibody.*

These autoantibodies are also found in some healthy individuals (5-10%), but their titres are usually low. Antinuclear antibodies also appear in blood in connective tissue diseases and autoimmune diseases.

Anti-smooth-muscle antibody and to a lesser extent antinuclear antibody may appear transiently in blood at a low titre in acute viral hepatitis, but they are present for long periods at relatively high titres in chronic liver disease. Antimitochondrial antibody is strongly associated with primary biliary cirrhosis and autoimmune disease. Since none of the autoantibodies damages hepatic tissue, they may not have any etiological importance.

VII. Liver biopsy

Needle biopsy of the liver is an useful tool to diagnose the cause of hepatocellular jaundice and of hepatomegaly and in demonstrating the presence of cirrhosis, alcoholic hepatitis, chronic hepatitis, biliary cirrhosis and carcinoma.

Chapter 46

Renal Function Tests

The progress of renal diseases can be ascertained based on the findings of azotaemia, proteinuria, hypertension, oedema, abnormal urinalysis, electrolyte disorders, abnormal urine values or infection. With the introduction of ultrasonography and other measures, the kidney function tests of the older days are of less significance.

Table 46.1 shows the list of laboratory investigations in disorders of kidney and urinary tracts.

Glomerular functions

The glomerulus is a network of capillaries surrounded by Bowman's capsule, which is an extension of the basement membrane and connective tissue of the proximal convoluted tubule (Fig. 46.1).

Glomerular filtration is the process whereby a fluid, that resembles plasma, passes across the glomerular membrane by bulk flow or diffusion. The glomerular filtration rate (GFR) in an average-sized normal man is approximately 125 ml per minute.

Tubular functions

The filtrate thus formed passes through the tubule and is modified according to the requirement of body by selective reabsorption of its constitutents and tubular secretion. About 180 litres of water are filtered normally in 24-hours through the glomeruli of kidney, while the output of urine is only 1.0 to 1.5 litres. Thus, 98-99% of filtered water is reabsorbed through the tubules; about 85% of this in proximal tubules. Dissolved solids are selectively reabsorbed by the tubular cells. Substances such as :

Table 46.1
Laboratory investigations in disorders of kidney and urinary tract

Physical basis	Measurement
R. E. urine	*Volume* / 24-hr. *Chemical exam / Dipstix* : Protein, Glucose, blood, bile, urobilinogen. *Microscopy* : RBC, WBC, Casts.
Special tests on urine	*Quantitative culture* : MSU or urine aspirated from bladder. *Urine pH* : Urine acidification after administration of NH_4Cl or $CaCl_2$. *Urine sp.gr.* or *osmolality* (Na^+, K^+, BUN, etc.). *Overnight concentration test.* *Water loading test.* 24-hour *protein excretion* (Esbach's test) *Protein / creatinine ratio.* *Protein selectivity*
Exam. of blood to assess renal function	*Blood* : Urea, creatinine, Na^+, K^+, calcium, phosphate, uric acid, H^+, HCO_3^-, Pa_{CO_2}. Creatinine clearance, insulin clearance (measurement of GFR). 24-hour *output* : Na^+, K^+, Calcium, phosphate, urea, amino acids.

(i) Glucose, amino acids, sodium and calcium are actively reabsorbed to a great extent.

(ii) Phosphates and sulphates are reabsorbed to a less extent.

(iii) Potassium and uric acid are both reabsorbed and secreted.

(iv) Besides free glomerular filtration, creatinine in man is also actively secreted by renal tubular cells in minimal amounts, that results in overestimation of true GFR when compared to inulin clearance.

(v) Urea is passively reabsorbed.

Based on above facts, the renal function tests are conveniently divided into three groups : (i) *renal blood flow,* (ii) *glomerular filtration* and (iii) *renal tubular activity.*

KIDNEY FUNCTION TESTS

The important renal function tests include : (a) tests for renal blood flow, (b) tests for glomerular filtration and tests for tubular function. With the introduction of IVP, ultrasonography and scanning, these renal function tests have lost significance excepting the test for glomerular filtration rate and concentration test for tubular function.

A. Tests for Renal Blood Flow

Fifteen-minute P.S.P. (Phenolsulphonephthalein) excretion test

Phenolsulphonephthalein (phenol red) is mainly excreted by the tubules and PSP test is a simpler

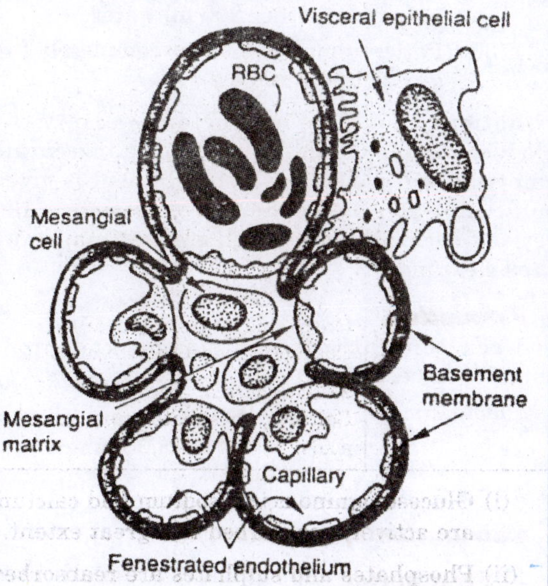

Fig. 46.1. Glomerular lobule in cross section

measurement of secretory ability of kidney and renal plasma flow. This test is no more done nowadays.

Reagents

1. Phenol red, 6 mg/ml in water in sterile ampoules.
2. Sodium hydroxide, 10%.

Technique

1. Breakfast is withheld.
2. Have the patient drink 500 ml water.
3. After 20 to 30 minutes inject intravenously exactly 1 ml phenol red solution (6 mg) avoiding extravasation into the tissues.
4. Collect urine specimen at exactly 15 min, 30 min, 60 min and 120 min, after injection in 500 ml, 250 ml and 100 ml volumetric flasks, respectively.

Estimation of PSP

(a) Add a few ml of 10% sodium hydroxide to the urine until maximum colour (reddish purple) develops and make to the marks with water.

(b) As a standard, add 1 ml 6% phenol red solution to 400 to 500 ml water in a litre volumetric flask. Add 5 ml 10% sodium hydroxide as above. Phenol red (an indicator) turns reddish purple on addition of alkali. Then add distilled water to the mark.

The diluted specimens are compared with artificial standards colorimetrically at 540 nm against a water blank, or visually.

Calculation

A standard curve can be prepared from the diluted standard (S).

% PSP in any specimen (T = test)

$$= \frac{T \times \text{volume of specimen in ml}}{S \times 1000}$$

For visual comparison, 6 test tubes of equal bore are taken and the standard is diluted as follows :

P. C. phenol red (PSP)	0%	20%	40%	60%	80%	100%
ml Standard (6 mg/litre)	0	2	4	6	8	10
ml dist. water	10	8	6	4	2	0

Interpretation

Volume of urine after 15 min should be over 100 ml, otherwise dye containing urine remaining in bladder results in a falsely low value.

1. Normal kidney excretes 30 to 50% of the dye during the first 15 min.

2. Excretion of less than 23% of the dye during the 1st 15 min, regardless of the amount excreted in 2-hour period, indicates impaired kidney function since the 15-min urine specimen is one of primary importance.

B. Tests for Glomerular Filtration Rate

Glomerular filtration is studied by estimating the concentration of a substance in both blood and minute volume of urine simultaneously. The formula of calculating renal clearance is given below :

$$\text{Clearance (ml / min)} = \frac{\text{U (mg / dl)}}{\text{P (mg / dl)}} \times \text{V (ml / min)}$$

U = concentration of measured substance in urine.

P = concentration of same substance in plasma.

V = urine volume expressed as ml/min.

If a small molecular substance in plasma passes freely through the glomerular filter, and is neither reabsorbed nor excreted by the tubules, the amount excreted in urine (UV) is identical with the quantity filtered by the glomeruli. The renal clearance of such a substance, therefore, equals the glomerular filtration rate (GFR). *Inulin,* a polysaccharide with Mol. wt. 5,100, is an ideal substance to measure GFR as it appears to be excreted in this way. The GFR for inulin is 120 ml/min. Inulin clearance test is commonly done in experimental conditions. It is not routinely employed in clinical practice because of the necessity of continuous intravenous infusion. In clinical practice the clearance of an endogenous substance creatinine, which approximates to that of inulin, is usually measured. The *urea clearance* test is also done in measuring GFR.

I. Urea clearance test

Urea — the nitrogen containing waste product of protein metabolism — is filtered by the glomerulus and then a portion (about 40%) is reabsorbed by the tubules. The ratio between the urea content of blood and the quantity of urea excreted remains constant regardless of the blood urea level when urine flow is 2 ml or more per minute. In normal kidney, this is equivalent to the excretion per minute of the amount of urea in 75 ml of blood. This figure is called *maximal clearance* (C_m).

When the urine flow is less than 2 ml/minute, the rate of excretion of urea in relation to the blood urea level decreases in proportion to the square root of the urine volume. Normally, this is equivalent to the excretion per minute of urea in 54 ml of blood, which is called the *standard clearance* (C_s).

These values for maximal clearance (75 ml) and for standard clearance (54 ml) are regarded as 100%. Kidney function and the findings are expressed as percentage of these figures in any urea clearance test. According to Van Slyke, the normal range is 75-130%.

Test procedure

The test is traditionally carried out during a 2-hour period following a normal breakfast between 9 a.m. to 12 noon. Two accurately timed specimens of urine over 1 hour periods and a venous blood sample in mid-point are collected. The concentration of urea in plasma and urine is measured. The following protocol is usually followed :

0925	Patient drinks 200-400 ml water.
0930	Patient empties bladder completely, urine is discarded.
1030	Patient again empties bladder completely to give urine (sample 1).
1035	Take a specimen of blood and give the patient a further 200 ml water.
1130	Patient empties bladder completely to give urine (sample 2).

Patient should be instructed to empty the bladder completely during test since inaccurate emptying will yield false result. Patient is given sufficient water before the test to promote a diuresis of over 2 ml/min which ensures maximum urea clearance.

Estimation

Urea concentration of plasma and urine samples are estimated colorimetrically, say

Plasma urea	24.0 mg%
Urine 1 (58 min)	95 ml, urea 350 mg%
Urine 2 (62 min)	165 ml, urea 312 mg%.

Calculation of urea clearance

(i) **First period** (applying the standard clearance formula, as the per unit excretion of urine is less than 2 ml).

Standard urea clearance (C_s)

$= (U/B) \times \sqrt{V} = (350/24) \times \sqrt{(95/58)}$

$= 14.58 \times \sqrt{1.638}$

$= 14.58 \times 1.28 = 18.66.$

Per cent of normal clearance

$= C_s/54 \times 100 = (18.66/54) \times 100$

$= 34.55\%.$

(ii) **Second period** (applying the maximum clearance formula, as the per unit excretion of urine is 2 ml or more than 2 ml).

Maximal clearance (C_m)

$= (U/B) \times V = (312/24) \times (165/62)$

$= 13 \times 2.66 = 34.58,$

where U = urine urea mg per 100 ml, B = blood urea mg per 100 ml, and V = volume of urine excreted as ml per minute.

Per cent normal clearance

$= (C_m/75) \times 100 = (34.58/75) \times 100$

$= 46.10\%.$

II. Creatinine clearance test

Creatinine, a degradation product of creatine, is formed by a relatively constant rate by muscle, which is the principal storage site of creatine phosphate. Thus, production and excretion of creatine is directly related to muscle mass. Creatinine clearance is near to the GFR as measured by inulin clearance. Besides free glomerular filtration of creatinine, small amount is also secreted by tubules. Measurement of the 24-hour excretion of creatinine is done.

Procedure

(1) A 24-hour urine specimen, such as 7 a.m. to 7 a.m. next day is collected.

(2) Blood sample collected for serum creatinine estimation.

(3) Serum and urine creatinine concentrations are determined.

Calculation of creatinine clearance

$C_{creatinine} = (U/P) \times V,$

where U = urine creatinine concentration in gm/ litre, P = serum creatinine concentration in mg per 100 ml ÷ 100, V = 24-hour urine volume in ml ÷ 1000.

Interpretation

The average normal 24-hour endogenous creatinine clearance is 170 litre for an adult male.

III. Inulin and p-aminohippurate (PAH) clearance tests

Inulin and PAH are absent from normal blood and are completely filtrable by glomerulus and are not reabsorbed or secreted by the tubules. Combination of inulin for GFR and PAH for renal plasma flow is used. The test has a disadvantage that estimation of inulin is an intricate procedure.

Procedure

(1) An initial intravenous dose is followed by continuous I.V. infusion or

(2) A large dose is injected subcutaneously into the loose tissue of axilla. It is a less satisfactory method.

Materials

(1) Inulin injection, BP, a sterile 10% solution of inulin in saline, pH 5.5 to 6.5. When deposit is formed on storage, it is redissolved completely by heating for 15-20 minutes. After cooling, the injection should be given at once.

(2) Sodium p-aminohippurate injection, USP, 20% (Merck) is a sterile solution in water at pH 7 to 7.6.

(3) Injectable normal saline (0.9% NaCl).

(4) *Priming solution* : An amount of 30 ml of insulin injectable is mixed with 4 ml of sodium PAH aseptically in a syringe.

(5) *Maintenance solution* : Remove 90 ml of saline from a saline infusion bottle of 500 ml and replace by 70 ml inulin injection and 20 ml sodium PAH injection aseptically.

(6) *Mixture for subcutaneous injection*

Inulin injection — 50 to 75 ml
Sodium PAH injection — 10 ml
Injection lignocaine (2%) — 5 ml.

These are mixed in a large syringe with aseptic precautions.

Technique

1. **Fasting is unnecessary**. Patient is given a litre of water to drink during the hour before test starts.

2. A bladder catheter is introduced and urine is allowed to drain continuously. A venous canula is

then inserted and a sample of blood is collected. The blood sample and portion of urine act as blanks.

3. **In the infusion technique**, the priming solution is injected intravenously through the canula over a few minutes. This is followed by a sustaining infusion through the canula at about 4 ml/min.

After 30 min of the sustaining infusion, three accurately timed urine specimens are collected, each of 20-min duration. At the end of each collection, the bladder is rinsed with 20 ml of sterile normal saline and 20 ml of air.

Blood specimens are drawn from opposite arm 3 min before midpoint of each urine collection.

4. **In single dose axillary subcutaneous injection**, the solution is slowly introduced over several minutes. After one hour, three accurately timed urine specimens and blood samples are collected as in infusion technique.

5. **Determination** of inulin and PAH in plasma and urine is made colorimetrically.

Calculation of inulin or PAH clearance

C_{Inulin} or $C_{PAH} = (U/P) \times V$.

It is corrected to a standard body surface area of 1.73 sq. m.

Interpretation

Diminished urea, creatinine and inulin clearance result from impairment of glomerular filtration due to :

1. Alteration of glomerular basement membrane with reduction of GFR occurs in glomerulonephritis.

2. Reduction of GFR also occurs due to decreased renal blood flow as in hypertensive nephrosclerosis.

C. Tests for Tubular Function

Diminished tubular function results from renal ischaemia, direct action of substances on tubular cells and biochemical defects impairing transfer of substances across tubular cells. An early sign of impaired tubular function is decreasing ability to secrete a concentrated urine.

Arteriolar nephrosclerosis, or other diseases diminishing blood flow in kidney, causes inability of kidney to concentrate or dilute the urine with resultant *isosthenuria* (fixation of sp. gr. at 1.010). The concentration test is simple and useful in evaluating the ability of tubules to handle water.

A. Concentration test

Principle : This test of impairment of water reabsorption is based on the ability of tubule to concentrate urine. Impairment of concentrating ability occurs early in renal disease (e.g., arteriolar nephrosclerosis and interstitial nephritis), but the diluting capacity is also affected later in renal disease.

Contraindication : The concentration test should not be undertaken in patients with significant nitrogen retention (high blood urea and creatinine), as that may precipitate symptoms of uraemia.

Tests for concentrating capacity

There are several techniques for performing the concentration test to measure the solute concentration of urine and specific gravity.

Water deprivation :

1. **Maximum concentration** is attained when the patient is deprived of water for 24 hours. Such a long deprivation of water is not only unpleasant but also dangerous for some patients. The specific gravity of urine passed during last 12 hours should not be less than 1.022 but may increase up to 1.040 in normal young adults.

2. **Examination of single random specimen** : According to de Wardener, if specific gravity of random urine (especially the first one passed in the morning on wakening after withdrawal of fluid during night) is above 1.018, it is most unlikely that the water deprivation test will show an abnormally low result.

3. **Fishberg concentration test** : It is the frequently used test. In this technique, the specific gravity of normal urine is 1.023 or higher in one or more specimens.

Procedure :

(i) Patient takes a good protein meal at 6 p.m. with not more than 200 ml water;

(ii) Patient is allowed no fluids from 8 p.m. until 10 a.m. next morning;

(iii) Discard the night urine;

(iv) Collect urine next day at 8 a.m. and 10 a.m. and determine specific gravity and osmolality (a measure of the number of dissolved solute particles in solution).

4. **Tests using posterior pituitary extract**: ADH is less effective in impaired tubular function.

Procedure

(i) Patient is allowed no fluids from 18-00 hr to 10-00 hr in the following day.

(ii) Inject 5 units vasopressin tannate in oil subcutaneously at 20-00 hr and the bladder is emptied at 22-00 hr.

(iii) Specific gravity of urine passed at 20-00 hr on the second day is determined.

Interpretation

A specific gravity over 1.020 or higher is considered normal and lower value indicates renal damage. The test is contraindicated in hypertensive and late kidney diseases.

B. Dilution test

It is less sensitive than concentration test. Loss of capacity to dilute urine is a later consequence of renal damage. It is contraindicated in cardiac failure or incipient renal failure.

Procedure

1. Patient withholds breakfast.
2. Patient drinks 1200 ml water during an interval of 30 minutes.
3. Urine is collected hourly thereafter for 4 hours.

Interpretation

1. In normal individual, 1200 ml urine is excreted during the 4 hr. period.
2. Largest part is passed during first 2 hours. Specific gravity of one of the sample of urine should fall to 1.003.
3. In kidney disease with functional impairment, (a) quantity of urine voided in the 4 hr. period is much smaller and (b) specific gravity of urine may not fall below 1.010.

AZOTEMIA

Azote literally means nitrogen. The term *azotemia* refers to any significant increase in the plasma concentration of non-protein nitrogenous compounds, principally urea and creatinine. The principal conditions in which blood urea nitrogen (BUN)) may be increased are the same as those for creatinine.

Acute renal failure (ARF)

It is a syndrome characterised by an acute and usually reversible deterioration of renal function which develops over a period of days, or, rarely, weeks and retention of nitrogenous waste products (BUN, creatinine), called *azotemia*. In oliguria — a rate of urine flow less than 400 ml/24 hr — is usual but not invariable. Many of the disorders giving rise to ARF carry a high mortality due to their severe nature, but when the patient survives, renal function usually returns to normal or near normal. ARF is divided into three categories for the purpose of diagnosis and management : *pre-renal, renal* and *post-renal* azotemia or acute renal failure.

Pre-renal azotemia (pre-renal ARF)

The kidneys are inadequately perfused (hypoperfusion) in which the kidney is intrinsically normal. It is responsible for about 50% incidence.

Causes

1. *Absolute decrease in relative volume* : Haemorrhage due to trauma; GIT bleeding; loss of plasma as in burns and crushing injuries; renal fluid loss (diuretics, diabetes mellitus).
2. *Relative decrease in blood volume* (ineffective arterial volume) : Congestive heart failure, dehydration, septic shock, liver failure.
3. *Arterial occlusion* : Thrombosis of arteries, occlusive embolism of the aorta or renal arteries, aortic aneurysm.

Intrarenal azotemia

Causes

1. *Renovascular obstruction* : Renal artery obstruction, atherosclerotic plaque, malignant hypertension, eclampsia.
2. *Glomerulus* : Acute glomerulonephritis.
3. *Tubules* : Tubular necrosis due to ischaemia, drugs or toxins.
4. *Acute interstitial nephritis* due to infection or drug reactions.
5. *Nephrosis* from precipitation of crystals or protein.

Post-renal azotemia

It is usually the result of urinary tract obstruction so that urea is reabsorbed into circulation.

Causes

1. *Ureteric* : Calculi, blood clot, cancer.
2. *Bladder neck* : Neurogenic bladder, prostatic hyperplasia, calculi, cancer, blood clot.

3. *Urethra* : Stricture, congenital valve, phimosis.

Chronic renal failure (CRF)

Chronic renal failure is a syndrome characterised by a progressive and irreversible deterioration in renal function due to progressive destruction of nephron mass. Reduction of nephron mass causes an alteration in function of virtually every organ leading to the development of clinical syndrome of uraemia.

Causes

1. *End stage disease* : Diabetes mellitus, hypertension.
2. *Glomerulonephritis* in its several forms.

URIC ACID

Metabolism of uric acid

Uric acid is formed by the breakdown of purines (adenine and guanine). Urates (monosodium salt), the ionised form of uric acid, predominate in plasma, extracellular fluid and synovial fluid.

The upper limit of normal plasma uric acid level is 6.8 mg/dl (415 μmol/l), which is also the saturation point. At higher concentration, plasma is, therefore, supersaturated with urate and potential exists for urate crystal precipitation in soft tissue and joints forming deposits called *tophi*. This causes acute gouty arthritis, which can progress to chronic gouty arthritis.

Although purine nucleotide synthesis and breakdown occur in all tissues, uric acid is produced in tissues that contain *xanthine oxidase*, primarily liver and small intestine. In addition to endogenous source, uric acid is also formed from dietary purine containing (foods rich in cell nuclei) compounds.

The uric acid pool in the body is about 1200 mg (7.2 m mol), of which there is a turnover of about half daily, i.e. about 600 mg is formed daily and the same amount lost, of which 75% is excreted in urine and 25% destroyed by bacteria in the colon.

In the kidney, urate is filtered at the glomeruli and 98 to 100 per cent of the same is reabsorbed. About half the reabsorbed urate is secreted back into the proximal tubule, and 40-44% of that is again reabsorbed. Thus, approximately 8-12 per cent of urate filtered by glomeruli is excreted in urine as uric acid. The ionized forms of uric acid in urine include mono- and disodium, potassium ammonium and calcium urates.

Normal values

Normal concentration of uric acid in male is 4.0 to 7.5 mg/dl serum and that in women is 2.5 to 6.5 mg/100 ml.

Increased concentration

1. The serum uric acid is often raised in gout, mostly in the range of 7 to 12 mg/dl (420 to 720 μ mol/l), though higher figures have been reported. The uric acid level does not always correlate with the severity of gouty arthritis.

Gouts are classifed as primary and secondary. In *primary gout,* there is a lack of the enzyme hypoxanthine guanine phosphoribosyl transferase which takes part in the reutilisation of hypoxanthine. Then the hypoxanthine not so reutilised serves as a principal source of excessive formation of urate. Congenital absence of the enzyme is found in *Lesch-Nyhan syndrome* where all the symptoms of gout are present.

Secondary gout arises from increased production or decreased excretion of urate due to certain diseases other than primary abnormality of purine metabolism. Increased turnover of uric acid due to increased cell breakdown occurs in leukaemia, pernicious anaemia and chronic haemolytic anaemia and the serum uric level may reach 20 mg/100 ml.

2. *Kidney disease,* e.g., acute and chronic renal failure, uraemia also causes deficient elimination of uric acid.

Decreased concentration : Decreased concentration is of no clinical significance and is found after administration of ACTH, uricosuric drug and allopurinol. Allopurinol, an analogue of hypoxanthine, which inhibits the enzyme xanthine oxidase and thus reduces the amount of urate formed from hypoxanthine and xanthine.

Chapter 47

Lipid Metabolism:
Lipid and Lipoproteins

PLASMA LIPIDS

The principal lipids found in human plasma are *cholesterol, triglycerides, phospholipids* and *non-esterified fatty acids* (NEFA). Ester is a compound formed from an alcohol or acid by removal of water.

1. **Cholesterol** : It is an unsaturated sterol alcohol. It is an essential constituent of cell plasma membranes, and a precursor of the steroid hormones and bile acids. Two thirds of the plasma cholesterol is esterified, and one third is free. About 60-70% of cholesterol is transported by low density lipoproteins (LDL), 20-30% by high density lipoproteins (HDL) and 5-12% by very low density lipoproteins (VLDL). Total desirable concentration of blood cholesterol in adults ranges from 140-200 mg/dl.

Cholesterol is found only in animals. Most of the dietary source of preformed cholesterol is contained in egg yolks and animal fat. Related sterols that occur in plants (plant cholesterols), are negligibly absorbed from the gut if at all. The liver and other tissues also synthesize cholesterol endogenously.

2. **Triglycerides** (Triacyl glycerol) : Triglycerides are esters of glycerol and, usually, three different fatty acids. These are neutral fat. They constitute about 95% of fat stored in the adipose cells of deposits, the chief fuel reserve of the body. Triglycerides are transported in plasma in the form of chylomicrons and VLDL. The depot fat is active dynamic tissue undergoing continuous breakdown and resynthesis. In the depot, glucose is metabolised to fatty acids, and neutral fats are synthesized. Neutral fat is also broken down and free fatty acids are released into the circulation. The normal range of triglycerides in blood of adults is 50-160 mg/dl.

3. **Phospholipids** : Phospholipids are inherent part of the membranes and other parts of cells. These are esters of glycerol, two acyl groups, and phosphatidic acid. The main plasma phospholipids are lecithin, cephalin and sphingomyelin. Lecithin and cephalin are structural materials required by all types of living cells, while sphingomyelin is found chiefly in brain and nerve cells. Phospholipids comprise 25% of LDL mass (lecithin : sphingomyelin ratio 2 : 1) and about 30% of HDL (lecithin : sphingomyelin ratio of 5 : 1).

4. **Non-esterified fatty acids (NEFA)** : These free fatty acids do not circulate in the plasma in free form, but are bound to albumin. They constitute a very important source of energy. Quantitatively, NEFA are a very small fraction of total plasma lipids. Several grams of the rapidly turning over NEFA complexed with albumin are transported in the plasma everyday.

PLASMA LIPOPROTEINS

Fat from diet absorbed in the intestine, lipids synthesized by the liver and adipose tissue must be transported between the various tissues and organs for utilisation and storage (Fig. 47.1).

The lipids are mostly insoluble in water, but are soluble in fat solvents (ether, chloroform, benzene, light petroleum). The problem of transporting the lipids in aqueous environment of plasma is solved by certain proteins, which form macromolecular complexes composed of a hydrophobic lipid core

Table 47.1
Characteristics of the major classes of lipoproteins in human plasma

Lipoprotein class (normal range)	*Major lipids*	*Other constituents*	*Density*	*Diameter*	*Electrophoretic mobility*
Chylomicrons and remnants	Dietary triglycerides – 90% (Origin – intestine)	Cholesterol (free) – 2% Cholesteryl esters – 2% Phospholipid – 3% Apoproteins – 2%	< 1.006	800–5000 (Remnants 30-80)	Remains at origin
VLDL (< 33 mg/dl)	Endogenous triglycerides – 55% (Origin – liver and intestine)	Cholesterol (free) – 4% Cholesteryl esters – 16% Phospholipid – 17% Apoproteins – 8%	< 1.006	300-800	Pre-β
IDL	Cholesteryl esters – 25% Triglyceride – 40% (Origin – VLDL)	Cholesterol (free) – 5% Phospholipid – 20% Apoproteins – 10%	< 1.019	250-350	Slow pre-β
LDL (< 190 mg/dl)	Cholesteryl esters – 48% (Origin – LDL)	Cholesterol (free) – 7% Triglyceride – 6% Phospholipid – 21% Apoprotein – 18%	1.019-1.063	180-280	β
HDL (> 35 mg/dl)	Cholesteryl esters – 16% (Origin – liver and intestine)	Cholesterol (free) – 4% Triglyceride – 5% Phospholipid – 25% Apoprotein – 50%	1.063-1.210	50-120	α

and a hydrophilic phospholipid and protein surface. Lipids are transported primarily as lipoproteins with the exception of transport of NEFA as albumin complexes. The protein constituents of the lipoproteins are called *apoproteins*.

Five major classes of lipoproteins have been identified on the basis of particle size, chemical composition, physicochemical and floatation characteristics, and electrophoretic mobility (Table 47.1).

1. **Chylomicrons** : The dietary triglycerides and cholesterol are incorporated into large lipoprotein particles within intestinal epithelial cells, called *chylomicrons*. They enter the circulation via thoracic duct. After meals, high chylomicron content results in milky plasma. Chylomicrons contain apoenzymes B, C, A and E. The chylomicrons pass into the capillaries of adipose tissue and muscle, where they adhere to binding sites on the capillary walls and are exposed to the enzyme *lipoprotein lipase*. This enzyme catalyses the breakdown of the triglyceride in the chylomicrons to free fatty acid and monoglyceride, which enter the adipose cells or muscle cells, where they are reesterified to triglycerides or oxidised (Fig. 47.1).

Chylomicrons depleted of their triglycerides remain in the circulation as cholesterol-rich lipoprotein called chylomicron remnant particle (30-80 nm diameter). This remnant travels to the liver, where they bind to chylomicron remnant receptors on hepatocytes, and are immediately internalised by receptor-mediated endocytosis, and are degraded within the lysosomes. The overall result of the chylomicron transport system is to deliver dietary triglyceride to adipose cells and cholesterol to the liver.

Some of the cholesterol that reaches the liver is converted to bile acids that passes into bile, and some to tissues by the endogenous pathway.

2. **Very low density lipoproteins (VLDL)** : In the endogenous pathway, synthesis of triglyceride is enhanced when the diet contains excess carbohydrate. The liver converts the carbohydrates to fatty acids and esterfies the latter with glycerol to form triglycerides, and secretes the

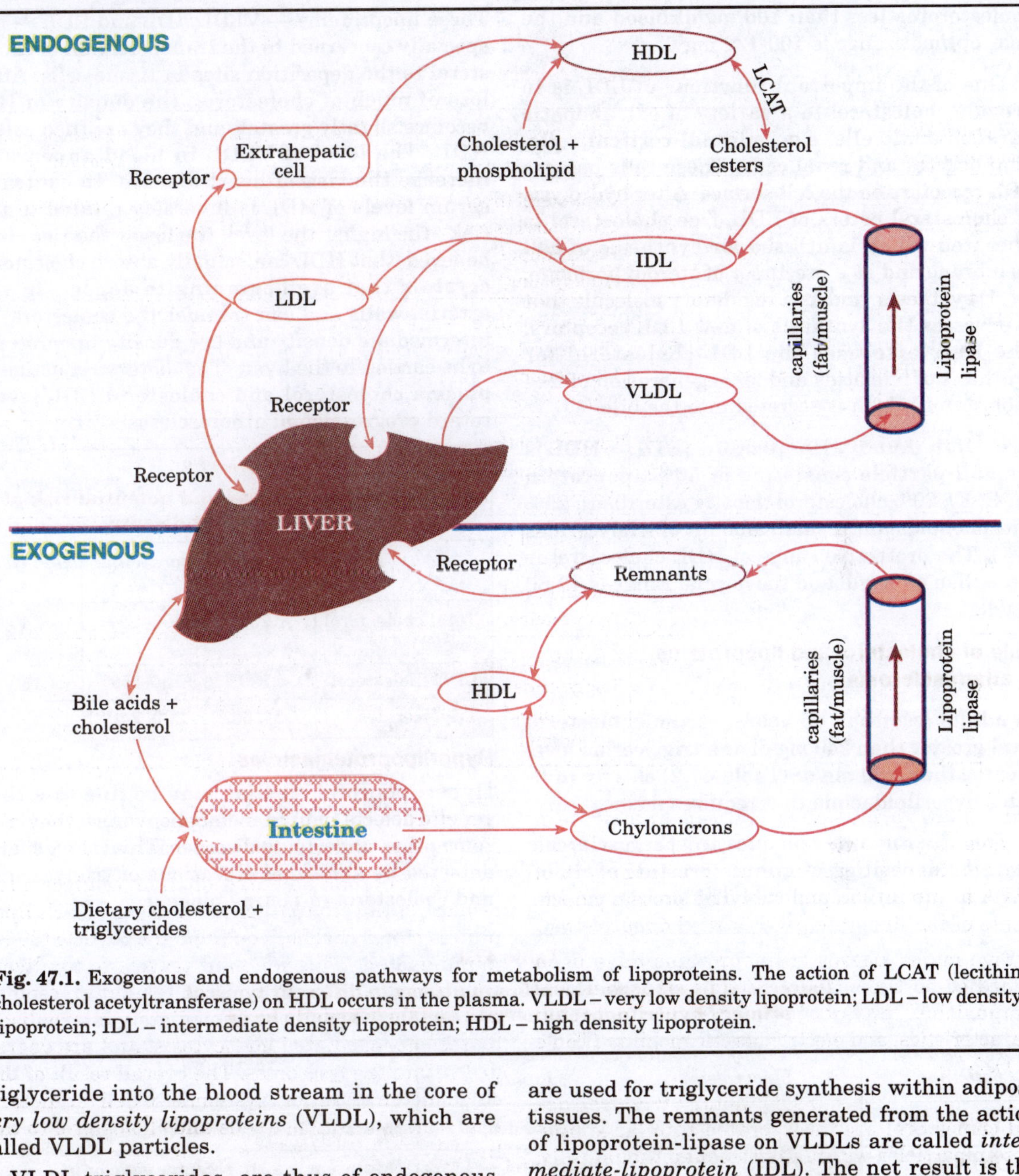

Fig. 47.1. Exogenous and endogenous pathways for metabolism of lipoproteins. The action of LCAT (lecithin cholesterol acetyltransferase) on HDL occurs in the plasma. VLDL – very low density lipoprotein; LDL – low density lipoprotein; IDL – intermediate density lipoprotein; HDL – high density lipoprotein.

triglyceride into the blood stream in the core of *very low density lipoproteins* (VLDL), which are called VLDL particles.

VLDL triglycerides, are thus of endogenous origin, mainly from the hepatic cells and constitute 60 to 70% of the particle mass. Cholesterol and phospholipids form only minor constituents, and about 8% of the mass is protein — mostly apoprotein B and C with some E.

The VLDL particles are transported to the tissue capillaries, where they are exposed to the enzyme *lipoprotein lipase* which catabolises the VLDL liberating free fatty acids. The fatty acids are used for triglyceride synthesis within adipose tissues. The remnants generated from the action of lipoprotein-lipase on VLDLs are called *intermediate-lipoprotein* (IDL). The net result is the transformation of IDL particle into LDL.

3. **Low density lipoprotein (LDL)** : LDL constitute about 50% of the total lipoprotein mass in human plasma. The core of LDL is composed almost entirely of cholesteryl esters, and the surface core is made up of only one apoprotein, apoprotein B100. About three-fourth of total cholesterol in normal individual plasma is contained within LDL particles. The optimal level of LDL

cholesterol is less than 100 mg/dl blood and the near optimal range is 100-129 mg%.

One of the important functions of LDL is to provide cholesterol to a variety of extrahepatic parenchymal cells, e.g., adrenal-cortical cells, lymphocytes and renal cells. These cells possess LDL receptors on the cell surface. After hydrolysis of cholesteryl esters of LDL, free cholesterol is liberated which is utilised for synthesis of cell membrane and as a precursor of steroid hormone, vit. D synthesis, and as a regulatory molecule that suppresses the synthesis of new LDL receptors. The liver also uses the LDL-cholesterol for synthesis of bile acids and for regeneration of free cholesterol, which is secreted into the bile.

4. **High density lipoprotein (HDL)** : HDL is a small particle consisting of 50% apoprotein (A, C, E), 20% cholesterol (mostly esterified), 25% phospholipids and a small amount of triglycerides (5%). The protective range of HDL-cholesterol is more than 40 mg/dl and the normal range is 40-60 mg/dl.

Role of cholesterol and lipoproteins in atherosclerosis

In adults less than 65 years, serum cholesterol level greater than 240 mg/dl or a triglyceride level greater than 250 mg/dl (Table 47.2) clearly indicates hyperlipidaemia that requires medical care.

The atheromatous plaques in atherosclerosis begin by deposition of minute crystals of cholesterol in the intima and sublying smooth muscle. Three lipoproteins — VLDL, IDL and LDL — are specially concerned to the transportation of cholesterol to the deposition sites in tissue cells. After loss of much of cholesterol, the density of IDL becomes slightly greater, and they are then called HDL. The level of VLDL in blood appears to increase the risk of heart disease. In contrast, serum levels of HDL is inversely related to the risk : the higher the level, the lower the risk. It is believed that HDL can actually absorb cholesterol crystals that are beginning to deposit in the arterial walls and can transfer the cholesterol to intermediate density and low density lipoproteins to be carried to the liver. The dietary reduction of plasma cholesterol and cholesterol LDL levels retard progression of atherosclerosis.

Table 47.2
Blood cholesterol level and potential risk of ischaemic heart disease

	Desirable	*Borderline risk*	*High risk*
Total cholesterol (mg/dl)	< 200	200–239	> 240
LDL cholesterol	< 130	130-159	> 160
Triglycerides	50–160	200–249	> 250

Hyperlipoproteinaemias

Hyperlipoproteinaemias may be due to either genetic defects in lipid metabolism or secondary to some other underlying disorder. This is in general detected by abnormal elevations of triglycerides and cholesterol in fasting plasma.

Table 47.3
Patterns of lipoprotein elevation in plasma in different types of primary hyperlipoproteinaemia and their genetic basis

Lipoprotein pattern	*Major elevation in plasma* Lipoproteins	Lipids	*Genetic defects*
Type 1	Chylomicrons	Triglycerides	Mutation in lipoprotein lipase gene.
Type 2a	LDL	Cholesterol ++++	Mutation in LDL receptor gene or in apolipoprotein B gene.
Type 2b	LDL and VLDL	Cholesterol ++ and triglycerides ++	Mutation in LDL receptor gene or in apolipoprotein B gene.
Type 3	Chylomicron and VLDL remnants	Triglycerides ++ and cholesterol +++	Mutation in an apolipoprotein E gene.
Type 4	VLDL	Triglycerides ++	Unknown.
Type 5	VLDL and chylomicrons	Triglycerides ++++ and cholesterol ++	Mutation in apolipoprotein C II gene.

A. Primary hyperlipoproteinaemia

These are usually classified into 5 main types, type 1 to type 5; type 2 has 2 subtypes — type 2a and type 2b. The patterns of lipoprotein elevation and genetic basis of the 5 main types are shown in Table 47.3. Most types cause premature atherosclerosis.

B. Secondary hyperlipoproteinaemias

This occurs secondary to some underlying diseases :

1. *Nephrotic syndrome*
2. *Alcoholism* (alcohol abuse)
3. *Hypothyroidism* : Both LDL and HDL are increased.
4. *Diabetes mellitus* : VLDL is often increased in diabetes mellitus.
5. *Obstructive liver disease,* either intra or extra-hepatic, increase in serum cholesterol associated with *β-lipoprotein* occurs.
6. Chronic renal failure.

Rare causes : Anorexia nervosa, glycogen storage disease, drugs (thiazide, corticosteroids, anabolic steroids, progesterons, oestrogen).

Hypolipoproteinaemia (Primary)

1. *Abetaliproteinaemia* : It is a rare inherited autosomal recessive trait and results in defective synthesis of apolipoprotein B. Chylomicrons and VLDL are absent in the serum.

2. *Familial hypobetalipoproteinaemia* : LDL is reduced to about 10% of normal.

3. *Familial HDL deficiency* : It is inherited as an autosomal recessive trait. HDL is reduced due to a failure to synthesize one of the HDL apoprotein.

4. *LCAT deficiency* : There is a marked deficiency of HDL with increase in free cholesterol and triglyceride concentration.

Chapter 48

Estimation of Blood Glucose Folin and Wu Tube

INTRODUCTION

Diabetes mellitus is due to an absolute or relative lack of insulin activity. All forms of diabetes mellitus share **hyperglycaemia**. The American Diabetic Association suggest the following classification of diabetes mellitus.

(i) *Type* 1 *diabetes* : Immune mediated *β cell* dysfunction → absolute insulin deficiency, also called Juvenile immune-mediated diabetes (10% cases).

(ii) *Type* 2 *diabetes* : Adult onset, caused by a combination of resistance to insulin and inadequate secretory response (80-90% cases).

(iii) *Type* 3 *diabetes* : A range of causes including pancreatic defects of *β cell* function and diseases of exocrine pancreas.

(iv) *Type* 4 *gestational diabetes* (GDM) : It is important to detect mild gestational diabetic women because of birth of overweight babies and perinatal mortality of infants of these patients. In non-pregnant state as well as throughout pregnancy, the fasting blood glucose concentration is lower and normal, but glucose tolerance increases during the second and third trimesters. Most of these women revert to normal glucose tolerance after delivery of baby, but have a substantial risk (30-50%) of diabetes mellitus later in life.

A one-hour plasma glucose concentration exceeding 155 mg/dl following a 50 gm oral administration of glucose has generally been taken as the screening criterion for carrying out GTT in pregnant women. Insulin resistance in these cases is related to the metabolic changes of late pregnancy. GTT in 2nd and 3rd trimester increases in these women with glycosuria.

The diagnosis is established by detecting elevation of blood by any of the following methods.

FOLIN AND WU TUBE

Identification :

Folin-Wu tube is a long wide-mouthed, thick walled glass tube with a long narrow neck below and a bulb at the bottom (Fig. 48.1). The tube has two markings, 12.5 at middle and 25.0 above.

Use : Estimation of sugar in blood, CSF and other body fluids by alkaline copper reduction method.

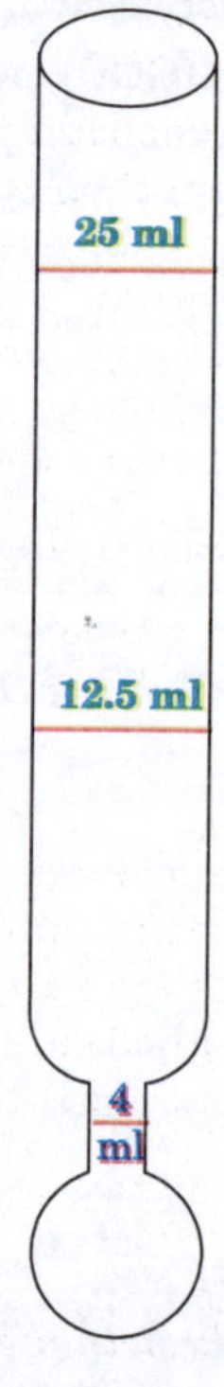

Fig. 48.1. Folin-Wu tube

BLOOD GLUCOSE DETERMINATION

Choice of blood specimen

1. *Plasma or Serum* : A volume of 2–3 ml blood is collected in a fluoride vial (10 mg/ml), and plasma is separated.

2. *Whole blood* : Whole blood is convenient for old method of Folin and Wu.

Anticoagulant :

Sodium fluoride	1 part	... 5 mg
Pot. oxalate	3 parts	... 15 mg

20 mg of anticoagulant mixture is adequate for 5 ml blood. Excess of anticoagulant interferes with the estimation.

Methods

Glucose estimation methods can be divided into two groups :

(a) *Enzymatic method* : Oxidase method.

(b) *Chemical method* : Orthotoluidine method and Folin-Wu method.

GLUCOSE OXIDASE METHOD

The enzymatic methods yield maximum specificity for estimation of glucose. It is the most widely employed method of blood glucose estimation.

Principle : Glucose is oxidised by glucose oxidase (GOD) forming gluconic acid and hydrogen peroxide. Hydrogen peroxide formed in this reaction, then in presence of peroxidase (POD), couples with 4-amino antipyrine/phenol or other chromogenic oxygen acceptors (phenylamine-phenazone) to produce red quinoneimine dye. The intensity of the colour complex is directly proportional to the concentration of glucose in specimen.

$$\text{(1) Glucose} + O_2 + H_2O \xrightarrow[\text{Oxidase}]{\text{Glucose}} \text{Gluconic acid} + H_2O_2$$

$$\text{(2) } H_2O_2 + \text{Phenylamine phenazone or orthodianisidine} + \text{phenol}$$
$$\text{(Chromogenic } O_2 \text{ acceptor)}$$
$$\xrightarrow{\text{Peroxidase}} \text{Colour chromogen} + H_2O$$
$$\text{(Red dye)}$$

Commercial reagent kits for glucose oxidase and orthotoluidine methods with instruction manual are now available. However, some standard methods are described below.

Trinder's glucose oxidase method

A. Manual method

Reagent

1. *Protein precipitant* :

Sodium tungstate	...	10.0 gm
Sodium chloride	...	9.0 gm
Disod. hydrogen phosphate (Na_2HPO_4)	...	10.0 gm
1.0 mol/l HCl (approx)	...	125 ml.

Adjust pH 3.0 using narrow range indicator paper.

Then add :

Phenol	...	1.0 gm
Distilled water to	...	1000 ml.

The solution keeps indefinitely.

2. *Colour reagent* :

4% Na_2HPO_4	...	75.0 ml
Distilled water	...	215.0 ml
Glucose oxidase (Fermacozyme of Hughes & Hughes Ltd)	...	5.0 ml
Peroxidase (1.0 gm/1, Sigma)	....	5.0 ml
Sodium azide	...	300 mg
4-aminophenazone	...	100 mg.

This reagent when stored at 4°C keeps up to 8 weeks.

3. *Standard glucose* solution 1.0 gm per litre in saturated solution of benzoic acid.

Procedure

Take 2.9 ml protein precipitant in a small tube and add 0.1 ml blood/serum/plasma and mix well. Allow to stand for 5 minutes and then centrifuge.

Prepare working standard by mixing 0.1 ml glucose stock standard with 0.9 ml of protein precipitant (1 ml contains 100 μg glucose).

Pipette into test tubes labelled Blank (B), Standard (S) and Test (T) as follows :

	B	S	T
Supernatant	—	—	1.0 ml
Glucose working standard	—	1.0 ml	—
Precipitation reagent	1.0 ml	—	—
Colour reagent	3.0 ml	3.0 ml	3.0 ml

Mix and incubate for 10 minutes at 37°C or for 15 minutes at room temperature (RT).

Read the test and standard against blank 415 nm or with green filter (500-540 nm).

Calculation :

$$\text{Glucose conc. in mg / dl} = \frac{\text{Abs. of T}}{\text{Abs. of S}} \times 100.$$

Note : Absorbance = Abs.

B. Manual technique without protein-precipitation

Reagent : Identical to that of manual method except reagent 1 (Sod. tungstate) which is omitted.

Procedure

	B	S	T
Distilled water	1.0 ml	1.0 ml	1.0 ml
Plasma	—	—	25 μl
Working standard (100 μg/ml)	—	25 μl	—
Distilled water	25 μl	—	—
Colour reagent	3.0 ml	3.0 ml	3.0 ml

Mix and incubate at 37 °C for 15 min shaking briefly two or 3 times. Read at 515 nm with water blank.

Calculation : As above.

Note : When blood glucose > 200 mg %, dilute the plasma and calculate accordingly.

Glucose oxidase/Peroxidase method

(Readymade Commercial kits available)

(1) Glucose + O_2 + H_2O $\xrightarrow{GOD}$ Gluconic acid + H_2O_2

(2) H_2O_2 + 4 - aminoantipyrine + Phenol $\xrightarrow{POD}$ Red dye + H_2O

Reagents

1. *Enzyme reagent* :
   - (a) Glucose oxidase (Fermacozyme 653 AM, Fermaco Laboratories, USA) 5.0 ml
   - (b) Peroxidase (1.0 gm/l, Sigma, USA) 5.0 ml
   - (c) Sodium azide 300 mg
   - (d) 4-aminophenazone 100 mg

The enzyme reagent is mixed; some commercial firms distribute the same in vials.

2. *Buffer solution* :
   - (a) 4% Sod. diydrogen phosphate solution 75.0 ml
   - (b) Distilled water 215.0 ml

3. *Glucose standard* :

   100 mg/dl in benzoic acid solution.

Storage : All reagents to be stored at 2-8°C and are stable for about 6 months.

Specimen

Serum/Plasma/CSF

Serum should be separated as soon as possible.

For plasma, collect venous blood in bulbs containing oxalate-fluoride (2 + 2 mg/ml of blood). Mix well by repeated inversions.

Working reagent preparation

(a) Bring buffer solution to R.T. before use.

(b) Dissolve one vial of enzyme reagent in one bottle of buffer solution and mix immediately.

This working reagent is stable up to 8 weeks at 2-8°C.

Procedure

(a) *Manual assay procedure*

Pipette into test tubes labelled Blank (B), Standard (S) and Test (T) as follows :

	B	S	T
Working reagent	1.0 ml	1.0 ml	1.0 ml
Glucose standard	—	0.01 ml	—
Specimen (serum/plasma)	—	—	0.01 ml

Mix well and incubate for 10 min at 37°C or 15 min at R.T.

Mix well and read absorbance (Abs.) of Standard (S) and Test (T) against Blank (B) at 605 nm or with green filter (500-540 nm).

Linearity : Up to 400 mg/dl.

The final colour is stable for 2 hours at R.T.

Calculation

$$\text{Glucose conc. in mg / dl} = \frac{\text{Abs. of T}}{\text{Abs. of S}} = 100.$$

(b) *For kinetic assay*

Prewarm at 37 °C the required amount of working solution before use.

1.0 ml procedure:	
Standard/specimen	... 0.01 ml (10 µl)
Working solution	... 1.0 ml

First take reading of the standard. Mix and start stop watch simultaneously. The absorbance is recorded at exactly 20th second after standard addition and then again at 60th second. Subsequently the assay of the specimen is carried out following exactly the same procedure mentioned above.

Calculation

Calculate the change in absorbance of (Δ Abs.) of Std. and Specimen.

$$\text{Factor} = \frac{\text{Concentration of Std}}{\Delta\text{ Abs. of Standard}} = \frac{100}{\Delta\text{ Abs of Standard}}$$

GLUCOSE in mg % = Abs. of Specimen × Factor

Note: The specimen to working solution can be altered proportionally without affecting the results.

Normal range : (i) Plasma/Serum — 70-100 mg/dl, (ii) CSF — 40-70 mg/dl.

Dextrostix

Strips *(dextrostix)* made by Aimes Company measure approximate glucose in blood by glucose oxidase technique. A drop of blood is placed on the printed side of the strip and immediately after one minute, the strip is quickly washed off under a fine jet of cold water. The strip is compared immediately with the colour chart that contains concentration of glucose as 50-120, 120-200, and over 200 mg/100 ml blood.

ORTHOTOLUIDINE METHOD

Principle

Orthotoluidine reacts quantitatively with the aldehyde group of aldohexoses (e.g. glucose) and condenses the same with an aromatic amine and glacial acetic acid. This stable green colour of the newly formed glycosylamine is measured colorimetrically.

In this method, galactose and mannose also react as glucose, but other aldosaccharides, such as lactose, maltose, sucrose and fructose react, but to a much lesser extent. Technique of test is supplied with the commercial reagent kits.

FOLIN AND WU METHOD OF ALKALINE COPPER REDUCTION

The technique of Folin and Wu (1920) was the most widely used test for many years. The technique of Folin and Wu has been superceded by the latest enzymatic methods, and is now practised by only few laboratories. The method has got simplicity and economy.

Disadvantages

The test detects the entire range of aldosaccharides and hence does not provide true glucose level. Moreover, reduction of copper also occurs with uric acid, creatine and creatinine.

Principle

Blood is deproteinised by 10% sodium tungstate and 2/3 N sulphuric acid. The glucose in the filtrate reduces the cupric salt solution to cuprous oxide on boiling. The amount of cuprous copper formed is determined colorimetrically by reacting with phosphomolybdic acid. The cuprous copper is oxidised to cupric and the phosphomolybdic acid is reduced to molybdenum blue (copper molybdate) which is dark blue solution. The intensity of the colour is compared with that obtained from a standard glucose solution colorimetrically and the glucose level is then calculated accordingly.

Reagents

1. *Sodium tungstate* ($Na_2 WO_4 2H_2O$) — 10% solution in water.

2. *Sulphuric acid* 2/3 N — Add 20 ml conc. H_2SO_4, slowly and with stirring, into 200-250 ml water and make to 1000 ml with water. Standardise by titration with sodium hydroxide solution.

3. *Alkaline copper solution*

Anhydrous sodium carbonate	...	40 gm
Tartaric acid	...	7.5 gm
Cupric sulphate	...	4.5 gm
Distilled water to	...	1000 ml

Dissolve sod. carbonate in 400 ml water and transfer to a 1000 ml volumetric flask. Then add tartaric acid till dissolved. Then transfer copper sulphate solution (dissolved in 100 ml water) quantitatively while mixing with a stirrer. Mix and make to 1000 ml by adding water. The fluid is decanted if precipitate forms on standing.

4. *Phosphomolybdic acid reagent*

Dissolve 35 gm molybdic acid and 5 gm sodium tungstate in 200 ml of 10% sodium hydroxide in a litre beaker. Add 200 ml distilled water and boil for 30-40 minutes to remove ammonia present in the molybdic acid. After cooling, the solution is transferred to a volumetric flask washing with sufficient water to make the volume 350 ml. Add 125 ml 89% phosphoric acid (Sp. gr. 1.75) and make up to 500 ml and mix well.

5. *Stock standard glucose*

Dissolve 1 gm of pure dry glucose in 100 ml saturated benzoic acid. Saturated benzoic is prepared by adding 2.5 gm powder to 1000 ml boiling water and then allowed to cool. Stock standard glucose keeps for at least 6 months. Benzoic acid serves as preservative of glucose. It does not interfere in the test.

6. *Working standard*

Dilute stock solution : (a) 1 in 100, (b) 2 in 100 with saturated benzoic acid to make low and high standard.

Technique

1. *Deproteinisation* (50 × 12 mm tube)

Distilled water	...	3.5 ml

Whole blood (anticoagulated by sod. fluoride)	...	0.5 ml
10% Sod. tungstate	....	0.5 ml
2/3 N Sulphuric acid	....	0.5 ml

Mix well by inversion (2 to 3 times), leave for 5 minutes and then filter.

2. *Boiling with alkaline copper solution (Folin & Wu tube)*

	T	S
Filtrate	1.0 ml	—
Glucose working std.	—	1.0 ml
Alkaline copper solution	1.0 ml	1.0 ml

Mix by shaking and boil for 10 minutes. Then cool in cold water for about 2-3 minutes.

3. *Developing the colour*

Add to each of the Folin tubes 1.0 ml phosphomolybdic acid reagent and wait for one minute to allow time for all the cuprous oxide to go into solution. Finally, the solutions are diluted with distilled water up to the mark 12.5 on the tube and read in a colorimeter at 680 nm or using a red filter with water as blank.

Calculation : Blood glucose (mg %)

$$\frac{\text{Reading of unknown}}{\text{Reading of standard}} \times \text{Multiplication factor}$$

(Factor, 100 with low standard and 200 with high standard)

GLYCOSYLATED HAEMOGLOBIN

Definition

Glycosylated (or Glycated) haemoglobin is a form of haemoglobin bound to glucose molecule.

Background information

Normal haemoglobin in blood is HbA. In very small quantities variation of HbA is found in blood. These are Hb A_{1a}, Hb A_{1b}, Hb A_{1c}. Hb A_{1c} has affinity for glucose molecule, and if available, is glycated.

In normal 120 days life span of RBC, haemoglobin in it may form stable glycated haemoglobin. Once formed HbA1c may remain in RBC throughout its life span. Thus a measure of Hb A_{1c} within RBC is a reflection of average glucose level in blood, to which the cell has been exposed.

Methods of measurement

(1) Hb A_{1c} is separated from the haemolysate of micro-column-chromatography, followed by spectrophotometric estimation of elutes containing Hb A_{1c}. This value is compared with the value of total haemolysate. The result is expressed as the percentage of the absorbance of Hb A_{1c} in total haemolysate.

(2) Hb A_{1c} in a haemolysate may be measured by HPLC and immunoassay. But these methods are cumbersome, time consuming and costly. So fallen in disfavour.

(3) Haemolysate is digested with proteases to yield fructosyl amino acid. Using oxidase, H_2O_2 is generated from it. H_2O_2 is subjected to react with a chromogenic substance in presence of oxidase. Colour developed is measured by spectrophotometer.

Significance

Measure of glycosylated haemoglobin is an assessment of the effectiveness in controlling long term glucose level in previous 4-12 weeks.

Interpretations :

Hb A_{1c} (%)		In last 12 weeks, average blood glucose (mg/dl)
5	......	80
6	......	120
7	......	150
8	......	180
9	......	210
10	......	240
11	......	270
12	......	300

Estimation of haemoglobin A_{1C}

Principle

At fast haemolysate is prepared and after preparing the hemolysate, where the labile fraction is eliminated, hemoglobins are retained by a cationic exchange resin. Hb A_{1c} is specifically eluted after washing away the hemoglobin A_{1a+b} fraction[1] (HbA_{1a+b}). Then HbA_{1c} is quantified by direct photometric reading at 415 nm.

Reagents

1. *Reagent* : Potassium phthalate 50 mmol/L, detergent 5 g/L, pH 5.0, sodium azide 0.95 g/L.

2. *Reagent* : Phosphate buffer 30 mmol/L, pH 6.5, sodium azide 0.95 g/L.

3. *Reagent* : Phosphate buffer 72 mmol/L, pH 6.5, sodium azide 0.95 g/L.

4. *Microcolumns* : Contain a pre-weighted amount of resin equilibrated with phosphate buffer 72 mmol/L, pH 6.5, sodium azide 0.95 g/L.

Reagents are stored at 15–30°C.

Sample

EDTA or heparin is used anticoagulants. HbA_{1c} is stable at 2–8°C for 7 days.

Procedure

(a) *Preparation of haemolysate* and elimination of labile fraction is done as follows :

1. The columns and reagents are brought to room temperature (21–26°C).

2. Blood and reagent (1) are pipetted into a test tube :

Blood	....	50 μL
Reagent (1)	....	200 μL

3. The mixture is shaken thoroughly and let it stand at room temperature for 10-15 minutes. This hemolysate is used in steps 6 and 11.

(b) *Column preparation* :

4. Remove the upper cap of the column and then snap the tip off the bottom.

5. By the aid of flat end of a pipette, push the upper disc down to the resin surface taking care not to compress it. Let the column drain completely to waste.

(c) *Separation and reading of HbA_{1c} fraction*

6. The Hb_{1c} fraction is carefully pipetted on the upper filter :

Hemolysate	50 μL	Allow the column drain to waste

7. In order to drain any sample residue left above the upper disc pipette :

Reagent (2)	200 μL	Allow the column drain to waste

8. Pipette :

Reagent (2)	2.0 μL	Allow the column drain to waste

9. Place the column over a test tube and add :

Reagent (3)	4.0 ml.	The eluate is collected (HbA_{1c} Fraction)

10. The mixture is thoroughly shaken and read the absorbance (A) of the HbA_{1c} fraction at 415 nm against distilled water (A_{HbA1c}). The absorbance is stable for at least one hour.

Reading of Hb_{TOTAL}

11. Blood and reagent are pipetted into a test tube :

Reagent (3)	12.0 ml.
Hemolysate	50 μL

12. The mixture is shaken thoroughly and the absorbance (A) is read at 415 nm against distilled water ($A_{HbTOTAL}$). The absorbance is stable for at least one hour.

Calculations

Calculation of HbA_{1c} percentage in the sample is made using the following general formula :

$$\frac{A_{HbA1c} \times V_{HbA1c}}{A_{HbTOTAL} \times V_{HbTOTAL}} \times 100 = \% \text{ HbA1c}$$

The volume of HbA_{1c} (V_{HbA1c}) in the test is 4 mL, the volume of Hb total ($V_{HbTOTAL}$) is 12 mL. The formula is deduced for the calculation of the concentration is as follows :

$$\frac{A_{HbA1c}}{A_{HbTOTAL}} \times \frac{100}{3} = \% \text{ HbA1c}$$

Conversion of result into equivalent to a US National Glycohemoglobin Standardization Program Certified method (NGSP) or equivalent to the International Federation of Clinical Chemistry standardized method (IFCC) is done by the following fomulas :

%HbA1c-NGSP = 0.86 × %HbA1c-BioSystems + 0.24

%HbA1c-IFCC = 0.94 × %HbA1c-BioSystems – 2.09

Reference values

The undermentioned cut-off points have been established by the Diabetes Control and Complications Trial Research Group (DCCT). It has been adopted by many countries for a reference population (Non diabetic) and also for the evaluation of the degree blood glucose control in diabetic patients.

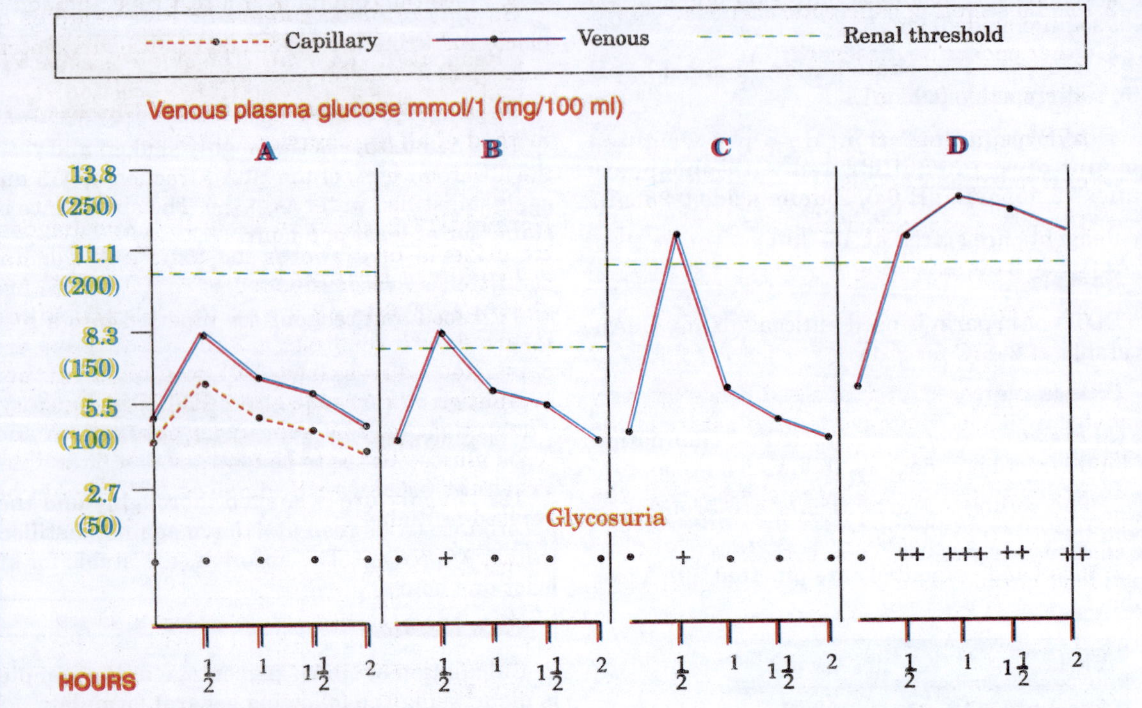

Fig. 48.2. **Glucose tolerance test** after 75 gm oral glucose. (A) normal curve, (b) renal glycosuria, (C) alimentary (lag storage) glycosuria and (D) diabetes mellitus of moderate severity.

DCCT/NGSP	IFCC	BioSystems	Degree of control
4.0–6.0	2.0–4.2	4.4–6.7	Non-diabetic
6.0–6.5	4.2–4.8	6.7–7.3	Goal
6.5–8.0	4.8–6.4	7.3–9.1	Good Control
> 8.0	> 6.4	> 9.1	Action suggested

Normal range of blood glucose

A. *By glucose oxidase and orthotoluidine method,* true glucose level is estimated.

(1) Fasting — 60-100 mg %

(2) Post-prandial (2 hours) — 90-120 mg %

B. *By other methods (Folin and Wu),* where variable amounts of non-glucose reducing substances are included.

(1) Fasting — 70-120 mg %

(2) Post-prandial (2 hours) — 80-139 mg %

Hyperglycaemia

Hyperglycaemia is a condition in which blood glucose level is above 120 mg/100 ml by oxidase method or blood sugar level above 140 mg/100 ml by method including non-sugar reducing substances.

Causes

1. Diabetes mellitus
2. Pancreatitis and carcinoma pancreas
3. Other endocrine diseases :
   (a) Hyperthyroidism
   (b) Cushing's syndrome
   (c) Hyperaldosteronism
4. Liver disease :
   (a) Chronic liver failure
   (b) Virus hepatitis
5. Intracranial injury

Hypoglycaemia

Hypoglycaemia may be considered to be present when the blood glucose level is below 40 mg/100 ml by glucose oxidase method or sugar below 60 mg/100 ml by method including non-sugar reducing substances.

Causes

1. Insulin induced (over-dosage with insulin) hypoglycaemia.

2. Insulin secreting pancreatic adenoma — rare.
3. Other endocrine diseases :
   (a) Hypothyroidism
   (b) Hypopituitarism
   (c) Hypoadrenocorticism
4. Glycogen storage disease
5. Ackee fruit poisoning

Glucose tolerance test (GTT)

Indication :

GTT is indicated in suspected cases of early diabetes mellitus who have family history of the disease.

In order to define diabetes chemically, the ability of an individual to regulate a glucose load or challenge is studied. This is done by determining blood glucose concentrations after either an oral meal or an intravenous glucose.

Post-prandial blood sugar determination is advantageous as the patient does not have to fast and blood is collected 2 hours after usual meal or 75 gm glucose meal only once. Moreover, the test is completed in a relatively short time.

Following ingestion of carbohydrate food, there is a temporary rise of blood glucose, which in normal persons does not exceed 160 to 180 mg/100 ml (renal threshold 180 mg/100 ml). Then there is return to normal level at the latest within 2 to 3 hours after taking food (Fig. 48.2).

Intravenous GTT is occasionally done to avoid effects arising from defective absorption of the glucose. About 20-30 gms glucose is injected intravenously over a few minutes and then blood for glucose is collected at ½-1 hour intervals in 3 hours. It has been observed that there is a greater insulin response to oral glucose meal than intravenous injection.

Oral glucose tolerance test

The patient, who should have been taking an unrestricted carbohydrate diet for at least 3 days or more prior to the test, fasts overnight. The patient should be ideally at rest for at least half an hour before starting the test.

After collecting fasting blood in the morning, 75 gm of glucose dissolved in 250-300 ml water is fed. The test can also be done 4 to 5 hours after the last meal.

Sample of blood collected : Five samples of blood and urine are collected at half hourly intervals up to 2½ hours after glucose meal.

Testing : Glucose is estimated by oxidase method of all the samples.

Interpretation

Normal GTT is shown in Table 48.1. The diagnostic criteria of diabetes mellitus and normal condition as recommended by WHO (1985) are shown in Table 48.2 and Fig. 48.2D. When intermediate readings are obtained, these are classified as impaired GTT and need further evaluation by cortisone-stressed GTT and history. The patient may be kept under observation and blood glucose test is to be repeated at a later date. Pregnant women with impaired GTT should be treated as diabetic.

Table 48.1 : Normal glucose tolerance curve

Time	*Fasting*	*After taking glucose*				
		½ h	1 h	1½ h	2 h	2½ h
Blood glucose mg/100 ml	75	130	140	100	65	70
Urine glucose		Negative in all samples				

Chemical diabetes mellitus : When post-prandial blood glucose is high and exceeds 180 mg% with glycosuria, but having normal fasting blood glucose level, it is referred to as chemical diabetes.

Single test diagnosis : When post-prandial blood glucose exceeds 160 mg%, it is suggestive of diabetes mellitus. It should be remembered that the fasting blood glucose level may not be high in early diabetes mellitus.

Renal threshold for glucose

Normal renal threshold value of blood glucose is 180 mg/100 ml blood. When blood glucose level exceeds renal threshold, glycosuria takes place.

1. ***Decreased renal threshold***

Apart from diabetes mellitus, glycosuria may occur when the renal threshold is low for glucose, which commonly may occur in pregnancy and in young adults after carbohydrate meal. This is termed *renal glycosuria* which is a benign condition (Fig. 48.2).

2. ***Raised renal threshold***

Renal threshold is sometimes raised over 200 mg glucose/100 ml blood in long-standing diabetes mellitus, arteriosclerosis and cerebrovascular accidents.

Alimentary (lag storage) glycosuria

In some individuals, there may be an unusually rapid but transitory rise of blood glucose after ingestion of high carbohydrate meal, and the concentration exceeds the renal threshold; glucose appears in the urine during this time. This is called *alimentary glycosuria* (Fig. 48.2). It may occur after gastric surgery and in hyperthyroidism or hepatic disease. It is a benign condition. Blood glucose level after 2 hours is normal.

Cortisone-stressed GTT

Fajans and Conn, 1954)

Principle

It is useful for detecting latent diabetes. Administration of a large dose of ACTH or of a glucocorticoid reduces glucose tolerance leading to glycosuria in normal individuals, while smaller doses of the same reduce the glucose tolerance only in latent diabetics.

Technique

Cortisone acetate, 50 mg (62.5 mg when body weight exceeds 160 lb or 72 kg) is given by mouth in two divided doses, the first 8½ hours, the second 2 hours before 50 gm glucose tolerance test is performed. Nowadays prednisolone is used which is given 0.4 mg per kg body weight in two divided doses, half at midnight and half at 06-00 hours. Fasting sample of blood is collected at 08-00 hours and then 50 gm glucose is given for GTT.

Result : The test is considered positive when two hour blood glucose level is higher than 140 mg/100 ml by oxidase method.

Complications of diabetes mellitus

1. **Diabetic coma** : two types —

(a) *Keto-acidotic coma* : It is a common complication of Type 1 (juvenile type) diabetes mellitus. If the disease is uncontrolled, there is hyperosmolarity, hypovolaemia, acidosis and loss of electrolytes which may lead to coma.

(b) *Hyperosmolar non-ketotic coma* : This complication slowly develops in Type 2 (adult onset) diabetes mellitus. There develops hyperglycaemia leading to profound dehydration.

2. **Hypoglycaemic coma** : This occurs when the quantity of insulin intake is excessive for the amount of food consumed.

3. **Cardiovascular lesions**

(a) *Atheroma* : Patient develops atheroma at early age with increased severity. Coronary thrombosis is commonly observed.

(b) *Microangiopathy* of arterioles and capillaries causing occlusion which are responsible for cardiac failure, retinopathy, neuropathy, Kimmelstiel-Wilson lesions in kidney and gangrene of limbs.

4. **Renal failure**

5. **Infections**

6. **Neuropathy**

Peripheral and autonomic neuropathy as a result of direct metabolic damage and also due to microvascular occlusion.

QUESTIONS

1. *What is the principle of estimation of blood glucose by glucose oxidase method?*
2. *What is Dextrostix test?*
3. *What is the normal range of blood glucose?*
4. *Name the causes of hyperglycemia.*
5. *What are the causes of hypoglycaemia?*
6. *What is chemical diabetes mellitus?*
7. *Which single test helps in detection of a case of diabetes mellitus?*
8. *What is renal glycosuria?*
9. *What is alimentary glycosuria?*
10. *What is the usefulness of determining glycosylated haemoglobin Hb A_{1c}?*
11. *Name the kidney diseases in diabetes mellitus.*
12. *What is KW syndrome?*
13. *Name a disease in which glucose, protein and ketone bodies are present in urine.*
14. *What is gestational diabetes mellitus?*

Chapter 49

Estimation of Nitrogenous Constituents

Nitrogen-containing compounds comprise of two types : **proteins** and **non-proteins**.

The term **non-protein nitrogen** (NPN) in blood is applied to a heterogeneous group of substances of relatively small molecular size which are not precipitated by protein precipitants (e.g., tungstic acid, trichloroacetic acid), which include *urea, creatine, creatinine, uric acid, amino acids* and *ammonia*.

SERUM CREATININE

Determination (Alkaline picrate method)

The endogenous substance creatinine — a degradation product of creatine — is formed at a relatively constant rate by muscle, the major storage site of creatine phosphate. Creatinine production and excretion is directly related to muscle mass.

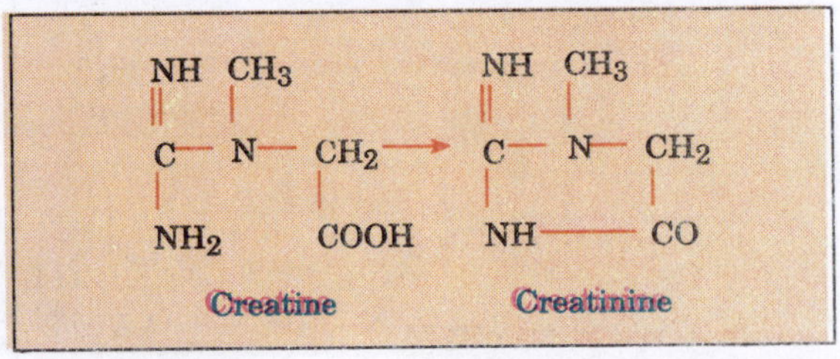

Principle

Creatinine in a protein-free solution reacts with alkaline picrate producing red coloured complex. This red coloured complex is measured colorimetrically.

Sample

1. *Serum/plasma* (1 ml is required).
2. *Urine* : 24-hour urine is preferred. Dilute urine 1 : 25 with distilled water.

Reagents

1. *Picric acid* (saturated picric acid solution) : Wash 13 gm picric acid into a measuring cylinder and add water to 1 litre. Allow the excess to remain in contact with water, shaking time to time. The solution is filtered and kept in a polythene bottle.
2. *Sodium hydroxide,* 0.75 N (3 gm/100 ml).
3. *Stock creatinine standard* (150 mg%) : Dissolve 150 mg pure dry creatinine in 10 ml concentrated hydrochloric acid and make to 100 ml with the acid. This keeps indefinitely.

Preparation of working standard : Dilute 0.1 ml stock creatinine standard to 10 ml with distilled water freshly before use. All other reagents are ready for use.

Storage and stability : Reagent 3 (stock standard) is stable at 2-8°C and reagents 1 and 2 are stable at room temperature (RT) for 4 to 6 months.

Precautions

1. Clean and dry glassware to be used.
2. All solutions to be brought to R.T. before use.
3. Prepare one blank and one standard for each series of estimations.
4. Mark the test tubes properly as Blank (B), Standard (S) and Test (T) before starting testing so that markings do not fade in the boiling water bath during deproteinisation (step A).
5. Remember to dilute the urine during urinary creatinine estimation.

Procedure

I. For colorimeter

Step A. Deproteinisation :

Serum/Plasma/Diluted urine	–	1.0 ml
Distilled water	–	1.0 ml
Reagent 1 : Picric acid	–	6.0 ml

Mix well, keep in a boiling water bath exactly for one minute. Cool immediately under tap water and centrifuge or filter.

Step B. Colour development :

	Blank (B)	Standard (S)	Test (T)
Filtrate/supernatant (From Step A)	–	–	4.0 ml
Working standard	–	1.0 ml	–
Distilled water	1.0 ml	–	–
Reagent 1 : Picric acid	3.0 ml	3.0 ml	–
Reagent 2 : Sodium hydroxide (0.75 N)	1.0 ml	1.0 ml	1.0 ml

Mix well and allow to stand at R.T. for exactly 20 minutes. Measure immediately O.D. of B, S and T against Distilled water using green filter or at 520 nm.

II. For spectrophotometer

All the volumes mentioned above can be halved. Read O.D. at 520 nm.

Calculations

$$\text{Serum creatinine in mg / 100 ml} = \frac{OD_T - OD_B}{OD_{Std} - OD_B} \times 3.0$$

$$\text{Urine creatinine in gm / litre (A)} = \frac{OD_T - OD_B}{OD_{Std} - OD_B} \times 0.75$$

Urine creatinine in gm / 24 hours collection

= A × 24 hour urine volume in litres.

Note :

1. When OD exceeds 0.8, the test is to be repeated after diluting the serum 1 : 2 and urine 1 : 50 and the final result is obtained by multiplying with dilution factor.
2. Optical density should be measured exactly 20 minutes after addition of NaOH.
3. Filtrate should be crystal clear.

Normal values

Serum creatinine :

Men	–	0.9 to 1.4 mg/100 ml
Women	–	0.8 to 1.2 mg/100 ml

Urine creatinine :

Men	–	1.1 to 2.8 gm/24 hours
Women	–	0.9 to 1.6 gm/24 hours

Clinical significance

1. Creatinine estimation in renal disease has advantage over urea determination in that unlike urea, creatinine is not affected by high protein intake.

2. Serum creatinine is increased in renal failure, up to 20 mg/100 ml.

3. In addition to kidney disease, elevated serum and urine creatinine may be seen in extensive muscle destruction.

4. Creatinine clearance test is useful to estimate glomerular filtration rate while studying kidney functions.

BLOOD UREA

Determination

I. Phenol-Hypochorile Method using the Berthelot Reaction (*Modified* : Fawcell and Scott, 1960; Chaney and Marbach, 1962)

Principle

Urease splits urea into ammonia and CO_2. The ammonia formed further reacts with phenolic chromogen in presence of hypochlorite producing a green coloured complex. Intensity of the colour formed is directly proportional to the concentration of urea in specimen.

$$\underset{\text{(urea)}}{NH_2\text{-}CO\text{-}NH_2} \xrightarrow{\text{urease}} 2NH_3 + CO_2$$

$$NH_3 + \text{Hypochlorite} + \text{phenolic chromogen} \rightarrow \text{Green colour}$$

Reagents	Concentration
1. Phosphate buffer, pH 7.0	
2. Urease	35 m Mol/L
3. Phenolic chromogen	15 K U/L
4. Hypochlorite	2 m Mol/L
5. Activators and preservative	4 m Mol/L

(All reagents are commercially available in the form of Kit)

Sample

Blood is collected in any of the undermentioned anticoagulants :

EDTA ... 2 mg/ml of blood

Citrate ... 6 mg/ml of blood
Sod/Pot Oxalate ... 3 mg/ml of blood
Heparin ... 200 IU/ml of blood

Note : Ammonium salts and sod. fluoride should not be used as anticoagulant.

Test procedure

Take three clean tubes and label Blank (B), Standard (S) and Test (T)

Reagent	B (ml)	S (ml)	T (ml)
Buffer reagent	1.0	1.0	1.0
Enzyme reagent	0.1	0.1	0.1
Distilled water	0.01	–	–
Urea standard	–	0.01	–
Sample (serum/plasma)	–	–	0.01

Mix well and incubate the mixture at 37°C for 5 minutes. Measure the absorbance of standard (Abs S) and Test sample (Abs T) against blank at 578 nm (570-620 nm) within 60 min.

Calculation

$$\text{Urea in mg\%} = \frac{\text{Abs T}}{\text{Abs S}} \times 40$$

Urea nitrogen in mg% = Urea in mg% × 0.467

Normal reference values :

Serum/Plasma .... 14-40 mg%
Urine .... upto 20 gm/L

II. Diacetyl Monoxime Method

Principle

In the determination of urea, diacetyl monoxime decomposes to give hydroxylamine and diacetyl which then condenses with urea.

When urea is heated with diacetyl monoxime in presence of thiosemicarbazide, coloured compounds (rose-purple) are produced which is measured colorimetrically.

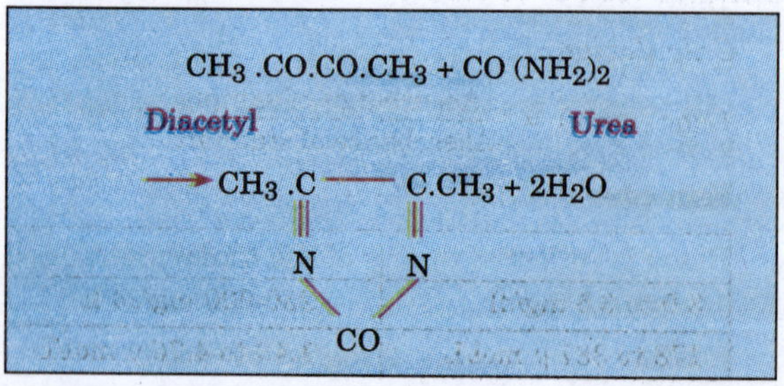

Sample

1. Serum or plasma (0.2 ml is required).

Note : Do not use anticoagulants containing ammonium salts.

2. Urine : Dilute 1 : 20.

Reagents

1. *Trichloroacetic acid (10 gm %).*
2. *Stock diacetyl monoxime 2.5 gm %* in water.
3. *Stock thiosemicarbazide 2.5gm%* in water.
4. *Acid ferric chloride solution* : Add 1 ml sulphuric acid to 100 ml of a 5% ferric chloride solution in water.
5. *Acid reagent* : Add 10 ml orthophosphoric acid (sp. gr. 1.75), 80 ml sulphuric acid and 10 ml acid ferric chloride solution to 1 litre of water and mix.
6. *Colour reagent* : To 300 ml acid reagent add 200 ml water, 10 ml stock diacetyl monoxime and 2.5 ml stock thiosemicarbazide.
7. *Urea standard* : Make two standards containing 30 mg/100 ml water (low standard) and 60 mg/100 ml water (high standard).

Procedure

Step A

	Test (T)
Serum/plasma	0.2 ml
Distilled water	1.0 ml
Trichloroacetic acid	1.0 ml
Mix well and centrifuge	

Step B

	Blank (B)	Test (T)	Standard (S)
Supernatant (from step A)	–	0.2 ml	–
Working urea standard (30 mg%)	–	–	0.2 ml
Distilled water	0.2 ml	–	–
Colour reagent	3.0 ml	3.0 ml	3.0 ml

Mix well and keep the tubes in a boiling waterbath exactly for 20 min. Cool to R.T. in cold water and read Test and Standard against blank at 520 nm or using a green filter within 15 min.

Calculations

Serum / Plasma :

1. Urea in mg / 100 ml, (A) = $\frac{OD_T}{OD_{Std}} \times 30$

2. Urea nitrogen in mg / 100 ml = A × 0.467.

Urine :

1. Urea in gm / l, (B) = $\frac{OD_T}{OD_{Std}} \times \frac{30 \times 20}{100}$

2. Urea nitrogen in gm / l = B × 0.467.

Normal values

Serum : 20-40 mg urea (10-20 mg urea nitrogen)/100 ml.

Urine : 20 gm urea (10 gm urea nitrogen)/litre.

Note :

1. If values are more than 60 mg urea/100 ml serum or 60 gm/litre urine, repeat the test after diluting the serum 1 : 2 and urine 1 : 40 (instead of 1 : 20) with normal saline and multiply the final result so obtained by 2.
2. In case of high urea values, 60 mg stock (high) standard to be used, and the multiplication factor will be 60 instead of 30.

III. Stick tests

Ammonia formed from urease action is detected by an indicator. *Urastrat* (Warner), is a strip of chromatography paper with several bands of reagent. It gives a semiquantitative measure of urea in blood. The end of strip is dipped in 0.2 ml serum/plasma in a 10 × 75 mm test tube. Serum rises by capillary action and passes first into a band of buffered urease. Ammonium salt formed reacts with potassium carbonate in the next band liberating ammonia gas which moves upwards. The upward migration of liquid is stopped at this point by a plastic barrier, above which lies an indicator band of bromocresol green acidified with tartaric acid that traps the ammonia. The height of colour change attained in 30 min at R.T. is proportional to the urea concentration in the sample. A hair breadth line indicates 6 mg/100 ml (4 mmol/l). Values up to 150 mg/100 ml (25 mmol/l) are covered.

SERUM URIC ACID

Determination

(A) Enzymatic method

Principle

Uricase converts uric acid into allantoin and hydrogen peroxide. Under the influence of peroxidase, hydrogen peroxide oxidatively couples with phenolic chromogens (2 hydroxy–3, 5 dichlorobenzene sulfonic acid and 4-aminoantipyrine) to form a red coloured compound which has got a maximum absorbance at 510 nm (500-530 nm). Concentration of the red coloured compound is proportional to the amount of uric acid in the sample.

$$\text{Uric acid} + H_2O \xrightarrow{Uricase} \text{Allantoin} + H_2O_2$$

$$H_2O_2 + \text{Phenolic chromogen} \xrightarrow{Peroxidase} \text{Red coloured compound.}$$

Reagents

- R1. *Buffer enzymes* :

Phosphate buffer pH. 7.4 ... 150 mmol/L

Peroxidase ... 450 U/L

4–aminoantipyrine ... 0.225 mmol/L

Uricase ... 120 U/L

- R2. *Chromogen* :

2–Hydroxy–3, 5 dichlorobenzene sulfonic acid ... 2 mmol/L

- R3. *Standard* :

Uric acid ... 10 mg/dl

Store reagents at 4°C.

Reagent preparation : The entire contents of vial R1 (buffer enzymes) is transferred to vial R2 (chromogen) and then mixed thoroughly.

Procedure : 1.0 ml procedure.

	Serum/plasma	Standard	Blank
	0.025 ml (25 μl)	0.025 (25 μl)	—
Reagent	1.0 ml	1.0 ml	1.0 ml

Mix well and incubate assay mixture for 5 minutes at 37°C or 10 minutes at room temperature (25°–30°C). Measure absorbance of sample and standard against Blank at 510 nm within 30 minutes (colour is stable for 30 minutes).

Calculation

$$\text{Conc (mg\%)} = \frac{\text{Absorbance of sample}}{\text{Absorbance of standard}} \times 6$$

Expected values :

Serum	Urine
3.0 to 6.5 mg/dl	250-800 mg/24 h
178 to 387 μ mol/L	1.49 to 4.76 μ mol/L

(B) Phosphotungstic acid method (Caraway, 1963)

Principle

Uric acid reacts with phosphotungstate and reduces it to tungsten blue which is measured colorimetrically and is proportional to the concentration of uric acid in the test sample.

Specimen : Serum/plasma.

Reagents :

1. *Sodium tungstate* : 10% aqueous solution.
2. *Sulphuric acid* : 0.33 mol/l.

*3. *Tungstic acid* : Add 50 ml sodium tungstate, 50 ml diluted sulphuric acid and a drop of phosphoric acid with mixing to 800 ml water. Keep in brown bottle. To be discarded when it becomes cloudy.

*4. *Sodium carbonate solution* : 10% of anhydrous salt solution. Keep in a well-stoppered polythene bottle.

*5. *Phosphotungstate reagent* (stock) : Dissolve 50 gm sodium tungstate (molybdate-free) in 400 ml water, then add 40 ml orthophosphoric acid (sp. gr. 1.75) and reflux gently for 2 hr. Cool, transfer to 500 ml flask and make to the mark with water. It keeps for months in brown bottle.

Working reagent : Dilute 1 : 10 before use.

*6. *Standard solution of urate* (stock) : 100 mg/100 ml water. Keep in brown bottle.

Working standard solution of urate : Dilute stock standard 1 ml to 100 ml with dist. water. Alternatively, dilute 0.1 ml stock standard to 10 ml distilled water and mix well. Prepare fresh working standard everyday.

Procedure

Step A : Deproteinisation of serum

	Test (T)
Serum	0.5 ml
Tungstic acid	4.5 ml
Mix well, keep for 10 minutes and then filter/centrifuge	

Step B :

	Test (T)	Standard (S)	Blank (B)
Supernatant (from step A)	3.0 ml	–	–
Uric acid standard (5 mg/100 ml)	–	3.0 ml	–
Distilled water	–	–	3.0 ml
Sodium carbonate	1.0 ml	1.0 ml	1.0 ml
Mix thoroughly and keep for 2-5 min at R.T.			
Working phospho-tungstic acid	1.0 ml	1.0 ml	1.0 ml

Step B contd. next column

Step B contd....

Mix the contents of each tube thoroughly until no further bubbles are seen to form, and leave in dark for 20 minutes at 25 (±5) °C at room temperature. Read the O.D. of test and standard against blank at 660 nm (range 660-700) or using a red filter.

Calculations

Serum urate/uric acid in mg/100 ml

$$= \frac{OD(T)}{OD(S)} \times 5$$

For the conversion into S.I. units use the formula, mg/dl × 59.5 = μ mol/l (S.I. units).

Note : The procedure with standard linear upto 10 mg/dl of uric acid. In specimens with higher uric acid concentration, dilute the serum with distilled water 1 : 2, and the value so obtained is multiplied by the dilution factor, i.e., 2, in this case.

Calibration curve

Dilute 0.1 m stock standard (100 mg/dl) in a test tube with 9.9 ml dist. water. Dilute the diluted standard to get different corresponding uric acid concentration to the calibration curve.

Tube No	Diluted 1 : 100 dilution of stock std (100 mg/dl)	Distilled water	Corresponding concentration of uric acid in mg/dl
1	1.0 ml	3.0 ml	2.5 mg
2	2.0 ml	2.0 ml	5.0 mg
3	3.0 ml	1.0 ml	7.5 mg
4	4.0 ml	–	10.0 mg

Carry out the uric acid estimations following testing procedure outlined above and plot a graph tabulating corresponding optical density. Prepare a graph with every batch of reagent.

Normal values

Men : 3.1-7.0 mg/dl (SI units 0.18-0.41 μmol/l)

Women : 2.5-6.0 mg/dl (SI units 0.16-0.36 μmol/l)

Children up to puberty : Values are lower than those of normal women.

Significance

1. **Gout** : Level increases in gout (range 7-12 mg/100 ml). Uric acid level does not always correlate with severity of gouty arthritis.

2. **Other conditions** : Uric acid levels are also increased in renal failure, uraemia, leukaemia and following radiotherapy of lymphomas.

Note :

1. Since RBCs contain sulfydryl compounds that give false high results, therefore, unhaemolysed serum should be used.

2. Filtrate/supernatant should be crystal clear.

3. Serum is preferable. In case plasma to be tested, pot. oxalate should not be used as anticoagulant as it forms insoluble potassium phosphotungstate.

PLASMA PROTEINS

Determination

A. Total protein (Biuret method)

Principle : Proteins and peptides containing at least two peptide bonds react with cupric ions of copper sulphate in alkaline solution forming blue to purple coloured compound having absorption of 540 nm.

Protein + Cu^{++} → Blue-violet complex.

Type of reaction : End point.

The reaction (biuret reaction) takes its name from the fact that the simple substance, biuret ($CONH_2$-NH-$CONH_2$), gave the same type of colour with cupric ions.

Reagents

1. *Stock biuret reagent* : Add 45 gm sodium potassium tartarate to 600 ml distilled water and mix well. Then add 8 gm sodium hydroxide and stir to dissolve. While stirring, add 15 gm copper sulphate ($CuSO_4$, $5H_2O$) gradually and mix until solution is complete. Then add 5 gm potassium iodide, and when dissolved make to a litre with distilled water. Filter the solution.

2. *Potassium iodide solution* 5 gm/l in 200 m mol/l sodium hydroxide. Add 8 gm sodium hydroxide to 800 ml distilled water and dissolve by shaking. Add 5 gm potassium iodide and dissolve. Then make to a litre with water. Filter the solution.

3. Brij 35, 35 gm/litre in water. It is a preservative.

4. *Standard serum* : Pooled human serum (HBsAg negative) – 6 gm/dl.

Preparation of biuret reagent for use : Add 200 ml stock biuret reagent to about 500 ml potassium iodide solution, mix, dilute to a litre with further potassium iodide solution and add 1 ml Brij 35.

Storage and stability : All reagents are stable at 2-8°C for at least 6 months.

Specimen : Serum should be collected freshly from a fasting individual and must not be haemolysed. The total protein value is slightly affected by meals but, more importantly, the presence of lipemia interferes with the direct total protein test by causing turbidity in the final reaction mixture.

Procedure : Pipette the following into 3 test tubes as B = Blank, S = Standard, T = Test. (Table 49.1).

Table 49.1 : Procedure of determination of total protein

Reagent	For 3 ml cuvette			For 1.5 ml cuvette		
	B	S	T	B	S	T
Working biuret reagent	3.0 ml	3.0 ml	3.0 ml	1.5 ml	1.5 ml	1.5 ml
Distilled water	50 μl	–	–	25 μl	–	–
Total protein standard (6 gm/dl)	–	50 μl	–	–	25 μl	–
Specimen (serum/plasma)	–	–	50 μl	–	–	25 μl
Mix by lateral shaking and allow to stand at R.T. (30°C) for 15 minutes. Measure OD against blank.						

Calculation

Total proteins in gm/dl

$$= \frac{OD(T)}{OD(S)} \times \text{concentration of standard}$$

$$= \frac{OD(T)}{OD(S)} \times 6$$

(Conc. of standard is 6 gm/dl in this case).

Normal values :

Serum : 5.5–8.0 gm/dl.

Linearity : When read at 550 nm, linearity is up to 15 gm/dl.

B. Serum albumin determination

(Using bromocresol green, Doumas, 1971)

Principle : In an acidic medium, albumin binds with bromocresol green (BCG) forming coloured complex. The blue-green complex formed has an absorption maximum at 630 nm, and intensity of colour of the complex solution is proportional to the concentration of albumin present in sample.

Albumin + BCG → BCG Albumin Complex.

Type of reaction : End point.

Reagents

1. *Stock succinate buffer* (pH 4.1; 0.5 mol/l) : Add 10 gm sodium hydroxide and 56 gm succinic acid in 800 ml water. Adjust to pH 4.10 ± 0.05 at 20°C with 1 mol/l sodium hydroxide (40 gm/l sodium hydroxide) and make up to 1 litre with water. Store at 4°C.

2. *Stock BCG dye solution,* 10 mmol/l : Dissolve 1.75 mg BCG (indicator grade) in 5 ml 1 mol/l sodium hydroxide and make up to 250 ml with water. When diluted 1:1000 with succinate buffer, pH 5.3, 0.2 mol/l, and read against water at 615 nm in a 1 cm cell this solution should have an extinction of 0.315 ± 0.015.

3. *Stock sodium azide,* 40 gm/litre.

4. Stock Brij 35, 250 gm/l : Warm 25 gm Brij 35 in 50 ml water to dissolve and then make up to 100 ml with water.

5. *Buffered dye reagent* : Add the following to 2000 ml water in a 5 litres volumetric flask :

(i) Stock succinate buffer ... 500 ml
(ii) Stock dye solution ... 40 ml
(remove all dye from pipette by washing with water)
(iii) Stock sodium azide ... 12.5 ml
(iv) Stock Brij 35 ... 12.5 ml

Make to volume (2,000 ml) adding water and the reagent is tested to see whether it fulfils the following criteria :

(a) ph–4.15 ± 0.05 at 20°C.

(b) Extinction — 1.347 ± 0.068 at 430 nm and 0.202 ± 0.023 nm in 1 cm cells.

6. *Stock standard albumin solution,* 4 gm/dl. Dissolve 4 g human albumin corrected for moisture content and 20 mg sodium azide in water and make up to 100 ml with water.

Caution : The buffered dye reagent is corrosive. Do not pipette by mouth. Avoid contact with skin or clothing.

Specimen : Serum should be collected from a fasting individual and must not be haemolysed.

Table 49.2 : Procedure of determination of serum albumin

Reagent	For 3 ml cuvette			For 1.5 ml cuvette		
	B	S	T	B	S	T
Buffered dye reagent	4.0 ml	4.0 ml	4.0 ml	1.5 ml	1.5 ml	1.5 ml
Distilled water	0.02 ml	–	–	0.01 ml	–	–
Albumin standard (4 gm/dl)	–	0.02 ml	–	–	0.01 ml	–
Specimen	–	–	0.02 ml	–	–	0.01 ml

Mix well by lateral shaking and allow to stand at R.T. for 1 minute. Measure the absorbance of standard and test at 600 nm or with a red filter against blank.

Procedure

Pipette into 3 test tubes labelled as B–Blank, S–Standard, T–Test (unknown) (Table 49.2).

Calculations

1. Serum albumin in gm / dl

$$= \frac{OD(T)}{OD(S)} \times \text{concentrate of albumin. (Here it is 4)}$$

2. Serum globulin in gm / dl

$$= \text{Total protein gm / dl} - \text{Albumin gm / dl}$$

3. $$\text{A / G ratio} = \frac{\text{Albumin gm / dl}}{\text{Globulin gm / dl}} = x : 1.$$

Normal values :

Total proteins : 5.5-8.0 gm/dl

Serum albumin : 3.5-5.0 gm/dl

Serum globulin : 2.0-3.5 gm/dl

Albumin-globulin ratio = 1.75 : 1.

Clinical significance

1. Total proteins and albumin levels decrease in various clinical conditions like cirrhosis, acute chronic hepatitis, nephrotic syndrome, various malignancies, nutritional deficiency, and certain chronic protracted conditions like ulcerative colitis.

2. Total protein levels may be increased in multiple myeloma and conditions associated with hyperglobulinaemia. High values reflect one or more of globulin fractions.

Chapter 50

Estimation of Serum Bilirubin

The Van den Bergh (VDB) Reaction

The DIAZO reagent consists of two parts :

Reagents

1. *Diazo A*

Sulphanilic acid	...	1 gm
Concentrated HCl	...	15 gm
Distilled water	...	1000 ml

Dissolve sulphanilic acid in HCl and make up to litre with water.

2. *Diazo B*

Sodium nitrite	...	0.5 gm
Distilled water	...	100 ml

Prepare freshly at intervals.

Procedure

Diazo reagent : Prepare freshly before use by adding 0.3 ml solution B to 10 ml solution A in a clean dry tube.

Direct reaction :

		Test tubes	
		T	B
Serum (ml)	....	0.2	–
Distilled water (ml)	....	–	0.2
Diazo reagent (ml)	....	0.2	0.2
Mix and observe colour change			

Interpretation

1. *Immediate direct reaction* : Colour (violet) develops immediately and progress rapidly almost to a maximum. Little change in colour occurs after 3 to 4 min.

2. *Delayed direct reaction* : Colour begins to appear only from 5 to 30 min after mixing. It then develops slowly to a maximum.

3. After 30 min add 4.6 ml distilled water in each of two tubes and mix well. For estimating total direct bilirubiin read at 540 mm against water blank.

4. *Calculation* : Total direct bilirubin mg %.

$$= \frac{T - B}{S} \times 4$$

(when artificial methyl red std is used)

I. Estimation of bilirubin

(Malloy and Evelyn method)

Principle

Direct : (Conjugated) Bilirubin couples with diazotized sulfanilic acid, forming a red-purpled colour product (azobilirubin) in acidic medium.

Indirect : (Unconjugated) Bilirubin is diazotized only in the presence of its dissolving solvent (methanol). Thus, the red-purple colour azobilirubin produced in presence of methanol originates from both *direct* and *indirect* fractions and thus represents total bilirubin concentration. The difference between total and direct bilirubin gives indirect (unconjugated) bilirubin.

The intensity of the red-purple colour of the azobilirubin so developed is measured colorimetrically and it is proportional to the bilirubin concentration of appropriate fraction. This reaction can be represented as :

Bilirubin + Diazotized Sulfanilic acid $\longrightarrow$ Azobilirubin $\xrightarrow{H^+}$ Red-Purple colour (λ max : 540 nm)

Sample

Serum (0.8 ml) is required.

Although serum is recommended, plasma from blood collected in heparin as anticoagulant can also be used for the test. Freshly collected serum samples should only be used for estimation of direct bilirubin, since direct reacting bile pigments — that may appear in serum under certain conditions — are reported to be unstable.

Note : Serum samples must be kept away from both artificial and sunlight during processing and storage. If sample cannot be assayed freshly, it should be stored in dark in the refrigerator. Bilirubin in serum/plasma is stable for one week when refrigerated in dark. About 50% decrease in bilirubin content may be caused by direct sunlight.

Reagents

1. *Diazo A* : Same as in VDB reaction.
2. *Diazo B* : Same as in VDB reaction.
3. *Diazo blank* : 15 ml conc. hydrochloric acid in 1000 ml water.
4. *Methanol* (absolute)
5. *Standard* :

(a) *Artificial methyl red standard* : Dissolve 0.29 gm pure methyl red in 15-20 ml glacial acetic acid and make to 100 ml with the acid (*stock standard*).

Working methyl red standard : To 1.25 ml of the stock standard add 0.5 ml acetic acid and wash in 1.44 gm sodium acetate (the trihydrate) and dissolve and make to 100 ml with water. This solution corresponds to 4.0 mg bilirubin/100 ml.

(b) *Bilirubin standard* : Bilirubin standard may be used in place of artificial methyl red standard.

Stock standard — 11.7 mg/100 ml in chloroform.

Working standard — (0.94 mg/100 ml). It is prepared by diluting 4 ml stock standard to 50 ml 95% ethanol.

Precautions :

1. Bring all solutions to R.T.
2. Prepare blanks (T_2 and D_2) for each sample.
3. Prepare diazo reagent fresh everyday before test : Diazo A 3.3 ml + Diazo B 0.1 ml and mix.
4. Mark the tubes properly as Direct (D_1), Direct Blank (D_2), Total (T_1) and Total Blank (T_2) before starting the test.
5. Tubes T_1 and T_2 must be kept under dark to avoid erroneous results.

Box 1 **Colorimetric procedure for estimation of serum/plasma bilirubin**

	T_1	T_2	D_1	D_2
Serum/plasma (ml)	0.2	0.2	0.2	0.2
Distilled water (ml)	1.8	1.8	1.8	1.8
Diazo blank (ml)	–	0.5	–	0.5
Diazo reagent (ml)	0.5	–	0.5	–
Distilled water (ml)	–	–	2.5	2.5
Methanol (ml)	2.5	2.5	–	–
Total (ml)	**5.0**	**5.0**	**5.0**	**5.0**
	Mix well and keep tubes T_2 and T_1 in dark at R.T. for 30 minutes and read the O.D. against water with yellow-green filter.		Mix well and read O.D. of contents of tubes D_2 and D_1 after 1 minute against water with yellow-green filter.	

Procedure (Box 1)

A. *For colorimeter — Vide Box 1*

B. *For spectrocolorimeter*

All the volumes mentioned under colorimetric procedure can be halved, rest of the procedures remain unchanged. Read at 540 nm.

Standard : Read the OD against water blank and discard once used. Artificial methyl red standard is equivalent to 4.0 mg bilirubin/100 ml, but that of natural bilirubin standard is 4.68 mg/100 ml.

Calculations

Bilirubin conc. in mg / 100 ml

Total (A) = $\frac{OD_{T1} - OD_{T2}}{OD_{Std}}$ × 4.68 when bilirubin standard is used (4.0 with methyl red standard)

Direct (B) = $\frac{OD_{D1} - OD_{D2}}{OD_{Std}}$ × 4.68 when bilirubin standard is used (4.0 with methyl red standard)

Indirect = (A) – (B)

Normal range : *Adults —*

Total bilirubin : 0.2-1.0 mg/100 ml serum or plasma,

Direct bilirubin : 0.1-0.3 mg/100 ml serum or plasma,

Indirect bilirubin : 0.2-0.7 mg/100 ml serum or plasma.

Notes :

1. When OD of Tubes D_1 or T_1 exceeds 0.8 or bilirubin level exceeds 8 mg% repeat the test after diluting the sample in water or saline and multiply the final result so obtained with the dilution factor.
2. When the serum to be tested is dark yellowish in colour, dilute the serum 1 : 2 or 1 : 4 in distilled water before test and multiply the final result so obtained with dilution factor.

Calibration curve (Box 2)

For a standard curve dilute the stock standard of bilirubin 1 to 5 with methanol to give a solution containing 2.34 mg per 100 ml, and set up a series of tubes as follows and read as for the test.

2. Estimation of bilirubin

(Method of Jendrassik and Grof, 1938)

Principle

Total bilirubin in blood (serum or plasma) is determined by coupling with diazotised sulfanilic acid after addition of caffeine, sodium benzoate and sodium acetate. A blue azobilirubin is formed in alkaline Fehling Solution II, which is photometrically measured.

The direct bilirubin is measured as a red azo dye at 546 nm using method of Schellong and Wende (1960) without the addition of alkali.

Calculation of indirect bilirubin is made from the difference between total and direct bilirubin.

Reagents

Reagent 1 : *Sulfanilic acid solution* :

$C_6H_7NO_3S$	29 mmol/l
HCl	170 mmol/l

Reagent 2 : *Sodium nitrite solution* :

Sodium nitrite	29 mg/dl

Reagent 3 : *Accelarator :*

Caffeine	130 mmol/l
Sodium benzoate	156 mmol/l
Sodium acetate	460 mmol/l

Reagent 4 : *Fehling solution II :*

Potassium sodium tartarate	930 mmol/l
Sodium hydroxide	1.9 mmol/l

The reagent is stored at 15-25°C.

Reagent preparation

Reagent 1 is mixed with Reagent 2 in the ratio

Box 2 Calibration curve

	Tubes					
	1	2	3	4	5	6
Serum bilirubin (mg/ml)	0	2.9	5.8	11.7	17.6	29.3
Standard solution	0	0.5	1.0	2.0	3.0	5.0
Methanol (ml)	9.0	8.5	8.0	7.0	6.0	4.0
Diazo reagent	1.0	1.0	1.0	1.0	1.0	1.0

of 4 + 1 (e.g. 400 µl of sulfanilic acid solution and 100 µl of sodium nitrite solution) to make a diazo solution. Freshly prepared diazo reagent is always to be used.

Sample

Serum, heparin-plasma.

Bilirubin is stable in serum or plasma for 2 days at 15-25°C, 7 days at 2–8°C. Sample must be protected from light.

Total Bilirubin (Box 3)

Box 3	Sample Blank	Sample
Diazo solution	–	100 µl
Sulfanilic acid	100 µl	–
Accelerator	500 µl	500 µl
Serum/Plasma	100 µl	100 µl
Mix and incubate for 30 min. at 37°C		
Fehling solution II	500 µl	500 µl
Mix well and incubate for 15 min. at 37°C. Absorbance is read against sample Blank at 578 nm.		

Calculation

Total bilirubin concentration = A × 10.3 mg/dl.

Direct Bilirubin (Box 4)

Box 4	Sample Blank	Sample
Diazo solution	–	100 µl
Sulfanilic acid	100 µl	–
Normal saline	1000 µl	1000 µl
Serum/Plasma	100 µl	100 µl
Mix well and incubate for 5 min. at 37°C. Absorbance is read against sample Blank at 546 nm.		

Calculation

Direct bilirubin concentration = A × 14.0 mg/dl.

Normal range : Serum/Plasma

Total bilirubin	Up to 1.0 mg/dl	Up to 17 mol/l
Direct bilirubin	Up to 0.25 mg/dl	Up to 4.3 mol/l

Dilution Limit : When the absorbance exceeds 1.0, samples should be diluted 1+5 with NaCl solution (9 g/l) and the result to be multiplied by 6.

Chapter 51

Estimation of Lipid and Lipoproteins

SERUM CHOLESTEROL

Normal level of total serum cholesterol is 150-240 mg/100 ml, being a little higher in men than women. About 30 per cent (range 20-40%) of total cholesterol in blood is free cholesterol and the rest is cholesteryl ester.

Cholesterol oxidase obtained from the bacterium *Nocardia erythropolis* reacts only with free cholesterol, so, for the determination of total cholesterol, the ester cholesterol has to be hydrolysed. This can be done either by using ethanolic potassium hydroxide or cholesterol ester hydrolases.

Determination of total cholesterol

(Enzymatic method of Allian *et al.*, 1974)

Principle

Cholesterol esterase hydrolyses esterified cholesterols to free cholesterols (Box 51.1). The free cholesterol is oxidised by cholesterol oxidase to cholestenone and H_2O_2. Now hydrogen peroxide reacts with phenol and 4-aminoantipyrine by the catalytic action of peroxidase producing a red coloured quinoneimine dye complex. The intensity of the pink/red colour formed is directly proportional to the cholesterol concentration in the specimen.The absorbance of the dye is measured at 505 nm. The reaction is end point.

Reagents

1. Single reagent solution (Enzyme reagent 1):

Sodium cholate	...	3 mmol/l
4-aminophenazone (4-amino antipyrine)	....	0.82 mmol/l
Phenol	....	14 mmol/l
Na_2HPO_4	....	50 mmol/l
NaH_2PO_4	....	50 mmol/l
Carbowax (6000)	....	0.17 mmol/l
Cholesterol ester hydrolase	....	33 U/l
Cholesterol oxidase	....	117 U/l
Peroxidase	....	6700 U/l

Adjust pH to 6.7

2. **Reagent blank (Enzyme reagent 2)** : Similar to single reagent solution but the cholesterol esterase and oxidases are omitted.

Box : 51.1

(i) $\text{Cholesteryl ester} \xrightarrow[\text{esterase}]{\text{cholesterol}} \text{Free cholesterol + fatty acids}$

(ii) $\text{Cholesterol} + O_2 \xrightarrow[\text{oxidase}]{\text{cholesterol}} \text{cholestenone} + H_2O_2$

(iii) $2\,H_2O_2 + \text{Phenol} + \text{4-aminoantipyrine} \xrightarrow[\text{Quinonimine dye } + 2\,H_2O \text{ (Red coloured)}]{\text{peroxidase}}$

3. **Cholesterol standard**, 200 mg/dl (5.17 mmol/l) in isopropanol.

Store at 2°–8°C.

Specimen

Serum or heparinised plasma (fasting sample)

Procedure (Box 51.2)

Box : 51.2	Blank (B)	Standard (S)	Test (T)
Single reagent solution	–	3.0 ml	3.0 ml
Distilled water	30 µl	–	–
Standard	–	30 µl	–
Sample	–	–	30 µl
Reagent blank	3.0 ml	–	–
Mix well incubate at 37°C for 5 min. or at R.T. (25°C) for 15 minutes			
Measure the OD at 505 nm (range 492-550 nm) or by using a yellow-green filter.			

Note:

(1) Anticoagulants like fluorides and oxalates result in false lower values.

(2) When less volume of the reactant is required, everything may be taken in half the amount.

Calculation

Serum cholesterol mg/100 ml (or mmol/l)

$$= \frac{OD(T) - OD(B)}{OD(S) - OD(B)} \times 200 \text{ (or } \times 5.17 \text{ m mol / l)}$$

Linearity : Upto 500 mg/dl.

Determination of total cholesterol

(Wybenga Pileggl's Method)

Principle

Cholesterol reacts with hot solution of ferric perchlorate in presence of ethyl acetate and sulfuric acid (cholesterol reagent) when heated in a boiling water bath to produce a lavender colored complex, which is measured colorimetrically.

Sample

Serum/Plasma (0.05 ml is required).

Reagents (commercial kit)

1. *Cholesterol reagent* (ethyl acetate and sulfuric acid).
2. *Working cholesterol standard* – 200 mg/dl.

Procedure (Box 51.3)

Pipette into clean dry tubes labelled Blank (B), Standard (S) and Test (T).

Box : 51.3	(B)	(S)	(T)
Cholesterol reagent (ml)	5.0	5.0	5.0
Distilled water (ml)	0.05	–	–
Working standard (ml)	–	0.05	–
Serum/Plasma (ml)	–	–	0.05

Mix well and keep the tubes immediately in a boiling water bath exactly for 90 seconds ($1^1/_2$ minutes). Cool immediately in running tap water. Measure the OD of Standard and Test against Blank on a colorimeter with a yellow green filter or on a spectrophotometer at 560 nm.

Calculation :

Serum/Plasma Cholesterol in mg/dl

$$= \frac{OD(T)}{OD(S)} \times 200$$

Normal values

Adults : 130–250 mg/100 ml serum/plasma

Children : Lower values are found

Clinical significance

(a) *Elevated levels* of cholesterol are found in hypercholesterolaemia, hypothyroidism, diabetes mellitus, nephrotic syndrome, obstructive jaundice, biliary cirrhosis, atherosclerosis etc.

(b) *Decreased levels* of cholesterol are found in hyperthyroidism, Gaucher's disease and malnutrition.

SERUM TRIGLYCERIDES

Determination (Enzymatic method)

Principle : Serum triglycerides are esters of fatty acids and are hydrolysed to glycerol and free fatty acids by *lipase (Box 51.4). Glycerol kinase* acts on glycerol in presence of ATP, and glycerol is converted to glycerol–3–phosphate. The glycerol–3–phosphate is then oxidised by glycerol–3–phosphate oxidase to yield hydrogen peroxide. Hydrogen peroxide (H_2O_2) reacts in the presence of peroxidase with chlorophenol ESPAS (N-ethyl-N–sulfopropyl–m–anisidine) and 4 aminoantipyrine to form a coloured complex. The intensity of the colour of the complex is proportional to the concentration of triglycerides and is measured photometrically at 546 nm (range 530-570 nm) or with green filter.

The enzymatic determination of triglycerides is done according to the following reaction :

Box : 51.4

(i) Triglycerides + H_2O $\xrightarrow{\text{Lipoprotein lipase}}$ Glycerol + Free fatty acids

(ii) Glycerol + ATP $\xrightarrow[\text{Mg}^{++}]{\text{Glycerol kinase}}$ Glycerol–3–phosphate + ADP

(iii) Glycerol–3–phosphate + O_2 $\xrightarrow[\text{oxidase}]{\text{Glycerol–3–phosphate}}$ H_2O_2 + Dihydroxyacetone phosphate

(iv) H_2O_2 + Amintoantipyrine + phenol $\xrightarrow{\text{Peroxidase}}$ Red quinoneimine + H_2O

Specimen

1. Serum (fasting) is preferred to plasma.
2. Plasma collected with heparin may be used.
3. Plasma collected using fluoride or oxalate should be avoided.

Interfering substances

Haemolysis and high bilirubin contents inferfere marginally with the test only when present in high concentrations.

Reagents

Reagent 1 *(Enzymes)* : It contains the active ingredients —

(i) Lipoprotein lipase ... 1500 U/L
(ii) Glycerol kinase ... 1000 U/L
(iii) Glycerol-3-phosphate oxidase ... 4000 U/L
(iv) Peroxidase ... 1800 U/L
(v) 4-aminoantipyrine ... 0.30 m mol/L
(vi) ATP Na (Adenosine triphosphate Na) ... 1.72 m mol/L

Since these enzymes are unstable in solution, they are conveniently stored in dry form as tablets and preserved at 2-8°C.

Reagent 2 *(Buffer)* : It contains —

(i) Pipe's buffer (pH 7.0) ... 100 m mol/L
(ii) Chlorophenol ... 3.5 m mol/L
(iii) Magnesium chloride ... 6 m mol/L

Reagent 3 : *Standard* :

Glycerol ... 2.28 m mol/L

Corresponding to 200 mg/dl of trioleine and 2.28 m mol/L of triglycerides.

Preparation of working solution (Chromogen)

Dissolve contents of one bottle of *Reagent* 1 with contents of one bottle of *Reagent* 2. Mix well and store at 2-8°C. This chromogen is stable for 3 days at 20-25°C and 4 weeks at 2-8°C.

Procedure

A. For spectrophotometer (Box 51.5)

Box : 51.5 Reagent	Blank (B)	Standard (S)	Test (T)
Chromogen reagent	1.0 ml	1.0 ml	1.0 ml
Standard	–	0.02 ml	–
Sample	–	–	0.02 ml
Mix and incubate at 37°C for 10 min or at RT (25-30°C for 20 min).			
Distilled water	2.0 ml	2.0 ml	2.0 ml
Mix and read the OD of Test, Standard and Reagent Blank againt distilled water at 546 nm (range 530-570 nm) or using green filter.			

B. For colorimeter (Box 51.6)

Sample and standard : Dilute 0.1 ml of sample and standard with 0.4 distilled water or saline and then proceed as follows :

Box : 51.6 Reagent	Blank (B)	Standard (S)	Test (T)
Chromogen reagent	1.0 ml	1.0 ml	1.0 ml
Diluted standard	–	0.02 ml	–
Diluted sample	–	–	0.02 ml
Mix and incubate at 37°C for 10 min or at RT (25-30°C for 20 min).			
Distilled water	4.0 ml	4.0 ml	4.0 ml
Mix and read the OD of Test, Standard and Blank against distilled water at 546 nm or using green filter.			

The colour developed is stable for one hour at room temperature, if protected from direct light.

Calculation

Triglyceride concentration (mg/dl)

$$= \frac{OD(T) - OD(B)}{OD(S) - OD(B)} \times 200$$

Note : To convert into mmol/l multiply by 2.28.

Normal values

Men : 60-165 mg/dl (0.68-1.88 mmol/l).

Women : 40-140 mg/dl (0.46-1.60 mmol/l).

Linearity : The method is linear up to 600 mg/dl for procedure A. For samples greater than that, dilute the samples suitably with normal saline and apply proper dilution factor to calculate the final result.

Clinical significance

1. Serum triglyceride level is of significant importance in primary hyperlipoproteinaemia.

2. Levels are increased in atherosclerosis, diabetes mellitus, glycogen storage disease like Von Gierke's disease, alcoholism, nephrotic syndrome.

HDL-CHOLESTEROL

Determination (Enzymatic PEG-PAP method)

Cholesterol, cholesterol esters, triglycerides and phospholipids are present in blood linked with varying proportion of apoproteins, called lipoproteins. They are grouped under five classes :

(i) Chylomicrons — Large lipoproteins.

(ii) Very low density lipoproteins (VLDL), which contain high concentration of triglyceride (90%) and low concentration of cholesterol and phospholipid.

(iii) Intermediate density lipoproteins (IDL), which are very low density lipoproteins from which a large share of triglycerides have been removed (triglyceride content 40%) so that the concentration of cholesterol (25%) and phospholipids (20%) are increased.

(iv) Low density lipoproteins (LDL) : The greater part of cholesterol circulating in plasma — about 55% — is in the form of LDL.

(v) High density lipoprotein (HDL) is a small particle with a density of 1.063 to 1.210, that contains a very high concentration of protein, about 50% but smaller concentration of phospholipid (25%) and smallest concentration of cholesterol and triglyceride (5% each).

Clinical significance

Ratio of total serum cholesterol to HDL–cholesterol (HDL-C) has a predictive value in determining the risk of coronary heart disease (CHD). Inverse relationships exist between the levels of HDL-cholesterol and CHD, that is, lower the HDL-C concentration, greater the risk of CHD and vice versa. Ratios of total cholesterol and HDL-C over 5 : 1 in males and 4.5 : 1 in females is indicative of risks of CHD. Approximately 20-25% of total cholesterol is represented by HDL-C.

Usually the values of LDL-C and HDL-C are examined simultaneously and compared to study CHD risk assessment. LDL-C can be calculated by using Friedwald and Fredrickson's formula :

$$\text{LDL-Cholesterol} = \text{Total Cholesterol} - \left[\frac{\text{Triglycerides}}{5} + \text{HDL-Cholesterol}\right]$$

Principle

Chylomicrons, very low density lipoproteins (VLDL) and low density lipoproteins (LDL) of serum are precipitated using buffered polyethylene glycol (PEG-6000), or by phosphotungstate magnesium method.

After centrifugation, high density lipoproteins (HDL) are in the supernatant. The cholesterol content in the supernatant (HDL fraction) is then determined by the enzymatic method using cholesterol esterase, cholesterol oxidase, peroxidase, 4-aminoantipyrine and phenol.

$$\text{Serum / Plasma} \xrightarrow[\text{Mg}^{++}]{\text{Phosphotungstate}}$$

$$= \underset{\text{(supernatant)}}{\text{HDL fraction}} + \underset{\text{(precipitate)}}{(\text{LDL} + \text{VLDL} + \text{Chylomicrons})}$$

Reagents

1. **Precipitating reagent** : There are several precipitating agents of which two are most commonly used — polyethylene glycol 6000 or phosphotungstate/magnesium.

Phosphotungstate / Magnesium method :

(i) Dissolve 22.5 gm phosphotungstic acid AR grade in 200 ml water, add 80 ml 1 mol/l sodium hydroxide and make to 500 ml with water.

(ii) Magnesium chloride solution, 2 mol/l. Dissolve 101.7 gm $MgCl_2 . 6H_2O$ in water and make to 250 ml.

(iii) Tris buffer, 10 mmol/l, pH 7.6. Dissolve 1.21 gm Tris in 900 ml water, adjust to pH 7.6 with 1 mol/l hydrochloric acid and dilute to 1 litre.

Working reagent : Mix 100 ml reagent no. (i) with 50 ml reagent no. (ii) before use. Dilute 1 : 20 with Tris buffer.

2. **Enzyme reagent**

Sodium cholate ... 3 mmol/l

Cholesterol esterase (ester hydrolase) ... 33 U/l

Cholesterol oxidase	...	117 U/l
Peroxidase	...	6700 U/l
4-aminoantipyrine	...	0.17 mmol/l
Carbowax 6000	...	0.82 mmol/L

Since the enzymes are unstable in solution, they are conveniently stored in dry form as tablet or in lyophilised form and preserved at 2-8°C.

3. **Buffer solution**

Na_2HPO_4	...	50 mmol/l
NaH_2PO_4	...	50 mmol/l
Phenol	...	14 mmol/l

Adjust pH to 6.7.

4. **Standard**, 50 mg/dl cholesterol (BDH/AR grade) in isopropanol.

Preparation of working solution (Chromogen) : Transfer the contents of one vial of enzyme (reagent 2) into a bottle of buffer diluent (reagent 3). Mix gently to dissolve the contents and store at 2-8°C.

Reagent storage and stability

The enzyme kit is stable for 6-8 months when stored at 2-8°C. The working solution (chromogen) is stable for 15 days in dark bottle at 2-8°C.

Specimen collection and preservation

1. Serum fasting is preferred to plasma.
2. Plasma collected using heparin as anticoagulant may also be used.
3. Serum or plasma should be separated immediately.
4. Serum may be stable for 7 days if stored at 2-8°C.

Procedure

Step I : Precipitation (HDL-Cholesterol separation) — (Box 51.7)

Box : 51.7

Pipette into centrifuge tube	Quantity
Sample	0.3 ml
Precipitating reagent (Polyethylene glycol – 6000)	0.3 ml

Mix well. Leave it at room temperature for 10 min. and then centrifuge at 3000 rpm for 15 min. or 4000 rpm for 10 min, to obtain a clear supernatant. Take the clear supernatant for HDL-cholesterol estimation (step II).

Step II : HDL–Cholesterol estimation

A. For spectrophotometer requiring 3.0 ml volume (Box 51.8)

Box : 51.8

Reagent	Blank (B)	Standard (S)	Test (T)
Working solution (Chromogen reagent)	1.0 ml	1.0 ml	1.0 ml
Standard (50 mg/dl)	–	0.2 ml	–
Sample (Supernatant from Step I)	–	–	0.2 ml
Mix and incubate at 37°C for 10 min or at RT (25-30°C) for 20 min.			
Distilled water	2.0 ml	2.0 ml	2.0 ml

B. For colorimeter requiring 5.0 ml volume (Box 51.9)

Box : 51.9

Reagent	Blank (B)	Standard (S)	Test (T)
Chromogen reagent	1.0 ml	1.0 ml	1.0 ml
Standard (50 mg/dl)	–	0.4 ml	–
Sample (Supernatant from Step I)	–	–	0.4 ml
Mix and incubate at 37°C for 10 min or at RT (25-30°C) for 20 min.			
Distilled water	4.0 ml	4.0 ml	4.0 ml

Note : The read out requirement for most colorimeter is 4.0 ml, even though the specification is for 5 ml. In such situation, the distilled water volume may be reduced to 3.0 ml after the incubation step. This will increase the sensitivity proportionately.

Mix and read the absorbance of all the tubes (Blank, Standard, Test) at 500 nm (range 490-550 nm) wave length against water.

Calculation

HDL-Cholesterol in mg/dl

$$= \frac{OD(T) - OD(B)}{OD(S) - OD(B)} \times 100$$

To convert mg/dl to mmol/l, use factor : mmol/l = mg/dl × 0.026.

Linearity :

The method is linear up to 200 mg/dl.

***Reference values of HDL cholesterol* (Box 51.10)**

Box : 51.10	Expected values	Standard risk	High risk
Men Women	35-55 mg/dl 45-65 mg/dl	35 mg/dl 45 mg/dl	< 35 mg/dl < 45 mg/dl
Ratio : $\frac{\text{Total cholesterol}}{\text{HDL - cholesterol}}$		3 to 6	More than 6

Calculation of LDL–Cholesterol

$$\text{LDL-Cholesterol} = \text{Total Cholesterol} - \left[\frac{\text{Triglyceride}}{5} + \text{HDL - Cholesterol}\right]$$

Expected results

LDL-Cholesterol : Up to 150 mg%.

Chapter 52

Estimation of Enzymes

ENZYMES

There are at least 50 proteins with enzymatic activity circulating in plasma. These enzymes normally play a role in intracellular metabolism, but small quantities pass through the cellular membranes and appear in blood plasma. When an organ is diseased, greater amount of its enzymes escape into the blood.

Units

The International Clinical Enzyme Subcommission (1966) recommended that all enzyme activities should be expressed in terms of *International Units* (U), i.e., one such unit being of the activity which transforms one micromole of substrate per minute under defined conditions.

Isoenzymes

Many enzymes are present in variant forms in different tissues, which are termed *isoenzymes* or *isozymes*. They have got several structural differences and electrophoretic techniques have been used to separate the isoenzymes.

Specimen for enzyme determination

Serum is preferred. Sample of blood should be free from haemolysis, since red cells are much richer than plasma in several enzymes, for example lactate dehydrogenase and aminotransferases.

On storing, leakage of enzymes from red cells, platelets and leukocytes occur. Hence serum should be separated as early as possible after collection of blood.

SERUM GLUTAMATE PYRUVATE TRANSAMINASE, SGPT

(Also called Alanine Transaminase, ALT)

Determination

A. Method of Reitman and Frankel

(2, 4-DNPH method of Reitman and Frankel modified by Bergmeyer and Bernt, 1974).

Principle

ALT (SGPT) catalyses the following reaction :

α-ketoglutarate + L-alanine $\rightleftharpoons$ Glutamate + Pyruvate.

Pyruvate so formed is coupled with 2, 4-Dinitrophenyl hydrazine (2, 4-DNPH) to give the corresponding hydrazone which gives brown colour in alkaline medium and this can be measured colorimetrically.

Specimen

Venous blood in plain bulb, 0.1 ml unhaemolysed serum is required.

Reagents

1. **Buffered substrate** with alanine

K_2HPO_4	....	15.0 gm
KH_2PO_4	....	2.0 gm
2-oxoglutaric acid	....	300 mg

Dissolve the ingredients in 700 to 800 ml water. Then add 17.8 gm DL-alanine, dissolve and adjust to pH 7.4 with sodium hydroxide (reagent 3) and make to a litre with distilled water.

2. **2, 4-dinitrophenylhydrazine (DNPH colour reagent)** : DNPH, 1 mmol (200 mg/l) in 1 mmol/l hydrochloric acid.

3. **Sodium hydroxide solution**, 400 mmol (16 gm/l).

4. **Working pyruvate solution,** 2 mmol/l : Dissolve 22 mg sodium pyruvate (analytical grade) in 100 ml distilled water.

Storage and stability : All the reagents are stable at 2-8°C for 6-8 months.

Procedure

Standard curve: As the reaction proceeds with time, more amounts of products are formed and since the end products inhibit the enzyme, there is more of inhibition. This is the main problem of colorimetric method of determination of ALT/AST. On the other hand, by kinetic method, the enzyme activity is measured during the initial few minutes, the amount of products formed during that period is negligible to cause any inhibition.

For the above reason, it is necessary to standardise any colorimetric method against a standard kinetic technique.

A standard curve is prepared by diluting pyruvate solution (reagent 4). It is not necessary to plot standard curve every time a test is done. It should be performed initially when the first test is done with a new batch of reagent. Subsequently, periodic checking may be done by running only a few tubes, viz., tubes 1 and 3 of the following table and their OD is compared with the original curve (Fig. 52.1). Standard curves for ALT and AST using pyruvate standard is prepared as follows :

I. Standard curve (Box 52.1)

A. *For colorimeter*

Box : 52.1 Tube No.	1	2	3	4	5
Enzyme activty (units/ml)	0	28	57	97	150
Buffered substrate, ml	0.5	0.45	0.4	0.35	0.3
Working pyruvate standard, ml (2 mmol)	–	0.05	0.1	0.15	0.2
Distilled water, ml	0.1	0.1	0.1	0.1	0.1
DNPH colour reag., ml	0.5	0.5	0.5	0.5	0.5
Mix well and allow to stand at RT for 20 min.					
Sodium hydroxide solution (reagent 3)	5.0	5.0	5.0	5.0	5.0
Mix well by inversion. Allow to stand at RT for 10 min and measure OD of standards using green filter against distilled water.					
OD recorded	–	0.40	0.48	0.58	0.69

B. *For spectrophotometer* : All the volumes mentioned above are halved without any change in the rest of the procedure. Read OD at 505 nm against distilled water.

Plot a standard as in Fig. 52.1 taking enzyme activity on X-axis and OD on Y-axis.

II. Test technique (Box 52.2)

A. *For colorimeter*

Box : 52.2 Reagent	Test (T)	Standard–3 (S–4)
Buffered substrate, pH 7.4	0.5 ml	0.4 ml
Incubate at 37°C for 5 min.		
Serum	0.1 ml	–
Mix well, incubate at 37°C for 30 min.		
Distilled water	–	0.1 ml
Standard	–	0.1 ml
DNPH colour reagent	0.5 ml	0.5 ml
Mix well, allow to stand at RT for 20 min.		
Sod. hydroxide (reagent 3)	5.0 ml	5.0 ml
Mix well and allow to stand at RT for 10 min and read the OD against distilled water using green filter.		

B. *For spectrophotometer* : All the volumes mentioned under colorimetric method can be halved and the rest of the technique remains unchanged. Measure the OD at 505 nm against distilled water.

Calculations : Mark the optical density of test on the Y-axis of the standard curve and extrapolate it to the corresponding enzyme activity on X-axis. The OD of standard 3 is checked with the previous reading on the Y-axis.

B. *UV Kinetic (IFCC) method*

(Commercial kits available)

Principle

$$\text{L-Alanine} + \alpha\text{–ketoglutarate} \xrightarrow{\text{GPT}} \text{Pyruvate} + \text{L–Glutamate}$$

$$\text{Pyruvate} + \text{NaDH} + H^+ \xrightarrow{\text{LDH}} \text{Lactate} + NAD^+$$

There is a decrease in absorption at 340 nm during conversion of NADH to NAD. The rate of increase in absorbance is proportional in the SGPT activity in the sample.

Specimen

Serum or heparinised plasma. One is to avoid

AT LABORATORY (ON SPECTRONIC 20)

GPT (ALT)		GOT (AST)	
Units/ml	O.D.	Units/ml	O.D.
0	0.316	0	0.303
28	0.459	24	0.403
57	0.553	61	0.508
97	0.639	114	0.592
150	0.703	190	0.679

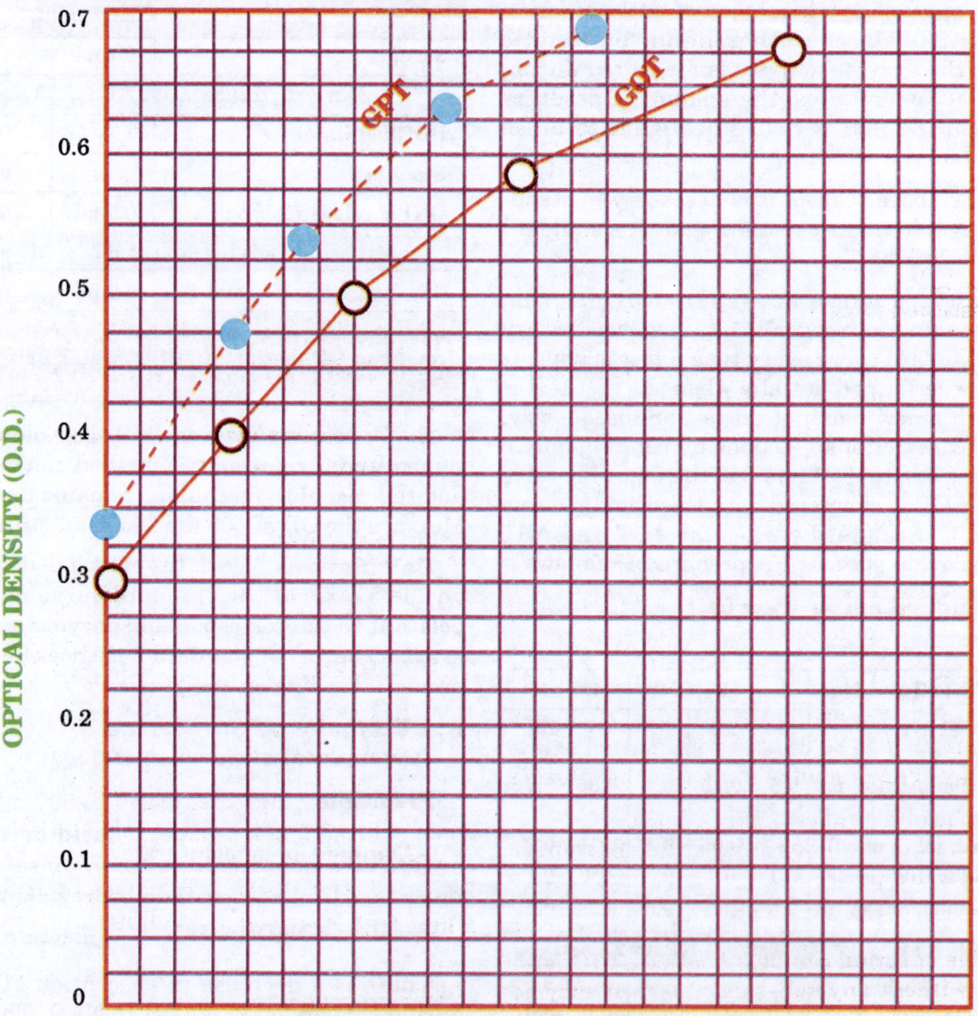

Fig. 52.1. Standard ALT and AST curves

using haemolysed plasma. ALT is stable in serum for 3 days at 2°C to 8°C.

Reagents

Reagent 1 (Working reagent)

LDH	≥ 1200 U/L
NADH	≥ 0.20 m mol/L
α-Ketoglutarate	... 16 m mol/L

Reagent 1A (Buffer)

Tris buffer, pH 7.5 ..	110 m mol/L
L–Alanine	.... 550 m mol/L

Reagents stored at 2–8°C and protected from light.

Reagent reconstitution (Box 52.3)

Bring reagents to room temperature. Dissolve contents of one vial or *Reagnt* 1 with one vial of *Reagent* 1A. Mix well by gentle whirling. To wait for 5 minutes before testing.

Procedure

Box : 52.3	Test
Reconstitued Reagent	1 ml
Sample	100 µl
Mix and read immediately	

Calculation

Units of SGPT per ml per minute = decrease in extinction in 5 minutes × 1000,

Or

GPT activity (IU/L) = (Δ A/min) × 1746

µKat/L = (Δ A/min) × 29.1.

Linearity

The assay is linear upto 250 IU/L. For higher values, sample is to be diluted with normal saline and reassayed and result is multiplied by diluting factor.

Normal values : 5-35 units per ml of serum or upto 40 U/L (37°C).

NOTES :

1. Sample of serum can be stored at 2-8 °C for 5 days without any substantial loss of enzyme activity.
2. When enzyme activity is more than 150, repeat the test after diluting serum 1 : 5 (or more, if necessary) with normal saline and multiply the final result so obtained with the dilution factor.
3. A separate blank is not necessary since tube no. 1 of standard curve substitutes the blank.
4. Glass wares used in the test should be clean and dry. Detergents are to be avoided.

Clinical significance of ALT (SGPT)

Elevated levels of ALT (SGPT) and AST (SGOT) are seen in many liver disorders and the increase of ALT is significantly higher than AST. Marked increase is observed in prodromal stage of acute viral hepatitis which persists during the early clinical phase.

SERUM GLUTAMATE OXALOACETATE TRANSAMINASE, SGOT

(Also called ASPARTATE Transaminase, AST)

A. Determination (2, 4-DNPH method)

Principle

AST (GOT) catalyses the following reaction.

α-ketoglutarate + L-aspartate $\rightleftharpoons$ L-glutamate + Oxaloacetate.

Oxaloacetate so formed is coupled with 2, 4-dinitrophenyl hydrazine (2, 4-DNPH) to give the corresponding hydrazone, which gives brown colour in alkaline medium and this is measured colorimetrically.

Specimen : Venous blood in plain vial : 0.1 ml serum is required.

Reagents

1. **Buffered substrate (aspartate)**

K_2HPO_4	.... 15 gm
KH_2PO_4	.... 2 gm
2-oxoglutaric acid	.... 300 mg

Dissolve the ingredients in 700-800 ml water. Then add 13.2 gm L-aspartic acid or 15.7 gm L-aspartate (monosodium salt), dissolve, and adjust to pH 7.4 with sodium hydroxide. Make to a litre with distilled water.

2. **2, 4-dinitrophenyl hydrazine (DNPH) :** Colour reagent (same as in ALT).

3. **Sodium hydroxide solution,** 400 mmol/l (4N).

4. **Working pyruvate standard,** 2 mmol/l (22 mg sodium pyruvate per 100 ml).

Procedure

I. Standard curve (Box 52.4)

A. *For colorimeter*

Box : 52.4 Tube No.	1	2	3	4	5
Enzyme activty (units/ml)					
Buffered substrate, ml	0.5	0.45	0.4	0.35	0.3
Working pyruvate standard, ml (2 mmol)	–	0.05	0.1	0.15	0.2
Distilled water, ml	0.1	0.1	0.1	0.1	0.1
DNPH colour reag., ml	0.5	0.5	0.5	0.5	0.5
Mix well and allow to stand at RT for 20 min.					
Sodium hydroxide 400 mmol/l ml	5.0	5.0	5.0	5.0	5.0
Mix well by inversion. Allow to stand at RT for 10 min read OD of all five tubes against distilled water using green filter or at 505 nm.					

B. *For spectrophotometer*

All the volumes mentioned above are halved without any change in the rest of the procedure. Measure OD at 505 nm against distilled water.

Plot a standard graph by taking enzyme activity on X-axis and OD on Y-axis (Fig. 48.1).

II. Test (Box 52.5)

A. *For colorimeter*

Box : 52.5 Reagent	Test (T)	Standard-3 (S-4)
Buffered aspartate	0.5 ml	0.4 ml
Incubate at 37°C for 5 min.		
Serum	0.1 ml	–
Mix well, incubate at 37°C for 60 min.		
Distilled water	–	0.1 ml
Working standard	–	0.1 ml
DNPH colour reagent	0.5 ml	0.5 ml
Mix well and allow to stand at RT for 20 min.		
Sod. hydroxide, 400 mmol/l	5.0 ml	5.0 ml
Mix well and allow to stand at RT for 10 min and read the OD of T and S–4 against distilled water using a green filter.		

B. *For spectrophotometer* : All the volumes mentioned above are halved and the rest of the procedure remains unchanged. Measure the OD at 505 nm against water.

Calculations : Mark the OD of Test (T) on the Y-axis of the standard curve and extrapolate it to the corresponding enzyme activity on X-axis. The OD of standard-3 (S-4) is checked with the previous reading of OD on the Y-axis.

B. SGOT determination UV Kinetic IFCC method

Principle

$$\text{L–Aspartate} + \alpha\text{-ketoglutarate} \xrightarrow{\text{GOT}} \text{Oxaloacetate} + \text{L-Glutamate}$$

$$\text{Oxaloacetate} + \text{NaDH} + \text{H}^+ \xrightarrow{\text{MDH}} \text{L-Malate} + \text{NAD}$$

MDH = Malate dehydrogenase.

IFCC = International Federation of Clinical Chemistry

At 340 nm, there is decrease in absorption as NADH is converted to NAD. The rate of decrease in absorbance is measured and is proportional to AST in the sample.

Reagents

- *Reagent 1 (Enzymes)*
  - MDH .... 600 U/L
  - LDH .... 900 U/L
  - NADH .... 0.20 m mol/L
  - α-Ketoglutarate .... 12 m mol/L
- *Reagent 1A (Tris buffer)*
  - Tris buffer (pH 7.8) .... 88 m mol/L
  - L-Aspartate .... 264 m mol/L

Store reagents at 2°–8°C and protected from light.

Working reagent

Both reagents 1 and 1A are brought to room temperature. Now dissolve reagent 1 (enzymes) in reagent 1A (Tris buffer) and mix by gentle shaking. This reconstituted reagent is stable for 4 weeks when stored at 2°–8°C.

Procedure (Box 52.6)

Pipette into tubes :

Box : 52.6	Test
Reconstituted Reagent	1 ml
Sample	100 µl

Mix and read immediately

or

Read initial absorbance after 1 minute and

start a timer. Read again after exactly 1, 2 and 3 minutes.

Calculation

GOT activity (IU/L) = (Δ A/min) × 1746

µkat = (Δ A/min) × 29.1

Linearity

The estimation is linear upto 350 IU/L. When (Δ A/min) is higher than 0.200, dilute sample and reassay and multiply result by dilution factor.

Normal values : 8-40 Karmen units/ml of serum or upto 35 IU/L.

Clinical significance : Elevated levels of AST (SGOT) are found in myocardial infarction but ALT level is normal. The duration and extent of increase is related to the size of the infarct. In the differentiation of myocardial infarction from other cardiac disorders, AST (GOT) determination is of great importance. AST levels are also increased in various types of liver disease, in skeletal muscle trauma and sometimes in renal disease.

ALKALINE PHOSPHATASE

A. Estimation by 4-aminophenazone method (King & Kings, 1954)

Principle : Alkaline phosphatase from serum converts phenyl phosphate to inorganic phosphate and phenol at pH 10.0. Phenol thus produced reacts in alkaline medium with 4-aminophenazone (4-aminoantipyrine) in presence of the oxidising agent potassium ferricyanide and forms an orange-red coloured complex, which can be measured colorimetrically. The colour intensity is proportional to the enzyme activity. This technique does not require deproteinisation of serum. Colour development is rapid and lasts longer.

Reaction can be represented as follows :

$$\text{(i) Phenyl phosphate} \xrightarrow[\text{pH 10.0}]{\text{Alk. phosphatase}} \text{Phenol + Pi}$$

$$\text{(ii) Phenol + 4–aminoantipyrine} \xrightarrow[\text{OH}^-]{\text{Pot. ferricyanide}}$$

Orange-red coloured complex (λ-max = 510-520 nm)

Reagents

1. **Disodium phenyl phosphate, 100 m mol/l** : Dissolve 2.18 gm (2.541 gm of the dihydrate) in water and make to a litre. Bring quickly to boil, cool, add a little chloroform and keep in the refrigerator.

2. **Sodium carbonate-sodium bicarbonate, 100 mmol/l** : Dissolve 6.36 gm anhydrous sodium carbonate and 3.36 gm sodium bicarbonate in water and make to a litre.

3. **Buffered substrate for use** : Prepare by mixing equal volumes of solutions 1 and 2. This should have a pH of 10.0 and adjust, if required.

4. **Stock standard phenol solution, 1 gm/l** : Dissolve 1 gm pure crystalline phenol in 100 m mol/l hydrochloric acid and make to a litre with the acid.

5. **Working standard phenol solution, 10 mg/100 ml** : Dilute 1 ml of the stock to 10 ml distilled water.

6. **Sodium hydroxide solution**, 500 mmol/l.

7. **Sodium bicarbonate solution**, 500 mmol/l.

8. **4-aminophenazone**, 6 gm/l in water.

9. **Potassium ferricyanide**, 24 gm/l in water.

Note : Buffered substrate (Reagent 3) is supplied in commercial test kit in powder form in a vial which is to be reconstituted in distilled water.

Sample

Serum : Venous blood collected aseptically in a clean dry vial/tube.

Procedure

A. *For colorimeter (Box 52.7).*

B. *For spectrophotometer* : All the volumes mentioned for colorimetric procedure can be halved and rest of the procedure remains unchanged. Measure the OD at 510 nm.

Calculations

Serum alkaline phosphatase activity in KA units/100 ml.

$$= \frac{\text{(OD) Test} - \text{(OD) Control}}{\text{(OD) Std} - \text{(OD) Blank}} \times 10$$

Notes :

1. KA units = mg phenol liberated/100 ml serum.
2. When OD of test exceeds 0.8, repeat the test after diluting the serum with normal saline.

Normal values :

Adults : 4-11 KA units (22-92 U/l).

Children : Higher values are found.

Box : 52.7 Reagent	Blank (B)	Standard (S)	Control (C)	Test (T)
Buffered substrate, ml	1.0	1.0	1.0	1.0
Distilled water, ml	1.1	1.0	1.0	1.0
Mix well and incubate at 37°C for 3 min				
Serum, ml	–	–	–	0.1
Phenol standard 10 mg%, ml	–	0.1	–	–
Mix well and incubate at 37°C for 15 min				
Sodium hydroxide, ml	0.8	0.8	0.8	0.8
Sodium bicarbonate, ml	1.2	1.2	1.2	1.2
4-aminophenazone, ml	1.0	1.0	1.0	1.0
Potassium ferricyanide, ml	1.0	1.0	1.0	1.0
Serum, ml	–	–	0.1	–
Mix well after the addition of each reagent and measure the OD of Blank (B), Standard (S) Control (C) and Test (T) against distilled water using a green filter.				

B. Estimation by p–NPP method

(Commercial reagent kits available)

Principle

In an alkaline solution, alkaline phosphatase hydrolyses paranitrophenyl phosphate into paranitrophenol and phosphate in the presence of magnesium ions. The rate of increase in absorbance of the reaction mixture at 405 nm is proportional to the alkaline phosphatase activity. Increase in absorbance of the reaction mixture is attributable to liberation of paranitrophenol i.e., alkaline phosphatase activity.

p–nitrophenyl phosphate + H_2O —Alkaline phosphatase→ p–nitrophenol + phosphate

Reagents

1. DEA buffer.
2. Substrate : para-nitrophenyl phosphate store reagents at 2°–8°C.

Reagent composition

DEA buffer .... 1 m mol/L

p–nitrophenyl phosphate .... 10 m mol/L

Reagent preparation

The entire content of reagent (substrate) vial 2 is transferred to reagent (DEA buffer) vial 1. Mix gently and allow to stand for 5-10 minutes.

Working reagent (buffer substrate) should be used on the same day. It may be stored at 2–8°C for 10 days in a dark coloured bottle.

Sample : Serum or heparinised or EDTA blood.

Procedure (Box 52.8)

Pipette into tubes :

Box : 52.8	Test
Reagent	1 ml
Sample	20 µl

Read the absorbance at 30, 60, 90 and 120 seconds at 405 nm. Determine the mean change in absorbance per minute and calculate the results of the test.

Calculation

Alkaline phosphatase activity (IU/L)
$= \Delta$ A/min × F

where F = 2713 (calculation is made based on molar extinction coefficient for *p*–nitrophenol and ratio of total assay volume to sample volume).

Normal range (IU/L) — Box 52.9

Box : 52.9	At 25°C	At 30°C	At 37°C
1. Children	150–470	183–573	245–768
2. Adults	60–170	73–207	98–279

Linearity

Procedure is linear upto 825 IU/L. If (Δ A/min) exceeds 0.250, sample is to be diluted with normal saline and reassayed. The result is multiplied by dilution factor.

Clinical significance

Alkaline phosphatase level is increased in the following conditions :

1. **Bone disease** when osteoid tissue is newly laid down, e.g., rickets, osteomalacia, osteitis deformans (Paget's disease), osteogenic sarcomas.

2. **Liver disease**: High values up to 40 KA units/ 100 ml (280 U/l) in cholestatic jaundice and primary biliary cirrhosis are seen. Blood level of 25-30 KA units/100 ml is seen in infective or toxic hepatitis.

ACID PHOSPHATASE

Estimation of serum acid phosphatase

(King's 4-aminoantipyrine method)

Principle

Acid phosphatase from serum converts phenyl phosphate to inorganic phosphate and phenol at pH 4.9. Phenol thus formed reacts in alkaline medium with 4-aminoantipyrine in presence of oxidising agent potassium ferricyanide and forms an orange-red colour complex, which is colorimetrically measured. The colour intensity of the complex is proportional to the enzyme activity.

As tartrate inhibits the prostatic fraction of the enzyme, the difference in acid phosphatase activity without and with tartrate represents the activity of prostatic fraction.

(i) Phenyl phosphate $\xrightarrow[\text{pH 4.9}]{\text{Acid phosphatase}}$ Phenol + Pi

(ii) Phenol + 4–aminoantipyrine $\xrightarrow[OH^-]{\text{Pot. ferricyanide}}$ Orange-red coloured complex (λ-max = 510-520 nm)

Sample : Venous blood in plain bulb/tube (0.6 ml of serum is required).

Reagents : Reagents are the same as in alkaline phosphatase estimation except :

(a) Buffer is substituted by citrate buffer (pH 4.9) and

(b) Additional reagent — Tartrate, 1.0 mol/l.

1. **Disodium phenyl phosphate, 10 mmol/l, 2.18 gm/l**: Bring the solution quickly to boil to sterilise, cool and add a little chloroform.

2. **Citric acid — sodium citrate buffer**: Dissolve 2.1 gm crystalline citric acid in water, add 188 ml 1 mol/l sodium hydroxide and make to 500 ml with water. Adjust to pH 4.9, if necessary, by adding drop by drop sodium hydroxide or hydrochloric acid. Alternatively, dissolve 58.82 gm sodium citrate dihydrate in 200 mmol/l hydrochloric acid and make to a litre with the acid. Check the pH and adjust, if necessary.

Keep solutions 1 and 2 in refrigerator.

3. **Buffer substrate** : Prepare freshly by mixing equal volumes of the above two solutions (Nos. 1 and 2).

4. **Stock standard phenol solution**, 1 gm/l (see alkaline phosphatase).

5. Phenol standard for use, 10 mg/100ml : Dilute the stock solution 1 to 10 in dist. water.

6. **Sodium hydroxide solution (0.5N)**, 500 mmol/l.

7. **Sodium bicarbonate (0.5N)**, 500 mmol/l.

8. **4-aminophenazone (antipyrine)**, 6 gm/l in water.

9. **Potassium ferricyanide**, 24 gm/l in water.

10. **L(+) Tartrate solution**, 1 mol/l. Dissolve 15 gm L(+) tartaric acid in 70 ml water, add 18.5 ml 1 mol/l sodium hydroxide to pH 4.9 and make to 100 ml. Store with a few drops of chloroform in the refrigerator.

Note : In commercially available kits reagent 3 (buffer substrate), 8 (4-Amino antipyrine), 9 (Potassium ferricyanide) are supplied in powder form which are to be reconstituted with distilled water before use as per manufacturer's instructions.

Procedure

A. *For colorimeter (Box 52.10 on p. 458)*

B. *For spectrophotometer* : All the volumes mentioned for colorimetric procedure are halved. Rest of the procedure remains unchanged. Measure the OD at 510 nm.

Calculations : Serum acid phosphatase activity in KA units/100 ml serum :

$$\text{Total} = \frac{OD(T) - OD(C)}{OD(S) - OD(B)} \times 5$$

$$\text{Prostatic fraction} = \frac{OD(T) - OD(Ts)}{OD(S) - OD(B)} \times 5.$$

Normal range

Total acid phosphatase : 1.0-4.0 KA units.

Prostatic fraction : 0.0-0.8 KA units.

Box : 52.10 Reagent	Blank (B)	Standard (S)	Control (C)	Test (T)	Tartrate stable (Ts)
Buffered substrate (pH 4.9), ml	–	–	1.0	1.0	1.0
Distilled water, ml	2.2	1.2	1.0	1.0	1.0
Mix well and incubate at 37°C for 3 min					
Working standard, ml	–	1.0	–	–	–
Tartrate, 1.0 mol, ml	–	–	–	–	0.05
Serum, ml	–	–	–	0.2	0.2
Mix well and incubate at 37°C for 60 min					
Sodium hydroxide 0.5N, ml	1.0	1.0	1.0	1.0	1.0
Serum, ml	–	–	0.2	–	–
Sodium bicarbonate 0.5N, ml	1.0	1.0	1.0	1.0	1.0
4-aminoantipyrine, ml	1.0	1.0	1.0	1.0	1.0
Potassium ferricyanide, ml	1.0	1.0	1.0	1.0	1.0
Mix well after the addition of each reagent and measure the OD of Blank (B), Standard (S), Control (C), Test (T) and Tartrate stables (Ts) against distilled water using a green filter.					

Notes :

1. When OD exceeds 0.8, repeat the test after diluting the serum suitably with normal saline and multiply the final result with the dilution factor.

2. The final colour is stable for at least an hour.

Clinical significance

Increase in serum acid phosphatase levels are observed in prostatic carcinomas with metastasis, Paget's disease of bone, hyperparathyroidism, metastasis in bone, Gaucher's disease and chronic renal disease.

Section VII

MISCELLANEOUS

Section VII contains

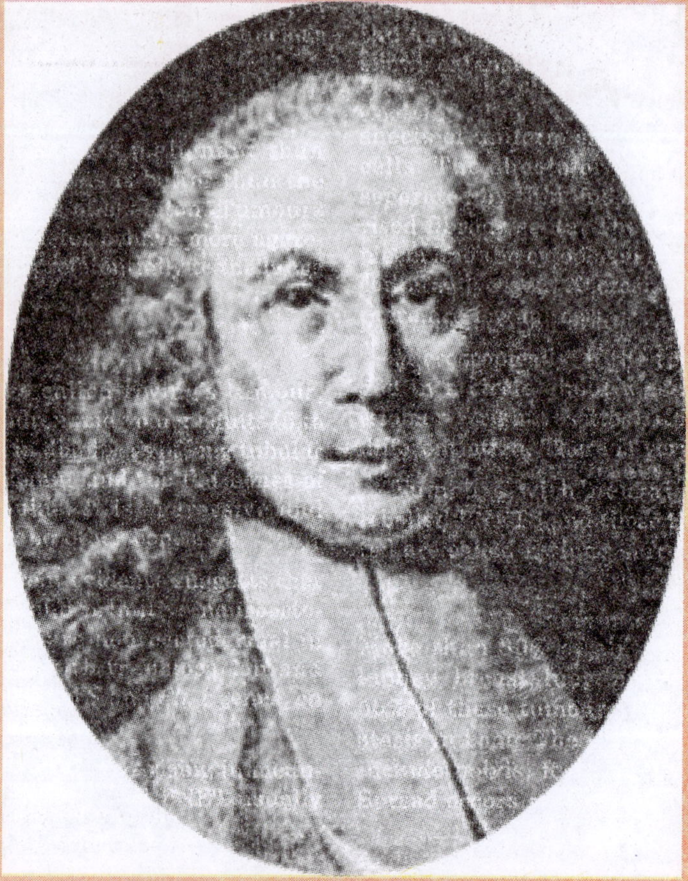

Giovanni B Morgagni (1682–1771)

Founder of CPCs — *is an Italian anatomist and pathologist, who for the first time made correlation between pathology found at postmortem and clinical findings. Virchow considered that Morgagni introduced modern pathology.*

Chapter 53

Autopsy Methods

Medical autopsy is the **postmortem** examination of the dead body for the purpose of ascertaining the cause of death.

Codes

1. Autopsy should be conducted in a place specially designed for the purpose (e.g., Mortuary).

2. A written permission of the person in charge of the body must be obtained.

3. Prosector must put on a pair of thick rubber gloves and an apron. There should be arrangement for smears, cultures and fixatives.

4. Examination should be done in *daylight* and not in artificial light, as far as practicable, because colour changes, such as jaundice, cannot be appreciated in artificial light. Postmortem examination may be conducted on the next day, as early as possible.

5. During postmortem examination, findings of examination should be recorded by an assistant.

6. Every organ must be examined and specimens collected.

7. The body should be reconstituted after postmortem examination.

Autopsy specimens

1. Gross materials of interest should be preserved for museum specimens.

2. Slices of tissue from organs are preserved in Zenker's fluid or 10% formalin.

3. Smears and cultures should be collected properly with asepsis.

Autopsy report

Autopsy report consists of three parts, mainly :

I. Introduction

This includes permission given by the incharge of the body, clinical history of the case, the date and place of examination, the name, age and sex of the deceased.

II. Report

This consists of a complete description of the external and internal examinations of the body including results of histopathological, cultural and chemical examination of specimens.

III. Conclusion

The clinical and anatomical diagnosis is made on the basis of postmortem findings.

External examination

The following are looked for :

1. Height, weight and general state of body build and nourishment.
2. Colour of skin—jaundice, pigmentation.
3. Lymph nodes—cervical, axillary, inguinal.
4. Presence of oedema legs, surgical emphysema around the chest.
5. Presence of any external wound or other signs of violence (together with marks of burns).
6. Presence of deformity, hernia, etc.
7. Conditions of natural orifices — mouth, nostrils, ears, anus, vagina, etc.
8. Conditions of eyes, pupils, tongue, lips, gums, etc.

Internal examination

All body cavities and viscera should be examined

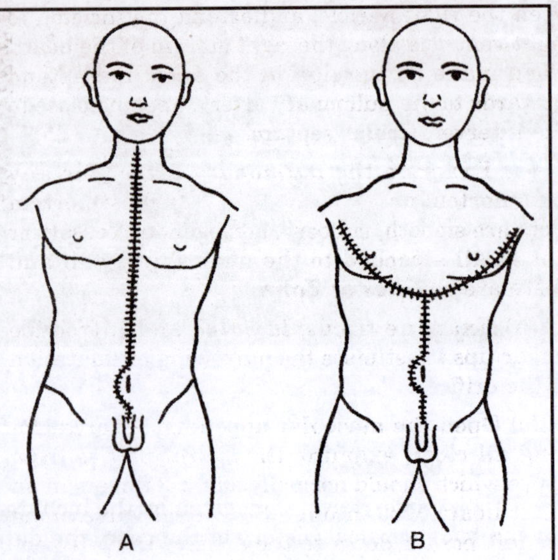

Fig. 53.1. A. Skin incision : From chin to symphysis pubis. B. Y-shaped incision

systematically. Stand on the right side of the body and give incision.

Incision

(i) Extend the chin, make a 'I'-shaped vertical incision from the chin (just above the prominence of thyroid cartilage) straight down to the symphysis pubis (Fig. 53.1A) passing on either side of the umbilicus. (ii) Y-shaped incision from near the acromial process of the clavicle extends down below the nipple and across to the xiphoid process (Fig. 53.1B).

In the neck, the skin and subcutaneous tissues should only be divided and the incision should go down to the bone over the sternum. The chest muscles are reflected towards the axillary line on each side.

1. Abdomen

The peritoneal cavity is opened cautiously by nicking through the peritoneum at the lower third of the abdomen. The contents of the peritoneal cavity and the pelvis *in situ* are inspected. Fluid, when present, to be collected aseptically for culture and cytology. The abdominal viscera are then examined.

(a) Oesophagus with stomach

Removal : These are removed after applying double ligatures at each end and are placed in a clean dish. The stomach is opened along the greater curvature and spread out.

Examination : Look for any helminths, mucus membrane is examined for haemorrhage, ulceration, neoplasm, stenosis and oesophageal varices.

(b) Intestine

For culture, intestinal fluid is aspirated by a sterile syringe and placed in culture media.

Removal : Small and large intestines are examined. Two ligatures are applied and cut between them at the junction of duodenum and jejunum. The small intestine is removed of the body by cutting the attachments of mesentery to the jejunum and ileum. Ascending colon is separated by incising the peritoneum along its right border and the descending colon by incising the peritoneum along its left border. Transverse and pelvic colons are removed from body by cutting the attachments of mesocolon as in small intestine. Two ligatures are applied at the junction of sigmoid colon and rectum and is cut between them, and the whole bowel is thus removed.

Examination : The small intestine is opened in a sink along the line of mesenteric attachment, and the large intestine along the anterior tenia. The contents are examined and cleansed in running tap water. The wall of the intestine is palpated and examined for congestion, inflammation, erosions, ulcers, perforation, growth, etc. The *ileocaecal* valve and the appendix are carefully examined.

(c) Spleen : The spleen is removed by cutting the vessels on the hilum. Weigh the spleen and note the presence of any accessory lobe. It is incised along its long axis towards the hilum and the cut surface is examined.

(d) Liver : Liver is taken out, weighed and examined. Whole organ is cut into slices (2 mm thick). The gall bladder is slit lengthwise, washed and the mucosa is examined. Examine for any enlarged lymph node at the portal fissure.

(e) Pancreas : The duodenum is examined *in situ* and see the pancreatic duct by passing a probe. The pancreas is usually taken out together with stomach and duodenum. The pancreas is incised and its main duct is opened.

(f) Kidneys : The vessels are cut at the hilum and the kidneys are removed with ureter still in place and weighed. The suprarenals are separated. Examine kidney surface and section the kidney longitudinally through the convex border into the hilum in one sweep of the knife, so as to divide into half along with its pelvis. The capsule is stripped off along the cut surface with forceps. Note the surface, adhesion, colour and measure the ratio of cortex to medulla and measure the thickness of each. The pelvis is examined for calculi and inflammation. Ureters are also slit open and looked for calculi or debris.

Adrenals are specially examined for the presence of haemorrhage. Abdominal aorta is opened down its anterior midline.

(g) Pelvic organs : Bladder, prostate, seminal vesicles, urethra and rectum are examined in the order. Catheter passed into bladder and any urine present is drawn out for analysis. In the female, tubes and ovaries are freed from the pelvis and uterus. The tubes and ovaries are taken out. The vagina and uterus are slit anteriorly or posteriorly up to the fundus. Also examine for signs of recent delivery. Testes and epididymis are cut longitudinally and examined.

2. Neck

Pharynx, larynx, trachea, thyroid and thoracic oesophagus are taken out together after the tongue is pulled down. They are cut open and examined.

3. Thorax

The thorax is opened by cutting through the costal cartilages and also sterno-clavicular joint — sternum and costal cartilages are removed in one piece. The anterior mediastinum is examined for enlarged lymph node and pleural cavities for the presence of adhesions, fluid or blood. The fluid, if present, is collected by sterile syringe and cultured and then measured. The hand is passed over the whole surface of each lung and brought the lungs forward breaking down any adhesion.

If there is fluid in pericardial cavity, collect aseptically for culture, and measure the fluid. Open the pericardium and examine outside of the heart for adhesions, etc.

Heart : Cut through the vessels from below up as far away as possible from the base of the heart, namely inferior vena cavae, the pulmonary veins, superior vena cavae, pulmonary artery and aorta. Weigh the heart.

The heart is opened with a straight scissors placing on the table with anterior surface up. Approach through the superior vena cavae and open the right auricle, and extend the incision to right ventricle along the right margin of the heart. Then make an incision in the apex and extend upwards to the pulmonary artery, keeping close to the interventricular septum.

(a) Examine the *pulmonary artery* for any antemortem or **postmortem clot**. Postmortem clots are smooth, rubbery, homogenous, loosely or not at all attached to the underlying wall and there are no ***lines of Zahn***.

(b) Examine *tricuspid valve* and introduce finger tips to estimate the narrowing or dilatation of the orifice.

(c) Open the auricular appendix. After removing all clots, examine the *mitral orifice* from above which should normally admit 2 fingers in an adult heart. Cut through the mitral valve along the left border down to the apex of the left ventricle.

(d) The *aortic valve* is palpated with fingers, then cut upwards from the apex of the left ventricle, keeping close to the inter-ventricular septum towards the aortic opening. One blade of the scissors is passed through the opening and extended, cutting across the pulmonary artery just above the pulmonary vein. Cut open the *aorta* above and below the thoracic duct. Inspect the walls of aorta and great vessels. Aorta is examined for any syphilitic aortitis, atheromatous plaques and narrowing of the coronary ostium.

Introduce a probe into the coronary arteries, cut the arteries by longitudinal incision and examine the interior.

The interior of the left ventricle is examined after removing all clots. The wall of myocardium is incised and its colour, consistency and thickness is noted.

Lungs : Both lungs are removed at their roots. Lungs are opened by a long deep incision from the apex to the base.

(a) Examine for pathological changes.

(b) Small pieces of lung are placed in water which float unless collapsed or consolidated.

(c) Look for pale area produced by minute infarcts.

4. Head

A wooden block is placed under the shoulders so that the neck remains extended and the head is fixed by a head rest. An incision is made in the

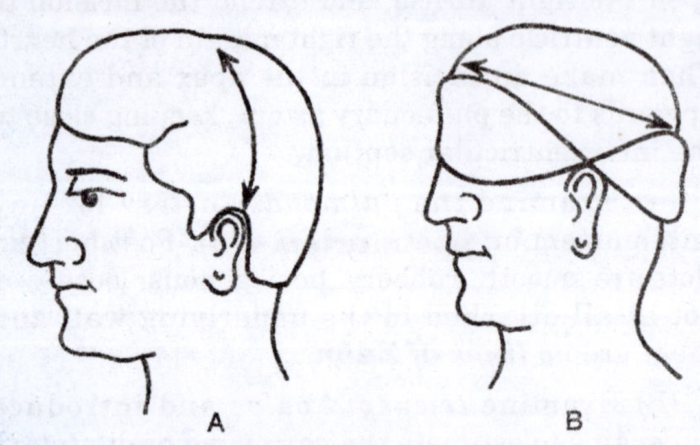

Fig. 53.2. A, B, Scalp incision

scalp down to the bone, extending from near the mastoid process of one side over the vertex of the scalp to the back of the opposite mastoid (Fig. 53.2A).

Reflect the scalp into anterior and posterior flaps. Then the skull cap is cut by sawing and using chisel and hammer through the bones along horizontal line passing through the centre of the forehead, base of the mastoid process and a point little above the external protuberance (Fig. 53.2B). Dura is incised along the line of the saw-cut. Meninges are inspected for congestion, extradural or subdural and intracranial haemorrhages. The skull cap is also examined. The superior longitudinal sinus is carefully examined for an antemortem thrombus.

The skull in newborn is opened in a different way (Fig. 53.3). An incision is made about 5-6 mm away from midline into anterior fontanelle and the knife is moved as shown in Fig. 53.3.

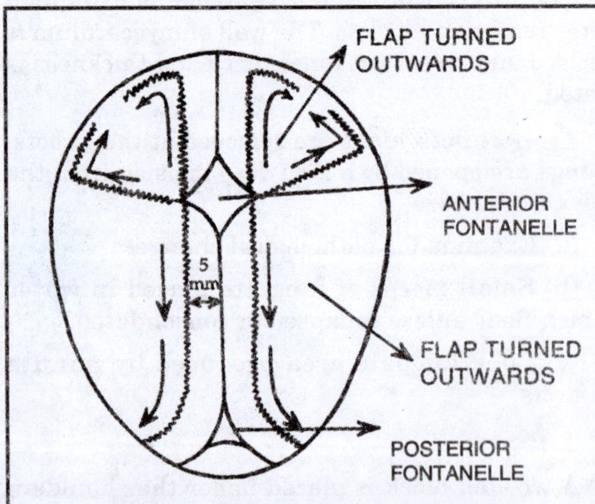

Fig. 53.3. Barr's technique of opening skull of newborn

Brain : Remove the brain by raising it gently from the frontal lobes backwards, dividing the nerves successively as they enter and the tentorial cerebelli is incised along its attachments.

Surface and base of brain are examined for haemorrhage, injury or disease. The brain is sectioned transversely and preserved in 10% formalin.

Pituitary is removed by cutting away the posterior clinoid processes with the chisel. The gland is carefully dissected out of the fossa.

Spinal cord : Spinal cord is taken out after cutting through the soft part ANT. FONTANELLEs in the midline. The laminae are cut using saw and the ensheathed cord is separated from all attachments from below upwards and lifted from its bed.

5. Limbs

Bones and blood vessels of limbs are examined. Marrow is obtained after cutting a window over cortex.

Laboratory procedure

A. Bacteriological

(a) Culture and smear from involved area (e.g., intestinal content, pleural, peritoneal fluid) should be made aseptically. Intestinal fluid is collected by sterile syringe or glass pipette for culture.

(b) Blood is obtained from right auricle aseptically by a sterile syringe or glass pipette with rubber teat.

(c) In case of a solid organ like liver or spleen, the surface of the organ is touched with a hot spatula and an incision is made into that area using a sterile scalpel and a quantity of juice is obtained with a sterile platinum loop to make direct films for smear and culture in suitable media.

B. Histopathological

Tissues removed from various organs are preserved in 10% formol saline.

C. Microscopical

Vaginal and anal swabs, urethral discharge, faeces and urine (deposit) are examined by preparation of stained smears when indicated.

D. Biochemical

Blood, CSF and other body fluids are used for biochemical examination.

POSTMORTEM-RECORD

MEDICAL COLLEGE HOSPITALS, KOLKATA

DEPARTMENT OF PATHOLOGY

P.M. No. .... Ward/OPD .... Reg. No............ Bed No..........................

Date and time of death ....

Date...and Time...(of holding P.M.)

Hours Postmortem ....

NAME ....Age..................Religion..........................Sex....................

Restriction (Partial/Complete) ....

Referred by ....

Clinical diagnosis...

Anatomical diagnosis..

Histological diagnosis...

Signature of Prosector ....

A. EXTERNAL EXAMINATION

(Body surface, nutritional status, height, weight, injuries if any, scars)

B. INTERNAL EXAMINATION

PRIMARY INCISION

PERITONEAL CAVITY

PLEURAL CAVITIES

MEDIASTINUM

PERICARDIAL CAVITY

HEART : Weight

Valves :	T.V.	M.V.	A.V.	P.V.
Measurements :	L.V.	Rt.V.	L.A.	Rt.A.

MUSCLES (Myocardium) :

VESSELS :

Aorta :

Portal veins and tributaries

LUNGS : Weight — R. L.

Spleen :

Wt. Size Cut surface

ORGANS OF NECK :

Tongue :	Larynx :
Tonsils :	Trachea :
Salivary glands :	Thyroid :

Contd.......next page

LYMPH NODES :

ALIMENTARY TRACT : Pharynx

Oesophagus :

Stomach :

Small intestine :

Appendix :

Large intestine :

Rectum :

PANCREAS :

LIVER :

Weight : gm, size :

Cut surface :

GALL BLADDER : BILE DUCT :

KIDNEYS :

Weight : Rt. Lt.

ADRENALS :

Weight : Rt. Lt.

PELVIC ORGANS : Urinary Bladder

MALE :

Prostate :

Testes :

Spermatic cords :

FEMALE :

Ovaries :

Uterus, cervix and vagina :

Fallopian tubes :

BONES : Ribs : Vertebrae : Sternum : Pelvis : Femora :

BRAIN :

Weight : Pituitary :

Middle ear and mastoid processes :

Air sinuses of skull :

SPINAL CORD :

Relevant Microscopic findings :

Chemical and Bacteriological Investigations :

Clinical Summary :

Pathological Summary :

Clinicopathological correlations :

REPORTING

MEDICAL COLLEGE HOSPITALS, KOLKATA

DEPARTMENT OF PATHOLOGY

Name..........................
Age/Sex.......................
Reg. No.......................
Ward/OPD.................
Date............ Income

Referred by

Clinical diagnosis

HIV status

Autopsy No....................

MICROSCOPIC DESCRIPTION (ORGANWISE) :

FINAL AUTOPSY DIAGNOSIS :

CAUSE OF DEATH :

Date of receiving ....

Date of reporting...............................

PATHOLOGIST

Chapter 54

Weights and Measurements of Normal Organs

• BRAIN

Weight (male)	....	....	1400 gm
Weight (female)	....	....	1250 gm
Cerebrospinal fluid (volume)	....	....	120-125 ml

• HEART

Weight (male)	....	....	300-350 gm
Weight (female)	....	....	250-300 gm
Thickness of ventricular wall (right)	....	....	0.3-0.5 cm
Thickness of ventricular wall (left)	....	....	1.3-1.5 cm
Circumference, mitral valve	....	....	10 cm
aortic valve	....	....	7.5 cm
pulmonary valve	....	....	8.5 cm
tricuspid valve	....	....	12 cm
Pericardial fluid (volume)	....	....	10-30 ml

• LUNGS

Weight, right lung	....	....	375-500 (450) gm
Weight, left lung	....	....	325-450 (400) gm
Volume, pleural fluid	....	....	< 15 ml

• OESOPHAGUS

Length, cricoid cartilage to cardia	....	....	25–26 cm
Distance from incisors to gastro-oesophageal junction	....	....	38–40 cm

• INTESTINES

Length, duodenum	....	....	30 cm
small intestine	....	....	550-650 cm
large intestine	....	....	150-170 cm

- **LIVER**

Weight (male)	....	....	1400-1600 gm
Weight (female)	....	....	1200-1400 gm

- **PANCREAS**

Total weight	....	....	60-100 (80) gm
Weight of endocrine pancreas	....	....	1-1.5 gm

- **SPLEEN**

Weight	....	....	125-175 (150) gm

- **THYMUS**

Weight (at birth)	....	....	10-35 gm
Weight (in adults)	....	....	5-10 gm

- **THYROID**

Weight	....	....	15-40 gm

- **KIDNEYS**

Weight each (male)	....	....	150 gm
Weight each (female)	....	....	135-140 gm

- **PROSTATE**

Weight	....	....	20-30 gm

- **OVARIES**

Weight (each)	....	....	4-8 (6) gm

- **UTERUS**

Weight (in non-pregnant woman)	....	....	35-40 gm
Weight (in parous woman)	....	....	75-125 gm

- **PLACENTA**

Weight at term	....	....	400-600 gm

Chapter 55

Laboratory Values of Clinical Significance

The laboratory values given below are divided into three sections — *haematologic values, clinical chemistry of blood* and *other body fluids.*

A. HAEMATOLOGIC VALUES

Analyte	Specimen		Conventional Units	S.I. Units
Erythrocytes and Haemoglobin				
Erythrocyte count	Blood			
males			$4.5\text{-}6.0 \times 10^{12}/l$	
females			$4.0\text{-}5.2 \times 10^{12}/l$	
Erythrocyte life-span	Blood		120 days	
Erythrocyte diameter			6.7-7.7 µm (mean 7.2 µm)	
Erythrocyte thickness				
peripheral			2.4 µm	
central			1.0 µm	
Erythrocyte indices (Absolute values)	Blood			
mean corpuscular haemoglobin (MCH)		....	29.5 ± 2.5 pg	
mean corpuscular volume (MCV)		....	85 ± 5 fl	
mean corpuscular haemoglobin concentration (MCHC)		....	33 ± 2 gm/dl	
mean corpuscular diameter (MCD)	Blood	....	6.7–7.7 µm	
Erythrocyte sedimentation rate (ESR)	Blood			
Westergren 1st hr, males			0-15 mm	
females			0-20 mm	
Wintrobe, 1st hr, males			0-8 mm	
females			0-15 mm	
Ferritin, serum	Serum			
males			16-250 ng/ml	16-250 µg/l
females			12-160 ng/ml	12-160 µg/l

Analyte	Specimen	Conventional Units	S.I. Units
Haematocrit (PCV)	Blood		
males		47 ± 7	0.47 ± 0.07 l/l
females		41 ± 5	0.42 ± 0.05 l/l
Haemoglobin (Hb)			
adult haemoglobin (HbA)	Whole blood		
males		13.5-18.0 gm/dl	130-180 gm/l
females		11.5-16.5 gm/dl	115-165 gm/l
haemoglobin A_2 (HbA_2)		1.5-3.1%	0.015–0.031
haemoglobin, foetal (HbF) in adults		0–2%	
HbF, children under 6 months		< 5%	
Iron, total	Serum	41-141 μg/dl	7–25 μmol/l
Total iron binding capacity (TIBC)	Serum	250-460 μg/dl	44.8-71.6 μmol/l
Iron binding capacity saturation	Serum	16-35%	0.16–0.35%
Osmotic fragility	Blood		
slight haemolysis	....	at 0.45 to 0.39 gm/dl NaCl	
complete haemolysis	....	at 0.33 to 0.36 gm/dl NaCl	
mean corpuscular fragility	....	0.35-0.45 gm/dl NaCl	0.0035–0.0045
Reticulocyte count	Blood		
adults	....	0.8-2.3%	0.008–0.023
infants	....	2-6%	
Reticulocyte haemoglobin content	Blood	> 26 pg/cell	
Leucocytes			
Total leucocyte count (TLC)	Blood		
adults	....	3.54-9.06 × 10^3/mm^3	
infants (full term, at birth)	....	10.0–20.0 × 10^3/mm^3	
Differential leucocyte count (DLC)	Blood film		
N (neutrophils or polymorphs)	....	40-70% (2000-7500/μl)	
L (lymphocytes)	....	20-50% (1500-4000/μl)	
M (monocytes)	....	2-10% (200-800/μl)	
E (eosinophils)	....	1-6% (40-400/μl)	
B (basophils)	....	< 1% (10-100/μl)	
Platelets and Coagulation			
Bleeding time (BT)			
Ivy's method	Prick blood	2-7 min	
Template method	....	2.5-9.5 min	
Clot retraction time	Whole blood		
qualitative	....	Visible in 60 min (complete in < 24 hours)	
quantitative	....	50-60%	
Bleeding time			
Ivy's method	Prick blood	2-7 min	
Template method	....	2-9 min	
Coagulation time (CT)	Whole bloood		
Lee and White method	....	4-9 min at 37 °C	

Analyte	Specimen	Conventional Units	S.I. Units
Partial thromboplastin time with kaolin (PTTK) or activated partial thromboplastin time (APTT)	Plasma	26.3-39.4 sec	
Plasminogen activator inhibitor 1	Plasma	4-43 ng/ml	4-43 μg/L
Prothrombin time (PT) (Quick's one-stage method)	Plasma	12-15.5 sec	
Thrombin time (TT)	Plasma	15.3–18.5 sec	
Platelet count	Blood	150,000-400,000/μl	

B. CLINICAL CHEMISTRY OF BLOOD

Analyte	Specimen	Conventional Units	S.I. Units
Acetoacetate	Plasma	0.2–1.0 mg/dl	20-99 μmol/L
Aminotransferases (transaminases)			
aspartate (AST, SGOT)	Serum	8-40 Karmen units	8-35 IU/l
alanine (ALT, SGPT)	Serum	5-35 Karmen units	5-40 IU/l
Ammonia, as NH_3	Plasma	19-60 μg/dl	11-35 μmol/l
Amylase	Serum	16-120 Somogyi units/dl	20-96 IU/l
Angiotensin-converting enzyme (ACE)	Serum	9-67 U/L	0.15-1.1 μkat/L
Arterial blood gases	Serum		
$[HCO_3^-]$	....	20-30 meq/L	20-30 mmol/l
PCO_2	....	32-45 mm Hg	4.3–6.0 kPa
pH	....	7.35–7.45	7.35–7.45
PO_2	....	72-104 mm Hg	9.6–13.8 kPa
Bicarbonate	Plasma	21-28 mmol/l	21-28 mmol/l
Bilirubin			
total	Serum	0.2-1.0 mg/dl	5.0-17 μmol/l
direct (conjugated)	Serum	0.1-0.3 mg/dl	1.7-5.1 μmol/l
indirect (unconjugated)	Serum	0.2-0.7 mg/dl	2-17 μmol/l
Calcium, ionised	Plasma	4.5-5.3 mg/dl	1.12-1.32 mmol/l
Calcium, total	Serum	9.2-11.0 mg/dl	2.3-2.7 mmol/l
Carcinoembryonic antigen (CEA)	Serum		
non-smokers	....	0.0-3.0 ng/ml	0.0-3.0 μg/L
smokers	....	0.0-5.0 ng/ml	0.0-5.0 μg/L
CO_2 content	Whole blood	22-30 mEq/L	22-30 mmol/l (arterial)
Chloride (Cl^-)	Serum	98-106 mEq/l	98-106 mmol/l
Cholesterol	Serum		
total desirable for adults	....	140-200 mg/dl	3.88-6.47 mmol/l
borderline high	....	200-239 mg/dl	
very high	....	> 240 mg/dl	

B. CLINICAL CHEMISTRY OF BLOOD contd...

Analyte	Specimen	Conventional Units	S.I. Units
LDL-Cholesterol desirable range		< 130 mg/dl	
HDL-Cholesterol, protective range		> 40 mg/dl	
Triglycerides		< 160 mg/dl	
Copper	Serum	70-140 µg/dl	11-22 µmol/l
Creatine kinase (CK)	Serum		
males	....	51-294 IU/l	0.87-5.0 µ kat/L
females	....	39-238 IU/l	0.66-4.0 µ kat/L
Creatinine	Serum	0.5-1.5 mg/dl	44-106 µmol/l
Glucose (fasting)	Plasma/serum		
Normal		75-110 mg/dl	4.2-6.1 mmol/l
Diabetes mellitus		> 125 mg/dl	
Glucose (2-hr post-prandial)	Plasma		
Normal	....	70-120 mg/dl	
Impaired glucose tolerance (IGT)	....	111-125 mg/dl	
Diabetes mellitus	....	> 125 mg/dl	
Lactate dehydrogenase (LDH)	Serum	115–221 U/L	
Phosphatases	Serum		
acid phosphatase	....	1.0-0.3 King-Armstrong units	2.2-10.5 U/l
alkaline phosphatase	....	4.0-13.0 King-Armstrong units	33-96 U/l
Phosphorus, inorganic	Serum	2.5-4.3 mg/dl	0.81-1.4 mmol/l
Potassium	Serum	3.5-5.0 mEq/l	3.5-5.0 mmol/l
Prostate-specific antigen (PSA)	Serum		
male, < 40 years	....	0.0-2.0 ng/ml	
male, > 40 years	....	0.0-4.0 ng/ml	
Proteins	Serum		
total	....	5.5–8 gm/dl	
albumin	....	3.5–5.5 gm/dl (50-60%)	
globulin	....	2.0-3.5 gm/dl (40-50%)	
A/G ratio	....	1.75 : 1	
Renal blood flow		1200 ml/min	
Sodium	Serum	136-146 mEq/l	136-146 mmol/l
Urea	Blood	15-40 mg/dl	
Urea nitrogen (BUN)	Blood	10-20 mg/dl	
Uric acid	Serum		
males	....	3.1-7.0 mg/dl	0.18-0.41 mmol/l
females	....	2.5-6.0 mg/dl	0.16-0.36 mmol/l

C. OTHER BODY FLUIDS

Analyte	Specimen	Conventional Units	S.I. Units
Cerebrospinal fluid (CSF)	CSF		
volume	....	120-150 ml	
pressure	....	60-150 mm water	
leucocytes	....	0-4 lymphocytes/mm^3	
pH	....	7.31-7.34	
glucose	....	40-80 mg/dl	
proteins (lumbar)	....	15-50 mg/dl	
cisternal	....	15-25 mg/dl	
ventricular	....	6-15 mg/dl	
Glomerular filtration rate (GFR)	Urine	180 l/day (about 125 ml/min)	
Seminal fluid	Semen		
liquefaction		Within 20 min	
sperm morphology	....	> 70% normal, mature spermatozoa	
sperm motility	....	> 60%	
pH	....	7.2-8.5 (averagee 7.7)	
sperm count	....	60-150 million/ml	
volume	....	1.5-4.0 ml	
Urine examination	24-hr volume	600-1800 ml (variable)	
specific gravity	urine (random)	1.001-1.035 (average 1.018)	
phosphate (phosphorus) (varies with intake)	24-hour urine	400-1300 mg/day	
protein excretion	24-hour urine	< 150 mg/day	
protein, qualitative	urine (random)	Negative	
glucose excretion	24-hour urine	50-300 mg/day	
glucose, qualitative	urine (random)	Negative	
porphobilinogen	urine (random)	Negative	
urobilinogen	24-hour urine	1.0-3.5 mg/day	
urobilinogen	Urine (random)	Present in 1:20 dilution	

Appendices

Appendix – I, Appendix – II, Appendix – III, Appendix – IV, Appendix – V, Appendix – VI

APPENDIX – I

Scheme for Second Professional MBBS University Examination in Pathology

A. Written Paper :

Paper I — General Pathology and Hematology

Paper II — Systemic Pathology and Clinical Pathology

Each paper will be of 40 marks. There will be four questions in each paper with the following distribution of marks.

Gr. A — Q. (1) One clinical problem-oriented question — Marks 10

Gr. B — Q. (2) One short essay-type question (out of two) consisting of 2-3 small segments and marks for each segment will be indicated separately. — Marks 10

Gr. C — Q. (3) One short essay-type question (out of two) consisting of 2-3 small segments and marks for each segment will be indicated separately — Marks 10

Gr. D — Q. (4) Short notes (five out of six) — Marks 10 (5 × 2)

Answer to each question should be given by the candidates in a separate answer book. Only one examiner will examine all the answer scripts to the same question of the paper in that centre. Preferably each external examiner will examine answer script of Q. 2 of one paper and Q.4 of the other paper. Each examiner will examine answers to one question of each paper.

B. Oral/Viva :

There will be two tables with 7.5 marks in each table — Marks will be 15 (7 ½ × 2)

Table I : General and Systemic Pathology

Table II : Hematology and Clinical Pathology

C. Practical :

- Urine – chemical tests (2 out of 3 — protein, reducing subs, ketone bodies) — 4 marks
- Staining a peripheral blood smear and identifying few cells — 5 marks
- Performing blood grouping/ESR/Hb estimation — 4 marks
- Problem card and its interpretation — 5 marks
- Identification (3 H/P slides, 1 hematology slide, 2 instrument, 1 specimen) — 7 marks

Distribution of Internal Assessment marks :

Total marks = 30

Theory = 15	Practical = 15
Class-tests (continuous I.A.) = 7.5	Item cards (continuous I.A.) = 7.5
1st Periodical I.A. – 40	1st Periodical I.A. – 25
2nd Periodical I.A. – 40	2nd Periodical I.A. – 25
3rd Periodical I.A. – 40	3rd Periodical I.A. – 25
Total – 120	Total – 75
120/16 = 7.5	10% of 75 = 7.5

Question pattern for Periodical Internal Assessment examination :

A.	Theory : One paper of 40 marks	Time – 2 hrs.
	1. One clinical problem-oriented question	10 marks
	2. Two short-answer questions (2—3 segments)	10 × 2 = 20 marks
	3. Five short notes	2 × 5 = 10 marks
B.	Practical (including oral) :	
	1st Periodical I.A. examination	25 Marks
	• Instruments (two)	5 × 2 = 10
	• Peripheral blood smear staining	5
	• Any two of the following three tests (ESR, TC, Hb estimation)	5 × 2 = 10
	2nd Periodical I.A. examination	25 Marks
	• Urine examination (two)	5 × 2 = 10
	• Problem card	5
	• Blood grouping	5
	• Instrument	5
	3rd Periodical I.A. examination	25 Marks
	• Urine examination	5
	• Peripheral blood smear	5
	• Blood grouping /ESR/TC	5
	• Problem card and its interpretation	5
	• Identification (4 HP and 1 Hematology slide)	5

APPENDIX – II

Theory Question Papers for MBBS Examination (Paper I and II)

Subject : Pathology — Paper I **Time : 2 Hours** **Full Marks : 40**

Use separate Answer Script for each group
Attempt all questions

Group – A

1. A 3 year old child presented with anaemia, fever, hepatosplenomegaly, lymphadenopathy and bony tenderness for the last one month. His peripheral blood smear shows some abnormality. What is your provisional diagnosis? How will you proceed to investigate the case in the laboratory? What are the prognostic factors in such a case?

2 + 6 + 2

Group – B

2. (a) What is jaundice? What are the different types of jaundice? Describe the different tests of laboratory diagnosis in jaundice.

OR

(b) Define Oedema. Discuss the important factors that regulate oedema. Describe the pathogenesis of oedema due to cardiac cause.

2 + 5 + 3

Group – C

3. (a) Define shock. Discuss the pathogenesis of hypovolemic shock. What do you mean by irreversible shock?

2 + 6 + 2

OR

(b) Define gangrene. Mention the different types of gangrene. What is the mechanism of gas gangrene?

Group – D

4. Write short notes on *any five* 5 × 2

(a) Granuloma. (b) Primary amyloidosis. (c) Reverse grouping

(d) Reticulocyte (e) Free radicals (f) Down's syndrome

Subject : Pathology — Paper II **Time : 2 Hours** **Full Marks : 40**

Use separate Answer Script for each group
Attempt all questions

Group – A

1. A 55 year old man presents with painless hematuria. Enumerate the causes. How do you investigate the patient to reach a diagnosis ?

3 + 7

Group – B

2. (a) Classify Bronchogenic Carcinoma. Discuss in brief the aetiopathogenesis of Bronchogenic Carcinoma. Describe the morphological features of small cell carcinoma.

3 + 4 + 3

OR

(b) Classify tumours of the stomach. Discuss the aetiopathogenesis of Gastric Carcinoma. Enumerate the differences between a benign and malignant gastric ulcer.

2 + 5 + 3

Group – C

3. (a) Classify Primary Glomerulonephritis. Describe the glomerular changes of Acute Proliferative Glomerulonephritis. What are the urinary findings in such case?

3 + 5 + 2

OR

(b) Write the pathogenesis of Osteomyelitis. Enumerate the pathogens. Mention complications that can occur in such diseased states.

4 + 3 + 3

Group – D

4. Write short notes on *any five* 5 × 2

(a) Barrett's esophagus.

(b) Jone's criteria.

(c) Serological diagnosis of Hepatitis B virus infection.

(d) Adult polycystic kidney disease.

(e) Ulcerative colitis.

(f) Flea-bitten kidney.

APPENDIX – III

Practical Question Papers for MBBS Examination

Total Marks : 25 **Time : 2 Hours**

1. Examine the supplied specimen of urine for protein, reducing substance, ketone bodies *(any two of them)* **4**
2. Stain the supplied peripheral blood smear and identify few cells. Show it to examiner. **5**
3. Perform any one of the following test in the supplied blood sample : Blood Group/ESR/Hb Estimation. **4**
4. Problem card and interpretation. **5**
5. Spotting. **7**

APPENDIX – IV

Regulation Related to Conduction of M.D. (Pathology) Examination

1. **Eligibility criteria for appearing for the final examination :**

   (a) 80% attendance in the tenure of the course.

   (b) Submission of thesis in time and its acceptance.

   (c) Attendance in at least 75 PG teaching session (seminars, journal clubs, CME etc.)

   (d) Satisfactory performance in the places of posting/training as recorded in the log book.

   (e) Attainment of at least 50% marks in the continuous assessment programme — to be implemented from 2006 admission year.

2. **Distribution of marks :**

Theory 4 papers (4 × 100)	....	400
Practical	....	400
Oral	....	200
Total	....	1000

3. **Gradation of marks :**

Candidate has to obtain 50% marks in Theory, Practical and Oral each.

Candidates obtaining less than 50% marks will not be awarded degree.

Candidates obtaining more than 50% marks on aggregate will be awarded grades as follows :

Grade D	51% – 60%
Grade C	61% – 70%
Grade B	71% – 80%
Grade A	more than 80%

4. **Theory examination : 400 marks**

There will be 4 papers 100 marks each

Paper I	General Pathology, Investigative techniques, Immunopathology
Paper II	Hematology, Cytology
Paper III	Systemic pathology, Clinical pathology, Immunopathology.
Paper IV	Recent advancements, Genetics and Molecular Biology.

In each paper there will be four (4) questions of 20 marks each (preferably broken up into shorter ones) and one (1) question of 20 marks, preferably short notes (5 × 4) or objective questions.

5. **Practical Examination 400 marks + Viva 200 marks**

DAY 1

• Biochemistry and Clinical pathology	1 hr. – 50 marks
• Blood examination	1 hr. – 50 marks
• Histology — grossing, section cutting, staining	2 hr. – 80 marks
• Postmortem exercise	1 hr. – 30 marks
• Viva on thesis works	1 hr. – 30 marks

APPENDIX – V

PLAN/PROGRAMME OF M.D. (PATHOLOGY)

PRACTICAL AND ORAL EXAMI NATION

Day 1 :

- Examination will start at 10 AM
- Candidates will be divided into 2 groups — A and B.
- 10 – 11 a.m. Group A will go for Biochemistry and Clinical Pathology
  Group B will go for Blood examination
- 11 – 12 a.m. Reversing of the work
- 12 – 1 p.m. Postmortem exercise for Group A
  Viva on thesis work for Group B
- 1 – 2 p.m. Lunch break
- 2 – 3 p.m. Reversing of Postmortem exercise & Viva (A+B)
- 3 – 4 p.m. Section cutting and staining for Group A
  Grossing for Group B
- 4 – 5 p.m. Reversing of the work
- 5 p.m. Lottery for the topic of Microteaching/Presentation

Day 2 :

- Reporting of slides (16 in numbers) 2 hr 160 marks
- Microteaching/Presentation session 2 hr 50 marks
- Grand Viva with slide reports 150 marks

Plan and distribution of work :

- Examination will start at 9 a.m.
- 9–10 a.m. Group A for 4 Cytology and 4 Hematology slides
  Group B for 8 Histology slides
- 10–12 a.m. Reversing of the work
- 12–1 p.m. Microteaching/Presentation common session
- 1–2 p.m. Lunch break
- 2–5 p.m. Grand viva with slide reports

N.B.

- Biochemical tests—estimation of any one of the following tests :
  (a) Glucose (b) Protein (c) Bilirubin (d) Urea (e) Cholesterol
- Clinical Pathology tests — examination, reporting and interpretation of any one of the following — (a) Urine (b) Stool (c) Unstained FNAC slide.
- Examination of blood — any two of the following — (a) Hb estimation (b) TLC (c) DLC (d) Reticulocyte count (e) PCV (f) Direct Coombs' test (g) Blood group and Rh.
- Histology section staining include performance of H & E staining and viva on special staining and immuno histochemistry.
- Grossing — one specimen will be allotted to each examinee and the grossing will be observed by the examiner who will also ask questions.
- In slide session the examinee has to draw a diagram and offer a diagnosis with points in favour.

APPENDIX – VI

M.D. (Pathology) Examination

Paper I **Full Marks : 100 Time : 3 Hours**

Attempt all questions

1. Mention briefly mechanism of tumourogenesis by oncogenes and role of tumour suppressor genes. 20
2. Outline the pathogenesis and pathology of oedema. 20
3. Write short notes on : 5 × 6
   (a) HPV – mediated cervical carcinogenesis.
   (b) Autoimmune hepatitis. (c) Apoptosis.
   (d) Endotoxic shock.
   (e) Defects in neutrophil function.
4. Answer in brief : $4 \times 7\frac{1}{2}$
   (a) Steatohepatitis
   (b) Pathophysiology of neonatal jaundice.
   (c) Assessing hormonal status in vaginal smear.
   (d) Pathogenesis of dengue fever.

Paper II **Full Marks : 100 Time : 3 Hours**

Attempt all questions

1. A 50 year old man has been suffering from essential hypertension since long. Describe the morphology of heart and kidney in this condition. Discuss the pathogenesis of essential hypertension. 12 + 8
2. Describe the pathology of common lung tumours. Discuss role of molecular markers in prognosis of the lesion. 15 + 5
3. Write short notes on : 5 × 6
   (a) Prognostic factors in malignant melanoma. (b) Myxoma.
   (c) Osteoid forming bone lesions. (d) Acromegaly.
   (e) Pathogenesis of peptic ulcer.
4. Answer in brief : $4 \times 7\frac{1}{2}$
   (a) Mantle cell lymphoma.
   (b) Placental site trophoblastic tumour and its differential diagnosis.
   (c) Stellate granuloma in lymph node.
   (d) Paget's disease of bone.

Paper III

Full Marks : 100 Time : 3 Hours

Attempt all questions

1. Outline the pathogenesis, classification and laboratory diagnosis of disseminated intravascular coagulation (DIC). **20**
2. Discuss classification of Myelodysplastic syndrome (MDS). **20**
3. Write short notes on : **5 × 6**
   (a) Cryoprecipitate and FFP.
   (b) Screening tests of β-thalassaemia in population.
   (c) Prognostic markers in acute lymphocytic leukaemia.
   (d) Paroxysmal nocturnal haemoglobinuria
   (e) Hairy cell leukaemia.
4. Answer in brief : **4 × 7½**
   (a) Antenatal diagnosis of haemophilia.
   (b) Non-immunological complications of blood transfusion.
   (c) Diagnosis of immune thrombocytopenia.
   (d) Informations from urinary sediment.

Paper IV

Full Marks : 100 Time : 3 Hours

Attempt all questions

1. Mention indications of stem cell transplantation. Discuss in brief the scope of adult stem cell transplantation in multiple somatic sites. **8 + 12**
2. Describe the recent advances in the pathogenesis of chronic obstructive pulmonary disease (COPD). **20**
3. Write short notes on : **5 × 6**
   (a) Microassay in mesenchymal tumours.
   (b) Castleman's disease.
   (c) Desmoid tumour.
   (d) Flurescent in situ hybridisation (FISH).
   (e) Splice variant proteins.
4. Answer in brief : **4 × 7½**
   (a) Immunohistological pattern of Gastrointestinal stromal tumour (GIST).
   (b) Pathogenesis of atherosclerosis.
   (c) Grossing of a panhysterectomy specimen in a case of carcinoma of uterine cervix.
   (d) Recent classification of cutaneous lymphoma.

Index